FIRST AID THE®

WARDS

Fourth Edition

TAO LE, MD, MHS
Assistant Clinical Professor of Medicine and Pediatrics
Chief, Section of Allergy and Immunology
Department of Medicine
University of Louisville

VIKAS BHUSHAN, MD
Diagnostic Radiologist

JULIA SKAPIK, MD, MPH
Resident, Department of Internal Medicine
University of Pittsburgh
Pittsburgh, Pennsylvania

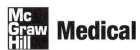 **Medical**

New York / Chicago / San Francisco / Lisbon / London / Madrid / Mexico City
Milan / New Delhi / San Juan / Seoul / Singapore / Sydney / Toronto

The McGraw·Hill Companies

First Aid for the® Wards, Fourth Edition

ISBN 978-0-07-159796-8
MHID 0-07-159796-4
ISSN 1557-4083

NOTICE

Medicine is an ever-changing science. As new research and clinical experience broaden our knowledge, changes in treatment and drug therapy are required. The authors and the publisher of this work have checked with sources believed to be reliable in their efforts to provide information that is complete and generally in accord with the standards accepted at the time of publication. However, in view of the possibility of human error or changes in medical sciences, neither the authors nor the publisher nor any other party who has been involved in the preparation or publication of this work warrants that the information contained herein is in every respect accurate or complete, and they disclaim all responsibility for any errors or omissions or for the results obtained from use of the information contained in this work. Readers are encouraged to confirm the information contained herein with other sources. For example and in particular, readers are advised to check the product information sheet included in the package of each drug they plan to administer to be certain that the information contained in this work is accurate and that changes have not been made in the recommended dose or in the contraindications for administration. This recommendation is of particular importance in connection with new or infrequently used drugs.

This book was set in Electra LH by Rainbow Graphics.
The editors were Catherine A. Johnson and Peter J. Boyle.
The production supervisor was Phil Galea.
Project management was provided by Rainbow Graphics.
Quebecor World Dubuque was printer and binder.

This book is printed on acid-free paper.

DEDICATION

To all our contributors, who took time to share their experience, advice, and humor for the benefit of students

and

To our families, friends, and loved ones, who endured and assisted in the task of assembling this guide.

CONTENTS

CONTRIBUTING AUTHORS

CHERYL ADACKAPARA

Resident, Department of Pathology
Brigham and Women's Hospital

HERMAN S. BAGGA

Resident, Department of Urology
University of California, San Francisco

DARCY K. WEIDEMANN

Johns Hopkins University School of Medicine
Class of 2009

MARISA L. CRUZ

Resident, Department of Internal Medicine
University of California, San Francisco

PUSHPA V. RAJA

Johns Hopkins University School of Medicine
Class of 2009

FACULTY REVIEWERS

JOSEPH COCOZZELLA, MD

Fellow in Child Psychiatry, Department of Child and Adolescent
  Psychiatry
Johns Hopkins Hospital

LEONARD FELDMAN, MD

Assistant Professor, Department of Internal Medicine
Johns Hopkins University School of Medicine

CYNTHIA HOLCROFT ARGANI, MD

Assistant Professor, Department of Obstetrics and Gynecology
Johns Hopkins University School of Medicine

FREDERICK LEVY, MD, JD

Assistant Professor, Department of Emergency Medicine
Johns Hopkins Hospital

MARTIN MAKARY, MD

Mark Ravitch Chair in Gastrointestinal Surgery, Department
  of Surgery
Johns Hopkins University School of Medicine

BARRY SOLOMON, MD, MPH

Assistant Professor, Department of Pediatrics
Johns Hopkins University School of Medicine

STEVE ZEILER, MD

Senior Neurology Resident, Department of Neurology
Johns Hopkins Hospital

PREFACE

The change from the passive and controlled environment of the classroom to the fast-paced and active world of the wards can be stressful, confusing, and downright frightening at times. The purpose of *First Aid for the® Wards* is to help ease the transition wards students must make as they begin their clerkship rotations. This book is a student-to-student guide that draws on the advice and experiences of medical students who were successful on the wards. It is our hope to familiarize you with life on the wards and to pass on some of the "secrets of success" that we picked up along the way in our training. The facts and wisdom contained within this book are an amalgam of information we, the authors, wish we had known at the beginning of our third year of medical school. *First Aid for the® Wards* has a number of unique features that make it an indispensable guide for MD, DO, and DPM students:

- Insider advice from students on how to succeed on your clinical rotations.
- Sample H&P notes, daily progress notes, procedure notes, postop notes, labor and delivery notes, and admission orders.
- Specific advice on how to give both concise and detailed oral patient presentations.
- Descriptions of typical daily responsibilities and interactions on each core rotation, including emergency medicine, medicine, pediatrics, obstetrics and gynecology, neurology, psychiatry, and surgery.
- A checklist of high-yield clinical topics in each chapter.

First Aid for the® Wards is meant to be a survival guide rather than a comprehensive source of information. It should supplement information and advice provided by other students, house staff, and faculty. It is designed not to replace reference texts as a source of information but rather to provide some essential background information for each core ward rotation. Although the material has been reviewed by medical faculty and students, errors and omissions are inevitable. We urge readers to suggest improvements and identify inaccuracies. We invite students and faculty to continue sharing their thoughts and ideas to help us improve *First Aid for the® Wards* (see How to Contribute, page xiii).

Louisville   Tao Le
Los Angeles   Vikas Bhushan
Baltimore   Julia Skapik

ACKNOWLEDGMENTS

This collaborative project would not have been possible without the thoughtful comments, insights, and advice of the many medical students and faculty whom we gratefully acknowledge for their support in the development of *First Aid for the® Wards.*

Special thanks to Andrea Fellows, our tireless editor; Selina Franklin; Louise Petersen; and the section editors, contributors, and faculty reviewers for bringing the book together under constant pressure. For continuing enthusiasm, support, and commitment to this project, thanks to our acquisitions editor, Catherine Johnson. For remarkable editorial and production support, we thank David Hommel, Susan Cooper, and the staff at Rainbow Graphics.

HOW TO CONTRIBUTE

First Aid for the® Wards is a work in progress—a collaborative project that was refined through the many contributions and changes received from students and faculty. The authors and McGraw-Hill intend to update *First Aid for the® Wards* so that the book grows both in quality and in scope while continuing to serve as a timely guidebook to survival and success on the wards. We invite you to participate in this process by passing on your own insights. Please send us:

- Tips for survival and success on the wards.
- New topics, diagrams, and tables that you feel should be included in the next edition.
- Mnemonics or algorithms you have used on the wards.
- Personal ratings and comments on books that you have used while on the hospital wards, including books that were not reviewed in this edition.
- Your medical school's handbook to the clerkships.
- Corrections and clarifications.

For each entry incorporated into the next edition, you will receive a **$10 Amazon.com gift certificate**, as well as a personal acknowledgment in the next edition. Significant contributions will be compensated at the discretion of the publisher.

The preferred way to submit suggestions and contributions is via the First Aid Team's blog at:

www.firstaidteam.com

Please also check **firstaidteam.com** for the latest updates and corrections.

NOTE TO CONTRIBUTORS

All entries become properties of the authors and are subject to review and edits. Please verify all data and spelling carefully. In the event that similar or duplicate entries are received, only the first entry received will be used. Include a reference to a standard textbook to facilitate verification of the fact. Please follow the style, punctuation, and format of this edition if possible.

INTERNSHIP OPPORTUNITIES

The author team is pleased to offer part-time and full-time paid internships in medical education and publishing to motivated physicians. Internships may range from three months (e.g., a summer) up to a full year. Participants will have an opportunity to author, edit, and earn academic credit on a wide variety of projects, including the popular First Aid series. Writing/editing experience, familiarity with Microsoft Word, and Internet access are desired. For more information, e-mail a résumé or a short description of your experience along with a cover letter to the authors at **www.firstaidteam.com**.

Introduction to the Wards

▶ Guide for Wards
  Success

▶ Practical Information
  for All Clerkships

Guide for Wards Success

INTRODUCTION

For the past two years, you have learned medicine in classrooms, labs, and libraries. Yet while you may well have shadowed a preceptor or practiced taking histories on the wards, you likely have not yet had any significant clinical experiences. That is all about to change. As a third-year medical student, you will be an integral part of a clinical team. You will now be given real responsibilities—and yes, your own patients.

The transition from classroom to wards will be one of the most exhilarating periods in your training, and the purpose of this book is to make that transition as smooth and stress-free as possible.

In this section, we will offer advice to help you avert **common pitfalls** that many students encounter when starting clinical rotations. Some of these pitfalls include:

- Not understanding the responsibilities and expectations associated with the rotation
- Not seeking timely feedback
- Not using appropriate pocket references and clinical texts
- Not knowing what to study
- Failing to be a team player
- Not efficiently organizing and executing daily work
- Not sufficiently preparing for oral presentations
- Scheduling key rotations too early or too late

To prevent these mistakes, you must first understand the wards experience itself.

WHO?

To succeed on the wards, you should understand how your team works and how you fit in. Toward this end, you should have three major goals:

- To function as a productive team member
- To care for your patients
- To learn

A medical team typically consists of the following members:

Attending

As the head of the team, the attending is usually involved in the most critical treatment decisions affecting your patients, while the logistics of patient care are typically left to the residents and interns. On certain surgical services, the chief resident acts as the head of the team and reports to several "attending" surgeons.

The attending is legally and morally responsible for the actions of each member of the team. He or she is therefore responsible for **educating and evaluating** the residents, interns, and medical students.

Your attending will interact with you primarily during morning rounds. In order to make a good impression, it is important to:

- Deliver buffed oral presentations.
- Submit a clear, **well-organized** admission note.
- Have a basic understanding of your patients' problems and the rationale behind the treatment plan of each.

Resident

The residents (PGY-2 and up) are house officers who have completed internship. They work closely with the attending to formulate and manage treatment plans for your patients, and they oversee your daily activities. Residents are also responsible for teaching medical students and interns through didactics or informal pimping. Subinterns often report directly to the residents. You can make a strong impression on your residents through your:

- **Concise** presentations on rounds
- Solid knowledge base concerning the illnesses commonly seen on the service
- Awareness of all changes in the status of your patient (e.g., new CXR results)
- Hustle and effort in scut work

Intern

The interns (PGY-1) carry out the practical aspects of patient care under the direct supervision of the residents. Because interns are generally overworked, they do little didactic teaching. Usually, however, they are excellent sources of information on how to get tasks done **quickly and efficiently.** Junior medical students usually report directly to the interns.

Intern rules: Eat when you can, sleep when you can, leave when you can.

Although interns are not always involved in grading, they will let the resident know how you're doing. You can score points with them by:

- Keeping your intern up to date on your patients
- Lightening the scut burden

Interns can be your best friends, so keep them informed.

Subintern

Subinterns are fourth-year medical students who carry the same responsibilities as interns. Subinterns do not evaluate or teach you, but they can often serve as a valuable source of clinical pearls and practical information.

Nurse

Ward nurses carry out physician orders and attend to the daily needs of the patient. They are often very knowledgeable about patient care and can give you the scoop on your patient when you preround in the morning. If nurses like you, they may also take the time to teach you important scut skills, like placing Foley catheters or IV lines. For these reasons, a **good rapport with the nursing staff is critical** to a successful and enjoyable rotation. So make sure that you:

- Learn the names of the nurses caring for your patients.
- Always be respectful in discussing patient care with nurses.

Nurses can make or break your rotation.

- Always double-check with your resident if you are unsure about how a treatment plan should be carried out.
- Never leave a mess for the nurse to clean up.
- Always let nurses know if there is an important change in treatment or discharge plans.

Ward Clerk

The ward clerk is usually in charge of administrative issues such as taking written orders off the charts, scheduling procedures, and completing discharge work on your patient. If a patient has been taken somewhere for a diagnostic study, the ward clerk often knows where that patient is and when he or she will return.

Pharmacist

Staff pharmacists or pharmacy residents may also round with the team. Do not hesitate to hit them up for valuable information regarding toxicity, drug interactions, dosing in different disease states, and efficacy.

Other Hospital Staff

Other members of the hospital staff include physician assistants, nurse practitioners, nutritionists, physical therapists, social workers, respiratory therapists, phlebotomists, radiology technicians, and laboratory technicians.

- Tagging along with the phlebotomy team can quickly improve your blood draw and IV placement skills.
- Social workers provide patient counseling, psychosocial assessment, and housing or transportation arrangements.
- Some hospitals conduct multidisciplinary rounds to make sure that all team members are aware of the treatment and discharge plans for each patient.

WHEN?

The Schedule—Medicine Wards

The following is a general outline of the daily schedule for **medicine, pediatrics, neurology, and psychiatry.** Please refer to the chapters that follow for specific advice and information on each rotation.

"SOAP" format:

Subjective status
Objective status
Assessment
Plan

Prerounds: 7:00–8:00 A.M. During prerounds, note and evaluate all events that have affected your patient since you left the hospital the previous day (see Table 1-1). Allow 15–20 minutes per patient at first, and write all information down to make sure you don't forget any details. Thorough prerounding in "**SOAP**" format (see mnemonic) will help you complete the progress note quickly and efficiently later.

Work rounds: 8:00–9:30 A.M. During work rounds, you will round with the team (minus the attending) and give a very brief (less than 30-second) presentation on your old patients to the resident. After you present your plan, the team will create a "to-do" list for the day. Toward this goal:

TABLE 1-1. Preround Checklist

☐ Ask the overnight nurse and cross-covering house officer for overnight events.

☐ Review the patient chart for any overnight events or consult notes.

☐ **Subjective:** Ask the patient how he or she feels.

☐ **Objective:** Check vital signs, perform a brief physical exam, and review new labs, culture results, study results, and radiographs.

☐ **Assessment:** Summarize the patient in one sentence (e.g., Mr. Smith is a 79 yo man with a history of ischemic cardiomyopathy, who presented on 9/12 for a CHF exacerbation and is now clinically improved after 4 L diuresis).

☐ **Plan:** Formulate a plan for the patient for today, breaking it down by problem.

- Have the patient charts available to write orders as you discuss the patient.
- Get your orders cosigned by the resident.
- Write down "to-do" tasks immediately to avoid later confusion.

Work time: 9:30–11:00 A.M. This is when you and the intern crank out the scut. Speed and efficiency during this period determine when you and the intern go home. Be sure to **call in consults and order studies as early in the day as possible,** because those requested later are often not done until the following day. Tasks often include:

- Scheduling studies (e.g., CT scans)
- Requesting consults
- Performing procedures (e.g., paracentesis)
- Completing discharge paperwork
- Writing progress notes

Attending rounds: 11:00 A.M.–noon. During attending rounds, the entire medical team will discuss new admissions and will follow up on current patients. These rounds may take place in a conference room, on walking rounds, or at bedside. On postcall days, you will formally present your patient with a four- to six-minute oral presentation to the attending.

- Make your presentation smooth, concise, and well organized!
- Read up on the illness you are presenting: presentation, differential diagnosis, and treatment.
- Volunteer to present a relevant topic to your team. Preparing a brief handout on your patient's disease will demonstrate your interest in the subject.

Noon conference: Noon–1:00 P.M. If your service offers a noon conference, you should attend it. Not only is there often free food, but the topics are generally bread-and-butter subjects geared toward house staff and medical students.

Afternoon work: 1:00 P.M.–? In the afternoon, you will finish your "to-do" list and your progress notes. On some days, there will be additional conferences or lectures geared toward medical students.

- Follow up on the results of any consults, studies, or labs that were ordered in the morning. Work with the intern to adjust your treatment plan accordingly.
- Be inquisitive. If you have some downtime and your resident has a few free moments, ask about a particular disease or diagnostic study you don't quite understand.
- Keep your patients informed. If you are following a particular patient, make sure he or she knows what the team is planning.

Signing out: Sign out at the end of the day to your intern or to the cross-covering intern on call.

A good sign-out is the mark of

a good student.

- Make sure you communicate current problems, medications, and allergies.
- Highlight any details that need follow-up overnight (e.g., "Please check the wound site at 10:00 P.M.").
- Document the patient's code status and relevant management issues. Does an IV need to be restarted overnight if it falls out? Do you need blood cultures to be sent if a patient spikes a fever overnight?

The Schedule—Surgery Wards

The surgery day starts earlier and ends later than a typical medicine day. One or more days per week may also include clinic with an attending surgeon.

Prerounds: 5:00–6:00 A.M. Just like medicine prerounds, except that your physical exam must include checking on wounds and drains for post-op patients. You may be expected to write progress notes before work rounds begin.

Work rounds: 6:00–7:30 A.M. Progress notes will be completed during work rounds. You may write a second round of progress notes during afternoon rounds. Surgical progress notes are typically much shorter than medicine progress notes.

Pre-op preparation: 7:30–8:00 A.M. You and a house officer will work with the anesthesiologist to prepare patients for surgery. Typical medical student duties include positioning the patient, placing urinary catheters, and prepping (e.g., shaving, cleaning) the operative area.

Surgery: 8:00 A.M.–5:00 P.M. During surgery, your role may range from observation to retraction, suctioning, and tying and cutting sutures. This will be your primary exposure to attending surgeons.

Pimp questions often fly fast

and furious in the OR.

- Read up on the patient history, the surgical indications, and the basics of the procedure the night before the surgery.
- Know your anatomy—the operating room is home to frequent pimping sessions.

Floor work: 8:00 A.M.–5:00 P.M. When you are not in the operating room, you will be doing daily scut work on your patients with the resident. This usually includes wound checks, pulling staples, pulling chest tubes, and getting consults.

- Decide on a fair distribution of cases with your fellow medical students so that everyone gets some operating-room time and some floor time.

■ Know your patients, and read up on their conditions. Understanding a disease and its treatment will help you anticipate the next steps in management.

"Afternoon" rounds: 5:00–7:30 P.M. These rounds generally start just after the last surgery of the day has ended. They are usually more casual and abbreviated than morning rounds, and they allow the team to review the day's events and plan the next day.

WHAT?

Procedures

You will typically learn procedures either by observing them as they are performed or by doing them under supervision (see Table 1-2). Reading about a procedure in a manual beforehand will maximize your learning, but remember that a procedure is not just technique. You should be familiar with the indications, contraindications, and potential complications. Other tips include the following:

■ Before performing any procedure, you must obtain a signed informed consent from the patient or patient representative. Informed consent includes explanations of the procedure, indications, risks, benefits, and alternative options. Check with your resident as to whether you are allowed to consent a patient.
■ Have **everything you will need** at the bedside, and gather enough materials for multiple tries.
■ Position the patient and yourself for comfort (e.g., bed height, lighting).
■ Remember universal precautions.
■ Use drop cloths, and **clean up after yourself.** Discard all sharps appropriately.
■ Write a procedure note for all procedures and place it in the chart.

Consults

Your team will often call consults from specialty services. Obtaining a consult requires filling out a request form and calling the consultant to tell them about the patient.

TABLE 1-2. Common Procedures for a Junior Student

BASIC	ADVANCED
ABGs	Arthrocentesis
Blood culture	Chest tube insertion
ECG	Central line placement
IV placement	LP
NG tube placement	Obstetrical delivery
Surgical knots	Paracentesis
Suturing	Thoracentesis
Urine (Foley) catheterization	
Venipuncture	
Wound dressing changes	

- **Have a clear question to ask the consultant.** If you don't understand the reason for the consultation, clarify it with your resident **before calling.**
- Request consultations **early in the day.**
- Give a concise, one-minute overview of the patient to the consultant. Include patient identification, pertinent past medical history, pertinent medications, allergies, physical exam findings, and key lab and study results.

Checking Labs and Studies

Check labs and study results during prerounds, in the afternoon, and whenever stat labs or important studies are expected back. If a patient is unstable, labs should be checked more frequently. Anything pertinent should be reported to the resident.

Communicating with Patients and Families

You will serve as the main communication link between the team and the patient. The following tips may be helpful in learning to communicate effectively:

- **Respect the privacy of patients,** and do not discuss patients in public spaces.
- **Be compassionate,** but at the same time honest and direct. If you do not know an answer, tell the family that you will check with the team and get back to them promptly.
- Immediately inform the patient of any upcoming studies or events.
- Have a resident or an attending help you break bad news to a patient or his or her family.
- Choose a quiet time and a private location to talk to a patient.
- **Minimize technical jargon** and explain any medical terms.
- Always finish by asking, "Do you have any questions?"

Independent Reading

Aside from didactic teaching sessions, you will be expected to learn through independent reading. You need to understand the rationale behind the treatment plan for your patients, so your first priority should be to read about the pathophysiology of their conditions. Next, you should read about other patients on your team who might have interesting and active issues. This will keep you involved in patient discussions during rounds. Sources of information include the following:

- **Handbooks.** When you have five minutes before rounds, use the time to quickly review a disease using a handbook. A classic example is *The Washington Manual of Medical Therapeutics.*
- **Review books.** These reference books cover diseases in moderate detail and are meant to be read cover to cover during the course of a rotation. Examples include the First Aid Clerkship series and the Blueprints series.
- **Textbooks.** These tomes are comprehensive, highly detailed references. An example is *Harrison's Principles of Internal Medicine.*
- **Electronic references.** These useful resources are designed to give you a quick answer to your question. Examples include UpToDate (www.upto-

date.com) and AccessMedicine (www.accessmedicine.com). Ask your medical institution which resources are available to you.

- **Journal articles.** Journal articles contain information 2–4 years more current than that found in a reference book. For constantly evolving diseases or recent therapeutic developments, literature searches are highly useful. If you find a relevant paper, it is very appropriate to photocopy the document for your team.

Human Supply Cabinet

Particularly for surgical rotations, students are often relied on to have common items on hand for the attending or house staff. Stocking your pockets with tape, tongue blades, extra gloves, and scissors will save time on rounds and earn you points with your team.

HOW?

Admission H&P

Third-year medical students are generally expected to admit anywhere from one to three patients on a call night. Patients can be admitted through the ER or directly through a clinic, or they can be transferred from another service or an outside hospital. The resident will receive a call with a one-line description of the patient, such as "33-year-old African-American female with abdominal pain." On the basis of this description, you should start formulating a differential diagnosis. Use mnemonics like **MINT CANDY** to ensure that you don't forget any categories.

Review objective data. This includes any paperwork from paramedics or the ER. Also do a brief chart biopsy, focusing on discharge summaries from recent admissions and studies such as ECGs, recent echocardiograms, and past blood work.

Interview the patient. The history and physical (H&P) may be conducted as a team, or you may interview the patient alone. Remember to keep the interview focused and ask about pertinent positive and negatives in the history. Start with open-ended questions (e.g., "What brought you to the hospital?") and then move toward more structured questions (e.g., "Was the pain sharp or dull?"). Always do a complete review of systems (ROS) with every patient you see, asking about symptoms relating to all of the major organ systems.

Conduct a thorough physical exam. Practice your physical exam skills, and try to use the same sequence at all times. Ask for supervision and feedback from your residents.

Present your patient. Give a short, three- to five-minute presentation to your resident, including your leading diagnoses. Your resident may be able to help you polish your presentation and flesh out your assessment and plan (A&P) for your admit note.

Quick framework for a differential diagnosis—

MINT CANDY

Metabolic
Infectious
Neoplastic
Trauma
Collagen vascular disease
Allergies
'N'ything else
Drugs
Youth (congenital)

Two reasons not to do a rectal exam: (1) you don't have a finger, or (2) the patient doesn't have a rectum.

Key:

ADA = American Diabetes Association

BNP = brain natriuretic peptide

CBC = complete blood count

CHF = congestive heart failure

CMP = complete metabolic panel

CT = computed tomography

CXR = chest x-ray

D5 = 5% dextrose

I/O = intake/output

KVO = keep vein open

MI = myocardial infarction

NG = nasogastric

NKDA = no known drug allergies

NPO = nothing by mouth

NS = normal saline

PRN = as required

RR = respiratory rate

SBP = systolic blood pressure

T = temperature

TED = thromboembolic deterrent (stockings)

Key:

IM = intramuscular

QD = every day

QHS = at bedtime

PO = by mouth

PR = by rectum

SAMPLE ADMIT ORDER

6/10/07 12:02 PM

ADMIT TO: Ward, service, your name/intern's name, beeper number.

DIAGNOSIS: If there is no clear diagnosis, give the two or three most likely suspects (e.g., pulmonary embolism vs. CHF exacerbation), the presenting complaint (e.g., chest pain), or the diagnoses you are trying to exclude (e.g., rule out MI).

CONDITION: Options include satisfactory, stable, fair, guarded, critical.

VITALS: Options include per routine, q 4 h, q 1 h, q shift.

ALLERGIES: Mention the specific reaction to the drug (e.g., rash); note NKDA if no allergies.

NURSING ORDERS: Consider strict I/Os, oxygen, daily weights, telemetry, glucose checks, Foley catheter, NG tube, TED stockings.

DIET: Options include regular, 1800-cal ADA, low sodium, soft mechanical, NPO.

ACTIVITY: Options include ad lib, out of bed to bathroom (with assistance), out of bed to chair, strict bed rest, ambulation with crutches.

LABS: Consider specific labs relevant to the patient's presenting complaint (e.g., pro-BNP, D-dimer). Most patients get routine A.M. labs (CBC, CMP, etc.).

IV FLUIDS: Specify hep lock, KVO, or type of solution (e.g., D5, NS, D5 1/2 NS) and rate of infusion (e.g., D5 1/2 NS + 20 mEq/L KCl at 125 cc/hr).

SPECIAL STUDIES: ECG, CXR, CT, etc.

MEDICATIONS: Don't forget antibiotics and PRN medications.

NOTIFY HOUSE OFFICER: T > 38.4°C, pulse > 120 or < 50, SBP < 90 or > 180, RR < 8 or > 30, O_2 sat < 90%.

COMMON PRN MEDICATION ORDERS

Acetaminophen (Tylenol) 650 mg PO q 4 h PRN temp > 101.5°F

Bisacodyl (Dulcolax) 10 mg PO/PR QD PRN constipation

Diphenhydramine (Benadryl) 25 mg PO QHS PRN insomnia

Maalox 10–20 cc PO q 1–2 h PRN dyspepsia

Lorazepam (Ativan) 1–2 mg IM/IV q 6 h PRN anxiety/agitation

Promethazine (Phenergan) 25 mg PO/IM/IV q 4 h PRN nausea

Admit Orders

Admit orders should be entered **before** your admit note is finished. Once you have a working diagnosis and a skeletal management plan, begin entering orders. Many hospitals with electronic order entry have automated admission order sets, but it is important to be able to write out admit orders as well. Use the mnemonic **ADC VANDALISM** as a guide to help formulate your orders. The previous page shows an example of an admit order for a patient admitted with pneumonia.

Admit Notes

The amount of time you have to complete your admit note will depend on the policies of your service. Regardless of the time and circumstance, however, you should have the admit note in the chart **before work rounds** the next morning. Use the time you have to learn more about the patient's condition and to develop a thorough management plan. The history of present ill-

> **Admission orders—**
> ## ADC VANDALISM
> **A**dmit to
> **D**iagnosis
> **C**ondition
> **V**itals
> **A**llergies
> **N**ursing orders
> **D**iet
> **A**ctivity
> **L**abs
> **I**V fluids
> **S**pecial studies
> **M**edications

Key:

A&O × 4 = alert and oriented to person, place, time, and situation

A&P = assessment and plan

Ab = antibody

abx = antibiotics

ALT = alanine transaminase

AST = aspartate transaminase

BID = twice a day

BP = blood pressure

BRBPR = bright red blood per rectum

c̄ = with

CC = chief complaint

C/C/E = clubbing/cyanosis/ edema

CN = cranial nerve

CTAB = clear to auscultation bilaterally

CV = cardiovascular

D/C = diarrhea/ constipation

DOE = dyspnea on exertion

SAMPLE ADMIT NOTE

MS-3 Admission H&P

Date and Time: 6/10/07, 1:30 P.M.

ID/CC: 42-year-old Caucasian woman, former IV drug user, HIV ⊕ c̄ CD4 count of 250, complains of 3 days of painful neck rash and diffuse itching.

HPI: Patient has been HIV ⊕ × 3 years, no opportunistic infections. She complains of sudden-onset painful neck rash 2 days prior to admission. Noted vesicle formation on L neck and deltoid c̄ pruritus, as well as severe burning/stinging pain. Used warm compresses for symptomatic relief. She felt "drained" and stayed in bed × 2 days, denies any F/C/S, no N/V, no abdominal pain, no diarrhea. No arthralgias/myalgias, no cough, no SOB, no HA. She denies any vesicles on face. No ear pain; no eye pain or visual changes. She is unaware of any childhood history of chickenpox and denies any chemical or plant contacts or contact with others with similar symptoms. Denies any recent changes in medication.

PMH:

1. HIV ⊕ × 3 years. Last CD4: 250, 3 months ago. Denies any opportunistic infections.

2. Pneumonia 3–4 × in past 3 years. Hospitalized but cannot relate dates, durations, or diagnoses. Recalls having a chest CT in past and has never had to take prophylactic abx. Chart currently unavailable for review.

3. Cellulitis of extremities several times in the past. Patient unable to recall details or dates.

4. HCV Ab ⊕.

Meds: Indinavir 800 mg PO QID.

Zidovudine 300 mg PO BID.

ddC 0.75 mg PO TID.

13

Key:

DTRs = deep tendon reflexes

EOMI = extraocular movements intact

EtOH = ethanol

F/C/S = fever/chills/ sweating

HA = headache

HCV = hepatitis C

HEENT = head, eyes, ears, nose, and throat

HIV = human immunodeficiency virus

h/o = history of

HR = heart rate

HSM = hepatosplenomegaly

INR = International Normalized Ratio

MAE = moves all extremities

M/R/G = murmurs/rubs/ gallops

MS = musculoskeletal

MVI = multivitamin infusion

NABS = normoactive bowel sounds

NC = nasal cannula

NC/AT = normocephalic/ atraumatic

ND = nondistended

NT = nontender

N/V = nausea/vomiting

O/P = oropharynx

o/w = otherwise

PE = physical exam

All: NKDA.

FH: Noncontributory.

SH: Patient is homeless. Moved from Chicago to San Francisco 4 years ago. She is unmarried and has 4 children, no family on the West Coast. She is intermittently followed by the HIV clinic at San Francisco General Hospital; ⊕ tobacco 1 ppd × 20 years; ⊕ EtOH 1 pint vodka per day; no h/o withdrawal; ⊕ h/o IV drug use, none × 6 years.

ROS:

Constitutional: No fatigue/weakness, no N/V, no F/C, no night sweats, no recent weight change.

HEENT: Denies headaches, visual changes, blurry vision, hearing changes, tinnitus, vertigo, rhinorrhea, nasal congestion, epistaxis, sore throat.

Neck: As noted above. No stiffness or masses.

CV: No chest pains, no palpitations, no DOE, no orthopnea.

Resp: No SOB, no cough, no wheezing.

GI: No recent change in appetite, no dysphagia, no jaundice, no abdominal pain, no D/C, no melena, no BRBPR.

GU: No sexual dysfunction, no dysuria, no hematuria, no polyuria, no stones, no nocturia, no frequency, no hesitancy; no genital sores, rashes, or discomfort.

Neuro: No seizures, no paresthesias, no numbness, no motor weakness, no difficulties with gait.

Extremities/MS: No edema, no joint stiffness, no change in ROM.

Endocrine: No heat/cold intolerance, no excessive sweating, no polyuria, no polydipsia.

Psychiatric: No depression, no change in sleep pattern, no change in motivation.

PE:

Gen: Somnolent, but arousable to alert state, in mild distress due to pain and pruritus.

VS: T 37.1°C BP 111/80 HR 112 RR 18, 99% O_2 sat on 2 L NC.

Skin/hair/nails: Vesicular rash $\bar{c}$ erythematous base, clustered, on L lateral and posterior neck and L deltoid, anterior to clavicle, stops at midline anterior and posterior.

HEENT: NC/AT, PERRL 4 → 3, EOMI, mild conjunctival injection bilat, TMs clear without vesicles, O/P is dry with poor dentition, no vesicles or open lesions, no thrush.

Neck: 1 posterior SCM node 1 × 1 cm, supple neck.

Breast: Deferred at this time per patient request.

Lungs: CTAB, no rales, no wheezes.

CV: Tachycardic, reg rhythm, normal S1/S2, no M/R/G. Good distal pulses.

Abd: Soft, NT, NABS, ND, no HSM.

GU: Deferred at this time per patient request.

Ext: No C/C/E. Cool and dry. Numerous old needle-track scars.

Neuro: A&O × 4. CN II–XII intact. MAE, DTRs 2+ and symmetric, sensation intact. Normal and symmetric strength, tone, and bulk throughout.

Labs:

$$8.2 \diagdown \begin{array}{c} 13.3 \\ 40.0 \end{array} \diagdown 297 \diagdown \begin{array}{c|c|c} 142 & 105 & 8 \\ \hline 4.0 & 29 & 0.8 \end{array} \diagdown 92 \diagdown \begin{array}{l} \text{T. bili 0.7; AST 38; ALT 20; alk phos 77} \\ \hline \text{PT/INR/PTT: 12.4/1.2/32.2} \end{array}$$

Ca 8.3; Mg 2.3; phos 3.9; albumin 3.6; amylase 82

CXR: Increased interstitial markings, o/w ⊖.

A&P: 42-year-old woman c̄ HIV, presenting with likely herpes zoster in L C3/C4 dermatomal distribution.

1. **Herpes zoster:** The differential in this case is rather narrow given the history and presentation. A contact dermatitis is unlikely although a possibility. Given the specific dermatomal distribution, which stops at the midline, reactivation is far more likely than a 1° varicella infection. The patient's HIV status places her at risk for zoster dissemination. Admit for involvement of 2 contiguous dermatomes and monitor for signs of dissemination.

   ▪ Acyclovir 500 mg IV q 8 h.

   ▪ Benadryl 25–50 mg PO q 6 h PRN pruritus.

   ▪ TyCo#3 1–2 tabs PO q 4 h PRN pain.

   ▪ Isolation protocol to protect other immunocompromised patients on floor.

2. **HIV:** CD4 > 200, no h/o opportunistic infections.

   ▪ Continue current medications as noted above.

   ▪ Will arrange follow-up appointment with HIV clinic.

3. **EtOH:** Monitor for signs of EtOH withdrawal.

   ▪ Thiamine 100 mg IV.

   ▪ Folate 1 mg IV.

   ▪ MVI 1 amp IV.

   ▪ Ativan 1–2 mg IV q 1–2 h PRN agitation.

4. **Code status:** Patient is Full Code.

5. **Disposition:** Patient is homeless. Will consult social worker for discharge planning.

Key:

PERRL 4 → 3 = pupils equal, round, and reactive to light from 4 mm to 3 mm

PO = by mouth

ppd = pack per day

PT = prothrombin time

PTT = partial thromboplastin time

QID = four times a day

ROM = range of motion

SCM = sternocleidomastoid

SOB = shortness of breath

T. bili = total bilirubin

TID = three times a day

TM = tympanic membrane

VS = vital signs

ness (HPI) and the A&P are the two most challenging portions of the admit note to write. A well-written admit note is a testament to your thought processes and fund of knowledge. Some helpful ground rules are as follows:

- As you write the admit note, try to identify all missing information before going back to the patient to ask more questions.
- Feel free to use common abbreviations, but avoid abbreviations that might be unrecognizable or easily mistaken for something else.
- All of your notes will become part of a legal record, so avoid making any unprofessional or opinionated comments that are not relevant to the patient's care.
- Each page of your note should include the date and time as well as your name and signature.
- Neat handwriting wins points. Messy handwriting can always be improved by slowing down. There is little point to writing an illegible note.

HPI. Deciding which pieces of information belong in the HPI can be a difficult task. Some tips for helping you formulate your HPI include the following:

- Do not forget to characterize the chief complaint. Use the mnemonic **OPQRST**: **O**nset, **P**rogression, **P**rovocation, **P**alliation, **Q**uality, **R**egion, **R**adiation, associated **S**ymptoms, **S**everity, **T**ime course.
- Include **pertinent** positives and negatives that support your diagnosis, and rule out the other main suspects.
- Tell a story. Information should be presented in chronological order and should lead the reader toward the most likely diagnosis.
- If information in the patient's past medical history (PMH), family history (FH), or social history (SH) is pertinent to the reason for admission, it should be included in the HPI.

A&P. In your A&P, start off with a brief summary of the case, including presenting complaint, relevant symptoms, pertinent lab or imaging results, and your presumed diagnosis. Take the time to read up on your patient's diagnosis and management as well as his or her other important medical problems. Ask your team if they would prefer that your A&P be presented by problem or by system. In general, problem-based approaches are used on general medical floors, while systems-based approaches are used in critical care settings.

For **each** problem, you should include a brief A&P. For the **primary** problem, explain (1) why you think this is the diagnosis, and (2) why the other possible diagnoses are less likely to be correct. Other incidental problems get a one-line assessment. In the plan for each problem, outline your initial treatment plans (e.g., medications, procedures) and any additional workup that needs to be done to further clinch the diagnosis.

Progress Notes

A progress note is a daily written record of all events pertaining to a patient. An example is provided below. On medical-type services (including pediatrics, psychiatry, and neurology), progress notes are typically written in the afternoon. On surgical-type services (including OB/GYN), progress notes are written before work rounds in the morning. Make sure your intern or resident reviews and cosigns your notes. Most students write progress notes in the SOAP format:

Characterizing the chief complaint—

OPQRST

Onset
Progression
Provocation
Palliation
Quality
Region
Radiation
Symptoms
Severity
Time course

SAMPLE PROGRESS NOTE

Date and Time: 6/11/07, 10:00 A.M.

Hospital Day #2: Medicine Service

S: No events overnight. Patient "feels OK"; reports continued pruritus, although significantly improved since yesterday. Good sleep last night; good pain control. No other complaints. Has not noticed any progression of rash.

O: VS: T 36.6°C BP 110/65 HR 90 RR 18, 97% O_2 sat on RA.

I/O: 950 cc/BR.

Skin: No change in distribution or size of vesicles on L neck/shoulder, although some have crusted over. No new vesicles on body.

HEENT: PERRL, EOMI, no conjunctival injection, TMs clear, no vesicles, O/P moist and clear.

Lungs: CTAB, no crackles, no wheezes.

CV: RRR, nl S1/S2, no M/R/G.

Abd: Soft, NT, ⊕ BS.

Labs:

$$\begin{array}{c} 7.9 \end{array} \diagdown \begin{array}{c} 12.8 \\ \hline 37.2 \end{array} \diagdown 260 \qquad \begin{array}{c|c|c} 134 & 103 & 8 \\ \hline 3.6 & 25 & 0.8 \end{array} \diagdown 90$$

A&P: 42-year-old woman with herpes zoster, afebrile and comfortable, doing well.

1. **Herpes zoster:** No evidence of dissemination or spread to other dermatomes. Good pain control; tolerating IV acyclovir well.

   - Atarax PRN pruritus.
   - Continue IV acyclovir, TyCo#3.

2. **HIV:**

   - Continue AZT, indinavir, and ddC.
   - Plan to speak with HIV clinic today to arrange follow-up care.

3. **EtOH:** No sign of alcohol withdrawal at this time. Continue to monitor.

4. **Dispo:** Social worker to speak with patient this afternoon re housing and $.

Key:

BR = bathroom

BS = bowel sounds

nl = normal

RA = room air

RRR = regular rate and rhythm

- **Subjective:** The patient's account of symptom changes, significant events over the last day, and physical complaints.
- **Objective:** Vital signs; a focused, brief physical exam; and any laboratory and study results.
- **A&P:** Your impression of the objective and subjective information and what the appropriate diagnostic and treatment regimen will be. Your plan should be concise and laid out so that someone else reading your note can easily understand the team's plan for your patient.

SAMPLE PROCEDURE NOTE

Procedure: Diagnostic LP.

Indication: Suspected meningitis.

Consent: Patient gave informed consent.

Complications: None.

Patient was placed in left lateral decubitus position with spine flexed, and the L4–L5 interspace was identified. Under sterile conditions, the area was prepared with Betadine and anesthetized with 1% lidocaine 5 cc. Spinal needle introduced into L4–L5 interspace without difficulty. Opening pressure 130 mm; 8 cc clear, nonturbid spinal fluid collected and sent for protein, glucose, Gram stain, cell count, culture. Patient tolerated the procedure well.

Procedure Notes

A procedure note must be written and placed in the chart for any invasive procedure that is performed, including an LP, thoracentesis, paracentesis, and central line placement. The note should be concise and should document the date and time, indications, consent, preparation of the patient, anesthesia used (if any), details of the procedure, yield, any studies sent, and any complications.

Daily Orders

Make it clear to your team that you would like to write orders for your patients when possible (they will be cosigned). This will give you valuable practice in prescription writing and drug dosing and will also help you stay current with your patient's treatment regimens. Tips include the following:

An intern will usually cosign everything you do—including orders and notes.

- Become familiar with your hospital's order entry system so that you can enter or write orders quickly and avoid slowing the team down.
- Before writing orders, always double-check to make sure you have the right chart.
- When writing drug orders, always remember to consider patient weight and any medical conditions that may alter drug dosing (e.g., hepatic or renal insufficiency).
- If the order is important, also pass it on verbally to the nurse or the ward clerk. Check nursing records frequently to be sure orders were properly carried out.

Prescriptions

Prescriptions are most frequently needed in outpatient settings and before discharge in a hospital. While you cannot sign prescriptions, ask to fill them in before they are signed. If you are not sure why a patient is being discharged on a particular medication, don't be afraid to ask. This will show that you are interested and are trying to understand the rationale behind the patient's care. When writing prescriptions:

> ### SAMPLE PRESCRIPTION
>
> **Name:** John Smith
>
> **Hospital ID:** 222-22-255
>
> **Rx:** Keflex 500 mg
>
> **Disp:** #40
>
> **Sig:** Take one tab PO QID × 7 days
>
> **Refills:** None
>
> Generic OK

- Make sure to include time and date, generic drug name, dose, route of delivery (PO, IV, IM, SQ), frequency, and signature. Include your printed name, title, and beeper number.
- Write legibly; do not use abbreviations.
- Have the prescription cosigned immediately by a house officer. Your signature alone is not sufficient.

The Formal Oral Presentation

During your clerkships, no skill is more important to master than the delivery of a focused, fluent, and concise oral presentation. You will be called on to present patients under varied circumstances and time constraints for the rest of your professional life, so getting a good handle on this skill early on is critical to success on the wards.

Confidence and brevity should be your goals for formal oral presentations. Most presentations can be given in **less than seven minutes,** with a focus on delivering only essential details. The presentation should follow the same format as your admit note but should omit any superfluous information.

In general, more emphasis can be placed on the patient's *current* state (CC, HPI, PE, labs, A&P) than on past events (PMH, FH, SH). Each detail should clue the audience in to your decision-making process such that a listener can anticipate your A&P. While the substance of your presentation is important, **do not forget about style.** Deliver your presentation with confidence, and pay attention to body language, eye contact, and posture.

Each attending will have specific preferences for the format and length of an oral presentation. Listen closely to the style and format of presentations given by the residents and interns over the first few days of your rotation. The categories that follow should be addressed in any oral presentation.

Chief complaint (CC). The presenting symptom *according to the patient.* If a patient presents with shortness of breath and you make the diagnosis of congestive heart failure, the chief complaint is "shortness of breath," not "congestive heart failure."

History of present illness (HPI). Begin with a **one-line** introduction that includes identifying information and the chief complaint (e.g., "Mr. X is a 71-year-old diabetic male with long-standing hypertension who presents with a two-day history of dyspnea, bilateral pedal edema, and chest pain"). Your oral HPI should be similar to your written HPI and should take the listener through the story of how a patient arrived at the hospital. Include only pertinent positives and negatives.

Review of systems (ROS). This should be very brief, as most pertinent information will already have been covered in the HPI.

Past medical history (PMH). Include all ongoing medical conditions and any pertinent past history (you do not need to mention a history of childhood chickenpox in an elderly man with an acute MI). Any past history that is relevant to the current admission should be included in the HPI.

Allergies/medications. You do not need to present the dosage for each medication, but have dosages written down in case you are asked for them.

Social history (SH). Include a brief social history, including history of tobacco, alcohol, and drug use. Sexual histories are generally included only if they are relevant to the present admission.

Family history (FH). This section includes both positive and negative findings and should be very short, as any relevant information should already have been mentioned in the HPI.

Physical exam (PE). Always present a **focused physical exam,** elaborating only on relevant sections (e.g., if you are rotating through neurology, your attending is unlikely to be interested in poor dentition). Avoid general, uninformative sentences such as "The cardiac exam was unremarkable." Instead, briefly cover your specific physical findings: "No murmurs, rubs, or gallops were present on cardiac exam."

Labs/imaging. Some attendings prefer thorough reports of lab and imaging results, while others favor just hearing the highlights. If you are unsure, ask your attending in advance of the presentation. Make sure you have personally reviewed all imaging and ECGs so that you feel comfortable pointing out your findings to the team.

Practice, practice, practice
your presentation.

Assessment and plan (A&P). Begin with a short summary of the patient, tying together the most relevant points of your presentation and concluding with your most likely diagnosis. For example, "Mr. Smith is a 58-year-old man with known coronary artery disease and hypertension who presents with one hour of substernal chest pain radiating to the left jaw and troponin elevations to 7.3 without ischemic changes on ECG, consistent with an NSTEMI." If the diagnosis is unclear, present the two or three most likely diagnoses on your differential.

Again, you can present the A&P in the form of a problem or according to organ system. In either format, you should generate a list of the issues facing your patient and should then develop plans for both acute and long-term management of each issue. Finally, if you want to be a star, it is always impressive to present a brief discussion of a recent journal article on a management or diagnostic technique related to the admission.

The Bullet Presentation

The one-minute bullet presentation is an extremely concise synopsis of the case presentation. You may give bullet presentations during work rounds as well as to consultants or other health care providers who are unfamiliar with your patient. Practicing this skill with each patient you write up will help you filter information more easily.

A well-done presentation is like a riveting story.

- Summarize the history, physical exam, laboratory findings, and A&P sections into one sentence each.
- Include only the most pertinent positive and negative findings, usually encompassing anywhere from 15 to 20 facts about the case.

TIPS FOR WARDS SURVIVAL

So now you know what to do, when to do it, how to do it, and whom to talk to when you have questions. Those are the basics, but to make the best use of your time on the wards, there are a few other tips that might be helpful.

Efficient Time Management

Although complicated patients will certainly make your days longer, getting out at a reasonable hour ultimately depends on your ability to work closely with your team and efficiently execute your duties. Some people will swear that they have a "black cloud" surrounding them, meaning that for some unknown reason they appear to be swamped with more work and more admissions than others. Believe it or not, studies have been done to determine whether so-called black clouds really exist, and they have found that people who claim to have them are just less efficient than others. Use the following tips to improve your time management skills:

Make a to-do list. Write down all tasks, even those that seem to be less important than others. Remember that you will be bombarded with multiple responsibilities while on the wards, so it is inevitable that you will forget something. Keeping a running list of all tasks, and checking them off as they are accomplished, will help ensure that everything gets done.

Prioritize your tasks. Think about what you need to do first to ensure that your patients do not stay in the hospital any longer than necessary. For example, consults and studies must be requested in the morning or they will not get done that day (see Table 1-3). If you plan to discharge a patient, take care of the paperwork and placement issues early.

Try to organize tasks by location. Always think about how to combine tasks on a single trip. If you happen to be in radiology following up on a CXR for Patient A, for example, you should also check off any other radiology chores you might have, like looking at a head CT for Patient B or abdominal films for Patient C.

Learn to maximize the hospital information system. A good hospital information system can be your friend. Some systems can handle custom patient lists, print labs and problem lists, and even perform literature searches.

Keep scut essentials on board. Supply carts are always in the third place you look. So if you do find a mother lode of supplies, stock up on suture removal

TABLE 1-3. Example of Prioritized Tasks

Do Now	Do Next
Request consults	Write progress notes
Schedule studies	Check routine labs
Do discharge paperwork	Follow up on consults
Check stat or crucial labs	Follow up on studies

kits, blood-draw supplies, and other essentials you need to get through your scut so that you don't have to hunt for a supply cart every time you go to a different floor. Also be sure to carry a beeper. The easier you are to reach, the more you will stay involved with patient care. There is nothing worse than hanging around waiting for an admission without a pager when you could be in the library or call room instead.

Organizational Aids ("Peripheral Brains")

If you can't fit your organizational aid in your pocket, you risk misplacing it.

Another key to being an efficient medical student is to have and use the right organizational aids. The pros and cons of the most popular organizational aids are discussed below.

Clipboard. Many students start out with a clipboard as their preferred mode of organization. The clipboard offers lots of surface area on which to organize patient information and tasks. It also gives you the ability to hold additional items such as progress notes, journal articles, and lab requests. Clipboards are easy to lose, however, and are also easy to overstuff with miscellaneous papers.

Binders. Three-ring binders can be extremely helpful, particularly on medicine services, where much patient information is accumulated. Tabs can help you locate patient information quickly without necessitating that you shuffle through papers or cards. Remember, however, that binders can be bulky and can also be easily misplaced.

Data sheets. Many people prefer $8^{1}/_{2} \times 11$ sheets that can be folded in half and put in the pocket. You can carry separate sheets for the patient's H&P and lab data. You can shop around for a format you like (ask your residents or fellow medical students) or make your own.

Note cards. Most house staff and senior students use note cards to organize their patients, scut lists, and clinical cheat sheets. Note cards are compact and slide easily into your pocket. Because of space considerations, note cards also force you to organize your thoughts and record only important information. In addition, they are much less obtrusive than other organizational aids when you are presenting. However, note cards may force you to use abbreviations and tiny print to the point at which they are barely legible. Here are some pointers regarding note cards:

■ Blank note cards can often be found at the nurses' station.
■ A ring binder or clip allows you to keep your cards together. You will need to punch holes in the cards. An alternative is to maintain a pocket-size spiral-bound notebook.

- Use a high-quality fine-point pen (e.g., a Pilot fine ballpoint) to minimize "microglyphics." Do not use felt-tip pens, as they may run if your cards get wet.
- Consider using a card of a different color for the patient's admission H&P.
- Create an "if found" card with your name and pager number written on it. Losing your cards is like having an unscheduled lobectomy. You have not known true fear until you have misplaced your patient cards.
- Create a card with key phone numbers on it (e.g., team pagers, lab, x-ray, nursing stations of each ward). This is critical, as it will save you time and will often help members of your team.

Personal digital assistants (PDAs). Also known as electronic organizers, these handheld computers are increasingly popular on the wards with students, residents, and attendings alike. Indeed, some medical schools now require that their medical students own PDAs. Electronic organizers are highly useful for their ability to hold personal addresses, phone numbers, and appointments. You can also use them to record as a document file the clinical pearls you pick up during conferences and on the wards. Perhaps more significantly, medical software is now available for the PDA. Resources range from medical calculators to full-text reference books. Most PDAs also have infrared ports so that information can be exchanged between PDAs.

Keep track of your PDA at all times. It can grow legs!

Some of the more current and useful PDA resources are discussed within the Top-Rated Review Resources section. Aside from this, the choice of a PDA should depend on personal preference, memory capacity, price range, and other features. Remember, too, that PDAs operating on the Palm operating system cannot interface with those running on a Pocket PC operating system. You should choose a PDA with at least 16 megabytes of memory and should inquire about the expandability of a PDA, especially with respect to memory. You may also consider a "smartphone" like Palm's Treo series, which combines a cell phone with a PDA. Unlike note cards and clipboards, PDAs require a significant investment in both time and money. Also, since PDAs are a small but valuable piece of equipment, they are always at risk of being misplaced or stolen.

Surviving Call Nights

The following tips will make call nights more pleasant and less stressful events:

- Bring a travel alarm, or use the alarm on your pager.
- Make an "on-call" bag with a toothbrush, a hairbrush, a razor, and a change of clothes if you are working in a clinic the next day.
- Bring snacks! Dried fruit or nuts are good options for late-night hunger.
- Bring a review/mini–reference book to learn about your patients' problems when you find you have downtime.

EVALUATIONS

Your third-year evaluations are critical, as they make up the majority of your dean's letter. Residency directors who are seeking to recruit the best medical students examine third- and fourth-year evaluations first. To do well on the wards, you will need to develop new skills: working with a team, communicating effectively, and understanding the nuances of clinical presentations. During the first two years, your fund of knowledge is everything—but during the clinical years, it is only one of many criteria by which you will be judged.

Written evaluations. Written evaluations are usually subjective assessments written by the attending or the senior resident. These assessments are intended to convey comments and observations of your performance on a given service. Because not all residents and attendings will be asked to evaluate you in writing, however, it may be useful to find out who will be evaluating you before you start your rotation. Written evaluations are easily influenced by personal factors and can be dangerous, since they are often quoted verbatim in the dean's letter. A single interaction (be it positive or negative) can easily be seen by an attending as representative of your performance during the entire rotation.

Third-year evaluations are crucial to a successful residency application.

Maximizing your evaluations. It is critical to stay on top of your evaluations by getting feedback from your attendings and residents at an early stage, before potentially negative material ends up in your written evaluations. At least one study has shown that asking for verbal feedback before the resident or attending completes your written evaluation results in higher written evaluation marks. At the beginning of the rotation, you should thus ask both your attending and your resident what their expectations are. Then, two weeks into the rotation, meet with your attending as well as with your resident to see if you are fulfilling their expectations and if there are any areas in which you can improve (e.g., notes, rounds, procedures, communication). Sit down with your attending and resident at the end to review your performance. Your persistence will not only provide invaluable feedback but also demonstrate initiative that will not go unnoticed.

Within weeks, the clerkship office should have written evaluations on file. Visit the office to review them; with any luck at all, the results will be pleasant. However, if you believe your evaluation is an inaccurate representation of your performance, now is the time to bring it to the attention of the clerkship director or the dean. It may be too late to change an evaluation by the time dean's letters are written during the summer of your fourth year.

Find out what your team expects of you on the very first day of the rotation.

Do not allow evaluations to affect your self-perception, as they can vary widely. However, do not ignore trends or patterns in your evaluations, as they more or less reflect the consensus perception of your performance.

Honors/Grades

Most schools have a grading system of one sort or another—such as "honors/pass/fail" or the traditional letter grading system—with which to gauge your clinical performance. Make sure you have a clear understanding of the criteria for achieving honors and top grades. Looking at an evaluation form can tell you what specific skills and performance criteria will be used to judge you. In addition, keep in mind that getting honors is not necessarily everything. Although honors are certainly helpful for residency (icing on the cake), it is more important to perform consistently well on rotations, as such performance will be reflected in your dean's letter.

Your final grade in a rotation is usually reflective of both your performance on the wards and your grade on a final examination. Basic clerkships usually use the National Board of Medical Examiners (NBME) subject test, also known as the shelf exam—a 100-question standardized test administered to students at medical schools throughout the country. Because you will not be judged on your clinical skills alone, it is important to make time to study independently for this exam.

Letters of Recommendation

If your attending wrote you a glowing evaluation or has given you very positive feedback, you may ask for a letter of recommendation while details of your valor are still fresh. Letters of recommendation are used when you apply for residency positions. If you ask for a letter early in the third year, have the attending update the letter when your career path becomes clearer.

DIFFICULT SITUATIONS

The junior student is faced with a host of new situations that may require social and political savvy. Unfortunately, medical students are typically at the bottom of the totem pole and have little political leverage. At the same time, however, failure to handle these situations can lead to anything from simple embarrassment to patient endangerment.

Do not hesitate to seek help if circumstances on the wards become overwhelming. The wards can be a very stressful environment, so bear in mind that getting help is not a sign of failure but rather a testament to your ability to understand your limitations. The three main areas of stress for medical students are academic pressures, social issues, and financial problems. Try to recognize your stressors. If necessary, seek help from your medical school, as this will not reflect negatively on your evaluations or dean's letter; schools are more concerned with your well-being than anything else. Most institutions will also have discreet counseling services available to you at little or no cost. Remember, too, that your fellow classmates are in the same situation and may be facing similar issues. So this is a time to reach out to others and talk about your feelings, concerns, and fears.

Confidential counseling is available.

Needlesticks

Being stuck by a needle or other sharp is a cause for significant concern in the health care field. Because you are inexperienced with handling sharps, you are at a higher risk of incurring needlesticks. Following these tips will reduce your chances of being stuck:

- Always practice universal precautions, treating all body fluids as if they are potentially infectious. Wear gloves when handling blood products, protect your eyes against splashes, and wear a gown to protect yourself from contamination. Substances that require universal precautions include blood; maternal milk, semen, and vaginal secretions; and cerebrospinal, synovial, peritoneal, pleural, pericardial, and amniotic fluids.
- Don't rush. Slow down and think about what you are doing. Be especially careful in the ER and in surgery, where needles and other sharps are being passed around you.
- Dispose of contaminated sharps immediately using the nearest sharps container. Remember that you are responsible for your own sharps. Never simply leave a needle on a table or a bed, as you may forget it is there or some-

Treat all body fluids as if they are potentially infectious. Never recap, bend, or break a sharp.

one else may be stuck by it. If you absolutely must put a contaminated sharp down, announce that you are doing so ("Sharp on the table") so that others can be made aware of it. If others are in the room when you are carrying a sharp to the disposal container, let them know you are carrying a sharp.

- Never recap, bend, or break any needles/sharps.
- Don't force a needle into a sharps container that is full.
- Get vaccinated against HBV!

Despite your best efforts, the unthinkable may still occur. So if you are ever stuck by a contaminated sharp, try to remember the following:

- Don't panic. Take a deep breath.
- Make sure the patient is safe, and discard the sharp properly.
- Wash the involved area with soap and water or Betadine.
- Call the Needlestick Hotline as soon as possible, and inform one of your team members. Report exactly what happened and follow the appropriate protocol. The hotline will give you information and will facilitate blood testing, counseling, and possible HIV prophylactic treatment.

Always report a needlestick.

Do not hesitate to speak with team members, fellow students, friends and family, or counselors about what happened. A needlestick can be extremely traumatizing (in many ways, it can be like a brush with death). If you feel you need to leave early to go home, tell your resident.

Abusive or Inappropriate House Officers

House staff typically work long hours and lead hectic lifestyles. However, that does not give them the right to vent their frustrations on you. Such issues can, of course, be problematic given that you are likely being evaluated by the offending team member—but if an abusive situation does not resolve, you should bring it to the attention of the clerkship director or the student dean. Avoid bringing the issue to the attention of the attending, as doing so can further disrupt the dynamics of the team.

On the other hand, you may receive unwanted attention from a coworker, such as being asked out for a drink by the resident. You may avoid an awkward situation by suggesting that the entire team go out for drinks. If the resident is insistent, you may have to be more direct. If this leads to a negative working relationship, you may need to bring it to the attention of the clerkship director or the student dean in order to resolve the situation and protect yourself from any unfair evaluations.

Inappropriate Procedures

Be aggressive in volunteering for any procedures that may be appropriate to your skill level (residents love highly motivated students). However, do not allow yourself to be pushed into performing any procedure with which you are not comfortable, as this can be dangerous both for you and for the patient and will not make for an optimal learning situation. If you do not feel comfortable performing a procedure, it is acceptable to say, "I'm not comfortable with this procedure. Can you walk me through it, or can I watch this one and perform the next one?"

Overly Competitive Classmates (aka "Gunners")

The desire to achieve recognition and to get good grades can cloud the better judgment of your classmates (and sometimes your own). When there is more than one student to a team, a sense of do-or-die competition may arise, leading to excessive "brown-nosing" or backstabbing behavior. This way of thinking must be curbed at the very start of any rotation. Your classmates are some of your most valuable resources, and their cooperation and support are key to learning and doing well on the rotation. Also remember that residents and attendings have all been junior students themselves and can thus spot brown-nosing and backstabbing behavior easily. So take the initiative—keep your classmates informed of scheduled events, share procedures and information, and teach one another. Address backstabbing behavior immediately and firmly. If the pattern persists, bring it to the attention of your intern or resident. Always maintain the moral high ground; you'll sleep better at night.

Learn to trust and depend on your classmates.

Patient Death

Despite the best efforts you and your team might make, some of your patients will inevitably die while under your care. The first patient death can be particularly disturbing, especially if you developed any personal attachments to the patient. You should thus consider discussing the patient's death with your team or with other students if they are receptive. Good social and family support can also be of benefit. Seek confidential counseling if necessary. As you continue your clinical training, you will learn to deal more effectively with patient death. However, do not distance yourself from the patient so much that you lose the human perspective.

The first few patient deaths can often be very difficult to deal with.

Sexual Harassment

The power structure of a medical team can lead to abuses of attending and house staff privileges. Female students are especially vulnerable to snide remarks and outright inappropriate behavior. However, confronting the offender immediately is an option you should exercise only if you feel that you can handle it. In any case, you should document the event(s) clearly and unambiguously, record the exact circumstances and nature of the incident(s), and identify any witnesses. Then make an appointment to see your student dean as soon as possible, and review the school's written policies on the subject. Your dean should be able to confidentially evaluate the information and determine the best course of action. Your school may also have a sexual harassment prevention office or a dean or ombudsperson in charge of a sexual harassment protocol.

Sexual harassment is a highly charged issue, so you will want to have as many backers as possible before you confront an offender. If you decide that the degree of harassment is mild, you may elect to tolerate the situation or wait until the rotation is finished for the sake of preserving your evaluation and team dynamics. This is a personal decision. However, it is advisable that you continue to document all offending incidents in the event that you do change your mind and decide to act. At the end of the rotation, consider using evaluation forms to state your case so that you can help prevent this behavior in the future.

Document harassment. Then see your student dean.

Difficult or Violent Patients

Not all patients are pleasant and enjoyable to work with. To the contrary, patients can sometimes be manipulative, hostile, verbally abusive, and even violent. Often, however, such negative behavior is a physical manifestation of the patient's anger and frustration. So do not take anything personally. You need not like every patient you care for, but each deserves your best efforts and respect. You should also use common sense when dealing with difficult patients. Never hesitate to call on more experienced house staff to intervene when situations escalate. And never, ever retaliate against a patient. When dealing with agitated or potentially violent patients, keep the following in mind:

Personal safety is a priority with potentially violent patients.

- Remember that your own safety must come first.
- Never let the patient get between you and the door.
- Keep the door open.
- Visit the patient only with a nurse or house officer.
- Assess restraint status.
- Rule out reversible causes of increased agitation and lability.
- Don't let your dislike for a patient compromise his or her care.

Difficult Family Members

Having a sick loved one in the hospital places considerable stress on family members and friends, and sometimes the anger, frustration, and sadness they feel are redirected toward you. So again, do not take anything personally. When dealing with family members, find out who the chief decision maker is, especially if the patient is incapacitated or is not competent to make his or her own decisions. Do not, however, let family members push you into speculating about a treatment course. If you are unsure about anything, check with your team before giving the family a definitive answer. Again, know when to seek help from your team or a social worker in order to defuse highly charged or emotional situations.

"Narcolepsy"

Do whatever it takes to stay awake.

During your preclinical years, no one ever noticed if you fell asleep after lunch in a roomful of people. On the wards, however, everyone will notice you if you doze off. Although falling asleep occasionally is understandable given your state of frequent exhaustion, constant snoozing will leave a bad impression. The best remedy is to get more sleep. Some students become staunch believers in coffee; however, be aware that caffeine withdrawal is a real clinical syndrome! Another option is to remain standing during rounds and conferences. Although this may raise a few eyebrows, remember that it is your learning (and to some extent your evaluation) that is at stake. If you can sneak in a quick nap (20–30 minutes), do so if you are having trouble concentrating. Do not drive home if you are unable to stay awake; automobile accidents are a major cause of morbidity and mortality in exhausted residents, and you are not immune.

Personal Illness

As students slip into the role of health care provider, they often come to believe that they themselves are not allowed to get sick. In fact, it is a wonder that students do not get sick more often given the long work hours and relentless stress they face. When you do get sick, however, your first priority must be your own health. You cannot provide good patient care while sick, and you may transmit your illness to your patients. With this in mind, do not dwell on your clinical responsibilities while you are ill; your team will likely get the job done just fine without your help. However, use your judgment when calling in sick, as some house staff will inevitably think less of your dedication to the team if you choose to do so. When sick, immediately page your resident or intern and let them know when you hope to return. If you are out for more than one day, try to keep track of events with your patients by speaking to your team once a day. This will help you slide back into the ward routine with minimal confusion. Use the downtime to catch up on reading.

No one can blame you for getting sick.

Time Off for Personal Obligations

When you need time off to attend to personal obligations such as a wedding, make arrangements with your resident as far in advance as possible, preferably at the beginning of the rotation. Arrange your call nights around the event if possible. If not, make up the call day elsewhere in the rotation. Try to limit major time off to once a rotation. Of course, there will also be situations in which you unexpectedly need time off, such as a family illness or a death. Here again, give your team as much advance notice as possible, even if it is just one day. Everyone will understand. As with personal illness, try to keep track of your patients' events if possible. Otherwise, come in the evening before or very early in the morning of your next workday to review patient notes.

Strategies for Mental and Physical Health

Clinical clerkships are highly taxing, but you must make a conscious effort to balance work and rest, as ignoring your body's needs will eventually compromise your clinical performance. Remember that your own health must come first, as you are no help to the team if you are ill. Most of the following advice is considered so basic that it is actually ignored.

Streamline and/or delegate household chores when possible. Consider using an automatic bill-payment service. Chip in for a bimonthly cleaning service. Schedule household chores while you are on an easier rotation in exchange for having your roommate or spouse do them during the more time-consuming services. Make sure your roommate or spouse understands how difficult your schedule will be on the wards.

Stay grounded in friends and family. Your friends and family have been there for you during the preclinical years, but you'll need their support and companionship more than ever during the clerkships. Given the hours you may be keeping, it can become difficult to stay in touch at times, especially since many of your friends may be classmates who are equally overwhelmed. Nonetheless, be sure to make a solid attempt to return phone messages and to remember birthdays, anniversaries, and the like.

Eat well. It is a well-known fact that hospital food and most lunches at noon conferences are considered risk factors for cardiovascular disease. You can still be picky without sacrificing speed. In addition, eat when you can. Being well fed is key to maintaining a high energy level. Load up with complex carbohydrates instead of fat and sugar snacks.

Exercise. "No kidding," you might say—but getting exercise can be especially tough when you're exhausted from a long day on the wards. It's even worse if you view exercise as yet another chore. You must find an activity that you enjoy, whether it be walking or basketball. Exercising with a friend can keep you more committed and can make the activity more social. Consider joining a 24-hour gym so that you can work out during the odd hours in which you are free. Another option is to keep a treadmill or a bike at home so that you can work out while watching TV or reading.

Practice what you preach—
stay healthy.

Find healthy ways to deal with stress. Unfortunately, the incidence of alcohol and substance abuse is higher among medical students and medical graduates than in the general population. This abuse grows most rapidly between the second and fourth years of medical school. You should thus recognize that you are entering a significantly vulnerable group and be prepared to deal with the stress in ways other than using alcohol and drugs. Find a nonmedical activity—such as reading, running, or painting—that can help you escape the stress of medical school every once in a while. Put it on your schedule and make sure to do it for your health!

MAXIMIZING YOUR POTENTIAL

Although you may think that starting on the wards is akin to getting tossed to the wolves, you are not going in empty-handed. Instead, you need to be aware of several advantages that you can maximize to work in your favor.

Enthusiasm

House staff may have a deeper fund of knowledge than you as well as more experience, but you can easily match or even surpass them when it comes to hustle, effort, getting there early, and staying late. Team members are often impressed by enthusiastic students, as are patients.

Time

The house staff's time is very precious. You, on the other hand, have plenty of time available. While the house officers have to do brief H&Ps, you have the opportunity and privilege to really learn about your patients. This often allows you to ferret out bits of information on H&Ps that can contribute to—or sometimes even drastically change—patient management. If your patients are frustrated at having to repeat their entire histories again, let them know that you will be able to give them more time than anyone else on the team.

Basic Science Knowledge

Not too long ago, you completed one of the most arduous tasks of medical school: passing the United States Medical Licensing Examination (USMLE) Step 1. Believe it or not, some of the minutiae that you memorized are still buried somewhere in your unconscious and will surface when you least expect it. By contrast, the interns and residents on your team are years away from their basic science classes, so don't be surprised if you can show them a thing or two on rounds in front of the attending (of course, don't make a habit of making your resident look dumb, or you may be less than happy with your evaluation). Discreetly feeding the tired intern or resident factoids for attending rounds helps them look good. This can build your reputation as a "team player."

"Low" Expectations

Remember that you are **not** expected to know the answer to every question, nor are you expected to know the set of orders written for a rule-out-MI protocol with your first patient. You will find to your surprise that residents are often impressed by your level of knowledge, even when you consider a question to be a relatively simple one. You are, however, expected to care about your patients and to make a sincere effort to be a contributing member of the team. As long as you show your resident that you are trying to be productive, he or she will be satisfied.

GETTING OFF TO A GOOD START

To further maximize your wards experience, here are some preparatory measures you can take in the months and weeks before your first rotation starts.

Scheduling Rotations

In the spring of your second year, you will go through the process of scheduling your third-year clerkships. Many schools have rotations prescheduled on tracks, in which case your only task is to choose a track, usually by lottery. Fortunately, there are only a few guidelines you need to know when scheduling your third-year clerkships.

Do not do your most likely specialty first. During the first few weeks of your clerkships, you won't even know where the bathroom is, let alone competently function as a health care provider. It is therefore important to give yourself a chance to get the general feel of the hospital wards, to understand the role you will play, and to become comfortable presenting patients and writing notes. With this in mind, your first rotation should be in a field that you are not likely to enter. For example, most students do not end up going into neurology; however, neurology (as opposed to psychiatry) has the look and feel of a medicine rotation. You should also make sure every member of your team knows that this is your first rotation; that way, they are likely to be more pleasant and forgiving.

Do not do your most likely specialty last. You will be scheduling your senior clerkships in the spring of your third year. If you're interested in pediatrics, you will want to have completed your junior pediatrics clerkship before that crucial scheduling period so that you can decide if and when you will be taking any senior pediatrics rotations.

Avoid back-to-back tough rotations. This is a soft rule, especially if you've decided that you have no career interests in one of those specialties. However, you should be concerned about the possibility of burnout when "killer" rotations get scheduled together. Strategically place vacation time after especially difficult rotations to give yourself a chance to unwind.

Schedule an easy rotation before your most likely specialty rotation. Also a soft rule, this gives you time to relax and do some preemptive reading before you start that big rotation. Some students even recommend taking a little vacation time before a key rotation to do some heavy-duty reading.

Choosing Rotation Sites

Your rotations occur in a variety of hospital and clinical settings. Each type of setting has characteristics that will color your clinical experience. Consult senior students regarding the pros and cons of each site, including key attendings to seek out or avoid. The generalizations below don't always apply but should give you an idea of what to expect.

County. The county hospital is typically very busy yet understaffed. Chaos seems to be the baseline rule as interns and residents battle high patient loads and constant fatigue. County hospitals usually serve the urban poor. In this "all hands on deck" state, you can expect to have increased responsibility and more hands-on procedures but less guidance and didactic teaching. You can excel in this environment by being the perfect "scut monkey," taking care of all those little (but necessary) patient-care tasks. This will help get your team's census down before the next on-call onslaught. The discharge of county hospital patients tends to be more difficult and time-consuming owing to their social situations, so social workers will often become your best allies as you struggle to get your patients out of the hospital.

Department of Veterans Affairs (VA). The VA system personifies the U.S. government in that things take twice as long to get done at twice the cost. Indeed, things sometimes don't get done at all without a little political back-scratching and schmoozing. Therefore, being savvy with regard to the political hierarchy definitely helps. The VA population is also unique, consisting mostly of older men. Female students should thus be prepared, if necessary, to be a bit more cautious with these patients. Because the population is somewhat demographically restricted, you will also see the same diseases over and over again, including the following:

At the VA, know how to work the system.

- CHF
- MI
- COPD
- Lung cancer
- Diabetes
- Arrhythmias
- GI bleeding
- Peripheral vascular disease

You should definitely read up on these diseases before you go to the VA. You should also be aware that VA patients often remain in-house because of placement issues (where will the patient go after discharge) rather than medical issues. So if you neglect discharge planning, you may end up with a large yet inactive census.

Academic/university center. Ivory-tower medicine has its own unique approach toward treating patients. Medical and surgical services are top-heavy with consultants and fellows. As a result, residents and interns are often deprived of procedures, leaving even less for you to do. In addition, university hospitals are often tertiary and quaternary referral centers; thus, they get the patients that stump the community physicians. This is where you will see those "zebra" cases, so be prepared to spend some quality time with PubMed.

The high staff-to-patient ratio at academic centers also means that a lot of time is spent rounding and discussing the latest treatment for your patient's disease. You can stay ahead of the game by pulling current review papers in the literature for yourself and for the team. The quality of didactics is typically best in the academic center but can sometimes stray into the realm of cutting-edge research and basic science. Finally, a lot of the bigwigs at your school can be found in the academic center. Many students schedule key core and senior rotations there to rub elbows with the academic gods. Scoring an enthusiastic letter of recommendation from them can help make your residency application more impressive.

Community hospital. Community hospitals are the antithesis of academic centers in that the focus here is on the patient's treatment and the bottom line. Patients thus tend to come in with bread-and-butter diagnoses, and the populations tend to be more skewed toward the middle class. Many of the physicians are, in addition, private community types—so if residents are present, they are sometimes relegated to "water boy" status, carrying out orders rather than formulating treatment plans. In many cases, you will be working with a different private physician for each patient. Here again, schmoozing is key to participating in a meaningful learning experience as well as to getting things done. Teaching is also more relaxed and deals with the practical treatment approach. Nobody really cares if the long-QT syndrome is linked to the Harvey ras (H-ras-1) oncogene on the short arm of chromosome 11, so long as you know what to do when a patient with a more common problem walks (or rolls) through the door.

Outpatient clinic. Reforms in medical education will lead to more time spent seeing patients in the outpatient clinic. In an outpatient setting, residents can blow through half a dozen patients in an afternoon; you'll be lucky if you manage to see three patients in the same amount of time. Keys to being a well-regarded outpatient clerk include obtaining a focused H&P guided by past clinic notes and studies, as well as making a succinct presentation with pertinent positives and negatives that allow your resident or attending to clearly assess the problem. It is also crucial to learn the important things to ask and document as well as the nonessential information that is better left out, since time and efficiency are of the essence. Outpatient medicine is very different from inpatient care in that the patients are not "prisoners," so you cannot order all the tests at once and expect to get them back the same day. In this setting, you will also learn the frustration of patient noncompliance and missed appointments (think about that the next time you decide to blow off your dental appointment).

Before You Start on the Wards

Months before starting on the wards. A few months prior to your rotation, you should consider the following:

- Order an extra white coat or two from the AMA catalog. These coats have huge pockets both inside and out.
- Gather your medical supplies. Find a stethoscope that is light, yet one you can actually hear with. Test them out in the bookstore on your own heart, lungs, and belly; you're sure to get some strange looks, but doing so will

help you decide whether you really need the Littmann Cardiology III.

■ Remember, too, that equipment is less costly when ordered in bulk through medical schools. You may also want to buy a cheap stethoscope to have as an "extra" in case your good one walks off one day and you have no time to go to the bookstore to replace it. You should also buy a clip-on name tag for your stethoscope so that if it does happen to walk off one day, you may eventually be reunited.

One week before. You will feel less lost on the first day if you follow these general rotation-specific guidelines:

■ If you're starting neuro, practice the neuro exam.
■ If you're starting psych, practice or review the psych interview.
■ If you're starting medicine, review normal values and the H&P.
■ If you're starting surgery, review knots, sutures, and what goes in a pre-op, brief-op, post-op, and progress note.
■ Read the appropriate chapter in *First Aid for the® Wards*.

The night before. On the night before your rotation starts, you should observe the following guidelines:

■ Set out everything you will need to bring with you. Chances are that there is no safe place to leave anything in the hospital on your first day, so don't bring too much. Remember to bring your ID, your white coat, your name tag, some money, extra pens, your stethoscope, a pharmacopoeia (for all rotations, because it is tiny and will quickly translate all those brand names into generic names), and your beeper (memorize the number so that you can give it out).
■ Set your alarm half an hour early, especially if you're not sure how to get either to the hospital or to your floor.
■ Make sure you know where to go and when to get there. If in doubt, ask classmates who are on your team, or page a resident on the team.
■ Recheck your alarm, especially the volume and the A.M./P.M. settings.

The first day. On the first day of your wards experience, be sure to do the following:

■ Arrive early.
■ Make sure every member of your team knows that this is your first rotation. That way, they are likely to be more tolerant toward you and to pay more attention to teaching you hospital basics, such as how to read a nursing chart, get labs or cultures off the computer, or page someone.
■ Don't leave until the chief resident says to leave.
■ If in doubt, ask when and where rounds will be the next day. Especially for surgery and medicine, bring an on-call bag with a toothbrush and toothpaste, underwear, socks, any medication you are on, and earplugs. Leave this gear in your car in case you are on call that first night.

Practical Information for All Clerkships

This chapter reviews some key high-yield skills and information that you will need regardless of the rotation you are on. Topics include how to read a chest x-ray (CXR), how to make sense of an ECG, how to manage your patients' fluids and electrolytes, and how to interpret acid-base problems. The final section outlines key abbreviations with which you should be familiar as well as key formulas that you may need to use in order to solve common clinical problems.

The most important thing you can do when learning the high-yield skills and knowledge presented in this chapter is to create a systematic approach. Whether you are solving an acid-base problem or interpreting a CXR, you will be far less likely to miss something essential if you are systematic. There are many different ways to approach each of these skills, so find one that you are comfortable with and stick to it. Consistency is key to comprehensive and accurate readings. Your residents and attendings will be impressed!

Be systematic in clinical problem solving.

READING KEY STUDIES

The CXR

Many of your patients in the hospital and emergency room will require a CXR. Although a formal reading will be completed by a radiologist, it is important that you learn the basics of CXR interpretation.

There are many different ways to approach a CXR. Again, the key here is to be systematic. When your attending asks for your impression of the study, you will earn points by walking through it step by step. One basic approach will be discussed below. First, however, you should become familiar with a few common ways of making a chest film. Most of the studies you see will be one of the following:

- **Anteroposterior (AP):** X-rays pass through the patient from front to back (anterior to posterior). Since the heart is farthest from the film (the film is placed behind the patient as the x-ray is taken), AP films often falsely enlarge heart size. For this reason, these films are less than ideal and are typically used when the patient cannot stand up (e.g., when portable films are obtained in an ICU patient).
- **Posteroanterior (PA):** X-rays pass through the patient from back to front (posterior to anterior). These films yield a more accurate estimate of heart size.
- **Lateral:** Typically, the patient's left side is facing the film to prevent cardiac distortion. The lateral projection is named according to the side closest to the film (e.g., left lateral). These films are used to pinpoint the location of abnormalities seen on AP/PA films; to assess AP diameter; and to check the posterior costophrenic angles for small (< 250-cc) effusions.
- **Decubitus:** Patients are lying on their sides (e.g., in a left decubitus film, the left side faces down). These films are used to evaluate the presence of free air or fluid (e.g., pleural effusion or pneumothorax).

When you set out to interpret a CXR, you should always begin by checking the patient's name and the date to ensure that you are looking at the correct film. No matter how stellar your interpretation may be, it won't count for much if you have the wrong patient! Next, begin to assess the film systematically using the A-B-C-D sequence (see Table 2-1).

The ECG

Many books teach a detailed approach toward interpreting an ECG (see Top-Rated Review Resources). However, it is important to have a basic method for quickly scanning an ECG on the spot. There are many different methodolo-

Each small box on an ECG is 0.04 second and each large box is 0.2 second.

TABLE 2-1. The A-B-C-D Sequence

STEP	PROCESS
Assessment	■ Assess the quality of the film using the mnemonic **PIER**: 　■ **P**osition: Is this a supine AP film? PA? Lateral? 　■ **I**nspiration: Count the posterior ribs. You should see 8–9 ribs with a good inspiratory effort. 　■ **E**xposure: Well-exposed films have good lung detail and show a detailed outline of the spinal column. Overpenetration → a dark film with more spinal detail. Underpenetrated films are whiter with little spinal detail. 　■ **R**otation: The space between the medial clavicle and the margin of the adjacent vertebrae should be roughly equal on each side. ■ Also look for indwelling lines or objects (e.g., endotracheal tube, feeding tube, airway obstruction), which may reveal clues to the pathology in the film.
Bones and soft tissues	■ Scan the bones for symmetry, fractures, osteoporosis, or metastatic lesions. Evaluate the soft tissues for foreign bodies, edema, or subcutaneous air.
Cardiac	■ Evaluate heart size. The heart should be < 50% of the chest diameter on PA films and < 60% on AP films. ■ Check for heart shape, calcifications, and prosthetic valves.
Diaphragms	■ Check the diaphragms for position (the right is slightly higher than the left due to the liver) and shape (they may be flat in asthma or COPD). ■ Look below the diaphragms for free air (a sign of bowel perforation).
Effusions	■ Pleural effusions may be large and obvious or small and subtle. Always check the costophrenic angles for sharpness (blunted angles may indicate small effusions). ■ Check a lateral film for small posterior effusions.
Fields/Fissures	■ Check lung fields for infiltrates (interstitial vs. alveolar), masses, consolidation, air bronchograms, pneumothoraces, and vascular markings. Vessels should taper and should be almost invisible at the lung periphery. ■ Evaluate the major and minor fissures for thickening or fluid.
Great vessels	■ Check aortic size and shape and the outlines of pulmonary vessels. The aortic knob should be clearly seen.
Hilar/mediastinal area	■ Evaluate the hila for lymphadenopathy, calcifications, and masses. The left hilum is normally higher than the right. Check for widening of the mediastinum (which may indicate a mass effect or tension pneumothorax). In children, be careful not to mistake the thymus for a mass.
Impression	■ Always formulate a preliminary impression of the film. Even if it is incorrect, it will show that you have been thinking.

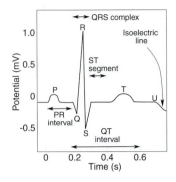

FIGURE 2-1. Sample ECG tracing.

gies with which to accomplish this objective, so again, pick one you like and stick with it. One basic approach is presented in Table 2-2.

Most studies you see will be 12-lead ECGs. Before you begin your reading, check the standardization mark. In a standard ECG set at 25 mm/sec, each small box represents 0.04 second, and each large box (composed of five small boxes) represents 0.2 second. See Figure 2-1 for the identification of the elements of an ECG tracing. Table 2-3 outlines the three degrees of atrioventricular (AV) block.

FLUIDS AND ELECTROLYTES

On the wards, you will be managing your patients' fluids and electrolytes from the outset. Although no one will expect you to be a pro at this on day one, you will benefit greatly from an understanding of some key terms and concepts. At

TABLE 2-2. ECG Interpretation

VARIABLE	METHOD OF ASSESSMENT
Rate	▪ Estimate the rate by counting the number of large boxes between consecutive R waves. The rate is roughly equal to 300 divided by this number. ▪ Rates over 100 are tachycardia; rates under 60 are bradycardia. ▪ For tracings in which the rate appears irregular, you can count the number of RR intervals in six seconds and multiply that number by 10 to estimate the rate.
Rhythm	▪ Identify the basic rhythm and look for abnormal waves, irregularities, or pauses. ▪ Check for sinus rhythm. Is there a single P wave before each QRS complex? Is there a single QRS after each P wave? Do all the P waves look alike? Are the P waves upright in lead II and inverted in lead aVR? ▪ Check for ectopic beats (premature atrial or ventricular contractions). ▪ Check the RR intervals for regularity of rhythm. If the baseline appears jagged and consecutive RR intervals vary in duration (an irregularly irregular rhythm), the tracing suggests atrial fibrillation.
Axis	▪ For a quick assessment of the axis, look at the QRS complexes in leads I and aVF. If both are upright, the axis is normal. See Figure 2-2 for the diagnosis of axis deviation.

Intervals	▪ Check the PR interval for AV block (> 0.2 second). The classification of AV blocks is discussed in Table 2-3.
	▪ Check the QRS for bundle branch block (> 0.12 second).
	  ▪ Right bundle branch block (RBBB): RSR′ ("rabbit ears" pattern) in V_1 and V_2; wide S in I and V_6.
	  ▪ Left bundle branch block (LBBB): RR′ ("slurred" pattern) in I and V_6; wide S in V_1.
	▪ Check the QT interval using the corrected interval: QTc = QT/RR. For a quick check, the QT interval should be less than half of the RR interval.

Hypertrophy	▪ Right atrial abnormality (RAA): Biphasic P in V_1, peaked first portion, > 2.5-mm height, or > 1 × 1 mm = "p pulmonale." Remember, **right** is **height.** ▪ Left atrial abnormality (LAA): Biphasic P in V_1, wide/negative terminal portion, > 0.8-mm duration = "p mitrale." Remember, **left** is **length.**

TABLE 2-2. ECG Interpretation *(continued)*

VARIABLE	METHOD OF ASSESSMENT
Hypertrophy	▪ Right ventricular hypertrophy (RVH): R > S in V_1; S persists in V_5 and V_6; right axis deviation; widened QRS interval. ▪ Left ventricular hypertrophy (LVH): Amplitude of S in V_1 + R in V_5 > 35 mm; left axis deviation; wide QRS; inverted/asymmetric T wave.

Infarction	▪ Look for Q waves (old transmural infarct), inverted T waves, and ST-segment elevation or depression.
	 ▪ Significant Q wave = 1 mm wide or more than one-third the amplitude of QRS.
	 ▪ An inverted T wave may point to ischemia—may be difficult to rule out without an old ECG.
	 ▪ ST-segment depression may mean ischemia or subendocardial infarct (non-ST-elevation MI).
	 ▪ Localize the infarct:
	   ▪ Inferior MI (dominant coronary, usually right): II, III, aVF.
	   ▪ Lateral MI (left circumflex): I, aVL, V_5, V_6.
	   ▪ Anterior MI (left anterior descending): V_1–V_4.
	   ▪ Posterior MI (right coronary): Large R and ST depression in V_1, V_2.
	   ▪ Septal MI: V_2, V_3.

Electrolyte abnormalities	▪ Hyperkalemia: Peaked T waves → short PR interval → loss of P wave → wide QRS → sine wave. ▪ Hypokalemia: Flat T wave → U wave → prominent U wave. ▪ Hypercalcemia: Short QT interval ▪ Hypocalcemia and hypomagnesemia: Prolonged QT interval → torsades de pointes.

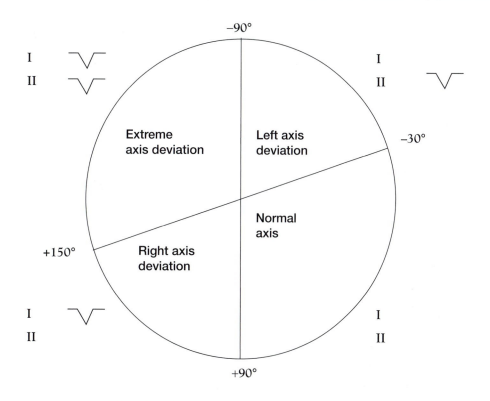

FIGURE 2-2. Quick method of axis determination.

TABLE 2-3. Degrees of AV Block

DEGREE	CHARACTERISTICS
First degree	Prolonged PR interval (> 0.2 second) with normal tracing.
Second degree	
Mobitz type I (Wenckebach)	Progressive lengthening of PR interval until a QRS is dropped.
Mobitz type II	Consistent ratio of conducted to dropped QRS complexes. Requires a pacemaker.
Third degree	Complete dissociation between atrial and ventricular rates. Requires a pacemaker.

a minimum, you should become familiar with the basic fluid and electrolyte composition of the body, the types of fluids available, and the phases of fluid therapy. Keep in mind that the approach will differ somewhat from service to service and for adult and pediatric patients, but the basic principles will remain the same.

Total Body Water

To order fluids, you will often need to estimate a patient's total body water (TBW). As a general rule, more body fat means less TBW. For calculations, use the following guidelines:

- 50% of lean body weight in adult females and the elderly.
- 60% of lean body weight in young adult males.
- 75–80% of lean body weight in infants.

Fluid Compartments

The TBW is distributed between the intracellular (two-thirds) and extracellular (one-third) compartments. Extracellular fluid is further distributed between the interstitial (three-fourths) and intravascular (one-fourth) spaces. Fluid distribution can also be calculated as a percentage of body weight (BW):

- Intracellular water accounts for 40% of BW.
- Extracellular water accounts for 20% of BW.
- Interstitial water accounts for 15% of BW.
- Blood volume in adults accounts for 7% of BW.
- Blood volume in children accounts for 8% of BW.

NS and LR are used for acute resuscitation.

IV Fluids

You will have different types of fluids from which to choose in the hospital. Isotonic fluids include normal saline (NS) and lactated Ringer's (LR), which are frequently used for acute resuscitation; these are the best fluids to use for increasing intravascular volume. Note that resuscitation fluids do not contain dextrose, which can cause hyperglycemia and osmotic diuresis. Typically, LR is also a maintenance fluid of choice on surgical services. The lactate is converted by the liver into HCO_3. As a result, **this fluid should be avoided in patients with metabolic or respiratory alkalosis.**

In general, maintenance fluids contain added dextrose and potassium. Dextrose prevents the breakdown of muscle for energy needs, provides fuel for the Krebs cycle, and prevents ketoacidosis. "D5" means 5% dextrose solution, and "D5W" means dextrose in water. Potassium should be added only if the patient has adequate urine output. The components of common fluids are listed in Table 2-4, expressed in milliequivalents per liter (mEq/L). Normal plasma osmolarity ranges from 280 to 300.

Don't add potassium until you know that the patient's kidneys work.

Fluid and Electrolyte Therapy

The important elements of complete fluid therapy are acute resuscitation, provision of maintenance fluids, replacement of ongoing losses, and replacement of deficits. Some patients will present in an acutely dehydrated state and will require resuscitation and deficit replacement, while others may be admitted for an elective surgical procedure and will require only maintenance fluids. Keep in mind that fluids are ideally maintained by mouth; don't add fluids just because a patient is in the hospital.

Fluid resuscitation. If a patient is significantly volume depleted, the first goal will be to rapidly replenish intravascular volume. It is important to recognize that the extent of clinical symptoms will depend not only on the volume lost but also on the rate of loss. Patients who have a gradual volume contraction may be well compensated, while those with rapid volume loss may go into hypovolemic shock. Signs of dehydration are not obvious until a patient has lost a significant volume, so make sure to assess volume status in all patients routinely, especially those who are vulnerable populations or have altered mental status. Remember that patients with burns or infections are likely to be more severely dehydrated at baseline and will need much more fluid than the average patient.

TABLE 2-4. Components of Common Fluids

FLUIDS	Na	Cl	K	HCO$_3$	Ca
Crystalloids					
NS	154	154			
D5NS	154	154			
½ NS	77	77			
D5 ½ NS	77	77			
D5 ¼ NS	39	39			
D5W					
LR	130	109	4	28	3
3% NaCl	513	513			
Colloids					
Hespan	154	154			
Plasmanate	145	100	0.25		
25% albumin	130–160	130–160	1		

In adults, the standard resuscitation fluid is LR or NS. In a severely dehydrated adult, a 1- to 2-L bolus may be given over 30–120 minutes. If the patient has a history of cardiac disease with a ↓ ejection fraction, a slower rate is recommended, and the patient should be monitored for signs of heart failure.

In children, you can ask parents about recent intake (bottle- or breast-feeding) and output (fewer than 4–5 wet diapers in 24 hours suggests dehydration). You should evaluate physical signs of dehydration, which are outlined in Table 2-5.

Mild to moderate dehydration in children may be treated with oral rehydration therapies such as Pedialyte or Ricelyte, which contain approximately 45–90 mEq/L of sodium, 20 mEq/L of potassium, 20 g/L of glucose, and 30 mEq/L of citrate or bicarbonate. IV fluid boluses with isotonic crystalloid (NS or LR) are used to rapidly expand intravascular volume within the following guidelines:

- **Mild dehydration:** 10 cc/kg bolus over one hour.
- **Moderate dehydration:** 20 cc/kg bolus over one hour.
- **Severe dehydration or shock:** 30–50 cc/kg over one hour.
- Reassess urine output and clinical status and rebolus as necessary.

KEY POINT

THREE-FOR-ONE RULE

To replace 1 L of intravascular volume, you should give 3 L of isotonic solution. After 1–2 hours, 1 L of isotonic solution redistributes such that only 300 mL remains in the intravascular space. Colloid solutions remain in the intravascular space for a longer period but are quite expensive and should be used only in appropriate clinical settings (e.g., in edematous patients).

The second phase of fluid therapy involves the provision of maintenance fluids, the replacement of ongoing losses, and the replacement of existing deficits.

Maintenance fluids. People in the hospital often order IV fluids on the basis of average fluid requirements. For example, an average order for an adult is D5 ½ NS with 20 mEq/L of KCl at 125 cc/hr. You can also calculate the exact water and electrolyte needs of a given patient, which will be more accurate if your patient differs from the standard 70-kg male. Maintenance fluid requirements ↑ under certain conditions, such as burns, hyperventilation, sweating, fever, hyperthyroidism, renal disease, and GI losses. Water requirements are calculated using the following methods:

1. **Holliday-Segar method (100/50/20 rule):**
   - Administer 100 mL/kg/day for the first 10 kg of weight.
   - Add 50 mL/kg for the next 10 kg.
   - Add 20 mL/kg for each kilogram over 20.
   - **Sample calculation:** A 70-kg adult would need $(100 \times 10) + (50 \times 10) + (20 \times 50) = 2500$ mL/day.

TABLE 2-5. Clinical Manifestations of Dehydration

SIGNS/SYMPTOMS	MILD DEHYDRATION	MODERATE DEHYDRATION	SEVERE DEHYDRATION
Weight loss	5%	10%	15%
Pulse	Normal or slightly ↑	↑	Very ↑
Blood pressure	Normal	Normal to orthostatic	Orthostatic to shock
Tears	Present	↓	Absent; sunken eyes
Mucous membranes	Normal	Dry	Parched
Mental status	Normal	Altered	Depressed
Anterior fontanelle (in children)	Normal	Normal to sunken	Sunken
Skin	Capillary refill < 2 seconds	Delayed capillary refill 2–4 seconds; ↓ turgor	Very delayed capillary refill, > 4 seconds, cool skin, acrocyanosis
Urine specific gravity	1.020	> 1.020, oliguria	Maximal, oliguria or anuria
Estimated fluid deficit	< 50 mL/kg	50–100 mL/kg	> 100 mL/kg

2. **Hourly fluids (4/2/1 rule):**
   - Administer 4 mL/kg/hr for the first 10 kg.
   - Add 2 mL/kg for the next 10 kg.
   - Add 1 mL/kg for each kilogram over 20.
   - **Sample calculation:** A 70-kg adult would need $(4 \times 10) + (2 \times 10) + (1 \times 50) = 110$ mL/hr.
   - A shortcut is "40 plus the weight in kilograms." A 70-kg man would need $40 + 70 = 110$ mL/hr.

Electrolyte requirements for adults and children are shown in Table 2-6.

TABLE 2-6. Electrolyte Requirements

	ADULTS	CHILDREN
Na	80–120 mEq/day	3–5 mEq/kg/day or per 100 mL fluid
K	50–100 mEq/day	1–2 mEq/kg/day or per 100 mL fluid
Cl	80–120 mEq/day	3 mEq/kg/day or per 100 mL fluid
Glucose	100–200 g/day	100–200 mg/kg/hr

> ## SAMPLE MAINTENANCE FLUID CALCULATION
>
> - **Patient:** A 24-kg child is admitted for elective surgery.
>
> - **Maintenance fluids:** $(100 \times 10) + (50 \times 10) + (20 \times 4) = 1580$ mL/day = 65.8 mL/hr.
>
> - **Maintenance electrolytes:**
>
>   - Na = 3 mEq/100 mL × 1580 mL/day = 47.4 mEq/day.
>
>   - K = 2 mEq/100 mL × 1580 mL/day = 31.6 mEq/day.
>
> - **Answer:** ¼ NS provides 34 mEq/L of NaCl. If a child requires approximately 1.5 L/day, that child will receive 51 mEq of NaCl, which satisfies his requirement. The addition of 20 mEq of KCl to each liter (after the first void) will provide 30 mEq/day.
>
> - **Appropriate fluid order:** D5 ¼ NS + 20 mEq/L KCl to run at 65 mL/hr.

Replace ongoing losses. Evaluate the volume and composition of fluids lost through diarrhea, vomiting, chest tubes, or various other sources. Try to replace losses "cc for cc" with fluids of similar composition. The average composition of body fluids can be found in many pocket guides and textbooks.

Deficit therapy. The replacement of existing deficits will depend on the degree of dehydration (established by history and exam) and on the type of dehydration (established by serum sodium, and generally classified as isonatremic, hyponatremic, or hypernatremic). Although a complete discussion of volume and electrolyte imbalances lies beyond the scope of this book, there are some basic facts that you should know.

Deficit replacement generally takes place at a rate proportional to the rate of loss. In a patient with 2 L of acute blood loss, IV fluids should be given rapidly in the resuscitation phase. By contrast, in a patient with well-compensated chronic hypernatremic dehydration, replacement should be undertaken slowly to avert rapid fluid shifts and potential complications.

- **Isonatremic dehydration (Na 130–150 mEq/L):** This is the most common form of dehydration and involves a net loss of isotonic fluid. Begin treatment by estimating the fluid deficit based on the degree of dehydration (e.g., mild = approximately 5% BW). Some clinicians replace the entire deficit with isotonic solution; standard therapy is D5 ¼ NS in small children and D5 ½ NS in older children and adults. After urination, 10–20 mEq of KCl can be added. Half of the deficit should be replaced over eight hours and the remainder over 16 hours.

- **Hyponatremic dehydration (Na < 130 mEq/L):** There is a net loss of solute, so an additional sodium deficit must be replaced. The formula for calculating the sodium deficit is as follows:

  Na deficit (mEq) = (desired Na – measured Na) × 0.6 × weight (kg)

This sodium should be added to the patient's other fluid and electrolyte needs. Again, half of the deficit can be replaced over eight hours and the remainder over 16 hours. In chronic, severe hyponatremia, however, the serum sodium should not be ↑ by > 2 mEq/L/hr or 10–12 mEq/L/day because of the risk of central pontine myelinolysis. In a symptomatic patient (e.g., one who has CNS symptoms), 3% NaCl may be given in an ICU setting to ↑ Na to > 120 mEq/L. The remainder of fluid replacement should proceed slowly with NS. In general, free water should also be restricted.

- **Hypernatremic dehydration (Na > 150 mEq/L):** There is a net loss of water relative to solute. This is typically due to ↓ fluid intake in the presence of ↑ insensible losses (e.g., fever, burns) but may also be due to excess salt intake. Treatment involves replacement of the free-water deficit, which is calculated using the following formula:

$$\text{Water deficit (L)} = \text{TBW} \times (\text{actual Na} - \text{desired Na})/\text{desired Na}$$

Correction must be undertaken cautiously, as cerebral edema, seizures, and CNS injury may result if sodium is corrected too rapidly (> 0.5–1.0 mEq/L/hr). Sodium may be lowered by 10–15 mEq/L/day, not to exceed 25 mEq/L/24 hr. General guidelines suggest using D5 ½ NS, D5 ¼ NS, or D5W to correct half of the free-water deficit over 24 hours. The remaining deficit may then be corrected over the following 48–72 hours. Begin replacing potassium after the patient urinates, and remember to replace ongoing losses and to provide maintenance fluids.

ACID-BASE CALCULATIONS

On almost every rotation you embark on, you will be asked to evaluate the acid-base status of a patient. You will be sure to impress your residents and attendings if you can rapidly interpret your patient's acid-base status as well as provide a differential diagnosis for your patient's condition. Presented below is one systematic approach to acid-base problems.

Two essential laboratory results are necessary for interpreting acid-base problems: an arterial blood gas (ABG) and an electrolyte panel. Using these studies, you will ask yourself four major questions:

1. **Does the patient have an acidemia (pH < 7.36) or an alkalemia (pH > 7.44)?** Normal pH is 7.40.
2. **Is the 1° disturbance metabolic or respiratory?** First, look at the P_{CO_2} (normal value 40). If the P_{CO_2} has shifted in the opposite direction of pH (e.g., P_{CO_2} ↑ when pH ↓), then you know that the 1° disturbance is respiratory. If not, look at the HCO_3 (normal value 24). If the HCO_3 has shifted in the same direction as the pH, then the 1° disturbance is metabolic. See Table 2-7 for an algorithm with which to define the 1° disturbance.

TABLE 2-7. Method for Defining 1° Acid-Base Disturbances

pH	P_{CO_2}	HCO_3^-	1° DISTURBANCE
< 7.36	↑	↑ or ↔	Respiratory acidosis
	↓ or ↔	↓	Metabolic acidosis
	↑	↓	Combined respiratory and metabolic acidosis
> 7.44	↓	↓ or ↔	Respiratory alkalosis
	↑ or ↔	↑	Metabolic alkalosis
	↓	↑	Combined respiratory and metabolic alkalosis

Compensating mechanisms never overcompensate or compensate completely.

3. **Is compensation for the 1° disturbance appropriate?** See Table 2-8.
4. **Is there an anion-gap (AG) acidosis?** Regardless of whether you initially identified a metabolic acidosis, always check for an AG acidosis. A normal anion gap is 12.
   a. Calculate the patient's AG.
   b. Calculate ΔAG: ΔAG = calculated AG – normal AG.
   c. Calculate ΔHCO_3^-: $\Delta HCO_3^- = [HCO_3^-]_{plasma} - [HCO_3^-]_{normal}$.
   d. Refer to Table 2-9 to determine if the patient has AG acidosis, non-anion-gap (NAG) acidosis, or combined metabolic acidosis.

Some examples are as follows:

1. **Lab values:** pH = 7.11, P_{CO_2} = 16, HCO_3^- = 5, Na^+ = 140, K^+ = 4.0, Cl^- = 115.

   Step 1: Does the patient have an acidemia or an alkalemia?
   pH = 7.11, so the patient is acidemic.

   Step 2: Is the 1° disturbance metabolic or respiratory?
   P_{CO_2} = 16, which is lower than normal. P_{CO_2} has moved in the same direction as pH (i.e., down), so the 1° disturbance is not respiratory but metabolic. Consistent with a metabolic etiology, we see that HCO_3^- = 5, which indicates that the major base, bicarbonate, is ↓. We conclude that this patient's 1° disturbance is a metabolic acidosis.

TABLE 2-8. Methods of Compensation for 1° Disturbance

1° DISTURBANCE	COMPENSATORY MECHANISM	CALCULATING APPROPRIATE COMPENSATION	COMPENSATION IS INAPPROPRIATE
Metabolic acidosis	P_{CO_2}	▪ $P_{CO_2} = 1.5 \times HCO_3^- + 8 \pm 2$ (Winter's formula) ▪ P_{CO_2} = last two digits of pH ▪ P_{CO_2} ↑ by 10 for every ↓ in HCO_3^- by 10	If actual P_{CO_2} is: ▪ Higher, there is also a respiratory acidosis ▪ Lower, there is also a respiratory alkalosis
Metabolic alkalosis	P_{CO_2}	▪ $P_{CO_2} = 0.9 \times HCO_3^- + 9$ ▪ $\Delta P_{CO_2} = 0.6 \times HCO_3^-$ ▪ P_{CO_2} ↑ by 7 for every ↑ in HCO_3^- by 10	If actual P_{CO_2} is: ▪ Higher, there is also a respiratory acidosis ▪ Lower, there is also a respiratory alkalosis
Respiratory acidosis	HCO_3^-	▪ Acute: HCO_3^- ↑ by 1 for every ↑ in P_{CO_2} by 10 ▪ Chronic: HCO_3^- ↑ by 4 for every ↑ in P_{CO_2} by 10	If actual HCO_3^- is: ▪ Higher, there is also a metabolic alkalosis ▪ Lower, there is also a metabolic acidosis
Respiratory alkalosis	HCO_3^-	▪ Acute: HCO_3^- ↓ by 2 for every ↓ in P_{CO_2} by 10 ▪ Chronic: HCO_3^- ↓ by 5 for every ↓ in P_{CO_2} by 10	If actual HCO_3^- is: ▪ Higher, there is also a metabolic alkalosis ▪ Lower, there is also a metabolic acidosis

TABLE 2-9. Determination of Acidosis Type

ΔAG	ΔHCO_3^-	TYPE
0 ± 2	$> \Delta AG$	NAG acidosis
> 2	$= \Delta AG$	AG acidosis
> 2	$> \Delta AG$	Combined NAG and AG acidosis

Step 3: Is the compensation for the 1° disturbance appropriate?

For a metabolic acidosis, we expect $P_{CO_2} = 1.5 \times HCO_3^- + 8 +/- 2$. So in this case, we would expect that $P_{CO_2} = 1.5 \times 5 + 8 +/- 2 = 15.5 +/- 2$. We therefore conclude that the compensation is appropriate.

Step 4: Is there an AG acidosis?

First we calculate the AG: $140 - 115 - 5 = 20$. ΔAG therefore equals 8. $\Delta HCO_3^- = 19$. Since ΔHCO_3^- is greater than ΔAG, we conclude that there is a combined AG and NAG metabolic acidosis.

SOLUTION: Combined AG and NAG metabolic acidosis.

2. **Lab values:** pH = 7.67, $P_{CO_2} = 30$, $HCO_3^- = 34$, $Na^+ = 140$, $K^+ = 3.0$, $Cl^- = 94$.

Step 1: Does the patient have an acidemia or an alkalemia?

pH = 7.67, so the patient is alkalemic.

Step 2: What is the 1° disturbance?

$P_{CO_2} = 30$, which is lower than normal. P_{CO_2} has moved in the opposite direction from pH, so we can conclude that the 1° disturbance is respiratory. We also check HCO_3^- to determine if there is a combined 1° disturbance. $HCO_3^- = 34$, which indicates that the major base, bicarbonate, is ↑. We therefore conclude that there is also a 1° metabolic alkalosis.

Step 3: Is the compensation appropriate?

For a respiratory alkalosis, we expect HCO_3^- to ↓ 2–5 mEq/L for every 10-mmHg ↓ in P_{CO_2}. We would therefore expect HCO_3^- to be between 19 and 22. $HCO_3^- = 34$, which is higher than expected, so we once again confirm that there is a metabolic alkalosis in addition to the respiratory alkalosis.

Step 4: Is there an AG acidosis?

First, we calculate the AG: $140 - 94 - 34 = 12$. ΔAG therefore equals zero, and we can conclude that there is no underlying AG metabolic acidosis.

SOLUTION: Combined 1° respiratory and metabolic alkalosis.

SLIDING-SCALE INSULIN

When patients are admitted to the hospital, you will often be asked to write a sliding-scale insulin (SSI) order in their admission orders. Scales differ significantly across institutions and may also be tailored to individual patients. Table 2-10 gives just one example of a scale you might see.

TABLE 2-10. Sliding-Scale Insulin Orders

VALUE[a]	SSI[b]
< 60	Give 1 amp of D50 (dextrose) and call house officer
61–150	None
151–200	2 units
201–250	4 units
251–300	6 units
301–350	8 units
351–400	10 units
> 400	Give 12 units and call house officer

[a] Result of finger-stick blood glucose measurement.
[b] Regular human insulin administered subcutaneously.

KEY POINT

REGULAR INSULIN DOSING

Some patients need a regular insulin schedule. Type 1 diabetics generally require 0.4–0.6 unit per kilogram of lean body weight. A typical dosing schedule is constructed in the following way:

- ⅔ total insulin in the A.M.:
    - ⅓ regular
    - ⅔ NPH
- ⅓ total insulin in the P.M.:
    - ½ regular
    - ½ NPH

PATIENT EMERGENCIES

In an emergency, immediately call for help.

One of a student's worst nightmares centers on the prospect of being all alone with a patient when something bad happens. In such a situation, the primary rule is, "Don't panic!" Immediately call for help (i.e., yell, "Nurse, I've got a problem!"). We cover basic CPR here, but please refer to the Emergency Medicine chapter for information on other patient emergencies.

Cardiopulmonary Arrest

In the event of cardiopulmonary arrest, check for patient responsiveness first. In a loud voice, ask the patient, "Are you okay?" while shaking him or her. If the patient is unresponsive and does not pass the "eyeball test" (i.e., the patient looks very sick), do not hesitate to call a code blue. Once you do this, you will get all the help you ever wanted.

By the time you check ABCs (airway, breathing, and circulation), there should be hordes of physicians and other health care professionals who will take over for you. The patient's code status will then be ascertained, and the resulting resuscitation will be driven by established advanced cardiac life support (ACLS) protocols. In a full-code situation, the medical student may do chest compressions, place an IV, or help defibrillate. The basic sequence of a code blue is outlined as "A-B-C / D-E-F" (see the boxed item below).

While the code is being activated, check **ABCs**:

- **Airway:** Determine if the patient is breathing. If not, adjust the patient's airway with a backward head tilt (if a C-spine injury is not suspected) or a forward jaw thrust (if a C-spine injury is suspected) and reassess breathing.
- **Breathing:** If the patient is still not breathing, give two slow breaths. Then check the patient's circulatory status.
- **Circulation:** Check the carotid pulses, one at a time, on both sides. Peripheral pulses are not reliable in these situations. If pulses are absent, initiate CPR. In adults and children, use the heel of your hand to compress the sternum one and one-half to two inches at the level of the nipples at a rate of 80–100 bpm. In infants, use the tips of the middle and ring fingers to compress the sternum one-half inch to one inch at a rate of at least 100 bpm. The ratio of compressions to breaths in adults is 30:2 if alone and 15:2 for two-person CPR; in children and infants the ratio is 5:1. Check the ECG pattern, as this may alter further treatment. If no ECG is present, ask the nurse to call for one immediately.

A-B-C / D-E-F SEQUENCE

Airway	Ensure airway patency (clear the bronchotracheal tree).
Breathing	If the patient is not breathing, begin intermittent positive-pressure ventilation.
Circulation	If the patient does not have a pulse, compress the chest at 80–100 compressions per minute.
Drugs/fluids	Place an IV line.
ECG	Monitor cardiac rhythms.
Fibrillation	Defibrillate.

If asystole is detected by ECG in more than one lead, continue CPR. In addition to chest compressions, transcutaneous pacing may be considered. The patient must be intubated. An IV is started immediately, and 1 mg of epinephrine or 1 mg of atropine (up to a maximum of 0.05 mg/kg) is pushed every 3–5 minutes.

If a ventricular fibrillation (VF) or ventricular tachycardia (VT) is detected with a ventricular rate of > 150 bpm, cardioversion is necessary. Although stable VT may be treated with medication, a patient with VF or unstable VT (i.e., low BP or no pulse) should be treated immediately with electrocardioversion. In addition, the patient should be given an oxygen face mask if he or she is not intubated. Defibrillation is attempted with incremental increases in energy: 200, 300, and 360 J.

APPENDIX

Formulas

- Mean arterial blood pressure (MAP) = DBP + [(SBP – DBP)/3], where DBP = diastolic blood pressure and SBP = systolic blood pressure.
- A-a (alveolar-arterial) oxygen gradient = $PAO_2 – PaO_2$
$$= [(pAtm – pH_2O) \times FiO_2 – (PaCO_2/RQ)] – PaO_2$$
$$= [(713 \times FiO_2) – (PaCO_2/0.8)] – PaO_2$$
Normal FiO_2 = 0.21; normal A-a gradient = 5–15 mm or the upper limit of (age/4) + 4.
- Cerebral perfusion pressure (CPP) = MAP – ICP.

Electrolytes

- Osmolality = 2 × serum Na + serum glucose/18 + BUN/2.8.
- Normal plasma osmolality = 275–295 mOsm/kg.
- Corrected Ca = Ca_{plasma} + 0.8 × (normal albumin – patient's albumin) = Ca_{plasma} + 0.8 × (4 – serum albumin).
- Corrected Na_{plasma} = Na_{plasma} + (glucose – 100) × 0.0016.
- Corrected Na_{plasma} = Na_{plasma} + 0.2 × triglycerides (g/L).
- Corrected Na_{plasma} = Na_{plasma} + 0.025 × protein (g/L).
- TBW = k × weight (kg), where k = 0.6 in men and 0.5 in women.
- Stool osmotic gap = stool osmolality – 2(Na_{stool} + K_{stool}), where < 50 osm is consistent with secretory diarrhea and > 125 osm is consistent with osmotic diarrhea.

Acid-Base Equations

- AG = Na_{plasma} – (Cl_{plasma} + $HCO_3^-_{plasma}$).
- Urine AG = Na_{urine} + K_{urine} – Cl_{urine}.
- pH = 6.1 + log (HCO_3^-/0.03 × PCO_2).

Renal Function

- Fractional excretion of sodium (Fe_{Na})
= (Na_{urine}/Na_{plasma})/(Cr_{urine}/Cr_{plasma}) × 100 or
= (Na_{urine} × Cr_{plasma})/(Na_{plasma} × Na_{urine}) × 100.
- Creatinine clearance (CrCl) = (Cr_{urine} × urine volume in mL)/(Cr_{plasma} × time in minutes).
- Expected CrCl = [(140 – age) × weight (kg) × 0.85 for females]/(72 × Cr_{plasma}), where Cr_{plasma} is in mg/dL.

Statistics

		Test	
		+	−
Disease	+	A	B
	−	C	D

- Sensitivity = A/(A + B).
- Specificity = D/(C + D).
- False positive rate = C/(A + C).
- False negative rate = B/(B + D).
- Positive predictive value = A/(A + C).
- Negative predictive value = D/(B + D).
- Positive likelihood ratio = sensitivity/(1 − specificity).
- Negative likelihood ratio = (1 − sensitivity)/specificity.
- Absolute risk reduction (ARR) = disease rate without intervention − disease rate with intervention = A/(A+B) − C/(C+D).
- Relative risk reduction (RRR) = ARR/disease rate without intervention = [A/(A+B)]/[C/(C+D)].
- Number needed to treat (NNT) = 1/ARR.

Common Abbreviations

NUMBERS

$\dot{\text{T}}$	one	
$\ddot{\text{TT}}$	two	
$\dddot{\text{TTT}}$	three	
s̄s̄	one-half	*semis*

DOSING SCHEDULE

bid	twice a day	(*bis in die*)
hs	at bedtime	(*hora somni*)
tid	three times a day	(*ter in die*)
÷	divided doses	
q	each, every	(*quaque*)
q6h	every six hours	(*quaque 6 hora*)
qac	before each meal	(*quaque ante cibum*)
qd	every day	(*quaque die*)
qh	every hour	(*quaque hora*)
qid	four times a day	(*quater in die*)
qod	every other day	
pc	after meals	(*post cibos*)
prn	as needed	(*pro re nata*)

ROUTES OF ADMINISTRATION

IM	intramuscular	
inj	injection	
IV	intravenous	
PO	by mouth	(*per os*)
PR	by rectum	(*per rectum*)
SL	sublingual	
SQ	subcutaneous	

MEDICATION PREPARATIONS

amp	ampule	(*ampulla*)
caps	capsules	(*capsula*)
gtt	drops	(*guttae*)
liq	liquid	(*liquor*)
sol	solution	(*solutio*)
supp	suppository	(*suppositorium*)
susp	suspension	
tab	tablet	(*tabella*)
ung	ointment	(*unguentum*)

PREPOSITIONS

a	before	(*ante*)
p	after	(*cum*)
s	without	(*post*)
x	except	(*sine*)

MISCELLANEOUS

ad lib	at pleasure	(*ad libitum*)
disp	dispense	(*dispensia*)
NPO	nothing by mouth	(*nil per os*)
OD	right eye	(*oculus dexter*)
OS	left eye	(*oculus sinister*)
OU	both eyes	(*oculus uterque*)
qs	to a sufficient quantity	(*quantum sufficit*)
Rx	prescription, take	(*recipe*)
sig	label, or let it be printed	(*signa*)
stat	immediately	(*statim*)

Core Clerkships

- Emergency Medicine
- Internal Medicine
- Neurology
- Obstetrics and Gynecology
- Pediatrics
- Psychiatry
- Surgery

Emergency Medicine

Welcome to the emergency department (ED)! Emergency medicine (EM) is a popular clerkship as well as a "hot" field in medicine. This rotation allows students to see a broad spectrum of patients and diseases while also giving them the opportunity to be the first to diagnose and treat those patients. In the course of this rotation, you will be given a chance to do procedures, practice primary and critical care, and participate in traumas and resuscitations. Regardless of the field you enter, aspects of it will be found in EM, and many of your patients will come from the ED—so take advantage of this learning opportunity and enjoy the rotation. You will see it all in the ED!

What Is the Rotation Like?

EM is usually a required clerkship or elective of three or four weeks' duration, depending on the medical school involved. Your prior rotations and experiences will prove particularly useful in this rotation. You will be the first to see the patient and will decide which tests to order, and you will also be the one who renders a diagnosis and determines whether the patient is sick enough to be admitted into the hospital. For these reasons, your experience and confidence level will to a large extent dictate your ability to contribute and get the most out of this rotation.

For many students, the EM rotation may present the most patient responsibility you will encounter during medical school. While on this rotation, you will see diseases affecting every system—be it neurologic, psychiatric, GI, endocrine, cardiac, respiratory, or urologic. You must therefore have a broad knowledge base if you are to communicate effectively with the various services to which you may admit or with which you may request a consultation. Depending on the ED at your institution, you may also see adult and pediatric patients in the same or separate areas. This wide variation in disease severity and patient population is perhaps why many students prefer to do this rotation after they have completed the majority of their other basic clerkships—especially if they are contemplating a career in EM.

Remember, anything can happen in the ED! As Dr. Frederick Levy of the Johns Hopkins Hospital states, "I think the most important point that a student or resident can learn in EM is the adage, 'Absence of proof is not proof of absence.' It's not the MI in a 70-year-old diabetic, hypertensive male with the Levine sign that we miss; it's the 40-year-old with one or two risk factors and a normal ECG. Similarly, many patients with appendicitis may have unexplained RLQ tenderness but may be hungry and afebrile with a normal WBC." With this in mind, here are some tips on how to maximize your efficiency on this rotation.

- Patient evaluations:
  - **Be thorough yet efficient.** Remember that working up a patient in the ED is unlike doing a history and physical (H&P) during an inpatient service. The difference lies in the fact that in the ED, you have a limited amount of time at your disposal as well as many more patients waiting to be seen. So while some patients may well have a long list of problems, it is critical that you **isolate their chief complaint** and identify their most acute issue, and then do a focused H&P.
  - **Develop a focused differential** even if the diagnosis seems obvious. Have an idea of the likelihood of each of the most life-threatening dis-

EM will challenge you to draw on your knowledge of a variety of specialties and patient populations.

orders on your differential. Your differential will drive the diagnostic tests you order, and having a sense of the degree of suspicion you might have for a serious diagnosis will help you utilize resources appropriately and efficiently.

- **Learn to prioritize.** You should work on prioritizing your patients by disease severity and on establishing when treatment is dictated in the face of diagnostic uncertainty.

■ **Presentations:** Presenting a patient in EM can be quite challenging at first. Unlike many other fields—in which meticulous attention to detail is key to taking an adequate history—the art of succinctly yet thoroughly communicating a chief complaint, pertinent positive and negative findings, and an appropriate assessment and plan is critical to success in this rotation. You will most likely be presenting to a resident and then, perhaps, to the attending—as well as to other services when you are admitting or calling for consults. So remember that emergency physicians pride themselves on being able to present data concisely. Your presentations should reflect your ability to rapidly weave pertinent positives and negatives into a coherent picture of the patient and then, having done so, to synthesize a cohesive treatment plan.

■ **Signing out:** Learning to sign out a patient is a valuable skill learned during the EM rotation. When your shift ends, you will be expected to give a quick and concise summary of your patients to the party taking over care for you. Be sure to efficiently describe the chief complaint, interventions thus far, pending work/lab results/consults, and disposition plans.

■ **Trauma:** You will probably be involved in traumas as they come into the ED. Although these may occur at any time, you should be alerted by overhead announcements or pagers with the estimated time of arrival for the trauma. If you are participating in trauma resuscitation, you should observe the following guidelines:

- Be sure to gown up properly, making appropriate use of eye shields and gloves.
- Be calm, gowned, and ready to help in any capacity you can.
- Although the situation surrounding a trauma may seem hectic, there should be a resident at the head of the bed giving orders. This may be an ER resident or a trauma surgery resident, depending on your institution. The student's role during a trauma may be very limited, but each case is an opportunity for you to learn, even if staying out of the way is your primary responsibility.
- Remember the ABCDEs and do what you can.
- During a trauma scenario, you can be a superstar if you are able to anticipate need and quickly offer supplies to the physician who is performing procedures. You may even be rewarded with an opportunity to perform a procedure yourself!
- Don't take things personally if people don't say "please" or "thank you" at this time. Treating a trauma can be a stressful event, and teaching comes secondary to saving a life during a trauma resuscitation.

How Is the Day Set Up?

Most EM rotations consist of a certain number of 8-, 10-, or 12-hour shifts. When you initially arrive, patients already in the ED will be signed out to you by other medical students or residents. When assuming the care of a patient, be sure you know that patient's history and pertinent exam findings so that changes in his or her condition can be assessed adequately should a change in disposition be required. In addition, make sure you are aware of all procedures that need to be done and labs that are pending.

You should also take steps to familiarize yourself with your ED's etiquette regarding sign-out. In virtually every institution, it is poor form to sign out the less glamorous procedures (e.g., rectal and pelvic exams). However, there is significant variability among institutions with regard to other procedures, with some facilities requiring that you perform all procedures before sign-out and others expecting you to leave outstanding procedures for the next shift. Of course, many students find it worthwhile to remain after their shift has ended to perform unfinished procedures, regardless of the prevailing norm. Depending on the ED, new patients may be triaged and assigned to a care area for which you are responsible or, alternatively, you may pick up new cases from a stack of unseen patients. Regardless of the procedure for acquiring new patients at your institution, you should be sure to make the attending, residents, and charge nurse aware of your presence, as they will often allow you to "cherry-pick" interesting patients, seek you out for procedures, and recommend the best area for you to work.

Never sign out a pelvic or rectal exam to a colleague.

How Do I Excel in Emergency Medicine?

For medical students, the key to excelling in EM is to be thorough yet efficient. Overcrowding is a major concern in EM, so moving patients through the ED is vital. For this reason, you will need to rapidly distinguish patients who require admission and immediate treatment from those who just need reassurance and outpatient referral. In your efforts to maximize your efficiency, much of your time will be spent "doing things" for your patients rather than "sitting and talking" about them. With this in mind, the paragraphs that follow offer guidelines on how to excel on this rotation.

Be thorough and efficient in the ED.

- **Get along with the team.** Maintain a positive attitude. During a long shift, remaining upbeat and helpful will make you shine. Also remember that in the ED, you may work one-on-one with the nurses more often than you do with your fellow students and residents. So be sure to get on their good side, as they will be able to teach you a great deal. Nurses not only can make or break your rotation but can also make you look great by updating you on your patients and helping you with ordering prior to presentations.
- **Know your patients.** Be sure you are aware of your patients' conditions and vitals at all times. You want to be the first to know if your patients are decompensating or improving. You should be writing progress notes every couple of hours if a patient is stable and awaiting a bed, but you should be writing them more often than that if a patient is unstable. Also remember to keep on top of the tests you ordered, as your approach toward management will often hinge on the results of those tests. In addition, residents will gain confidence in your abilities when you can keep them apprised of your patients' status. Bear in mind that you should be writing progress notes on your patients when these results arrive as well as when the patients' conditions change.
- **Be assertive.** Assertiveness is key to furthering your education as well as to scoring points with the people who evaluate you. So ask good and well-thought-out questions; know other patients on the service (for your own learning and in case you are asked to fill in); take the initiative to ask for demonstrations of procedures; volunteer for drawing blood (you need to practice anyway); and ask for feedback from your residents and chiefs both at the midpoint of the EM rotation and at the end.
- **Be on time.** EM physicians value their time off. Thus, few things upset them more than seeing a colleague show up late for sign-out. Likewise, when you sign out, remember that you are done; unless you want to stick

EM is a "doing" specialty. Be prepared to be moving and working throughout your entire shift, as there is generally little downtime.

around for something educational, you are expected to go home. There is no need to stay after your shift just to show your face (another reason EM is so popular).

■ **Be thorough and efficient.** Again, you don't have all day to work up a patient, so just go for it. At the same time, remember that your evaluation should also be complete enough to ensure that you don't send any sick patients home.

Challenges in the ED

The ED will provide you with exposure to a highly diverse group of people. Indeed, in the current U.S. health care system, it is the only place where many patients are able to receive medical treatment. For this reason, overcrowding and long wait times are major issues. In the ED, you will encounter not only interesting medical pathology but also challenging social issues. These encounters will test your ability to gather clinical data in difficult situations as well as your capacity to mold your history-taking skills to each individual patient. At some point, for example, you will come across patients who are drug seeking, homeless, or victims of abuse. In such cases, the chief complaint you hear may not reflect the reasons these patients are actually in the ED—so taking a carefully tailored and compassionate history will be vital to determining the best course of action to take. When deciding on a plan of care, you should remember that the emergency physician is often these patients' only advocate. Also bear in mind that the ED can be a chaotic and stressful environment for physicians and patients alike. Because of this, you may encounter violent patients as well. It is important to remain aware of your environment, predict when extra safety precautions might be necessary, and ask for help early.

Key Procedures

■ Phlebotomy
■ IV line placement
■ Central line placement
■ Arterial line placement
■ Arterial blood gas
■ Foley placement
■ Lumbar puncture
■ Intubations
■ Chest tube placement
■ Suturing
■ Incision and drainage
■ Splinting
■ Paracentesis
■ Thoracentesis
■ Arthrocentesis

What Do I Carry in My Pockets?

❑ Stethoscope
❑ Penlight
❑ Pocket drug reference
❑ Antibiotic guide

- ❏ Calipers for ECG reading
- ❏ Trauma shears

Read about these topics before you start the rotation. Most are discussed in this chapter. A full list of common clerkship topics can be found at the end of this chapter.

- ❏ Angina
- ❏ Acute MI
- ❏ Arrhythmia
- ❏ Appendicitis
- ❏ Ectopic pregnancy
- ❏ Intracranial hemorrhage
- ❏ Pneumothorax
- ❏ Pulmonary embolism
- ❏ Drug overdose/antidotes
- ❏ Resuscitation

ALLERGY, IMMUNOLOGY, DERMATOLOGY

Anaphylaxis

A severe allergic reaction due to reexposure to an allergen after prior sensitization. Etiologies include drugs (penicillin, cephalosporins, ASA, NSAIDs), IV contrast, food, and latex exposure.

SIGNS AND SYMPTOMS

- **Dermatologic: Urticaria**, erythema, pruritus, angioedema.
- **Respiratory:** Nasal congestion, sneezing, coryza, cough, tachypnea, hoarseness, and a sensation of throat tightness may indicate **airway obstruction**.
- **Cardiovascular:** Tachycardia, hypotension.

DIFFERENTIAL

- **Dermatologic:** Angioedema, urticaria.
- **Respiratory:** Asthma, epiglottitis.
- **Psychiatric:** Anxiety.

WORKUP

- Obtain an H&P; diagnosis is clinical.
- Although never done in the ED, diagnostic tests include ↑ total tryptase drawn 1–4 hours after the event and ↑ serum histamine drawn < 1 hour since the event.

TREATMENT

- **Epinephrine.**
- **β-agonists:** Albuterol to treat bronchospasm.
- **Antihistamines:**
  - Diphenhydramine (Benadryl, an H_1 receptor blocker) to treat the cutaneous effects of anaphylaxis.

- Cimetidine (an H_2 receptor blocker) to treat allergic reactions and urticaria.
- Methylprednisolone (Solu-Medrol) 125 mg IV × 1.

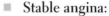

CARDIOVASCULAR

Angina

Originates from myocardial ischemia ($\uparrow O_2$ demand or $\downarrow O_2$ supply). Subtypes are as follows:

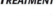

Major risk factors for CAD and acute coronary syndrome (ACS):

- *Age*
- *Male gender*
- *Hyperlipidemia*
- *Diabetes*
- *Hypertension*
- *Smoking*
- *Family history*
- *A personal history of ACS!*

- **Stable angina:**
    - Chest pain has an established character, timing, and duration.
    - Pain is transient, reproducible, and predictable.
    - Due to reduced coronary blood flow through fixed atherosclerotic plaques that narrow the blood vessel lumina; easily relieved by rest or sublingual nitrates.
- **Unstable angina:**
    - Angina that deviates from the normal pattern; rest angina lasting > 20 minutes; or new-onset angina that was previously undiagnosed.
    - Angina that $\uparrow$ in severity, frequency, or duration.
    - Remember that patients who present with chest pain rarely if ever have a working diagnosis of stable angina.
- **Variant (Prinzmetal's) angina:**
    - Has the same character as stable angina, but atherosclerosis is minimal.
    - Caused by vasospasm.
    - Treated with nitrates and calcium channel blockers.

SIGNS AND SYMPTOMS

- Exertional substernal chest pressure; pain that radiates to the lower jaw, left shoulder, or left arm.
- Nausea, vomiting, dyspnea, diaphoresis.
- Hypertension, tachycardia.

DIFFERENTIAL

Etiologies of chest pain include the following (see also the mnemonic **TAPUM**):

- **Cardiovascular:** Aortic dissection, unstable angina, MI, pericarditis.
- **Respiratory:** Tension pneumothorax, pulmonary embolism (PE), pneumonia.
- **GI:** Esophagitis, GERD, PUD, cholecystitis.
- **Musculoskeletal:** Costochondritis.
- **Neurologic:** Herpes zoster.

Deadly causes of chest pain—

TAPUM

Tension pneumothorax
Aortic dissection
Pulmonary embolism
Unstable angina
Myocardial infarction

WORKUP

- ECG may reveal ST-segment depression or T-wave flattening (see Figure 3-1).
- Serial cardiac enzymes, stress test, echocardiography, coronary angiography.

TREATMENT

- **Initial treatment:** Assume a possible infarction.
    - Give **ASA, sublingual nitroglycerin,** and **analgesics** (e.g., **morphine**).
    - O_2, cardiac monitoring.

HIGH-YIELD FACTS

EMERGENCY MEDICINE

- **Medical treatment:** β-blockers, long-acting nitrates, calcium channel blockers.
- **Coronary revascularization (CABG, PTCA):** ↑ O_2 delivery to the myocardium by increasing blood flow.
- **Risk factor modification:** Smoking cessation, dietary modification with exercise, treatment of underlying medical conditions (e.g., hypertension, diabetes, hypercholesterolemia).

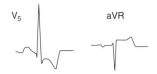

FIGURE 3-1. **ST-segment depression typical of ischemia.**

Note that the ST elevation in aVR is really depression, as it goes in the opposite direction of the QRS. (Reproduced, with permission, from Nicoll D et al. *Pocket Guide to Diagnostic Tests*, 2nd ed. Stamford, CT: Appleton & Lange, 1997: 294.)

KEY CARDIAC DIAGNOSTIC EXAMS

- **Exercise electrocardiography:**
  - **Method:** The patient's ECG is monitored while exercising. Exercise often takes the form of a treadmill according to the Bruce protocol—treadmill speed and elevation are ↑ every three minutes.
  - **Interpretation:** Angina, ST-segment changes on ECG, exercise intolerance, or ↓ systolic BP indicates myocardial ischemia. A ⊕ test should be further evaluated with cardiac catheterization.

- **Myocardial perfusion scintigraphy:**
  - **Method:** Radionuclides (e.g., thallium, Tc-MIBI) are injected into the blood. The amount of radionuclide uptake by the myocardium is directly related to the amount of blood flow.
  - **Interpretation:** Areas of ↓ uptake indicate relative hypoperfusion. With exercise or drug-induced vasodilation, coronary vessels vasodilate, giving the most blood flow to those vessels without lesions. If no areas of hypoperfusion are observed, the test is ⊖.
  - **Follow-up:** If defects are observed, a resting scan is done to determine if perfusion defects are reversible. Defects that normalize at rest indicate reversible ischemia, whereas fixed defects signify areas of dead tissue (i.e., post-MI). Areas of reversible ischemia may be rescued with PTCA or CABG surgery.

- **Echocardiography:**
  - **Method:** A real-time ultrasound of the heart, the echocardiogram ("echo") reveals abnormal wall motion due to ischemia or infarction.
  - **Interpretation:** Echo gives the additional benefits of assessing left ventricular function and estimating the ejection fraction (EF), an important predictor of prognosis. A normal EF is approximately 55–75%.

- **Coronary angiography:**
  - **Method:** An invasive procedure that visualizes the coronary vasculature by injecting dye into the vessels, coronary arteriography is the definitive diagnostic procedure for CAD.
  - **Interpretation:** Stenotic lesions in the vessels will be visualized and quantified with respect to the extent of obstruction (most lesions that lead to symptoms are > 70% stenotic) as well as their location. While this procedure

HIGH-YIELD FACTS

EMERGENCY MEDICINE

gives anatomical information, it does not indicate whether any given stenosis is clinically significant; that is, a 50% stenotic lesion may be the cause of the patient's symptoms as opposed to the 70% lesion in another vessel. This procedure also gives an estimate of the EF.

■ **Use:** Catheterization is typically used (1) to confirm the presence and map the extent of CAD, and (2) to define the method of revascularization (PTCA vs. CABG) if indicated.

Acute Myocardial Infarction (MI)

Usually caused by an occlusive thrombus or prolonged vasospasm in a coronary artery (see Figure 3-2). The most common cause is an **acute thrombus on a ruptured atherosclerotic plaque.** The time course and extent of vessel occlusion are key, as collateral circulation may help preserve some myocardial function.

Watch for "silent MIs" in elderly, diabetic, and post-orthotopic heart transplant patients.

SIGNS AND SYMPTOMS

■ Chest pain, pressure, or tightness that can radiate to the left arm, neck, or jaw.
■ Nausea, vomiting, dyspnea, lightheadedness.
■ Diaphoresis, anxiety, or an "impending sense of doom."
■ Tachycardia, heart failure/pulmonary rales, hypotension, gallop rhythms (especially an S4), mitral regurgitation 2° to papillary muscle dysfunction.

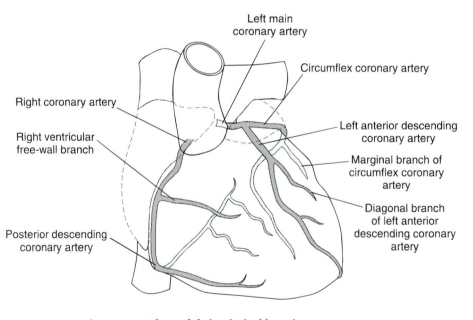

FIGURE 3-2. Coronary arteries and their principal branches.

(Reproduced, with permission, from Stobo JD et al. *The Principles and Practice of Medicine,* 23rd ed. Stamford, CT: Appleton & Lange, 1996: 17.)

DIFFERENTIAL

Refer to the discussion of angina.

WORKUP

- **ECG:**
    - **Wave morphology change sequence** (see Figure 3-3): Peaked T waves → T-wave inversion → ST-segment elevation → Q waves → ST-segment normalization → T waves return to upright.
    - **Lead location:**
        - **Changes in leads V_1–V_4:** Anterior MI.
        - **Changes in leads II, III, and aVF:** Inferior MI.
- **Cardiac enzymes:** The death of myocardium releases cardiac enzymes into the blood, and these enzymes can be measured (see Figure 3-4):
    - **Troponin-I/T:** Appears the **earliest** and is the **most sensitive and specific** of all the enzymes for the detection of MI.
    - **CK-MB:** Appears next.
    - **LDH:** Appears **last** and remains elevated for 3–6 days.
- **Imaging:** CXR may show signs of CHF.

KEY POINT

Q-WAVE VS. NON-Q-WAVE MI

- A Q wave on ECG in the presence of infarction indicates that the infarction extends through the full thickness of the myocardial wall **(transmural).**

- A non-Q-wave MI involves the **subendocardium,** not the full thickness. Non-Q-wave MIs are dangerous in the sense that the patient is still at risk for a full-thickness infarct in that area.

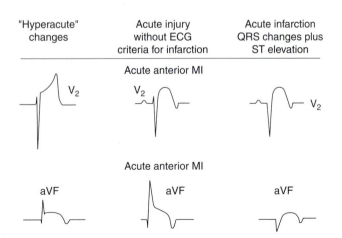

FIGURE 3-3. Classic evolution of the ECG in MI.

A normal waveform is seen in lead V_2. Following the ECG change from left to right, note the elevated ST segments and peaked T waves that evolve into rounded "tombstones" with new Q waves and T-wave inversions. (Reproduced, with permission, from Nicoll D et al. *Pocket Guide to Diagnostic Tests*, 2nd ed. Stamford, CT: Appleton & Lange, 1997: 291, 296.)

HIGH-YIELD FACTS

EMERGENCY MEDICINE

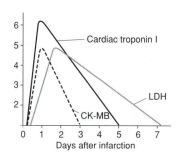

FIGURE 3-4. Myocardial enzymes.

The time course of serum enzyme concentrations after a typical MI. (Reproduced, with permission, from Harvey AM et al (eds). *The Principles and Practice of Medicine*, 22nd ed. Stamford, CT: Appleton & Lange, 1988.)

TREATMENT

- ↑ O₂ supply: Give **supplemental O₂**; emergent angioplasty vs. thrombolytics.
- ↓ O₂ demand: Treat with **β-blockers,** bed rest, pain medications (**e.g., morphine**), **nitrates, ACEIs,** and anxiolytics.
- **Thromboprophylaxis: ASA; heparin** to prevent stenotic lesions from enlarging.
- **Thrombolytics (tPA, urokinase, or streptokinase):** Yield the greatest benefit early (achieving 50% mortality reduction 1–3 hours after chest pain) but are still effective up to 10 hours after chest pain onset (10% mortality reduction). Thrombolytics are indicated for the following:
  - Patients < 80 years of age.
  - Those who present within 6–12 hours of chest pain onset.
  - Those with evidence of infarct on ECG (ST elevation > 1 mm in two contiguous leads).
- **Angioplasty:** Balloon angioplasty has been shown to be as good as or better than thrombolytics.
- **Cholesterol management:** Administer **statins** to ↓ LDL to < 100 mg/dL post-MI (shown to ↓ mortality).

REFERENCE

Aversano T et al. Thrombolytic therapy vs. primary percutaneous coronary intervention for myocardial infarction in patients presenting to hospitals without on-site cardiac surgery. *JAMA* 287:1943–1951, 2002. This study suggested that 1° percutaneous intervention at hospitals without on-site cardiac surgery was associated with better outcomes at six months.

Aortic Dissection

Defined as a "**false lumen**" created 2° to an intimal layer tear, allowing blood to enter the aortic media and subsequently splitting the medial lamellae. **Stanford type A** dissections involve the ascending aorta; **Stanford type B** dissections are distal to the left subclavian artery. Risk factors include the following:

- **Hypertension; coarctation of the aorta.**
- Syphilis, **Marfan's syndrome,** Ehlers-Danlos syndrome.
- Trauma, pregnancy.

What drugs have been shown to ↓ mortality in post-MI patients? ASA, β-blockers, ACEIs, and statins–not nitrates.

Treatment of unstable angina and MI–

MONA has HEP B

Morphine
Oxygen
Nitrates (e.g., nitroglycerin)
Aspirin
HEParin
Beta-blockers

- Severe **"tearing"** or **"ripping" chest** or **back pain.**
- Asymmetric or ↓ peripheral pulses.
- Syncope, stroke, shock, MI. Can rupture into the pericardium and cause cardiac tamponade.

DIFFERENTIAL

- **Cardiovascular:** Angina, MI, thoracic aortic aneurysm.
- **Respiratory:** Pulmonary embolus.
- **GI:** Esophageal rupture.

WORKUP

- ECG to evaluate for LVH and ischemic changes.
- CXR; CT with IV contrast; angiography.

TREATMENT

- **Stabilize BP.** For high blood pressure, use IV nitrates and β-blockers.
- Type A dissections require emergent surgery.
- Type B dissections may be managed medically in stable patients.

Arrhythmia

ASYSTOLE

Defined as a "flatline" rhythm that indicates no pulse and no electrical activity of the heart. Remember, you must always check for asystole in two separate leads!

SIGNS AND SYMPTOMS

- Patients are unconscious/unresponsive.
- Absent pulses; absent heart sounds.

DIFFERENTIAL

Detached lead/equipment malfunction; ventricular fibrillation (VF).

Never shock asystole (no matter what you see on TV).

TREATMENT

- ABCs, O_2, cardiac monitor, CXR, CPR.
- Identify and treat underlying causes.
- Consider transcutaneous pacing.
- **Epinephrine** 1 mg IV push q 3–5 minutes × 3.
- **Atropine** 1 mg IV push q 3–5 minutes × 3.
- Sodium bicarbonate (1 mEq/kg) in the presence of a known preexisting bicarbonate-responsive acidosis; if TCA overdose is suspected; or if attempts are being made to alkalinize urine for appropriate drug overdoses.

ATRIAL FIBRILLATION (AF)

See the Internal Medicine chapter.

What is the most common etiology of cardiac arrest?
Ventricular fibrillation.

VENTRICULAR FIBRILLATION (VF)

The most common arrhythmia in cardiac arrest patients. Associated with high mortality, so **early defibrillation** is the most important therapy.

SIGNS AND SYMPTOMS

Syncope, hypotension, pulselessness.

DIFFERENTIAL

Detached lead/equipment malfunction, ventricular tachycardia (VT), ventricular premature complexes.

WORKUP

ECG demonstrates a totally **erratic tracing** (see Figure 3-5).

TREATMENT

- ABCs.
- Initiate CPR until the defibrillator is attached.
- Defibrillate × 3 (200, 300, 360 J).
- Epinephrine 1 mg IV q 3–5 minutes **or** vasopressin 40 U IV × 1.
- If this fails, defibrillate again with 360 J.
- If there is still no response, the following may be tried:
    - Amiodarone 300-mg IV push; an additional 150-mg IV push may be given after 3–5 minutes.
    - Lidocaine 1.0–1.5 mg/kg IV; an additional 0.50- to 0.75-mg/kg IV push may be given in 3–5 minutes.
    - Magnesium sulfate 1–2 g IV.
    - Procainamide 30 mg/min for a maximum total dose of 17 mg/kg.

VENTRICULAR TACHYCARDIA (VT)

Consists of a heart rate > 100 bpm that arises distal to the bundle of His. This readily converts to VF.

SIGNS AND SYMPTOMS

- Tachycardia, hypotension, tachypnea.
- Pallor, diaphoresis.

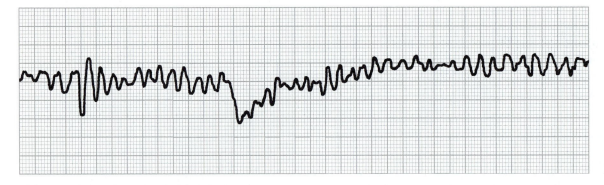

FIGURE 3-5. Ventricular fibrillation.

(Reproduced, with permission, from Stead L et al. *First Aid for the Emergency Medicine Clerkship*, 1st ed. New York: McGraw-Hill, 2002: 13.)

DIFFERENTIAL

AF, atrial flutter, atrial tachycardia, VF.

WORKUP

- ECG (see Figure 3-6) shows a **wide QRS complex and a rate > 100 bpm.**
- Cardiac enzymes; electrolytes.

TREATMENT

- **If unstable:** Immediate synchronized cardioversion (100, 200, 300, 360 J).
- **If stable:**
  - Amiodarone 150-mg IV bolus over 10 minutes or lidocaine 1.0- to 1.5-mg/kg IV push; then 0.50–0.75 mg/kg IV q 3–5 minutes (total maximum dose 3 mg/kg).
  - Procainamide 20–30 mg/min (maximum dose 17 mg/kg) may be used in patients with a normal EF.
  - Synchronized cardioversion (100, 200, 300, 360 J).

Cardiac Tamponade

Defined as fluid accumulation in the pericardium that prevents the heart from adequately filling or contracting efficiently, thereby decreasing stroke volume.

SIGNS AND SYMPTOMS

- Chest pain, dyspnea, fatigue.
- **Beck's triad:**
  - **Hypotension**
  - **JVD**
  - **Muffled heart sounds** with pulsus paradoxus (more than a 10-mmHg drop in SBP during inspiration)
- Electrical alternans on ECG; tachycardia.

DIFFERENTIAL

MI, tension pneumothorax, CHF.

Beck's triad for cardiac tamponade:

1. Hypotension

2. JVD

3. Muffled heart sounds

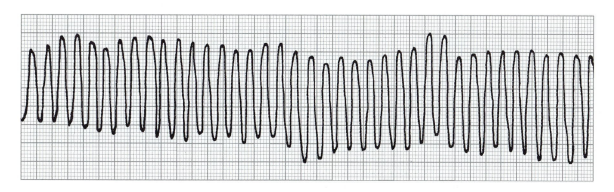

FIGURE 3-6. Ventricular tachycardia.

(Reproduced, with permission, from Stead L et al. *First Aid for the Emergency Medicine Clerkship*, 1st ed. New York: McGraw-Hill, 2002: 13.)

WORKUP

■ Echocardiogram if time permits.
■ CXR may show an enlarged, globular heart.
■ ECG may show ↓ amplitude and/or electrical alternans.

TREATMENT

■ **Pericardiocentesis.**
■ Pericardial window may be required.
■ Volume expansion with IV fluids.

What is the most common cause of hypertensive urgency? Noncompliance with medication.

Hypertensive Urgency/Emergency

Distinguished as follows:

■ **Hypertensive urgency: A BP > 220/ > 120 mmHg** that is asymptomatic (no end-organ damage).
■ **Hypertensive emergency:** Any evidence of **end-organ damage** regardless of BP.

SIGNS AND SYMPTOMS

■ **CNS:** Headache, blurred vision, mental status change, nausea/vomiting.
■ **Cardiovascular:** Angina, pulmonary edema, dyspnea.

DIFFERENTIAL

■ **Cardiovascular:** Angina, abdominal aortic aneurysm, CHF.
■ **Neurologic:** Headache (e.g., migraine, tension, cluster).
■ **Endocrine:** Thyroid storm.
■ **Preeclampsia.**

WORKUP

■ Cardiovascular, neurologic, ophthalmologic, and abdominal examinations.
■ ECG.
■ **Labs:**
  ■ **Blood tests:** CBC, electrolytes, BUN/creatinine.
  ■ UA to assess for RBCs, protein, and casts.
  ■ Cardiac enzymes if chest pain is present.
■ **Imaging:** CXR and head CT for hemorrhage or edema.

TREATMENT

■ ↓ mean arterial pressure by no more than 25% within minutes to hours.
■ **Oral agents:** β-blockers.
■ **IV agents:** Nitroglycerin, nitroprusside, or labetalol.

GASTROENTEROLOGY

Appendicitis

Acute appendicitis, or inflammation of the appendix, should **always** be near the top of your differential for an acute abdomen, as approximately 7% of the U.S. population will develop appendicitis at some point in their lives. Appendicitis peaks in the teens to the mid-20s, with atypical presentations including pregnant patients as well as those with retrocecal appendices. Its etiology can be traced to luminal obstruction of the appendix caused by hyperplasia of lymphoid tissue (55–65%), fecalith (35%), or foreign body (e.g., food, carcinoid tumor, parasites). The probable pathophysiology of appendicitis is as follows:

- Obstruction.
- Accumulation of fluid and mucus behind the obstruction.
- Distention of the appendix, inflammation, and 2° bacterial overgrowth.
- High intraluminal pressure, compression of the capillary blood supply, and resulting appendiceal ischemia.
- The inflammatory process may also become contained by the omentum or peritoneum, leading to a periappendiceal abscess.
- Both can lead to perforation of the appendix with subsequent peritonitis due to leaked intestinal contents. The mainstay of treatment for acute appendicitis is early diagnosis and operative intervention before perforation has occurred.

What is the most common surgical emergency? Appendicitis. In cases of abdominal pain, acute appendicitis must always be in the differential.

SIGNS AND SYMPTOMS

- Patients often present with a history of anorexia, low-grade fever, and **abdominal pain.**
- Patients often have a history of dull, vague periumbilical pain of 1–24 hours' duration that localizes to the RLQ at **McBurney's point** (two-thirds of the distance from the umbilicus to the right anterior superior iliac spine).
  - Discomfort progresses to a sharp pain as a result of irritation of parietal peritoneum from the progressively distended appendix.
  - This can be accompanied by rebound, guarding, high fever, hypotension, and a high WBC count. Associated symptoms include nausea, vomiting, and anorexia following the pain.
- Physical exam reveals the following:
  - **Rovsing's sign:** Referred pain in the RLQ elicited by deep palpation in the LLQ. This sign is specific but fairly insensitive.
  - **Iliopsoas sign:** RLQ pain elicited by passive extension of the hip (this is caused by stretching the iliopsoas tendon, which overlies the appendix). This sign is not sensitive (see Figure 3-7).

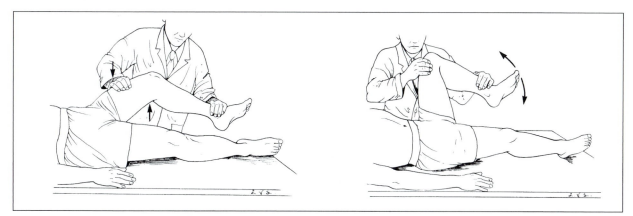

FIGURE 3-7. Iliopsoas test and obturator test.

(Reproduced, with permission, from Way LW (ed). *Current Surgical Diagnosis & Treatment,* 6th ed. Stamford, CT: Appleton & Lange, 1983.)

- **Obturator sign:** RLQ pain elicited by passive internal rotation of the hip. This sign is also insensitive (see Figure 3-7).
- A palpable RLQ mass may indicate an abscess.
- Rectal exam generally elicits pain on the right side.

DIFFERENTIAL

- **GI:**
  - Gastroenteritis (nausea and vomiting **before** the pain with no leukocytosis).
  - Intussusception (seen mainly in patients < 2 years of age); small bowel obstruction.
  - IBD, diverticulitis, mesenteric ischemia.
  - Perforated peptic ulcer, acute cholecystitis, pancreatitis.
- **Gynecologic:**
  - PID (cervical motion tenderness, discharge, bilateral lower abdominal tenderness, high fever).
  - Ovarian cyst torsion, ectopic pregnancy, mittelschmerz (due to a ruptured ovarian follicle in the middle of the menstrual cycle).
- **GU:** Testicular torsion, epididymitis, pyelonephritis, nephrolithiasis.
- **Endocrine:** DKA.

WORKUP

The diagnosis of acute appendicitis is based largely on the H&P. Other criteria are as follows:

- **Labs:**
  - CBC shows mild leukocytosis (11,000–15,000) with left shift.
  - UA may show RBCs or WBCs.
- **Imaging:**
  - AXR may demonstrate fecalith.
  - Ultrasound may show a noncompressible appendix. It is useful to rule out gynecologic abnormalities in female patients.
  - CT is 90–95% sensitive for appendicitis.

TREATMENT

Patients in whom appendicitis is strongly suspected should be taken to the OR immediately for **exploratory laparotomy and appendectomy.** Treatment is as follows:

- NPO, IV hydration.
- Administration of antibiotics.
- **Surgery:**
  - **Usually laparoscopic appendectomy (vs. open),** as the laparoscopic approach results in shorter hospital stays, reduces postoperative complication rates, and allows for definitive diagnosis by ruling out gynecologic diseases or other processes before the appendix is removed ("diagnostic laparotomy").
  - Normal appendices are removed approximately 15–20% of the time (this rate is higher in women owing to gynecologic disease). This is considered acceptable by virtue of the life-threatening potential of the disease.

COMPLICATIONS

The risk of perforation and mortality ↑ with the amount of time the appendicitis is present. This risk approaches 75% at 48 hours.

Ectopic Pregnancy

A medical emergency that occurs when the embryo implants outside the uterine cavity. Roughly 17 in 1000 pregnancies are affected. Etiologies include anything that contributes to abnormal tubal motility.

SIGNS AND SYMPTOMS

- **Amenorrhea; irregular vaginal bleeding**.
- Abdominal/pelvic pain (usually unilateral); nausea/vomiting; pelvic mass on physical exam.
- Signs of rupture (10% of cases) include orthostatic hypotension, tachycardia, abdominal tenderness, shoulder pain, syncope, and shock.

DIFFERENTIAL

- **Gynecologic:** Intrauterine pregnancy, threatened abortion, PID, endometriosis, ruptured ovarian cyst, ovarian torsion.
- **GI:** Appendicitis, diverticulitis.
- **GU:** Renal stones.

WORKUP

- **Quantitative β-hCG:** To check for subnormal doubling time and low levels (80% of ectopic pregnancies have a β-hCG < 6500 mIU/L).
- **Serum progesterone:** Ectopics usually have < 15 ng/mL.
- **Ultrasound:** Look for a noncystic adnexal mass or fluid in the cul-de-sac in the absence of intrauterine gestation.
- Correlate the β-hCG level with ultrasound findings and/or with time elapsed since the last menstrual period (LMP) (see Table 3-1).

TREATMENT

- **Medical management** (never appropriate for a patient with signs of ruptured ectopic pregnancy):
  - **Expectant management of serial β-hCG and ultrasound:** If the diagnosis of ectopic pregnancy is uncertain or β-hCG is in the "discriminatory zone" and reliable follow-up can be expected.
  - **Methotrexate:** For unruptured ectopic pregnancies < 3 cm with a β-hCG < 12,000 mIU/L.
- **Surgical management:** Choose with the reproductive plans, age, and clinical status of the patient in mind.

Risk factors for ectopic pregnancy:

- *A history of STDs or PID*
- *A prior ectopic pregnancy*
- *DES exposure*
- *Adhesions from prior abdominal, tubal, or pelvic surgery*
- *In vitro fertilization*
- *IUD use*
- *Use of exogenous progesterone or estrogen*

What is the classic presentation of ectopic pregnancy? A short period of amenorrhea leading to vaginal bleeding plus abdominal pain.

Always check a β-hCG level on a premenopausal woman with abdominal pain!

TABLE 3-1. Ultrasound Findings, β-hCG Levels, and Time Since LMP for a Normal Intrauterine Pregnancy

TRANSVAGINAL ULTRASOUND FINDINGS	β-hCG LEVEL	TIME ELAPSED SINCE LMP (DAYS)
Gestational sac[a]	1500	35
Fetal pole	5000	40
Fetal heart motion	11,000	45

[a] For transabdominal ultrasound, the gestational sac should be visualized at a β-hCG level of 6000–6500 mIU/L and/or 42 days since the LMP.

- **Salpingostomy:** The tube is incised and product of conception is removed.
- **Salpingectomy:** The entire tube is removed.
- **Salpingo-oophorectomy:** Both the tube and the ovary are removed.

Testicular Torsion

Twisting of the testicle on its root, usually in the horizontal direction, as a result of a weak connection of the gubernaculum. Most often occurs in young adults and infants < 1 year of age.

SIGNS AND SYMPTOMS

- Presents with sudden onset of pain in the lower abdomen, inguinal canal, or testicle that is constant, progressive, and unrelieved by changes in position.
- Usually occurs during strenuous activity, but may also occur during sleep.

DIFFERENTIAL

- Torsion of the appendix testis or the appendix epididymis.
- Epididymitis, orchitis.
- Hydrocele, varicocele.
- Inguinal hernia, appendicitis, kidney stone.

WORKUP

- **Doppler ultrasound:** To determine if there is blood flow to the testicle.
- **UA:** Usually normal.

TREATMENT

- Attempt manual detorsion.
- Request an immediate urology consult.
- Immediate exploratory surgery is warranted ("time is testicle!") when ultrasound is equivocal, when there is no alternative diagnosis, and even following manual detorsion to ensure full detorsion and to perform contralateral orchiopexy.

NEUROLOGY

Intracranial Hemorrhage

SUBARACHNOID HEMORRHAGE (SAH)

SAH typically occurs in patients 50–60 years of age and has a high mortality rate (35%). Ruptured aneurysms are reported to have a 50% one-month mortality rate. Etiologies include the following:

- **Ruptured aneurysm (e.g., berry, hypertensive): Berry aneurysms** are the **most common cause of SAH** and are associated with polycystic kidney disease and coarctation of the aorta (see Figure 3-8).
- **Other:** AVM; trauma to the circle of Willis (often at the middle cerebral artery).

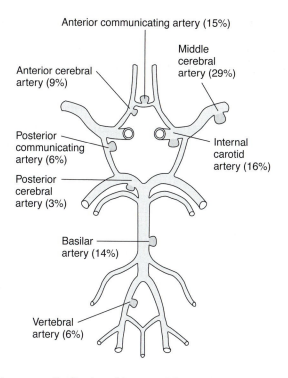

FIGURE 3-8. Frequency distribution of intracranial aneurysms.

(Reproduced, with permission, from Greenberg DA et al. *Clinical Neurology*, 5th ed. New York: McGraw-Hill, 2002: 77.)

Signs and Symptoms

- **Headache:**
  - Presents with a sudden-onset, intensely painful "thunderclap headache" in the occipital region. May be preceded by "sentinel headaches" in the weeks preceding the hemorrhage.
  - Sometimes associated with fever, nausea, vomiting, and a fluctuating level of consciousness.
- Signs of meningeal irritation (e.g., neck stiffness) may also be seen.
- Seizure may result from irritation of the cortex by blood.
- CN III palsy with pupillary involvement may be associated with berry aneurysms on the posterior communicating artery.
- Exam findings can range from normal to neurologic deficits and a depressed level of consciousness.

Differential

Hemorrhagic stroke, trauma, meningitis, first presentation of migraine headache.

Workup

- Emergent **head CT without contrast** to look for blood in the subarachnoid space, especially around the circle of Willis. Blood appears white on noncontrast CT.
- If the head CT is ⊖ but there is a moderate or high index of suspicion for SAH, obtain an immediate LP to look for red cells (must be in consecutive tubes to rule out traumatic tap), xanthochromia, and ↑ ICP.

What classically presents as "the worst headache of my life"? SAH.

Fifteen percent of head CTs will be falsely ⊖ in SAH. If the head CT is ⊖, an LP is needed to rule out SAH.

■ Four-vessel angiography once SAH has been confirmed to look for an aneurysm.

TREATMENT

Treatment should focus on preventing rebleeding, which is most likely to occur in the first 48 hours after SAH. Measures include the following:

■ ↓ ICP by raising the head of the bed and administering IV fluids.
■ Prevent hypo- and hypertension.
■ **Medications:**
  ■ Calcium channel blockers (nimodipine) to prevent vasospasm (start within 96 hours).
  ■ Dexamethasone for cerebral edema.
  ■ Antiseizure medication (phenytoin).
■ **Surgery:** Surgical treatment involves open or interventional radiologic clipping or coiling of an aneurysm or AVM.

COMPLICATIONS

■ **Neurologic deficits:** Caused by the mass effect of a large AVM or aneurysm impinging on brain parenchyma.
■ **Ischemic injury to the brain:** Vasospasm in the first week after SAH is the most common cause.
■ **Obstructive hydrocephalus:** 2° to intraventricular blood obstructing CSF drainage or interfering with CSF absorption through the arachnoid granulations.

CEREBROVASCULAR ACCIDENT (CVA)

See the Neurology chapter.

EPIDURAL HEMATOMA

What is the typical case scenario of epidural hemorrhage? A patient presenting several hours after blunt trauma to the head with altered consciousness, although the patient had seemed to return to baseline after the injury. Patients are said to "talk and die." Emergent neurosurgical evacuation is lifesaving.

Defined as a collection of blood between the dura and skull. Associated with temporal bone fractures due to blunt trauma with resultant tear of the **middle meningeal artery.**

SIGNS AND SYMPTOMS

■ Presents with loss of consciousness followed by a lucid interval ranging from several minutes to hours.
■ After the lucid interval, there is onset of headache, progressive obtundation, and hemiparesis.
■ Ultimately, epidural bleeding may lead to a **"blown pupil,"** in which the pupil becomes fixed and dilated as a result of uncal herniation and compression of CN III.

WORKUP

Head CT shows a **lens-shaped, convex** hyperdensity that is usually limited by the sutures of the cranium where the dura inserts onto the bone (see Figure 3-9).

TREATMENT

Emergent neurosurgical evacuation.

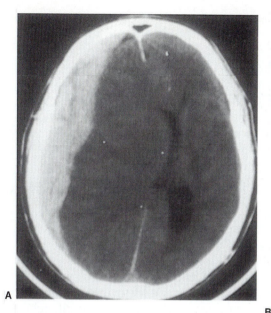
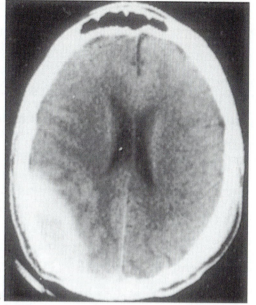

FIGURE 3-9. Head CT scans.

(A) Subdural hematoma. Note the crescent shape and the mass effect with midline shift. (B) Epidural hematoma with classic bi-convex lens shape. (Reprinted, with permission, from Aminoff MJ et al. *Clinical Neurology*, 3rd ed. Stamford, CT: Appleton & Lange, 1996: 296.)

SUBDURAL HEMATOMA

Defined as a collection of blood between the dura and the brain. Associated with tearing of the bridging veins between the cortex and dural sinuses. Often seen in the elderly and alcoholics, who have significant cortical atrophy that places the bridging veins under tension. Tearing usually occurs as a result of an acceleration-deceleration mechanism.

SIGNS AND SYMPTOMS

- Headache.
- Change in mental status or new-onset dementia. Changes can be acute (< 24 hours), subacute (24 hours to 2 weeks), or chronic (> 2 weeks).
- Contralateral hemiparesis or other focal deficit (the most common exam finding is nonfocality).
- A remote history of a fall.

WORKUP

- Head CT with and without contrast shows a **crescent-shaped, concave** fluid collection, with density depending on the age of the bleed (see Figure 3-9).
- In some cases, a hematocrit line may be observed in which the RBCs have settled down and separated from the plasma.

TREATMENT

- **If symptomatic:** Surgical evacuation.
- **If asymptomatic:** Observation, as subdural blood will frequently regress spontaneously.

Why is it important to establish the age of a subdural hematoma? Acute subdural hematomas have a high mortality. This is in contrast to chronic, asymptomatic subdural hematomas, which may be managed with observation.

AVMs are more likely than SAH to produce an intraparenchymal hemorrhage.

Look for mass effect and edema on head CT, as it may predict herniation.

Neuroleptic malignant syndrome has a 20% mortality rate.

INTRAPARENCHYMAL HEMORRHAGE

Etiologies include hypertension (usually in the basal ganglia), amyloid angiopathy (seen in the elderly), and vascular malformations (AVMs, cavernous hemangiomas).

SIGNS AND SYMPTOMS

Lethargy, headache, motor or sensory deficits.

WORKUP

Head CT without contrast to look for an intraparenchymal hemorrhage.

TREATMENT

- Raise the head of the bed to ↓ ICP.
- Institute seizure prophylaxis.
- Monitor for and prevent ischemic damage 2° to vasospasm.
- Surgical evacuation may be necessary and lifesaving if a mass effect is observed or if the hemorrhage occurs in the posterior fossa, thereby threatening vital brain stem function.

Neuroleptic Malignant Syndrome

Caused by central dopaminergic blockade. Most common in young men who are put on a **typical antipsychotic** for the first time, occurring during the **first 10 days of use.**

SIGNS AND SYMPTOMS

Hyperthermia, altered mental status, autonomic instability, muscular rigidity.

WORKUP

- Look for leukocytosis on CBC.
- Look for ↑ CK.

TREATMENT

- Discontinue the offending agent.
- Give benzodiazepines or dantrolene, or consider bromocriptine to ↑ dopamine activity.

Status Epilepticus

Defined as prolonged (≥ 30-minute) or repetitive seizures without a return to baseline consciousness. Seizures can be either convulsive or nonconvulsive (a distinction that can be made only by EEG). Etiologies include anticonvulsant/EtOH/sedative withdrawal, drug intoxication, metabolic disturbances, trauma, and infection.

SIGNS AND SYMPTOMS

On physical exam, look for the following:

- Signs of trauma, meningeal irritation, or systemic infection.
- Papilledema.

- Focal neurologic signs.
- Evidence of metastatic, hepatic, or renal disease.

WORKUP

- Check **ABCDs:** **A**irway, **B**reathing, **C**irculation, **D**-stick (to check blood glucose).
- **Establish access:** Insert an IV line.
- **Initial workup:** Treatment with anticonvulsants should be instituted immediately while the following measures are taken:
  - **Check vital signs:**
    - **BP:** To exclude hypertensive encephalopathy and shock.
    - **Temperature:** To exclude hyperthermia.
    - **Pulse:** To exclude life-threatening cardiac arrhythmia with cardiac monitoring.
  - **Labs:**
    - CBC, electrolytes, hepatic and renal function tests, calcium, ESR, toxicology, and PT/PTT (in case LP is necessary); ABGs.
    - **Calculate serum osmolality:** $2 (Na^+) + glucose/18 + BUN/2.8$ (normal range 270–290).
- **Poststabilization:** Once the patient is stabilized, obtain the following:
  - EEG and brain imaging (very rarely done in the ED).
  - LP in the presence of fever, meningeal signs, or **any** clinical suspicion (only after a CT has been done).

TREATMENT

- On admission, attend to cardiopulmonary status (ABCs).
- Give thiamine (100 mg) and glucose (50 mL 50% dextrose) IV.
- Administer anticonvulsants:
  - Give lorazepam (Ativan).
  - Then give a loading dose of phenytoin or fosphenytoin (see Table 3-2).
- If seizures continue, intubate and add IV phenobarbital.
- If the patient fails therapy, induce coma with an IV anesthetic such as midazolam and admit to the ICU with continuous bedside EEG monitoring.

RESPIRATORY

Asthma

A bronchial disorder characterized by inflammation, reversible smooth muscle constriction, and mucus production leading to airway obstruction and difficulty breathing. Most cases develop by age 40. Key asthma triggers include the following:

- **Airway irritants:** Cigarettes, air pollution, ozone.
- **Allergies:** Pollens, dust mites, pets, cockroaches, foods and food additives.
- **Drugs:** Aspirin, β-blockers.
- **Other:** Exercise, cold weather, stress; respiratory infections.

SIGNS AND SYMPTOMS

- **History:** Try to elicit a history that includes past severity, frequency, ER visits, hospitalizations, ICU admissions (including intubation history), and courses of steroids per year.

Status epilepticus is a medical emergency associated with a 20% mortality rate.

A woman on INH presents in status epilepticus and is unresponsive to treatment. What should she be treated with? Vitamin B_6.

Most clinicians start treating status epilepticus after 2–3 minutes of seizure activity, since brain damage begins after a short period of time.

What predicts a rapid and severe asthma exacerbation? Male gender, the absence of corticosteroid use, the absence of URI, and theophylline use.

TABLE 3-2. **Drug Treatment of Status Epilepticus**

DRUG	**DOSAGE/ROUTE**	**ADVANTAGES/DISADVANTAGES/COMPLICATIONS**
Lorazepam[a] or diazepam	10 mg IV over 2 minutes. 0.1-mg/kg IV rate ≤ 2 mg/min.	Fast-acting. Effective half-life is 15 minutes for diazepam and four hours for lorazepam. Abrupt respiratory depression or hypotension occurs in 5% of patients, especially when given in combination with other sedatives. Seizure recurrence affects 50% of patients; therefore, one must add a maintenance drug (phenytoin or phenobarbital).
Immediately proceed to phenytoin.		
Phenytoin or fos-phenytoin	1000–1500 mg (15 mg/kg), IV rate ≤ 50 mg/min (cannot be given in dextrose solution). Fosphenytoin at 100–150 mg/min.	Little or no respiratory depression. Drug levels in the brain are therapeutic at the completion of infusion. Effective as maintenance drugs. Hypotension and cardiac arrhythmias can occur, probably more often with phenytoin than with fosphenytoin.
If seizures continue following total dose, proceed immediately to phenobarbital.		
Phenobarbital	1000–1500 mg (18 mg/kg), IV slowly (50 mg/min).	Peak brain levels within 30 minutes. Effective as maintenance drug. Respiratory depression and hypotension are common at higher doses. (Intubation and ventilatory support should be immediately available.)
If the above is ineffective, proceed immediately to general anesthesia.		
Pentobarbital or midazolam[a]	15 mg/kg IV slowly, followed by 0.5–4.0 mg/kg/hr. 0.2 mg/kg IV slowly, followed by 0.75–10.0 mg/kg/min.	Intubation and ventilatory support are required. Hypotension is the limiting factor. Pressors may be required to maintain BP.

[a] Investigational in the United States for this application.

- **Symptoms:** Dyspnea, cough, wheezing, irritability, or feeding difficulties in young children.
- **Signs of increasing respiratory distress** include the following:
  - Tachypnea, tachycardia, prolonged expiration, cyanosis.
  - Intercostal and subcostal retraction; nasal flaring.
  - Inability to speak in full sentences owing to shortness of breath.

Why should you be concerned if an asthmatic stops wheezing? This may be a sign of ↓ air movement and respiratory failure.

DIFFERENTIAL

- **Children:** Aspiration, foreign body, bronchiolitis, bronchopulmonary dysplasia, vascular rings, CF, pneumonia.
- **Adults:** Foreign body, CHF, COPD, GERD, PE, sleep apnea, pneumonia.

All that wheezes is not asthma.

WORKUP

- **Peak expiratory flow (PEF):** < 50% of predicted indicates severe exacerbation.
- **Pulse oximetry.**
- **ABGs:** Look for hypoxia and respiratory acidosis during acute exacerbations.

- **CXR:** Shows bilateral hyperinflation and flattening of the diaphragms.
- **CBC:** WBC count demonstrates leukocytosis and/or eosinophilia.

TREATMENT

- A suggested algorithm for the emergent management of asthma is outlined in Figure 3-10.
- Bronchodilators are the drug of choice in an acute attack.
- Patients with moderate to severe attacks should receive systemic steroids such as PO prednisone or IV methylprednisolone (Solu-Medrol). Treatment with corticosteroids for < 10 days does not require tapering.
- All patients must get an ambulatory O_2 sat before they can be discharged.

Hemothorax

Blood in the pleural cavity caused by laceration of the lungs or intrathoracic blood vessels. Defined as follows:

- **Simple hemothorax:** < 1500 cc of blood in the pleural cavity.
- **Massive hemothorax:** > 1500 cc of blood.

SIGNS AND SYMPTOMS

- Dyspnea, tachypnea, tachycardia.
- ↓ or absent breath sounds on the affected side; dullness to percussion.
- Signs of hypovolemic shock can be seen if blood loss is severe.

DIFFERENTIAL

- ⊕ **history of trauma:** Consider pneumothorax, hemopneumothorax, tension pneumothorax, and communicating pneumothorax.
- ⊖ **history of trauma:** Consider other causes of pleural effusions (see the Internal Medicine chapter), chylothorax, and empyema.

WORKUP

CXR shows blunting of the costophrenic angle if > 200 cc of blood is present; there is complete opacification on the affected side in massive hemothorax (≥ 1500 cc).

TREATMENT

- **Simple hemothorax:** Usually self-limited.
  - Tube thoracostomy to control bleeding by apposition of the pleural surfaces.
  - If there is > 1500 cc of drainage from the initial chest tube, > 50% hemothorax, or 200 cc/hr continued drainage, or if the patient decompensates after initial stabilization, a thoracotomy is needed.
- **Massive hemothorax:** Thoracotomy followed by tube thoracostomy.

Pneumothorax

A collection of air in the pleural space that can lead to pulmonary collapse. Categorized as follows:

How long after corticosteroid administration will you see a response? Steroids target the late inflammatory response in asthma. You should not expect to see an improvement in symptoms for 4–6 hours.

HIGH-YIELD FACTS

EMERGENCY MEDICINE

The key determination to make in a hemothorax is whether the patient requires thoracotomy.

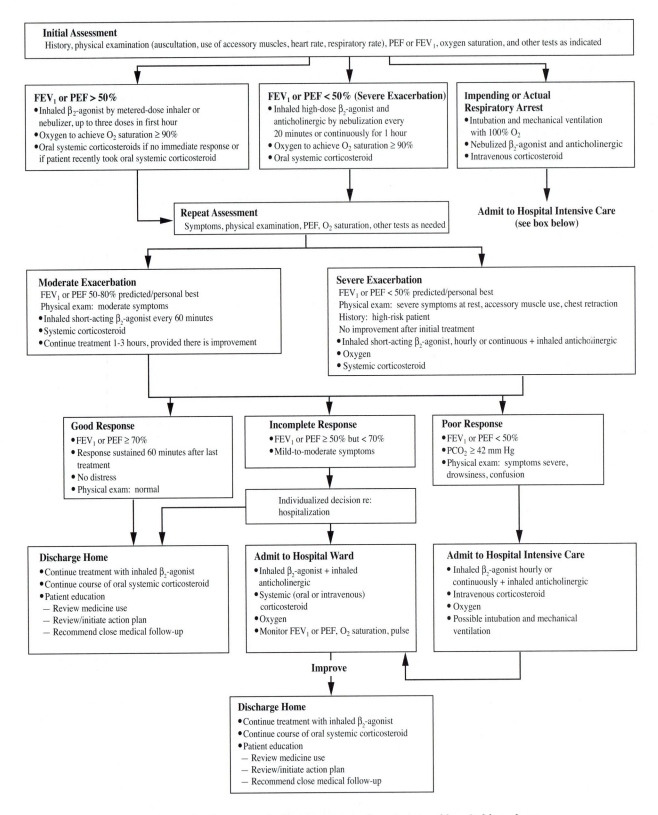

Initial Assessment
History, physical examination (auscultation, use of accessory muscles, heart rate, respiratory rate), PEF or FEV_1, oxygen saturation, and other tests as indicated

FEV_1 or PEF > 50%
- Inhaled β_2-agonist by metered-dose inhaler or nebulizer, up to three doses in first hour
- Oxygen to achieve O_2 saturation ≥ 90%
- Oral systemic corticosteroids if no immediate response or if patient recently took oral systemic corticosteroid

FEV_1 or PEF < 50% (Severe Exacerbation)
- Inhaled high-dose β_2-agonist and anticholinergic by nebulization every 20 minutes or continuously for 1 hour
- Oxygen to achieve O_2 saturation ≥ 90%
- Oral systemic corticosteroid

Impending or Actual Respiratory Arrest
- Intubation and mechanical ventilation with 100% O_2
- Nebulized β_2-agonist and anticholinergic
- Intravenous corticosteroid

Repeat Assessment
Symptoms, physical examination, PEF, O_2 saturation, other tests as needed

Admit to Hospital Intensive Care
(see box below)

Moderate Exacerbation
FEV_1 or PEF 50-80% predicted/personal best
Physical exam: moderate symptoms
- Inhaled short-acting β_2-agonist every 60 minutes
- Systemic corticosteroid
- Continue treatment 1-3 hours, provided there is improvement

Severe Exacerbation
FEV_1 or PEF < 50% predicted/personal best
Physical exam: severe symptoms at rest, accessory muscle use, chest retraction
History: high-risk patient
No improvement after initial treatment
- Inhaled short-acting β_2-agonist, hourly or continuous + inhaled anticholinergic
- Oxygen
- Systemic corticosteroid

Good Response
- FEV_1 or PEF ≥ 70%
- Response sustained 60 minutes after last treatment
- No distress
- Physical exam: normal

Incomplete Response
- FEV_1 or PEF ≥ 50% but < 70%
- Mild-to-moderate symptoms

Poor Response
- FEV_1 or PEF < 50%
- PCO_2 ≥ 42 mm Hg
- Physical exam: symptoms severe, drowsiness, confusion

Individualized decision re: hospitalization

Discharge Home
- Continue treatment with inhaled β_2-agonist
- Continue course of oral systemic corticosteroid
- Patient education
  — Review medicine use
  — Review/initiate action plan
  — Recommend close medical follow-up

Admit to Hospital Ward
- Inhaled β_2-agonist + inhaled anticholinergic
- Systemic (oral or intravenous) corticosteroid
- Oxygen
- Monitor FEV_1 or PEF, O_2 saturation, pulse

Admit to Hospital Intensive Care
- Inhaled β_2-agonist hourly or continuously + inhaled anticholinergic
- Intravenous corticosteroid
- Oxygen
- Possible intubation and mechanical ventilation

Improve

Discharge Home
- Continue treatment with inhaled β_2-agonist
- Continue course of oral systemic corticosteroid
- Patient education
  — Review medicine use
  — Review/initiate action plan
  — Recommend close medical follow-up

FIGURE 3-10. Management of asthma exacerbations: emergency department and hospital-based care.

(Reproduced from *Guidelines for the Diagnosis and Management of Asthma.* Expert Panel Report 2. NIH Publication No. 97-4051, July 1997.)

HIGH-YIELD FACTS

EMERGENCY MEDICINE

- **1° (spontaneous):** May involve rupture of subpleural apical blebs; most commonly seen in tall, thin young males.
- **2°:** Causes include COPD, asthma, TB, trauma, and PCP, or may be iatrogenic (thoracentesis, subclavian central line placement, positive-pressure mechanical ventilation, bronchoscopy).

SIGNS AND SYMPTOMS

- Unilateral pleuritic chest pain and dyspnea.
- Tachycardia.
- Respiratory physical exam reveals diminished/absent breath sounds, hyperresonance to percussion, and ↓ tactile fremitus.

DIFFERENTIAL

Suspect other deadly causes of chest pain (see the mnemonic **TAPUM** on p. 62) as well as pneumonia, pleural effusion, and pericardial tamponade.

WORKUP

CXR shows a visceral pleural line and/or lung retraction from the chest wall (best seen with an end-expiratory film in an upright position).

TREATMENT

- Small pneumothoraces are allowed to resolve spontaneously and may be treated with 100% O_2 by face mask.
- Large, severely symptomatic pneumothoraces are treated with a chest tube and/or pleurodesis.

TENSION PNEUMOTHORAX

A deadly variant of pneumothorax in which a pulmonary or chest wall defect acts as a one-way valve, drawing air into the pleural space during inspiration but trapping it during expiration. Etiologies include penetrating trauma, infection, CHF, and positive-pressure mechanical ventilation. The pathophysiology of tension pneumothorax involves the following:

- Ipsilateral lung collapse 2° to an ↑ amount of trapped air on the affected side.
- Shift of the mediastinum away from the injured lung.
- Impaired venous return leading to ↓ cardiac output.
- Shock and death occur unless the condition is immediately recognized and treated.

SIGNS AND SYMPTOMS

Suspect tension pneumothorax if you see signs of pneumothorax and the following:

- Respiratory distress; falling O_2 saturation.
- Hypotension.
- Distended neck veins.
- Tracheal deviation away from the side of the pneumothorax.

TREATMENT

- **Immediate needle decompression:** A large-bore needle (14 gauge) is inserted into the second or third intercostal space at the midclavicular line

Don't forget that a patient with pneumothorax may be asymptomatic!

How should you diagnose a tension pneumothorax on CXR? This is a trick question. Tension pneumothorax is a clinical diagnosis and should never be diagnosed by CXR. You should not delay needle decompression to confirm a suspicion of tension pneumothorax by CXR.

on the side of the pneumothorax. Watch for restoration of hemodynamics to determine successful intervention. Sometimes a hissing sound may also signal decompression of the pneumothorax, but this may be hard to discern in the noisy ED environment.

■ Once decompression is achieved, a chest tube (thoracostomy tube) can be placed.

■ Administer IV fluids to ↑ venous return to the heart.

COMMUNICATING PNEUMOTHORAX (SUCKING CHEST WOUND)

A pneumothorax due to an open defect in the chest wall that allows air to preferentially enter through the defect. This occurs when an open defect, often from a gunshot wound, is greater than two-thirds the diameter of the trachea. The affected lung collapses with inspiration as air enters through the wound, seriously impairing ventilation.

SIGNS AND SYMPTOMS

In addition to respiratory distress, air may be seen or heard bubbling through the wound.

WORKUP

This is immediately life-threatening, and the diagnosis is clinical.

TREATMENT

Cover the wound with an impermeable dressing on **three sides.** This allows air to escape during expiration and prevents it from entering during inspiration, effectively converting the defect into a simple pneumothorax.

Flail Chest

A free-floating segment of chest wall that moves paradoxically during respiration. This means that it moves inward during inspiration and outward during expiration in accordance with the ⊖ and ⊕ intrapleural pressure. The flail segment is created by consecutive rib fractures, with each having been broken in at least two places. This is caused by a mechanism of injury with significant force and is usually associated with significant injury to underlying lung tissue that leads to a pulmonary contusion.

SIGNS AND SYMPTOMS

Respiratory distress; pain associated with rib fractures; paradoxical movement of the flail segment.

WORKUP

The diagnosis is clinical and is made by seeing or palpating the paradoxical movement of the flail segment.

TREATMENT

Oxygenation; reexpansion of the lung; analgesia to improve ventilation.

Why don't you cover a sucking chest wound on all four sides? Covering the wound on four sides potentially converts it to a tension pneumothorax, which could be immediately life-threatening.

Pulmonary Embolism (PE)

An occlusion of the pulmonary vasculature, typically by a blood clot. Ninety-five percent of the time, the embolus originates from a DVT above the calf. PE often leads to pulmonary infarction, right heart failure, and tissue hypoxia. Risk factors for DVT and PE include Virchow's triad, which consists of the following:

- **Blood stasis:** Immobility, obesity, CHF, surgery.
- **Venous endothelial injury:** Surgery of the pelvis/lower extremity; trauma, surgery, recent fracture.
- **Hypercoagulable states:** Pregnancy or postpartum state, OCP use, coagulation disorder, malignancy, severe burns.

SIGNS AND SYMPTOMS

- Presents with sudden-onset dyspnea and pleuritic chest pain.
- Cough, hemoptysis (rarely), anxiety, syncope, and diaphoresis may be seen.
- Physical exam findings include the following:
    - **Unstable vitals:** Tachycardia, tachypnea, hypotension.
    - **Right heart failure 2° to pulmonary embolism:** Rales, bulging neck veins, a loud P2.
    - **DVT:** Erythematous, edematous, tender, warm lower extremity with a ⊕ **Homans' sign** (calf pain on forced dorsiflexion, which is neither sensitive nor specific for PE).

WORKUP

Table 3-3 outlines the diagnostic tests for PE.

TREATMENT

- **Anticoagulation:** Give heparin (for a PTT of 60–90) to prevent clot extension, and then give warfarin (INR goal of 2–3) for long-term anticoagulation (usually lasting 3–6 months).
- **IVC (Greenfield) filter:** Consider if anticoagulation is contraindicated or if PEs continue despite anticoagulation.
- **Surgical embolectomy:** Usually not successful, and attempted only if the patient is crashing.

TOXICOLOGY

Drug Overdose/Antidotes

Table 3-4 summarizes antidotes for substance overdoses.

Drug Withdrawal

Table 3-5 summarizes withdrawal symptoms and treatment.

Trust your clinical judgment. Even a patient with a low-probability V/Q scan still has a 40% chance of having a PE if the clinical suspicion is high.

What is the most common CXR finding in PE? A normal CXR. Hampton's hump and Westermark's sign are seen only rarely. Think PE in the setting of sudden-onset dyspnea and a clear CXR.

Substances that do not bind charcoal and need whole bowel irrigation—

PHAILS

Pesticides
Hydrocarbons
Alcohols/**A**cids/**A**lkalis
Iron
Lithium
Solvents

Toxins that can be dialyzed—

MUST BE Listed

Methanol
Uremia
Salicylates
Theophylline
Barbiturates
Ethylene glycol
Lithium

TABLE 3-3. Diagnostic Tests for Pulmonary Embolism

TEST	FINDINGS/COMMENTS
CXR	Usually normal. **Hampton's hump** (a wedge-shaped infarct) and **Westermark's sign** ($\downarrow$ vascular markings in embolized lung zone) are rarely seen.
ECG	Usually sinus tachycardia and/or nonspecific ST-T-wave changes. An **S1Q3T3** pattern is pathognomonic.
ABG	**Respiratory alkalosis** ($\uparrow$ pH, $\downarrow$ P_{CO_2}), P_{O_2} < 80 mm (90% sensitive). Not useful for predicting absence of pulmonary embolism.
D-dimer	Includes the latex agglutination and ELISA D-dimer tests, the latter being more sensitive. A low D-dimer might help rule out a low-suspicion pulmonary embolism. Neither assay is specific, as D-dimers $\uparrow$ in MI, sepsis, and other systemic illnesses. However, the ELISA D-dimer will be $\uparrow$ (> 500 ng/mL) in > 90% of patients with a pulmonary embolism.
Pulmonary angiogram	Gold standard. However, invasive and inherently risky.
V/Q scan	One or more segmental areas of mismatch in the lung (i.e., well ventilated but not perfused) suggest pulmonary embolism (see Figure 3-11). Results are reported as normal or as a low/intermediate/high probability of pulmonary embolism: ■ A normal result rules out pulmonary embolism. ■ **High probability:** 85–90% incidence of pulmonary embolism. ■ **Low probability:** Does not rule out embolism (14–31% incidence).
Spiral CT	Helical (spiral) CT (with IV contrast) is sensitive to pulmonary embolism in the proximal pulmonary arteries but less so in the distal segmental arteries.
Doppler ultrasound	Helps determine if DVTs are present in the lower extremities.

Adapted, with permission, from Tierney LM et al. *Current Medical Diagnosis & Treatment*, 36th ed. Stamford, CT: Appleton & Lange, 1997: 292.

TRAUMA AND SHOCK

The ABCDEFs of resuscitation:
Airway (with cervical spine precautions)
Breathing
Circulation
Disability (neurologic status)
Exposure
Foley

Resuscitation

The resuscitation of the trauma patient begins during the 1° survey with the ABCs. Life-threatening injuries are identified and treated, and assessment and resuscitation of vital functions occur. Rapid assessment, diagnosis, and stabilization in the period immediately following trauma—termed the "golden hour"—must occur in order to optimize the patient's prognosis. The **ABCDEFs** of resuscitation are as follows:

■ Airway:
  ■ Determine if the patient is breathing. Give supplemental O_2 to all trauma patients.
  ■ If the patient is not breathing, use a chin-lift or jaw-thrust maneuver to open the airway. Assume that all trauma patients have a cervical spine injury until proven otherwise. Do not manipulate the neck by putting patients in the sniff position.

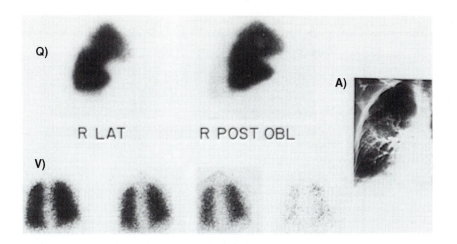

FIGURE 3-11. V/Q scan showing unmatched defects in the right midlung.

The perfusion scan (Q) of the right lung (seen from the right lateral view and the right posterior oblique view) shows defects in the right anterior midlung, while the ventilation scan (V) is normal. Pulmonary angiogram (A) of the right lower lobe shows an embolus to the right midlung field. (Reproduced, with permission, from Stobo JD et al. *The Principles and Practice of Medicine*, 23rd ed. Stamford, CT: Appleton & Lange, 1996: 174.)

- Clear foreign bodies and insert an oral or nasal airway as necessary.
- Patients with apnea, altered mental status, impending airway compromise, closed head injuries, or failed bag-mask ventilation should have early intubation.
- Surgical airway or cricothyroidectomy is used for patients who cannot be intubated or in whom there is maxillofacial trauma.
- **Breathing:** By inspecting, palpating, and auscultating the chest, identify and treat the five thoracic injuries that cause immediate death:
  - Tension pneumothorax
  - Cardiac tamponade
  - Communicating pneumothorax
  - Massive hemothorax
  - Airway obstruction
- **Circulation:**
  - Place two 14- or 16-gauge IVs in the antecubital fossae. Draw blood samples while placing IVs.
  - Assess circulatory status (check vitals, capillary refill, skin turgor).
  - Give a 1- to 2-L bolus of NS or LR for adults and 20 cc/kg in children. The need for further repletion is indicated by fluid status.
  - Replace blood loss with a 3:1 ratio (i.e., replace 1 L of blood with 3 L of crystalloid).
- **Disability:**
  - The patient's CNS dysfunction should be rapidly quantified with the Glasgow Coma Scale or with the **AVPU** scale (see mnemonic).
  - Establish pupil size and reactivity.
- **Exposure/Environment:**
  - Expose the patient completely so that he or she can be assessed from head to toe during the 2° survey and hooked up to monitors.
  - Be sure to keep the patient warm.

Why do you replace fluids in a 3:1 ratio? Crystalloid fluid redistributes into extravascular and interstitial spaces. Only about a third of the fluid volume remains in the intravascular space.

Assessing CNS function—

AVPU

Alertness
Verbal responsiveness
Pain responsiveness
Unresponsive

TABLE 3-4. Specific Antidotes

Toxin	Antidote/Treatment
Acetaminophen	N-acetylcysteine.
Anticholinesterases, organophosphates	Atropine, pralidoxime.
Antimuscarinic, anticholinergic agents	Physostigmine.
Black widow bite	Calcium gluconate.
Iron salts	Deferoxamine.
Methanol, ethylene glycol (antifreeze)	EtOH, fomepizole, dialysis.
Lead	Succimer, CaEDTA, dimercaprol.
Arsenic, mercury, gold	Succimer, dimercaprol.
Copper, arsenic, lead, gold	Penicillamine.
Cyanide	Nitrite, sodium thiosulfate.
Salicylates	Urine alkalinization, dialysis, activated charcoal.
Heparin	Protamine sulfate.
Methemoglobin	Methylene blue.
Opioids	Naloxone.
Benzodiazepines	Flumazenil.
Barbiturates (phenobarbital)	Urine alkalinization, dialysis, activated charcoal.
TCAs	Sodium bicarbonate for QRS prolongation, diazepam or lorazepam for seizures, cardiac monitor for arrhythmias.
Warfarin	Vitamin K, FFP.
Carbon monoxide	100% O_2, hyperbaric O_2.
Digitalis	Stop digitalis, normalize K^+, lidocaine (for torsades), antidigitalis Fab.
β-blockers	Glucagon.
Tissue plasminogen activator (tPA), streptokinase	Aminocaproic acid.
Phencyclidine hydrochloride (PCP)	NG suction.
Theophylline	Activated charcoal.
Acid/alkali ingestion	Upper endoscopy to evaluate for stricture.

HIGH-YIELD FACTS

EMERGENCY MEDICINE

TABLE 3-5. Management of Drug Withdrawal

Drug	Withdrawal Symptoms	Treatment
Alcohol	Tremor (6–12 hours), tachycardia, hypertension, agitation, seizures (in 48 hours), hallucinations, DTs (in 2–7 days).[a]	Benzodiazepines; haloperidol, thiamine, folate, multivitamins.[b]
Barbiturates	Anxiety, seizure, delirium, tremor, cardiac and respiratory depression.	Benzodiazepines.
Benzodiazepines	Rebound anxiety, tremors, insomnia.	Benzodiazepines and monitor for DTs.
Cocaine/amphetamines	Depression, hyperphagia, hypersomnolence.	Supportive treatment. Avoid β-blockers.
Opioids	Anxiety, insomnia, flulike symptoms, sweating, piloerection, fever, rhinorrhea, nausea, stomach cramps, diarrhea, mydriasis.	Clonidine and/or buprenorphine for moderate withdrawal; methadone for severe symptoms. Naltrexone for patients who are drug free for 7–10 days.

[a] DTs involve severe autonomic instability, including tachycardia, hypertension, delirium, and death.
[b] These will not affect withdrawal, but most alcoholics are malnourished.

- **Foley:**
    - The urinary catheter is necessary to monitor urinary output. Urine output is an accurate reflection of volume status and renal perfusion.
    - Perform a retrograde urethrogram if a urethral transection is suspected before placing the Foley.

Burns

Thermal burns are categorized according to depth and surface area.

- **First degree:** Involves the epidermis only. Painful and erythematous without blisters; will heal without a scar.
- **Second degree:** A partial-thickness burn that involves the epidermis and the dermis.
    - **Superficial partial-thickness burn:** Involves the dermis, sparing the follicles and glands. Characterized by pain, blistering, and erythema; heals in about two weeks with or without a scar.
    - **Deep partial-thickness burn:** Involves follicles and glands in the dermis. Characterized by pain, blistering, erythema, and charring (due to coagulation necrosis of the upper dermis); heals in 3–4 weeks, leaving a scar.
- **Third degree:** A full-thickness burn involving all skin layers. Painless and waxy white in a chemical burn or completely charred and black in flame injury. Requires skin grafts for healing and leads to significant scarring.
- **Fourth degree:** A burn involving skin, muscle, and bone that is severe and life-threatening.

WORKUP

- The size of the burn is estimated using guidelines similar to those in Figure 3-12 to determine the percentage of total body surface area (TBSA) burned.

Which burn patients are highest risk? Patients with diabetes, those with heart and lung disease, children < 10 years of age, and adults > 50 years of age.

Which are associated with higher mortality: acid or alkali burns? Although alkali burns result in more local tissue destruction through liquefactive necrosis, acid burns (which cause coagulative necrosis) are associated with higher mortality because they are absorbed systemically.

HIGH-YIELD FACTS

EMERGENCY MEDICINE

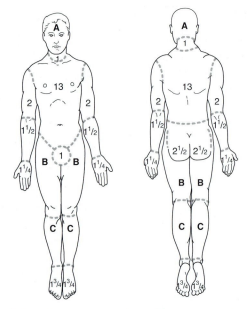
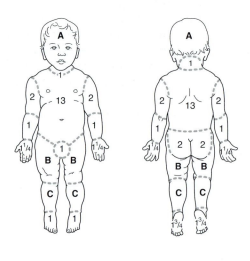

Relative Percentages of Areas Affected by Growth

Area	Age		
	10	15	Adult
A = half of head	5 1/2	4 1/2	3 1/2
B = half of one thigh	4 1/4	4 1/2	4 3/4
C = half of one leg	3	3 1/4	3 1/2

Relative Percentages of Areas Affected by Growth

Area	Age		
	0	1	5
A = half of head	9 1/2	8 1/2	6 1/2
B = half of one thigh	2 3/4	3 1/4	4
C = half of one leg	2 1/2	2 1/2	2 3/4

FIGURE 3-12. Rule of nines for adults, infants, and children.

(Reproduced, with permission, from Way LW, Doherty GM. *Current Surgical Diagnosis & Treatment*, 11th ed. New York: McGraw-Hill, 2003: 269.)

- Criteria for transfer to a burn unit are as follows:
  - Partial- and full-thickness burns affecting > 10% TBSA in patients < 10 or > 50 years of age.
  - Partial- and full-thickness burns affecting > 20% TBSA in patients between 10 and 50 years of age.
  - Full-thickness burns affecting > 5% TBSA in patients of any age.
  - Electrical or chemical burns.
  - Inhalational injuries.
  - Patients with preexisting medical problems.
  - Burns involving the face, hands, genitalia, perineum, or major joints.

TREATMENT

Do not be fooled by a small electrical burn. Nonvisible deep destruction may be present.

- The **ABCs** are critical:
  - **Airway:** Facial burns, singed nose hairs, wheezing, or hoarseness should raise suspicion for smoke inhalation. Early intubation may be needed, as upper airway edema can rapidly progress to complete airway obstruction.
  - **Breathing:** Provide humidified 100% O_2. Be sure that all burned areas have been doused with water, as O_2 can reignite a smoldering burn.

- **Circulation:** Fluid resuscitation is critical to the goal of maintaining 1 cc/kg/hr of urine output.
- The Parkland formula should be used as a guide for calculating fluid needs over the first 24 hours, and a Foley should be placed to monitor output.
- Escharotomy is needed for full-thickness and circumferential burns to prevent compartment syndrome. Blisters should be left intact.
- The patient should be covered with sterile sheets to prevent hypothermia and infection.
- Provide tetanus prophylaxis.

Hypothermia

A core temperature < 35° C. Usually caused by exposure, but one can be predisposed by conditions such as alcohol ingestion, hypoglycemia, and sepsis.

SIGNS AND SYMPTOMS

- Shivering.
- Initial tachycardia followed by bradycardia.
- J waves (Osborne waves) on ECG.
- Loss of DTRs.
- Confusion and lethargy.
- Diuresis leading to hypovolemia.
- Slow, shallow respirations.

TREATMENT

- ABCs.
- Remove wet or cold clothing.
- Rewarm (except in the setting of frostbite):
  - **Passive external rewarming:** Appropriate for patients with mild hypothermia (32.5°C–35.0°C). Apply warm clothing in a warm room.
  - **Active external rewarming:** Appropriate for patients with moderate hypothermia (27.5°C–32.5°C). Apply external heat from sources such as warm blankets, hot water bottles, or immersion in a hot bath.
  - **Active core rewarming:** Appropriate for patients with severe hypothermia (< 27.5°C) or hemodynamic instability. Involves the following:
    - Warm inhaled O_2.
    - Esophageal or rectal warm-water lavage.
    - Warm liquid peritoneal or pleural lavage.
    - Warm liquid femoral-arterial or cardiopulmonary bypass.

Shock

A physiologic state of circulatory failure leading to inadequate tissue perfusion and tissue hypoxia. The cardinal signs of shock are simultaneous tachycardia and hypotension. Subtypes are as follows:

- **Hypovolemic:** The two major causes are hemorrhage and dehydration.
- **Distributive:** Think of "misdistribution" of blood due to inappropriately low systemic vascular resistance (SVR). The major causes are septic, neurogenic, and anaphylactic.
- **Cardiac:** Due to inability of the heart to adequately pump blood to the body owing either to intrinsic dysfunction or to extrinsic factors.
  - **Intrinsic heart dysfunction:** Known as cardiogenic shock or CHF.

The Parkland formula is used to calculate the estimated fluid requirement of a burn victim over the first 24 hours. It is 4 cc/kg/% TBSA burned. Half is replaced over the first 8 hours and the other half over 16 hours.

Always check the core temperature of a patient with altered mental status to check for hypothermia or heatstroke!

Leave frostbitten lesions frozen until there is a definitive option for rewarming, such as submerging the frostbitten area in circulating hot (42°C) water until the extremity is flush. Also offer pain medications such as NSAIDs (frostbite hurts!).

A person cannot be pronounced dead until they are warm and dead. Always check core temperatures and resuscitate until the patient's temperature is > 32°C.

■ **Extrinsic factors:** Pericardial effusions leading to cardiac tamponade, tension pneumothorax, and massive pulmonary embolus.

WORKUP/TREATMENT

■ Considering the various etiologies of shock, the evaluation and management of the patient in acute shock involves assessment of volume status, SVR, and cardiac output (see Table 3-6).

■ The vast majority of shock cases are due to hypovolemia. Consequently, the treatment of shock in an emergency is the same as that described for hypovolemic shock below. Remember, the key to treating almost all types of shock is fluid resuscitation. If you do not give fluid to your patient, you are effectively making a diagnosis of cardiogenic shock.

HYPOVOLEMIC SHOCK

Due to any process that depletes intravascular volume. These include the following:

■ **Acute blood loss:** Hemorrhage in one of three compartments: the abdomen, pelvis (retroperitoneum), or thorax. Identifying the source of hemorrhage involves the following measures:
  ■ Direct peritoneal lavage or abdominal ultrasound.
  ■ NG tube to rule out upper GI bleed.
  ■ Stool guaiac to rule out lower GI bleed.
  ■ CXR to rule out intrathoracic bleed.
  ■ Pelvic x-ray to rule out pelvic fracture.
■ **Dehydration:** Most commonly 2° to protracted diarrhea, vomiting, overdiuresis, or fluid restriction (e.g., in elderly patients, who may not be able to drink adequate fluids).
■ **Third spacing:** Shifting of intravascular volume into the interstitial space or other compartments. Occurs 2° to burns, trauma, acute pancreatitis, and/or liver disease.

TABLE 3-6. Clinical Presentations of Shock

TYPE	CONDITION	SVR	SKIN	NECK VEINS
Hypovolemic	Hemorrhage	High	Cold, clammy	Flat
	Dehydration	High	Cold, clammy	Flat
	Third spacing	High	Cold, clammy	Flat
Distributive	Septic (early)	Low	Warm	Flat to normal
	Neurogenic	Low	Warm	Flat to normal
	Anaphylactic	Low	Warm	Flat to normal
Cardiac	Cardiogenic	High	Cold, clammy	Distended[a]
	Cardiac compression	High	Cold, clammy	Distended
	Tension pneumothorax	High	Cold, clammy	Distended
Hypoglycemic	Hypoglycemia	High	Cold, clammy	Flat to normal

[a] May be flat if the patient is also hypovolemic.

SIGNS AND SYMPTOMS

Presentation depends on the degree of volume loss.

- **Mild** (10–20% volume loss): The patient feels cold and exhibits orthostatic hypotension, flat neck veins, and pale and cool skin.
- **Moderate** (20–40% volume loss): The patient is thirsty, tachycardic/hypotensive, and oliguric.
- **Severe** (> 40% volume loss): The patient exhibits altered mental status (agitation leading to obtundation), severe hypotension, tachycardia, and tachypnea.
- ↓ central venous pressure and ↑ SVR are also seen.

TREATMENT

The goal in treating hypovolemic shock is to restore intravascular volume, treat the underlying cause of intravascular depletion, and restore tissue oxygenation. Emergency maneuvers in hypovolemic shock are as follows:

1. Place the patient in the Trendelenburg position.
2. Give the patient O_2.
3. Place two large-bore (14-gauge) IVs and rapidly deliver 2 L of crystalloid (bolus).
4. Reassess vitals. If vitals do not improve, give 1–2 L of additional crystalloid and reassess. If vitals still have not improved, consider initiating IV pressors and delivering blood products.
5. If a peritoneal bleed is identified, the patient must undergo emergent exploratory laparotomy.
6. If a pelvic fracture is identified, a pelvic bleed should be suspected and the patient should have angiography and embolization.
7. If a thoracic bleed is identified, a chest tube should be placed.

CARDIOGENIC SHOCK

Etiologies include arrhythmias and MI, vascular disease, myocarditis, and cardiomyopathy.

SIGNS AND SYMPTOMS

- Tachycardia, hypotension, tachypnea.
- Distended neck veins; peripheral edema.
- Patients may have S3 with rales.
- ↑ central venous pressure, ↓ pulmonary capillary wedge pressure, ECG abnormalities.

TREATMENT

Therapy should be directed at the underlying cause and at maintaining adequate BP.

- **Medical management:**
  - Inotropes (↑ contractility).
  - Vasodilators (↓ preload and afterload, leading to ↓ myocardial work).
  - Diuretics (↓ preload).
  - Antiarrhythmics should also be considered.
- **Surgical interventions:** Intra-aortic balloon pump (↑ CO, ↓ afterload, ↑ myocardial perfusion).

What is the most common cause of shock in the trauma patient? Hemorrhage.

Shock can be hypovolemic, distributive, or cardiogenic.

In which form of shock should you avoid fluid resuscitation? Cardiogenic shock is the only form of shock in which fluid may actually lead to further failure.

*Identify and treat the
underlying cause of septic
shock.*

SEPTIC SHOCK

Septic shock is 2° to the systemic effects of infection. Its pathophysiology is as follows:

- Toxins from both gram-$\oplus$ and gram-$\ominus$ bacteria as well as systemic inflammatory factors lead to vasodilation of the peripheral circulation and ↑ capillary permeability.
- This results in significantly ↓ SVR, redistribution of cardiac output, and massive fluid loss into the tissue.

SIGNS AND SYMPTOMS

- **Early septic shock:** Hyperdynamic phase. Marked by fever, tachycardia, and hypotension in a warm and pink patient; due to vasodilation.
- **Late septic shock:** Hypodynamic phase. Mimics hypovolemic shock due to ↑ capillary permeability and impaired cellular O_2 utilization.
- Leukocytosis with left shift and lactic acidosis support the diagnosis of septic shock.

TREATMENT

- Identify and treat the source of infection with IV antibiotics, surgical drainage, and central line changes.
- Aggressive IV fluid resuscitation (exercise caution with elderly patients), monitoring of cardiac function, pressors, and/or intubation to maintain adequate oxygenation.

NEUROGENIC SHOCK

Due to loss of vascular sympathetic tone, usually 2° to a high cervical spinal injury. Spinal anesthesia can also induce spinal shock.

SIGNS AND SYMPTOMS

- Hypotension; flat neck veins.
- Normal or slow pulse (no reflex tachycardia).
- Warm, dry skin.
- ↓ rectal tone; focal neurologic exam.

TREATMENT

- First rule out other etiologies of shock.
- Then proceed with IV fluid resuscitation, place the patient in the Trendelenburg position, and use vasoconstrictors.
- **Follow the protocols for spinal injury.** Give high-dose steroids in the form of a 30-mg/kg bolus of methylprednisolone, followed by 5.4 mg/kg/hr for 23 hours if steroids are initiated within 3 hours of injury, or for 47 hours if steroids are initiated 3–8 hours after injury.

Penetrating Wounds

The evaluation and treatment of penetrating wounds depend on the location and extent of the injury.

*What organs are most
frequently injured by
penetrating trauma? The liver
and then the small bowel.*

NECK WOUNDS

A penetrating neck injury is defined as any injury that violates the platysma.

WORKUP

- Protect the airway and intubate early. This can rapidly evolve into a difficult airway, so alternative airway management methods such as surgical airways should be available.
- Control of hemorrhage in the ED should be via direct pressure.
- Wounds should not be explored, as this may lead to bleeding in a tamponaded wound.
- **Surgery:** Indications for surgical exploration are as follows:
    - Zone 2 injury
    - Hemodynamic instability despite resuscitation efforts
    - An expanding hematoma
    - Subcutaneous emphysema
    - Tracheal deviation
    - Voice changes
- **Radiographic studies:** Films of the neck and a CXR should be ordered to evaluate for soft tissue hematoma, subcutaneous emphysema, and hemopneumothorax.

TREATMENT

The evaluation and management of a penetrating neck injury are dictated by zone (see Figure 3-13).

- **Zone 1:** May be evaluated with aortography.
- **Zone 2:** If the platysma is penetrated, the patient should be taken to the OR for exploration. Alternatively, angiography and triple endoscopy can be done.

Why should you leave impaled objects in place until a patient goes to the OR? They may be tamponading further blood loss.

HIGH-YIELD FACTS

EMERGENCY MEDICINE

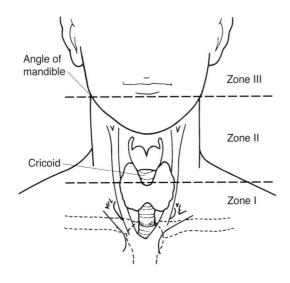

FIGURE 3-13. Zones of the neck.

(Reproduced, with permission, from Way LW, Doherty GM. *Current Surgical Diagnosis & Treatment*, 11th ed. New York: McGraw-Hill, 2003: 241.)

- **Zone 3:** May be evaluated with aortography, tracheobronchoscopy, and esophagoscopy.

CHEST WOUNDS

WORKUP

One must consider the possibility of aortic disruption, pneumothorax, hemothorax, cardiac tamponade, diaphragmatic tear, and esophageal injury in patients with penetrating thoracic injury.

TREATMENT

- Intubation and bilateral chest tubes are required for unstable patients with penetrating thoracic injuries.
- If the patient remains unstable despite resuscitative efforts, proceed with thoracotomy.

What should you suspect if a previously stable chest trauma patient suddenly dies? Air embolism.

ABDOMINAL WOUNDS

WORKUP/TREATMENT

- If the patient is hemodynamically stable with stab wounds or blunt trauma, obtain a CT scan or focused assessment with sonography for trauma (FAST) imaging.
- Otherwise, immediate exploratory laparotomy is indicated for the following:
  - Gunshot wounds
  - Removal of impaled instruments
  - Diaphragmatic injury (known or suspected)
  - Free air in the abdomen

What organ is most commonly injured in blunt abdominal trauma? The spleen. Be suspicious of this if you see left lower rib fractures.

MUSCULOSKELETAL INJURY

WORKUP/TREATMENT

- Do an arteriogram if you suspect neurovascular injury before proceeding with debridement and repair.
- Antibiotics and tetanus prophylaxis should be administered.
- However, early wound irrigation and tissue debridement are the critical steps in treating a contaminated wound.

COMMON CLERKSHIP TOPICS

The following is a list of core topics that you are likely to encounter in the course of your EM rotation and on a shelf examination.

- **Allergy, immunology, dermatology:**
  - Anaphylaxis
  - Necrotizing fasciitis
  - Erythema multiforme
  - Stevens-Johnson syndrome
  - Urticaria
- **Cardiovascular:**
  - Acute coronary syndrome
  - Acute myocardial infarction

- Abdominal aortic aneurysm (see Surgery)
- Aortic dissection
- Arrhythmia
  - Asystole
  - Atrial fibrillation (see Internal Medicine)
  - Ventricular fibrillation
  - Ventricular tachycardia
- Cardiac tamponade
- Congestive heart failure (see Internal Medicine)
- Hypertensive urgency/emergency
- **Gastrointestinal:**
  - Appendicitis
  - Cholecystitis (see Surgery)
  - Cholelithiasis (see Surgery)
  - Hernia (see Surgery)
  - Obstruction (see Surgery)
- **Genitourinary:**
  - Abnormal uterine bleeding (see Gynecology)
  - Ectopic pregnancy
  - Epididymitis
  - Fournier gangrene
  - Pelvic inflammatory disease (see Gynecology)
  - Sexually transmitted diseases (see Gynecology)
  - Testicular torsion
  - Urinary obstruction
  - Urinary tract infection
- **Neurology:**
  - Headaches (see Neurology)
  - Intracranial hemorrhage
    - Subarachnoid hemorrhage
    - Epidural hematoma
    - Subdural hematoma
    - Intraparenchymal hemorrhage
  - Neuroleptic malignant syndrome
  - Status epilepticus
  - Stroke (see Neurology)
    - Hemorrhagic
    - Ischemic
    - Transient ischemic attack
  - Temporal arteritis
- **Respiratory:**
  - Asthma
  - Hemothorax
  - Pneumothorax
    - Tension pneumothorax
    - Communicating pneumothorax (sucking chest wound)
  - Flail chest
  - Pulmonary embolism
- **Toxicology:**
  - Drug overdose/antidotes
  - Drug withdrawal
- **Trauma and shock:**
  - Resuscitation
  - Burns
  - Hypothermia

- Shock
  - Hypovolemic shock
  - Cardiogenic shock
  - Septic shock
  - Neurogenic shock
- Penetrating wounds
  - Neck wounds
  - Chest wounds
  - Abdominal wounds
- Musculoskeletal injury

Internal Medicine

The internal medicine clerkship, which usually lasts from 8 to 12 weeks, will expose you to a wide variety of fields, including cardiology, pulmonology, gastroenterology, endocrinology, nephrology, rheumatology, hematology, oncology, and infectious disease. Both outpatient and inpatient settings are significant to these disciplines. Given the broad scope of internal medicine, this clerkship will provide you with a strong foundation for your other rotations when done early—and when done later, it will help support your existing fund of knowledge.

Internal medicine addresses clinical issues practitioners face in all specialties.

Who Are the Players?

Attendings. Consisting of clinical and academic faculty, the attendings are in charge of the ward team and are ultimately responsible for patient care. Attendings are also the source of most of the didactic learning that takes place during attending rounds. Your interaction with attendings will consist primarily of making formal patient presentations in attending rounds and participating in didactic teaching. For this reason, it is crucial that you read up on your patients' problems before attending rounds, especially if you will be presenting a patient.

Residents. Since residents are at least a year ahead of interns, they supervise the ward team and help formulate patients' treatment plans. Residents also serve as a major teaching resource, dispensing clinical pearls on work rounds and bringing in pertinent review articles. Your interaction with the resident will vary depending on his or her style; some residents remain aloof and primarily answer questions, while others are more interactive, giving informal lectures and taking you to patients' bedsides to teach physical findings. Also remember that residents may "pimp" as a means of teaching and assessing your knowledge base. They may even take the time to give you organized lectures or quote recent trials or studies that are pertinent to patients assigned to the team.

Interns. Interns are the cogs that make the hospital machinery move by performing the bulk of primary patient care. Given that they will co-follow your patients, you will probably have the most interaction with your intern. For this reason, any questions and management issues you might have regarding your patients should initially be directed toward the intern. Remember, too, that interns were recently medical students themselves, so they can be an invaluable source of practical information as well as survival tips. You can use them for feedback on your progress notes and presentation style.

Try to consult with your intern before rounds to formulate a plan.

Support staff. The medicine team receives additional help from nurses, pharmacists, case managers, social workers, and members of the allied health professions, all of whom may also participate in team rounds. It is critical to maintain positive, respectful working relationships with these staff members. When you are swamped with work or are not sure how to accomplish a task, they can be lifesavers. The pharmacist associated with the team is an excellent source of information regarding medications and dosages to be administered, and he or she can also provide information about what is or is not on the hospital formulary. The case manager and social worker are outstanding resources when it comes to handling the difficult psychosocial issues or needs of your patients.

How Is the Day Set Up?

Although schedules vary by school and setting, the typical day on a medicine rotation starts at 6:30–7:00 A.M. and usually runs until 4:00–5:00 P.M. on non-call days. Prerounds are usually followed by team rounds and/or attending rounds. Sometimes only new patients are seen with the full team. Morning rounds are then followed by "work time" or the "hour of power." The noon or afternoon conference may be followed by additional work time, teaching sessions, or student lectures. Refer to Chapter 1 for more detail about the daily schedule.

What Do I Do During Prerounds?

Please refer to "The Schedule—Medicine Wards" in Chapter 1.

How Do I Excel in Medicine?

Learning the material well does not always correlate with doing well on the internal medicine clerkship. All too often, your grade will depend on subjective factors that lie beyond your control, such as whether your personality meshes with those of your residents. However, the following tips will help stack the deck in your favor.

- **Know your patient.** You should know the latest clinical information on your patient, whether it is the most recent laboratory values, the planned studies of the day, or simply how the patient is feeling. You should then relay this information to the intern so that management plans can be modified accordingly. You should also be sure to keep on top of consults and tests you have ordered. Speak with the consulting service about their recommendations, as consultants can give you valuable information and may even have time to give you short tutorials on your patients' disease processes. Another important part of knowing your patient lies in a daily check of the medication administration record (MAR). This check will allow you to ensure that the antibiotics you ordered were actually administered (which is not always the case) as well as to gauge whether a patient is receiving symptomatic relief. For example, is the patient's pain well controlled, or is he or she asking for additional pain medication? You should also be aware of a patient's social situation so that you can keep the family up to date regarding his or her progress. Finally, be aware of special circumstances to be considered on discharge (e.g., getting a hotel room or transportation for a homeless patient).
- **Develop a differential.** The search for the etiology of a patient's problem begins with knowing the differential diagnosis. Therefore, a critical goal of this rotation is to learn the basic differentials of common signs and symptoms. The differential can often be broken down into three groups: common etiologies, uncommon etiologies, and etiologies you don't want to miss (because they're either highly treatable or life-threatening). Mastering the differentials of common problems will serve you well in any specialty.
- **Care about your patients.** Perhaps the single most important thing you can do on any rotation is remain genuinely concerned about your patients. Nothing will elicit more respect from your faculty and team. Don't leave if there is important work remaining or if your patient is crashing.
- **Get along with your team.** It is important to remember that you are part of a team. Although you may be relatively low in the hierarchy, bear in mind that you still have an integral role to play. Also remember that medical students who make life easier for the interns and residents through dili-

You cannot diagnose what is not in your differential diagnosis.

gent and efficient work will ultimately be rewarded in their evaluations. It is therefore important that you remain personable and enthusiastic at all times so as to ensure that your team members can work as a cohesive unit. By contrast, fostering open conflict with others on your team should be avoided at all costs. If you feel uncomfortable with another team member or sense a personality problem developing, it is vital that you do whatever you can to avert such conflicts. A serious rift in the team is an uncommon situation, but when it does arise, it can be devastating to patient care, team morale, and your development.

- **Be early.** Never underestimate the importance of punctuality. Attendings and residents probably won't take notice when you show up on time, but they are certain to remember if you walk in late.
- **Work independently.** The easier you make your intern's life, the more he or she will appreciate your effort. If you can call the consults, order the lab tests, collect lab and radiology results, and determine if the patient is comfortable, you will go a long way. Expect to be dependent on others at first; this is perfectly normal. But as you gain more experience, you will feel the desire—and have the confidence—to work more independently.
- **Read, read, read.** Keep both a pocket manual and a more complete reference available. Try to read about your patients and their major issues. This will assist you in formulating a plan, save you when the pimping starts, and help you pose intelligent questions. Performing searches for current literature and reading hallmark papers may also be important; you will have to gauge how much you can do in relation to the time constraints you face.
- **Ask for feedback.** Midway through the rotation, ask your attending and resident to set aside some time so that they can give you feedback. "You're doing fine" is **not** a useful response. Be persistent and ask about your weaknesses. This will help you identify areas in which you need improvement while also making them aware that you are a responsible student. They may ask you how you think you are doing, so be prepared to explain what you are doing well and in what areas you are trying to improve.

If you are sincerely interested in pursuing a career in internal medicine, you will need to take some additional steps. First, let the members of your team know of your interests. If you do so, they may make a special effort to teach and help you. Do not lie, as insincerity is easily detected and is definitely frowned on. Second, the status of your attending becomes crucial; try to schedule (with the help of the course scheduler) at least one block of your clerkship with a senior or well-known attending. In a residency application, the person who writes your letter of recommendation can be almost as important as what is actually said about you. Doing well will help ensure a good letter of recommendation from a senior faculty member.

Presentations

Work rounds. Presentations during work rounds consist of an oral version of your **SOAP note** (see mnemonic). During these presentations, the team will focus on brevity and efficiency, with emphasis on the assessment and plan (A&P). A well-thought-out A&P takes extra time during prerounds, so start early and discuss your ideas with your intern. Do not be discouraged, however, if your A&P is occasionally in error; remember that you are there to learn, and bear in mind that the team will appreciate the fact that you are trying. In the final analysis, it is better to come up with a well-thought-out plan that is incorrect than to simply say "I don't know" when you are asked about your next move in patient management.

Remember why you decided to go to medical school in the first place. This is not a 9-to-5 job!

You should know the latest clinical information on your patient.

SOAP note—

Subjective
Objective
Assessment
Plan

Attending rounds. This is your time in the spotlight, when you really need to shine. So remember that your attending will probably want a more lengthy formal oral presentation than the ones you give on work rounds. Also keep in mind that while attendings will primarily want to learn about your patient, they will also be observing your presentation style and will note how well you understand your patient's problems. One key means of demonstrating your knowledge is to include pertinent positives and negatives relating to your patient's condition. This may be difficult at first, especially since it requires an understanding of the presentation of the other possibilities in the differential. It is okay, however, if you omit something from the history, since the attending will simply ask for additional information if it is important. Don't panic if your attending asks you several additional questions about your patient; instead, make a mental note of the specific tidbits your attending likes to hear so that you can include them in your next presentation. You should also make sure you understand why the attending considers certain pertinent positives or negatives to be relevant to your patient.

Remember, too, that your attending's comments weigh in your final grade. Formal oral patient presentations constitute a large part of how the attending perceives you, so you will want to shine in this arena. Ask the attending how he or she would like you to present the patient. Practice your presentation before attending rounds, even running it by your intern for feedback.

Key Notes

Admission notes and SOAP notes are key to your medicine rotation. Please review the sample notes in Chapter 1.

Key Procedures

Explanations for the basic procedures that follow can be found in any pocket ward manual:

- Phlebotomy
- Musculoskeletal injection
- IV line placement
- Arterial line placement
- Arterial blood gas draw
- Foley catheter placement

Your resident may also allow you to perform the following advanced procedures on your patient:

- Thoracentesis
- Paracentesis
- Lumbar puncture

What Do I Carry in My Pockets?

- ❑ Stethoscope
- ❑ Reflex hammer
- ❑ Tongue blades
- ❑ Patient-tracking PDA software and/or index cards and/or patient summary sheets (for recording history, vital signs, and tests)

- ❑ Normal-lab-value reference card
- ❑ Current pharmacopoeia and antibiotic guide (PDA software or handbook)
- ❑ Penlight
- ❑ Calipers for ECG reading
- ❑ Otoscope/ophthalmoscope (or know where to find one quickly)
- ❑ Eye chart

Read about these topics before you start the rotation. Most are discussed in this chapter. A full list of common clerkship topics can be found at the end of this chapter.

- ❑ Congestive heart failure
- ❑ Chest pain
- ❑ Hypertension
- ❑ Chronic obstructive pulmonary disease
- ❑ Acute renal failure
- ❑ Abdominal pain
- ❑ Anemia
- ❑ Diabetes
- ❑ Fever of unknown origin
- ❑ Systemic lupus

CARDIOLOGY

Atrial Fibrillation (AF)

AF is the most common arrhythmia besides sinus tachycardia. It is an irregularly irregular rhythm (i.e., irregular RR intervals on ECG) that is marked by the absence of P waves prior to every QRS complex. The atrial rate is 400–600 bpm (but there is no organized depolarization of the atria) and induces an irregularly irregular ventricular response rate of 80–160 bpm. AF may be idiopathic, especially in younger patients, but other etiologies are summarized in the mnemonic **PIRATES**. Pertinent epidemiologic data are as follows:

- The risk of developing AF doubles with each decade over the age of 55. By age 80, the prevalence of AF approaches 10%.
- The Framingham Heart Study showed that patients with AF have an ↑ risk of cardiovascular mortality as well as a 3- to 13-fold ↑ in the risk of embolic stroke.

SIGNS AND SYMPTOMS

- The clinical presentation of AF can vary from asymptomatic to severely symptomatic. Symptoms include the following:
  - Fatigue (most common).
  - Tachypnea, dyspnea.
  - Palpitations, "skipped beats," "racing heart," angina.
  - Lightheadedness, syncope (rare), or alterations in cognitive function (TIAs or stroke).
- A classic irregularly irregular rhythm will be palpated on physical exam. Irregular heartbeats of varying loudness can be heard on cardiac auscultation.

Etiologies of AF—

PIRATES

Pulmonary (COPD, pulmonary embolism), **P**heochromocytoma (rare), **P**ericarditis
Ischemic heart disease and hypertension
Rheumatic heart disease
Anemia, **A**trial myxoma (rare)
Thyrotoxicosis
Ethanol ("holiday heart") and cocaine
Sepsis (especially post-operative)

A normal echocardiogram (transthoracic, or TTE) has low sensitivity for identifying thrombi. A transesophageal echocardiogram (TEE) is preferred, as it affords better visualization of the left atrial appendage, the location where thrombi most commonly form.

DIFFERENTIAL

Paroxysmal atrial contractions, paroxysmal ventricular contractions, multifocal atrial tachycardia, atrial flutter with variable AV conduction.

WORKUP

- ECG shows a narrow-complex rhythm (QRS < 120 msec), variable RR intervals, and irregular or absent P waves (see Figure 4-1).
- Echocardiogram may show a thrombus in the left atrium but more often will show a dilated left atrium.
- Consider checking TSH levels (hyperthyroidism is a reversible cause of AF).
- Baseline coagulation studies (INR/aPTT) are usually performed prior to the initiation of anticoagulation therapy.

TREATMENT

- **Control ventricular rate** both emergently and nonemergently to ensure adequate ventricular filling and to maximize cardiac output.
  - **Emergent:** IV calcium channel blockers (e.g., diltiazem) or β-blockers (e.g., metoprolol). Hypotension is an adverse medication reaction that may require immediate DC cardioversion.
  - **Nonemergent:** Oral β-blockers (e.g., atenolol) and calcium channel blockers (e.g., verapamil or diltiazem) +/− digoxin. The goal is ≤ 80 bpm at rest and 110 bpm with activity.
- **Cardiovert rhythm:** Cardioversion to sinus rhythm is the definitive treatment for AF and includes the following:
  - **Pharmacologic conversion via amiodarone:** Prerequisites to successful treatment include recent onset (< 1 month is preferable) and lack of severe left atrial dilation (chamber < 46 mm by echocardiography).
  - **Electrocardioversion (starting with 100 J DC):** The most successful form of cardioversion. Note that if the arrhythmia has been present for > 48 hours, the patient must either be anticoagulated with warfarin for 3–4 weeks before cardioversion or receive transesophageal echocardiog-

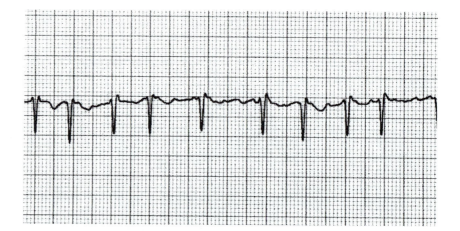

FIGURE 4-1. Atrial fibrillation in V₁.

Note the absence of P waves and the irregularly irregular rhythm. (Reproduced, with permission, from Stobo JD et al. *The Principles and Practice of Medicine*, 23rd ed. Stamford, CT: Appleton & Lange, 1996: 78.)

raphy (TEE) to exclude an atrial thrombus. Patients are always anticoagulated for at least four weeks after cardioversion.

- **Surgery:** Recurrence rates for AF may be as high as 75%. For symptomatic patients, the classical open Maze procedure or a catheter ablation approach may be indicated to interrupt electrical conduction pathways in the atria.
- **Anticoagulation:** The risk of stroke is approximately 4.5% per year in nonvalvular AF and is even higher in valvular AF. The most important risk factor is a prior history of stroke or TIA, followed by age > 65 years, hypertension, and diabetes. Stroke risk ↓ by 62% with warfarin administration and by 22% with aspirin use. If anticoagulation is required urgently (e.g., for cardioversion), use a heparin drip or low-molecular-weight heparin (LMWH) initially, as warfarin takes several days to take effect. The goal INR is 2–3.

REFERENCES

- Benjamin E et al. Impact of atrial fibrillation on the risk of death: The Framingham Heart Study. *Circulation* 98:946–952, 1998. A retrospective analysis of the first 40 years of the Framingham Heart Study showing that subjects with AF were significantly more likely than subjects without AF to have cardiovascular disease risk factors and preexisting disease at baseline; AF was associated with a statistically significant ↑ in risk of death (1.5 odds ratio in men; 1.9 odds ratio in women).
- Stroke Prevention in Atrial Fibrillation investigators. Adjusted-dose warfarin versus low-intensity, fixed-dose warfarin plus aspirin for high-risk patients with atrial fibrillation: Stroke Prevention in Atrial Fibrillation III randomised clinical trial. *Lancet* 348:633–638, 1996. A landmark study (double-blind randomized controlled trial [RCT]) that showed a statistically significant reduction of stroke in high-risk AF patients treated with warfarin (INR 2.0–3.0) when compared with those treated with aspirin alone.
- Wyse DG et al. The Atrial Fibrillation Follow-up Investigation of Rhythm Management Investigators. *NEJM* 347(23):1825–1833, 2002. The large-scale Atrial Fibrillation Follow-up Investigation of Rhythm Management (AFFIRM) study of patients ≥ 65 years of age, or with other risk factors for stroke or death, showed that rate control vs. rhythm control were no different for end points that included mortality and stroke, with fewer adverse effects observed in the rate-control group.

Congestive Heart Failure (CHF)

CHF occurs when the heart is unable to pump sufficient amounts of blood to meet the O_2 requirements of the heart and other body tissues. CHF is responsible for 300,000 deaths annually, with mortality rates greater in men than in women. Some five million people in the United States have CHF, including nearly 10% of Americans > 70 years of age, and 500,000 new cases are diagnosed each year. Most patients hospitalized for CHF are ≥ 65 years of age.

- Risk factors for developing CHF include MI, hypertension, valvular heart disease (e.g., mitral stenosis, endocarditis), pericardial disease, cardiomyopathy, AIDS, alcohol abuse, pulmonary hypertension, and, most commonly, chronic ischemic heart disease.
- CHF can be traced to problems in systolic or diastolic phases (see Table 4-1):

CHF exacerbation in previously stable patients–

"FAILURE"

Forgot medication
Arrhythmia, **A**nemia
Ischemia, **I**nfarction, **I**nfection
Lifestyle (e.g., excessive sodium intake; most common cause)
"**U**pregulation" (↑ cardiac output—e.g., pregnancy, hyperthyroidism)
Renal failure with fluid overload
Embolus (pulmonary)

TABLE 4-1. Physiologic Basis of CHF

ETIOLOGY	RELATED CONDITION
Systolic dysfunction	
↓ contractility	**Ischemic heart disease:** The most common cause of systolic dysfunction.
	Dilated cardiomyopathy: ↓ contractile functioning in the absence of pressure or volume overload. May be idiopathic or 2°—e.g., drug effect (ethanol, cocaine, heroin, doxorubicin), postmyocarditis, postpartum, or related to HIV, Chagas' disease, anemia, thiamine deficiency, or thyrotoxicosis.
	Hypertensive burnout or valvular heart disease: Both initially cause **diastolic** dysfunction, but after myofibrils stretch, the EF falls, and **systolic** dysfunction results.
↑ afterload	↑ systolic pressure (e.g., hypertension); ↑ pumping pressure (e.g., aortic stenosis).
	↑ chamber radius (e.g., ventricular dilation due to aortic insufficiency/regurgitation).
Diastolic dysfunction	
Abnormal active relaxation	**Ischemia.**
	Hypertrophic cardiomyopathy: Due to disorders causing LVH (e.g., hypertension, aortic stenosis, hypertrophic obstructive cardiomyopathy [HOCM]).
Abnormal passive filling	**Restrictive cardiomyopathy:** May be idiopathic or due to infiltrative disorders (e.g., sarcoidosis, amyloidosis, scleroderma, hemochromatosis, glycogen storage disease) that ↑ ventricular stiffness. The least common cardiomyopathy.
	Concentric hypertrophy from hypertension.

It is important to differentiate systolic from diastolic dysfunction because CHF treatment often depends on the 1° mode of failure. However, both types of dysfunction can coexist in the same patient.

- **Systolic dysfunction:** An ejection fraction (EF) < 40% leads to ↑ preload with ↑ left ventricular end-diastolic pressure (LVEDP) in a vain attempt to ↑ systolic contractility and cardiac output. Poor organ perfusion leads to a variety of compensatory mechanisms that are only temporarily effective and eventually result in ↑ myocardial work. In patients with CAD, the ↑ work can lead to cardiac hypertrophy and ventricular dilation and may even precipitate an MI.
- **Diastolic dysfunction:** ↓ LV compliance with normal contractile function. The ventricle is either unable to relax or unable to passively fill properly (↑ stiffness, ↓ recoil, concentric hypertrophy). There is an ↑ LVEDP, but with normal contractile function; cardiac output remains essentially normal, and the EF is either normal or slightly ↑.

SIGNS AND SYMPTOMS

CHF may be considered clinically as **right-sided** or **left-sided** in origin depending on which chambers fail first, but both types may be present simultaneously. Common to both are a ventricular heave, tachycardia, AF, and additional heart sounds. Subtypes are distinguished as follows:

- **Left-sided failure:**
  - **Early:** Dyspnea on exertion (DOE) and ↓ exercise tolerance.
  - **Late:** Orthopnea, dyspnea at rest, paroxysmal nocturnal dyspnea, chronic cough, nocturia, pulmonary congestion (pulmonary crackles, pleural effusion, "cardiac wheeze"), tachypnea, diaphoresis, cool extremities, and a laterally displaced PMI.
- **Right-sided failure:**
  - **Early:** Anorexia (due to hepatic congestion), cyanosis, and fatigue; ↑ JVP; pulsatile hepatomegaly (with possible transaminitis); peripheral edema on exam.
  - **Late:** Ascites and an abnormal hepatojugular reflex.

An S3 heart sound is present with systolic dysfunction. An S4 is present with hypertension, CAD, and diastolic dysfunction.

ASSESSMENT OF CHF PROGRESSION

- **New York Heart Association (NYHA) functional classification for CHF:**

  - **Class I:** No limitation of activities; no symptoms with normal activities.

  - **Class II:** Slight limitation of activities; patients are comfortable at rest or with mild exertion.

  - **Class III:** Marked limitation of activities; patients are comfortable only at rest.

  - **Class IV:** Patients are confined to complete rest in a bed or chair, as any physical activity brings on discomfort; symptoms are present at rest.

- **Heart failure staging by American College of Cardiology (ACC)/American Heart Association (AHA) Guidelines (2005):**

  - **Stage A:** High risk for developing heart failure, but no structural heart disorder is present. Includes patients with hypertension, CAD, and diabetes. Suggest lifestyle modification (smoking cessation, regular exercise, cessation of alcohol or illicit drug intake), antihypertensive medication, correction of dyslipidemias, and ACEIs/ARBs in appropriate patients (diabetics, those with peripheral vascular disease).

  - **Stage B:** No symptoms of heart failure, but structural disorder of the heart is present. Includes patients with a history of MI, LVH, low EF, or asymptomatic valvular disease. Treat with ACEIs/ARBs and β-blockers.

  - **Stage C:** Prior or current symptoms of heart failure associated with underlying structural heart disease. Treat with the full range of heart failure drugs (ACEIs/ARBs, β-blockers, and diuretics) and sodium restriction.

  - **Stage D:** Refractory heart failure requiring specialized interventions, such as mechanical circulatory support, continuous inotropes, cardiac transplantation, or hospice care.

What is the most common cause of right-sided heart failure? Left-sided heart failure.

What is the cause of pulmonary congestion in diastolic dysfunction? ↑ *hydrostatic pressure. (Note that activation of the renin-angiotensin-aldosterone system is usually not prominent.)*

DIFFERENTIAL

- **Cardiac:** Acute MI, myocarditis, high-output heart failure.
- **Pulmonary:** Pulmonary embolism, pneumonia.

WORKUP

- **Determine the underlying cause:** CBC, BUN/creatinine, and TSH can rule out severe anemia, renal failure, and thyrotoxicosis, respectively. ECG to evaluate for ischemia.
- **Assess severity:**
  - The physical exam is key.
  - CXR may show cardiomegaly and pulmonary vascular congestion (dilated vessels, interstitial or alveolar edema, Kerley-B lines).
  - Echocardiography provides information on the size and function (e.g., the EF) of both ventricles and valves and can also pinpoint an underlying cause (e.g., ischemia [segmental wall motion abnormalities], valvular disease).
- If concurrent MI is suspected, cardiac catheterization may be indicated.
- ↑ B-type natriuretic peptide (BNP) can be used to distinguish dyspnea due to heart failure from other causes of dyspnea.
- Systems for assessing CHF progression include the NYHA and ACC classifications (see above).

TREATMENT

- **Systolic dysfunction:**
  - ACEIs, β-blockers (carvedilol or metoprolol succinate), and diuretics are the cornerstone of treatment.

CHF TREATMENT: KEY DRUGS AND TRIALS

- ACEIs (e.g., enalapril) ↓ mortality and hospitalization in patients with class II–IV CHF (SOLVD trial, *NEJM* 325:293–302, 1991). However, 1% of people stop treatment because of cough. The CHARM study (*Lancet* 362:759–766, 2003) showed that ARBs have a similar effect on hospitalization and cardiovascular mortality.

- Carvedilol, a mixed α-/β-blocker, ↓ mortality and hospitalization in class II–IV CHF (COPERNICUS study, *Circulation* 106:2194–2199, 2002).

- Spironolactone ↓ mortality in patients with class III and IV CHF by 30% when given with ACEIs or diuretics +/– digoxin (RALES trial, *Am J Cardiol* 78:902–907, 1996). The EPHESUS trial (*NEJM* 348:1309–1321, 2003) showed that eplerenone confers similar benefits along with a ↓ incidence of gynecomastia or impotence (as may be seen with spironolactone).

- A combination regimen of hydralazine and isosorbide dinitrate has proven beneficial in patients with symptomatic CHF. A study of African-Americans demonstrated a 43% ↓ in one-year mortality (A-HeFT study, *NEJM* 351:2049–2057, 2004).

- Digoxin yields symptomatic relief in CHF but has no significant effect on ↓ mortality (DIG trial, *NEJM* 336:525–553, 1997) and may ↑ mortality in women (*NEJM* 347:1403–1411, 2002).

- Antiarrhythmics (e.g., amiodarone) with anticoagulants (e.g., warfarin) may be recommended when an arrhythmia is present.
- **Diastolic dysfunction:** Treatment aims to restore the heart's original relaxing and filling properties. Control of hypertension is paramount. Options are as follows:
  - **Diuretics:** ↓ afterload.
  - **Calcium channel blockers:** Induce bradycardia and facilitate myocardial relaxation.
  - **β-blockers:** Induce mild bradycardia and inhibit coronary remodeling.
  - **Nitroglycerin:** ↓ preload; dilates large coronary arteries.
  - **Antiarrhythmics** should also be used if indicated.
- Nonpharmacologic interventions include weight loss, sodium restriction (< 2 g/day), and fluid restriction (< 1.5 L/day).

In high-output heart failure, cardiac output is ↑ despite inadequate tissue oxygenation. Causes include thyrotoxicosis, severe anemia, Paget's disease, beriberi, and AV fistulas.

REFERENCES

In addition to those already mentioned, the list of significant CHF literature includes the following:

- The CONSENSUS Trial Study Group. The effect of enalapril on mortality in severe congestive heart failure: Results of the Cooperative North Scandinavian Enalapril Survival Study (CONSENSUS). *NEJM* 30:518–526, 1987. A double-blind RCT in which class IV CHF subjects were given placebo or enalapril. There was an overall reduction in mortality (27%), NYHA classification (symptoms), heart size, and CHF medication requirement in the enalapril group.
- Hunt SA. ACC/AHA 2005 guideline update for the diagnosis and management of chronic heart failure in the adult: A report of the American College of Cardiology/American Heart Association Task Force on Practice Guidelines (Writing Committee to Update the 2001 Guidelines for the Evaluation and Management of Heart Failure). *Circulation* 112(12): e154–e235, 2005. A comprehensive and updated version of the 2001 ACC/AHA practice guidelines. Developed in collaboration with the American College of Chest Physicians and the International Society for Heart and Lung Transplantation, and endorsed by the Heart Rhythm Society.
- Packer M et al. The effect of carvedilol on morbidity and mortality in patients with chronic heart failure. *NEJM* 334:1349–1355, 1996. A double-blind RCT with class II–IV CHF (EF 35%) subjects that demonstrated a ↓ in mortality (65% risk reduction), hospitalization (27% risk reduction), and combined death/hospitalization (38% risk reduction) in mild to moderate CHF.
- Pitt B et al (for the Randomized Aldactone Workup Study Investigators). The effect of spironolactone on morbidity and mortality in patients with severe heart failure. *NEJM* 341:709–717, 1999. A double-blind RCT in which CHF patients treated with spironolactone were found to have a 30% risk reduction in mortality, a 35% ↓ in hospitalization, and a significant ↓ in symptoms.

Hypertension

Hypertension is very common in both ambulatory and inpatient internal medicine settings, having a prevalence of 50 million patients in the United States and affecting > 40% of all men and women > 65 years of age. It has been estimated that up to one-third of those with high blood pressure go undiagnosed owing to the often "silent," asymptomatic nature of the disease. Some 95% of

Risk factors for essential hypertension:

- Age
- DM
- Obesity
- Family history
- Diet (salt, fat, alcohol intake)
- Lifestyle (inactivity, stress)
- Major depression
- Ethnicity–African-American > Caucasian = Hispanic > Asian

Why are calcium channel blockers not always first-line treatment for women? The Women's Health Initiative study indicates that calcium channel blockers significantly ↑ the risk of cardiovascular mortality in women.

hypertension cases are 1° ("essential"), having no identifiable cause. It is critical, however, to evaluate for 2° causes, which include the following:

- **Renal (4%):** Renovascular disease (e.g., renal artery stenosis, 2%), fibromuscular dysplasia in young women, atherosclerotic disease, renal parenchymal disease (polycystic kidney disease, renal cell carcinoma).
- **Drug effects:** OCPs, corticosteroids, COX-2 inhibitors, amphetamines, epoetin alfa (Epogen), lead poisoning.
- **Endocrine disorders:** Cushing's syndrome, hyperaldosteronism, pheochromocytoma, hyperthyroidism, hyperparathyroidism, polycystic ovarian syndrome, acromegaly.
- **Pregnancy:** Gestational hypertension, pregnant toxemia.
- **Other:** Aortic coarctation, obstructive sleep apnea.

WORKUP

- Diagnosis is based on the mean of two or more seated readings on each of three or more encounters. The diagnosis is valid if patients are > 18 years of age, have no acute illness, and have no 2° causes (e.g., diabetes, renal failure). See Table 4-2 for the stratification of disease severity.
- The goal of workup is to identify modifiable cardiovascular risk factors; to reveal 2° causes of hypertension (consider if the patient is < 20 or > 50 years of age, has sudden-onset or severe hypertension, has hypertension that is refractory to treatment, or has a suggestive H&P); and to assess for target-organ damage.
- Physical exam should focus on funduscopic, cardiac (listen for murmurs; look for signs of LVH such as LV heave), vascular, abdominal (pulsatile masses, bruits), and neurologic (TIA/CVA) factors.

TREATMENT

- Tables 4-2 and 4-3 outline basic treatment guidelines from the Seventh Report of the Joint National Committee on Prevention, Detection, Evaluation, and Treatment of High Blood Pressure (commonly referred to as the "JNC 7") for patients with classic and complicated hypertension. The goal is to reach a BP < 140/90 mmHg (unless the patent has diabetes or renal disease, in which case the goal is < 130/90 mmHg).

TABLE 4-2. Blood Pressure Classification

CLASSIFICATION	SYSTOLIC (mmHg)	DIASTOLIC (mmHg)	THERAPEUTIC RECOMMENDATION
Normal	< 120	< 80	
Prehypertension	120–139	80–89	Lifestyle modification.
Stage I hypertension	140–159	90–99	Thiazide diuretics are first-line treatment.
Stage II hypertension	> 159	> 99	Two-drug combination.

TABLE 4-3. Hypertension Management

CLINICAL HISTORY	RECOMMENDATIONS
Heart failure	Diuretics, β-blockers, ACEIs/ARBs, aldosterone antagonists.
Post-MI	β-blockers, ACEIs, aldosterone antagonists.
High risk for CAD	Diuretics, β-blockers, ACEIs, calcium channel blockers.
DM	Diuretics, β-blockers, ACEIs/ARBs, calcium channel blockers.
Chronic renal failure	ACEIs/ARBs.
CVA/stroke	Diuretics, ACEIs.
Osteoporosis	Thiazide diuretics.
BPH	α-blockers.

- Lifestyle modifications are recommended for all patients and include weight loss, sodium restriction (≤ 2.6 g/day), exercise, limited alcohol consumption (≤ 2 drinks/day in men; ≤ 1 drink/day in women), and eating a diet high in fruits and vegetables and limited in saturated fat.
- Thiazide diuretics are effective as first-line therapy for hypertension (ALLHAT study, *JAMA* 288:2998–3007, 2002).
- African-Americans may have ↓ nitric oxide levels and may be more sensitive to a high-salt diet than other groups. African-American patients should be treated with at least two medications if systolic or diastolic BP remains ↑ by > 15 mmHg.
- All patients with stage II hypertension will likely need a two-drug combination.
- Additional strategies may be guided by the Anglo-Scandinavian Cardiac Outcomes Trial (ASCOT) (*Lancet* 361:1149–1158, 2003):
  - Calcium channel blocker therapy (amlodipine) +/– ACEIs (perindopril) ↓ the risk of stroke and heart attack in comparison to β-blockers +/– thiazide.
  - Statin therapy ↓ cardiovascular events without regard to serum cholesterol level.

COMPLICATIONS

- **Neurologic:** TIA/CVA, ruptured aneurysms.
- **Retinopathy:** Arteriosclerotic narrowing, AV nicking, ischemic changes ("cotton–wool" spots), hemorrhages, exudates, papilledema, visual acuity loss (if the macula is involved).
- **Cardiac:** CAD, LVH, CHF, MI.
- **Vascular:** Aortic dissection, aortic aneurysm.
- **Renal:** Proteinuria, chronic kidney disease (CKD).

Risk factors for infective endocarditis include rheumatic heart disease, aortic valve disease, mitral valve prolapse, congenital valve abnormalities, the presence of foreign bodies (e.g., pacemakers, prosthetic valves), senile calcification, poor dentition, and a history of IV drug use.

Infective Endocarditis

Infective endocarditis is the most common endovascular infection, with 10,000–15,000 new cases diagnosed each year. Men are affected more frequently than women, with a mean age of onset at 60 years. The mortality rate is approximately 25%. Infection of the endothelial lining generally results from four factors: local hemodynamic abnormalities, the presence of endothelial damage, the presence of circulating bacteria, and the status of the host's immune system. Subtypes are as follows (see also Table 4-4):

- **Acute endocarditis:** Infection of normal heart valves with a virulent organism, most commonly S. *aureus*; infection leads to a rapid decline in valve function and death (depending on the valve involved).
- **Subacute endocarditis:** Infection of abnormal heart valves, often with a less virulent organism (primarily S. *viridans*). Characterized by a more insidious course and a gradual decline.

SIGNS AND SYMPTOMS

- Patients generally present with fever, chills, malaise, night sweats, anorexia, weight loss, arthralgia, and myalgia.
- On exam, patients may have a new or changing murmur, splenomegaly, and the classic findings outlined in the Duke criteria (see below).
- Later complications include CHF, embolization (especially from left-sided valvular disease), glomerulonephritis, anemia, and myocardial abscess formation.

TABLE 4-4. Causes of Infective Endocarditis

TYPE OF DISEASE	ETIOLOGIES
Culture-⊖ endocarditis	HACEK organisms: *Haemophilus, Actinobacillus, Cardiobacterium, Eikenella, Kingella* spp.
Native valve endocarditis (NVE)	The most common causes are *Streptococcus* spp. (e.g., α-hemolytic S. *viridans* or S. *bovis*) and *Enterococcus*.
Prosthetic valve endocarditis (PVE)	Early PVE is caused by perioperative seeding of endocarditis by *Staphylococcus epidermidis;* late PVE is generally caused by the same organisms as NVE.
Postsurgical endocarditis (most commonly GU and GI surgery)	The most common causes are gram-⊖ species or *Enterococcus*.
Endocarditis 2° to IV drug use	The most common cause is S. *aureus;* consider this agent in the presence of a tricuspid valve lesion.
Other	Fungi (*Candida* or *Aspergillus*, especially in the setting of an indwelling catheter); *Rickettsia, Chlamydia*.

DIFFERENTIAL

Endocarditis should always be suspected in patients with fever of unknown origin (FUO) and IV drug use. For those who fulfill the Duke criteria, the differential is limited to infective endocarditis and other endovascular abnormalities, including septic thromboemboli and mycotic aneurysms.

WORKUP

The Duke criteria constitute the standard for making a clinical diagnosis of endocarditis. A complete assessment includes the following:

- Funduscopy, skin exam, and clinical cardiac exam.
- At least two sets of blood cultures.
- **Labs:** CBC (an ↑ WBC count is seen in acute endocarditis vs. moderate anemia in subacute endocarditis), ESR (often ↑), UA (may see proteinuria and hematuria with glomerulonephritis), and RF (may be ⊕).
- **Echocardiography:** Start with TTE except in patients with an intermediate pretest probability, the presence of prosthetic valves, or suspected progressive or invasive infection, in which case TEE should be obtained. TEE has 90% sensitivity for mitral valve pathology (vs. the 60% sensitivity of TTE).

KEY POINT

DUKE CRITERIA FOR INFECTIVE ENDOCARDITIS

Requires two major criteria, one major combined with three minor criteria, or five minor criteria. These are as follows:

- **Major criteria:**
  - Persistently ⊕ blood cultures (two or more ⊕ cultures separated by at least 12 hours, three or more cultures at least one hour apart, or 70% of cultures ⊕ if four or more are drawn).
  - Evidence of endocardial involvement (through echocardiography demonstrating a vegetation, abscess, or prosthetic dehiscence) or new valvular regurgitation.
- **Minor criteria:**
  - Fever > 38° C.
  - **Vascular phenomena:** Arterial emboli, Janeway lesions (painless lesions on the palms and soles), pulmonary emboli, mycotic aneurysms, intracranial hemorrhage.
  - **Immunologic phenomena:** Osler's nodes (painful nodes on the tips of the fingers or toes), glomerulonephritis, ⊕ RF, Roth's spots (retinal hemorrhage).
  - Predisposing heart abnormality or IV drug use.
  - ⊕ blood cultures not meeting major criteria.
  - ⊕ echocardiogram not meeting major criteria.

Heart valvular dysfunction requiring surgery is common with which class of organism? Fungi.

TREATMENT

- Infective endocarditis requires 4–6 weeks of high-dose IV antibiotics. Since the prevalence of methicillin-resistant *S. aureus* (MRSA) is 50% or more in many areas of the country, vancomycin should be the empiric treatment until sensitivities are known. Antibiotic selection should then be guided by speciation and antibiotic sensitivities. Previously, treatment consisted of 4–6 weeks of an antistaphylococcal β-lactam (e.g., nafcillin), with the first two weeks including additional aminoglycoside therapy (e.g., gentamicin) for synergy. Synergy with an aminoglycoside is still a reasonable choice. In areas with a high prevalence of MRSA or in the presence of coagulase-⊖ *Staphylococcus* infection, vancomycin can be substituted for the β-lactam.
- Surgery is indicated if the patient has severe, refractory CHF, treatment-resistant infective endocarditis, infection of a prosthetic valve, suspected fungal infection, recurrent embolic events, or progressive intracardiac spread of infection.
- For patients with valvular abnormalities, prophylactic amoxicillin or clarithromycin is recommended one hour prior to dental procedures. Be aware that prophylaxis regimens were recently updated.

REFERENCE

Wilson W et al. Prevention of infective endocarditis: Guidelines from the American Heart Association: A guideline from the American Heart Association Rheumatic Fever, Endocarditis, and Kawasaki Disease Committee, Council on Cardiovascular Disease in the Young, and the Council on Clinical Cardiology, Council on Cardiovascular Surgery and Anesthesia, and the Quality of Care and Outcomes Research Interdisciplinary Working Group. *Circulation* 116(15):1736–1754, October 9, 2007. Outlines updated guidelines for the use of prophylactic antibiotics in the prevention of infective endocarditis.

Syncope

A sudden, transient loss of consciousness and postural tone due to cerebral hypoperfusion. More than 30% of people will experience at least one syncopal episode during their lifetimes. Patients usually have lightheadedness preceding the episode. Most people do not even remember falling. Prodromal symptoms such as diaphoresis, pallor, and abdominal discomfort may also occur. The mnemonic **SVNCOPE** and the descriptions below outline its etiologies.

- **Situational sources:** Include performing the Valsalva maneuver, defecation, coughing, sneezing, micturition, carotid sinus hypersensitivity (syncope with head turning, tight collars, or shaving), and subclavian steal (syncope with arm exercise).
- **Vasovagal responses, or the "common faint":** Usually occurs in young patients; precipitated by an emotional situation. Due to excessive vagal tone.
- **Neurogenic causes:** TIAs of the vertebrobasilar circulation, also known as "drop attacks" (technically not syncope). Very large strokes of the anterior circulation can also lead to loss of consciousness; these patients will also have neurologic deficits if and when they rouse.
- **Cardiac causes:** Include cardiac arrhythmias (e.g., bradycardia/tachycardia syndrome, or "sick sinus syndrome"), conduction disturbances (e.g., second- or third-degree AV heart block, torsades de pointes, ventricular tachycardia, ventricular fibrillation, Brugada syndrome, prolonged QTc), inflow/outflow obstruction (e.g., valvular stenosis, HOCM, pulmonary embolism, pulmonary hypertension, myxoma), and cardiac ischemia with ↓ contractility.

Etiologies of syncope—

SVNCOPE

Situational
Vasovagal
Neurogenic
Cardiac
Orthostatic hypotension
Psychiatric
Everything else

- **Orthostatic hypotension:** Caused by hypovolemia from diuretics (furosemide, alcohol), vasodilators (α-blockers, nitrates), or, in patients with DM, autonomic insufficiency. Systolic BP will ↓ at least 20 mmHg within 2–5 minutes after the patient changes position from supine to standing. Heart rate often ↑.
- **"Everything else":** Includes idiopathic causes as well as nonsyncopal events causing loss of consciousness (e.g., drug intoxication, hypoglycemia, hypoxia, psychogenic pseudosyncope, seizures/epilepsy).

WORKUP

- Taking a good history both from the patient and from witnesses (if available) constitutes the most important part of a syncope workup. Most importantly, try to determine if the event has a cardiac etiology.
- It is also important to distinguish syncopal causes of loss of consciousness from nonsyncopal causes. Focus on activity and posture prior to the incident, precipitating factors (exertion or positional changes), whether or not a prodrome occurred, any associated symptoms (incontinence, chest pain, palpitations, neurologic signs), and any medications taken.
- Diagnostic measures include the following:
  - Positional vital signs ("orthostatics") to rule out orthostasis.
  - Electrocardiography to evaluate cardiac conduction (although most are normal).
  - Conducting a tilt-table test to evaluate patients for autonomic insufficiency.
- Additional tests include Holter monitoring (20–50% sensitive for arrhythmias) or continuous-loop event monitoring, echocardiography, exercise (stress) testing, cardiac catheterization, subclavian ultrasound, and carotid massage (especially in the elderly—can be done at the bedside).

In what percentage of syncope cases does an EEG indicate the etiology? Fewer than 1%.

TREATMENT

Treatment is dependent on the cause and includes the following:

- **Subclavian steal:** Patients should be referred to a vascular surgeon.
- **Vasovagal syncope:** Avoidance of triggers in situational syncope. Patients may benefit from β-blockers and can be treated with anticholinergics (e.g., diphenhydramine) or pacemaker placement.
- **Cardiac causes:** If a cardiac condition is present, its treatment is of critical importance.
- **Orthostasis:** Patients should have their volume repleted and underlying conditions (e.g., anemia) corrected or offending drugs removed.

REFERENCES

- Brignole M et al. Guidelines on management (diagnosis and treatment) of syncope: Update 2004. *Europace* 6(6):467–537, 2004. A comprehensive guideline and expert-consensus document compiled by the European Society of Cardiology.
- Kapoor WN. Syncope. *NEJM* 343(25):1856–1862, 2000. A brief but helpful review article on the diagnosis and management of syncope.

Valvular Heart Disease

Valvular diseases can be divided into two general types: stenotic lesions and regurgitant/insufficient lesions. Most valvular heart disease is detected clinically in the seventh decade of life with the exception of mitral stenosis, which usually presents in the fourth and fifth decades. Causes of valvular disease include the following:

Etiologies of sudden death in patients < 35 years of age:
- *Usually exercise related (> 85%).*
- *There is an identifiable cardiac source in nearly half of all cases (e.g., HOCM, CAD, myocarditis), but more than one-third of cases remain idiopathic.*

- **Rheumatic fever:** Historically the most common cause of valvular heart disease in adults (usually mitral stenosis or aortic stenosis accompanied by aortic insufficiency). Incidence has ↓ precipitously with treatment of streptococcal infections.
- **Degenerative heart disease:** The leading cause of valvular heart disease; most commonly calcific stenosis (related to atherosclerosis).
- **Congenital abnormalities** (e.g., bicuspid aortic valve, CHD).

WORKUP/TREATMENT

- Listen to the murmur. Attempt to describe it in detail. Listen to it with the patient in multiple positions.
- Table 4-5 summarizes the management of major valvular lesions.

TABLE 4-5. Summary of Valvular Heart Diseases

VALVULAR LESION	RISK FACTORS/ SETTING	SYMPTOMS/SIGNS	MURMUR	TREATMENT
Aortic outflow obstruction	**Aortic stenosis (AS):** Rheumatic heart disease, congenital stenosis/bicuspid valve, age-related degeneration (e.g., calcific sclerosis). **Subvalvular stenosis** (e.g., HOCM).	The classic triad consists of angina, syncope, and heart failure. Remember them with the **"5-3-2" rule:** 50% mortality rates occur at **5, 3, and 2 years,** respectively, for angina, syncope, and heart failure. Pulsus parvus et tardus (weak and delayed carotid upstroke); sustained apical beat; S4 and soft S2 heart sounds.	**AS:** Midsystolic crescendo-decrescendo (diamond-shaped) murmur heard best at the second intercostal space; radiation to the carotids with a musical apical component (Gallavardin phenomenon); systolic ejection click. The intensity of the murmur does not necessarily relate to its severity (severe AS = ↓ cardiac output = quieter murmur). **HOCM:** Systolic, diamond-shaped, harsh murmur at the apex and left sternal border, poorly transmitted to the carotids (vs. AS); earlier and longer with ↓ left ventricle size (Valsalva or standing); ↓ with ↑ left ventricle size (squatting).	**AS: Avoid afterload reducers** (vasodilators, ACEIs) **and β-blockers.** Gentle diuresis for congestive symptoms. Consider prophylactic antibiotics for endocarditis. Aortic valve replacement is curative; balloon valvuloplasty (BV) is only palliative (for poor surgical candidates). The critical value for the aortic orifice area is < 0.5 cm², or a pressure gradient > 50 mmHg. **HOCM: Avoid strenuous exercise** (risk of sudden death). β-blockers may be used to ↓ outflow obstruction. Surgical myomectomy or pacemaker placement.

TABLE 4-5. **Summary of Valvular Heart Diseases** (continued)

VALVULAR LESION	RISK FACTORS/ SETTING	SYMPTOMS/SIGNS	MURMUR	TREATMENT
Aortic insufficiency (AI)	**Valve disease:** Rheumatic heart disease (mixed AS/AI + MS), endocarditis, congenital bicuspid valve. **Root disease:** Hypertension, Ehlers-Danlos syndrome, Marfan's syndrome, collagen vascular disease, vasculitis (Takayasu's, giant cell), aortic dissection, syphilitic aortitis, idiopathic aortic root dilation, subaortic VSD, trauma.	**Acute:** Pulmonary edema +/– hypotension. **Chronic:** Gradual-onset angina (due to reduced diastolic coronary filling); dyspnea, orthopnea, paroxysmal nocturnal dyspnea. **Signs of LVH and left heart failure due to volume overload:** ↑ in stroke volume, widened pulse pressure, laterally displaced PMI. Possible brachial pulsus bisferiens (twin pressure peaks).	1. **High-pitched, blowing diastolic murmur:** Left sternal border; loudest when leaning forward. 2. **Austin Flint murmur:** Low-pitched mid-diastolic rumble (similar to MS, but without opening snap). 3. **Midsystolic murmur at the base** (due to high volume flow).	**Aortic valve replacement is curative.** If not possible, treat with afterload reducers (e.g., vasodilators such as nifedipine and hydralazine), diuretics, and/or digoxin. Consider endocarditis prophylaxis. In the setting of acute decompensation, use afterload reducers (nitroprusside) and ⊕ inotropes (dobutamine).
Mitral stenosis (MS)	Rheumatic heart disease, congenital stenosis, cardiac myxoma, connective tissue disease (SLE).	**Left heart failure symptoms:** Exertional dyspnea, orthopnea, paroxysmal nocturnal dyspnea. **Right heart failure symptoms:** Edema, ascites, hepato-splenomegaly, ↑ JVP, hemoptysis. Often concomitant AF and embolic events. **Signs of left or right heart failure:** Pulmonary crackles, ↑ intensity of S1 and P2, right ventricular heave, AF.	Mid-diastolic rumble with opening snap at the apex; no change with inspiration (vs. tricuspid stenosis, which ↑ with inspiration).	Avoid inotropic agents for all grades. Consider endocarditis prophylaxis. **Grade I:** Sodium restriction, diuretics, anticoagulants, digitalis. **Grade II:** As with grade I plus BV if there is no improvement. **Grades III/IV:** BV or, for refractory disease, valve replacement.

HIGH-YIELD FACTS

INTERNAL MEDICINE

TABLE 4-5. **Summary of Valvular Heart Diseases** *(continued)*

VALVULAR LESION	RISK FACTORS/ SETTING	SYMPTOMS/SIGNS	MURMUR	TREATMENT
Mitral valve prolapse (MVP)	Idiopathic (found in 7% of the population, especially in young women or Marfan's syndrome patients). Can progress to mitral regurgitation.	Usually asymptomatic, but may lead to chest pain that is not associated with exertion or dyspnea. Echocardiography to assess severity.	Late systolic murmur with midsystolic click (Barlow's syndrome). Valsalva leads to an earlier and longer murmur.	Generally not necessary to treat unless symptomatic. Routine prophylactic antibiotics before dental procedures are no longer recommended and are reserved only for high-risk patients (e.g., those with prosthetic heart valves, a prior history of endocarditis, or certain kinds of CHD).
Mitral regurgitation (MR)	**Cusp disease:** Rheumatic heart disease, endocarditis, congenital cleft valve, myxomatous degeneration. Chordae tendineae dysfunction (2° to MI, Marfan's syndrome, MVP). Mitral annular expansion (e.g., dilated cardiomyopathy).	DOE, orthopnea, paroxysmal nocturnal dyspnea, fatigue. Left heart failure signs; can progress to right heart failure. Laterally displaced PMI with left ventricular heave, S3, AF.	High-pitched, holosystolic murmur at the apex radiating to the axilla; systolic thrill; laterally displaced, hyperdynamic PMI.	**Acute:** Afterload reduction (nitroprusside), inotropic support (dobutamine), and surgical repair. **Chronic:** ACEIs, vasodilators/nitrates, diuretics, digoxin, anticoagulants. **Endocarditis prophylaxis:** In severe mitral regurgitation, valve repair and/or replacement.

REFERENCE

Shipton B, Wahba H. Valvular heart disease: Review and update. *Am Fam Physician* 63(11):2201–2208, 2001. An excellent, concise review article with a useful table comparing the physical findings associated with the various valvular heart lesions.

PULMONOLOGY

Chronic Obstructive Pulmonary Disease (COPD)

A progressive disease characterized by a ↓ in lung function due to airflow obstruction. In contrast to asthma, COPD is not reversible and is the fourth most common cause of death in the United States. It is generally due to cigarette smoking and is pathologically divided into **chronic bronchitis** and **emphysema** (although most patients exhibit components of both). These are distinguished as follows:

- **Chronic bronchitis:** A clinical diagnosis of excessive bronchial secretion with productive cough for at least three months per year over two consecutive years.
- **Emphysema:** A pathologic diagnosis of terminal airway destruction due to smoking (**centrilobular**) or to an inherited α_1-antitrypsin deficiency (**panacinar**).

SIGNS AND SYMPTOMS

- Signs and symptoms of COPD are often absent until the disease is significantly advanced (with loss of > 50% of lung function).
- In both emphysema and bronchitis, patients may present with a barrel chest from high lung volumes, accessory chest muscle use, JVD, end-expiratory wheezing, prolonged expiration, and/or muffled breath sounds.
- Disease-specific presentations are as follows:
  - **Emphysema:** Patients are classically described as "pink puffers" who exhibit ↓ breath sounds, minimal cough, DOE, pursed lips, weight loss, rare cyanosis, and hypercarbia/hypoxia late in disease.
  - **Chronic bronchitis:** Patients are described as "blue bloaters" with severe (usually sterile) productive cough, crackles, early onset of hypercarbia/hypoxia and cyanosis, weight gain, lethargy, peripheral edema due to CHF, and late-onset dyspnea.

DIFFERENTIAL

Asthma, bronchiectasis, 1° ciliary dyskinesia, CF, CHF, congenital heart abnormalities, pulmonary hypertension.

WORKUP

- Obtain a CXR, PFTs, ABGs, and serum electrolytes.
- Spirometry is diagnostic (see Table 4-6).
- For both disorders, an ABG during an acute exacerbation could show hypoxemia with an acute respiratory acidosis (↑ P_{CO_2}; patients with COPD often have a baseline ↑ P_{CO_2}) as well as an ↑ alveolar-arterial (A-a) oxygen gradient.

Parenchymal bullae or subpleural blebs are pathognomonic for emphysema.

In emphysema, the CXR shows hyperinflation, hyperlucency, loss of the capillary-alveolar surface area, a flattened and depressed diaphragm, widened retrosternal air space, and an ↑ AP diameter (see Figure 4-2). There are no specific findings for chronic bronchitis on CXR or PFTs except those associated with the comorbid emphysema.

HIGH-YIELD FACTS

INTERNAL MEDICINE

TABLE 4-6. Pulmonary Function Parameters in Lung Disease

MEASUREMENT	OBSTRUCTIVE DISEASE	RESTRICTIVE DISEASE
Spirometry		
FEV$_1$	↓	↓ or normal
FEV$_1$/FVC	↓	↑ or normal
Lung volumes		
FVC	↓ or normal	↓
VC	↓ or normal	↓
TLC	↓ or normal	↓
RV	↑	↓ or ↑ or normal

Adapted, with permission, from Tierney LM et al. *Current Medical Diagnosis & Treatment,* 36th ed. Stamford, CT: Appleton & Lange, 1997: 239.

PULMONARY FUNCTION TESTS (PFTs)

PFTs consist of spirometry with flow volume loops, diffusion capacity for carbon monoxide (DL_{CO}), lung volumes, and ABGs. They are used primarily to detect the presence and quantify the severity of obstructive and restrictive pulmonary disease (see Table 4-6).

- **Obstructive dysfunction:** ↓ expiratory airflow and ↑ air trapping in the lung 2° to obstructed airways. Seen in asthma, chronic bronchitis, emphysema, and bronchiectasis.
- **Restrictive dysfunction:** ↓ lung volume. Seen in extrapulmonary (chest wall disorders, neuromuscular disease, pleural disease) and pulmonary diseases (pulmonary infiltrates and diffuse interstitial lung disease).

Anticholinergics are first-line therapy for COPD.

Indications for home O₂:

- $Po_2 < 55$ mmHg or $Sao_2 < 88\%$.
- Po_2 55–59 mmHg with symptoms of hypoxia (mental status changes, right-sided heart failure from cor pulmonale, polycythemia).

■ Blood and sputum cultures (with Gram stain) are warranted in the presence of fever or ↑ purulent sputum production.

TREATMENT

The management of COPD is akin to that of asthma and is similar for both emphysema and chronic bronchitis.

- Acute exacerbations:
  - Supplemental O_2, hydration, IV or oral steroids, anticholinergics (ipratropium is first line in COPD), β-agonists (e.g., albuterol).
  - Antibiotics (e.g., TMP-SMX, cefuroxime) in the presence of concurrent infection (controversial).
- Chronic management:
  - Anticholinergics (e.g., ipratropium, tiotropium) are preferred; long-acting β-agonists (e.g., salmeterol) may also be added.
  - Influenza and pneumococcal vaccines are recommended.
  - Make sure you have already discussed smoking cessation with your patients before your attending sees them. It is the only therapy that can slow the disease process.
  - Mucolytics are often used in chronic bronchitis, but their efficacy has not been conclusively established.
  - As with asthma, prophylactic antibiotics do not seem to be of use in preventing exacerbations.
  - Corticosteroids, while used in COPD, do not seem to yield the same symptomatic benefit as in asthma, although some data suggest that they may be helpful.
  - Home supplemental O_2 therapy does prolong life if the patient is hypoxemic.
  - PFTs when the patient is stable to assess disease severity.
  - Patients with α_1-antitrypsin deficiency should be given appropriate supplementation.

COMPLICATIONS

- **Chronic respiratory failure:** Chronic hypoxemia with a compensated respiratory acidosis (↑ Pco_2).
- **Destruction of pulmonary vasculature:** Leads to pulmonary hypertension and eventually to right heart failure (cor pulmonale).
- Pneumonia; bronchogenic carcinoma.

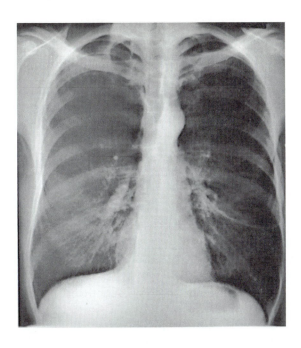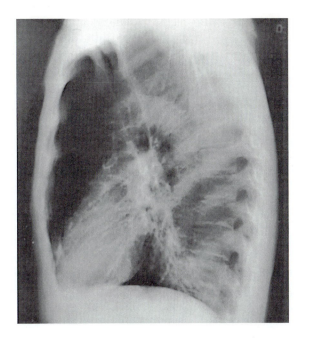

FIGURE 4-2. CXR with COPD.

Note the hyperinflated and hyperlucent lungs, flat diaphragm, ↑ AP diameter, and narrow mediastinum. (Reproduced, with permission, from Stobo JD et al. *The Principles and Practice of Medicine*, 23rd ed. Stamford, CT: Appleton & Lange, 1996: 135.)

REFERENCE

Hurst JR, Wedzicha JA. Chronic obstructive pulmonary disease: The clinical management of an acute exacerbation. *Postgrad Med J* 80(947):497–505, 2004. An excellent review of current management and treatment guidelines for COPD.

Lung Cancer

Solitary pulmonary nodules are discovered in 0.1–0.2% of CXRs. Of these, 60–90%, depending on demographics, do not represent a malignancy. Approximately half of all lung tumors are metastatic, and half are 1° to the lung. Etiologies are as follows:

- Smoking plays a role in 85% of 1° lung cancers. Nearly 15% of smokers develop lung cancer, with the risk proportional to the number of pack-years smoked (always calculate pack-years).
- Smoking in concert with asthma or vitamin E supplementation can further ↑ cancer risk.
- Smoking cessation ↓ risk in a time-dependent manner but does not completely return it to baseline.
- Other risk factors include radon exposure, environmental exposure (e.g., arsenic, asbestos, uranium, chromium), and first-generation familial history.

SIGNS AND SYMPTOMS

Only 10–25% of patients are asymptomatic at the time of diagnosis. Others present with the following:

Beware of "CO_2 retainers" who occasionally do worse with supplemental O_2 because, as some believe, they lose their hypoxemic drive to hyperventilate and acutely ↑ their P_{CO_2}

- Cough, dyspnea, hemoptysis, chest pain, and constitutional symptoms (fever, chills, weight loss, malaise, and night sweats).
- Physical exam may reveal ↓ breath sounds, crackles, ↑ fremitus with postobstructive pneumonitis, and pleural effusion.
- May present with dermatomyositis, anemia, DIC, eosinophilia, clubbing, thrombocytosis, or acanthosis nigricans. Specific syndromes may be associated with cancer subtypes (see Table 4-7).

DIFFERENTIAL

TB and other granulomatous diseases; fungal disease (aspergillosis, histoplasmosis); lung abscess; metastasis or benign tumor.

WORKUP

- CXR, CBC with differential, electrolytes, LFTs, calcium.
- CXR may show hilar and peripheral masses, atelectasis, infiltrates, or pleural effusion (see Figure 4-3).
- Chest CT can better characterize involvement of the parenchyma, pleura, and mediastinum.
- PET scan with CT is revolutionizing the staging process.
- For malignancy, a histologic diagnosis from fine-needle aspiration (FNA), bronchoscopy with biopsy, lymph node biopsy, thoracentesis, mediastinoscopy, or thoracotomy is necessary, as the treatment and prognosis for small cell lung cancer (SCLC) and non–small cell lung cancer (NSCLC) differ.

TREATMENT

Treatment depends on the type and extent of the lung cancer and includes surgery, chemotherapy, and radiation therapy.

- **NSCLC:** Surgical resection followed by radiation/chemotherapy. Early-stage NSCLC is curable.
- **SCLC:** Nonresectable but usually responsive to combination and radiation therapy; recurrence is common.

COMPLICATIONS

Complications include those outlined in the mnemonic **SPHERE.**

Chronic Cough

Defined as a cough that is present for > 3 weeks. For nonsmokers, the prevalence is 14–23%; for smokers, the prevalence ↑ with the number of packs smoked, from 25% with half a pack per day to 50% in those who smoke > 2 packs per day. Chronic cough may commonly have more than one etiology.

- Some 90% of cases are caused by the five most common etiologies: smoking, postnasal drip, asthma, GERD, and chronic bronchitis.
- Other causes include medication (e.g., ACEIs), airway hyperresponsiveness 2° to URI, malignancy, TB, aspiration, foreign bodies, occupational irritants, psychogenic factors, CHF, and irritation of cough receptors in the ear.

SIGNS AND SYMPTOMS

Presentation varies according to the etiology:

- **Asthma related:** Coughing that worsens at night, a family history of atopy, wheezing, worsening around specific irritants (e.g., pollen, smoke, temperature).

TABLE 4-7. Malignant Pulmonary Lesions

LESION TYPE/ INCIDENCE	MOST COMMON LOCATION	RISK FACTORS	RELATED CONDITIONS	FIVE-YEAR SURVIVAL
SCLC (15–25%)	Central hilum.	Strong association with smoking (99%).	Cushing's syndrome, SIADH, hypercalcemia, ectopic ACTH, peripheral neuropathy, Lambert-Eaton syndrome, SVC syndrome.	5–10%.
NSCLC (60–70%)				
Squamous cell carcinoma (20%)	Central or in main bronchus.	Strong association with smoking (> 90%).	Hypercalcemia from PTH-related peptide (PTHrP), hypertrophic pulmonary osteoarthropathy (HPO), SVC syndrome.	Varies with stage.[a]
Adenocarcinoma (60%)	67% peripheral subpleural; 33% central; bronchoalveolar subtype in airways.	Weak association with smoking; the most common type in non-smokers. Ras gene mutations (30%).	HPO, thrombophlebitis.	Varies with stage.[a]
Large cell carcinoma (20%)	Peripheral.	Moderate association with smoking.	Gynecomastia, galactorrhea, HPO.	Varies with stage.[a]
Mesothelioma (3–5%)	Pleural-based.	Asbestos exposure 20–40 years prior (80%).	Pleural effusion.	20%.
Carcinoid of the lung (6%)	Subsegmental bronchi.	All groups except African-Americans.	Tachycardia, flushing, bronchial constriction, diarrhea, Cushing's syndrome.	60–95%.
Metastasis (most commonly colon, breast, renal, osteosarcoma, melanoma) (2–8%)	Random (may be vascular or lymphatic in distribution).			Varies by 1° site.

[a] Five-year survival is stage dependent: I = 50–60%; II = 30–50%; III = 5–10%; IV = < 5%.

HIGH-YIELD FACTS

INTERNAL MEDICINE

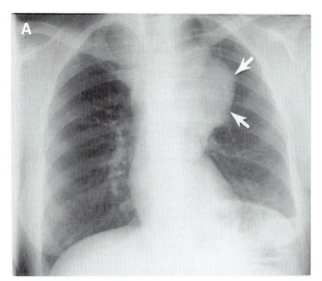

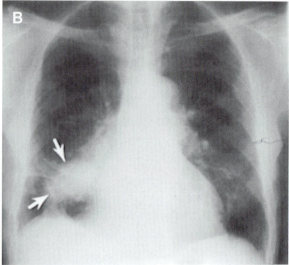

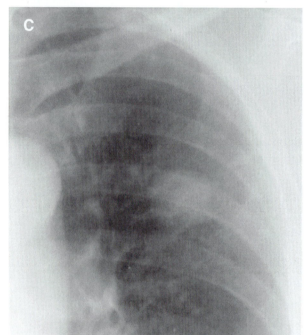

FIGURE 4-3. **CXRs in lung cancer.**

(A) Small cell cancer in the left hilum. Note the left hemi-diaphragm paralysis 2° to phrenic nerve involvement. (B) Squamous cell cancer in the right lower lobe. (C) Adenocarcinoma in the left upper lobe. (Reproduced, with permission, from Stobo JD et al. *The Principles and Practice of Medicine*, 23rd ed. Stamford, CT: Appleton & Lange, 1996: 180.)

- **GERD:** Sour mouth, heartburn, or worsened symptoms while supine.
- **Postnasal drip:** Mucus draining from the nose or down the throat and, on exam, cobblestone mucosa.
- **Malignancy:** Constitutional symptoms such as fever, chills, unintentional weight loss, malaise, fatigue, and night sweats.

WORKUP/TREATMENT

A workup should proceed in a stepwise manner to rule out the various causes:

- Treat postnasal drip with a combination antihistamine-decongestant; if symptoms persist, consider adding a steroid and/or obtaining a CT of the sinuses.
- Evaluate and treat for asthma (see the Pediatrics chapter); avoid suspected irritants (e.g., medications, allergies) or triggers.

- If postnasal drip and asthma are ruled out, treat for GERD with H_2 blockers or PPIs; consider endoscopy or 24-hour pH monitoring if refractory.
- If all of the above are $\ominus$, consider bronchoscopy.

Pleural Effusion

Defined as an abnormal accumulation of fluid in the pleural space. It is normally classified as **transudative** or **exudative**.

SIGNS AND SYMPTOMS

- Frequently presents with dyspnea and pleuritic chest pain, but often asymptomatic.
- Physical exam reveals ↓ breath sounds, dullness to percussion, and ↓ tactile fremitus.

 TRANSUDATIVE VS. EXUDATIVE EFFUSION

- **Transudative effusion:**
  - **Mechanism:** ↑ hydrostatic pressure and/or ↓ oncotic pressure, with intact capillaries leading to protein-poor pleural fluid that is an ultrafiltrate of plasma.
  - **Causes:** CHF, cirrhosis, nephrotic syndrome, peritoneal dialysis, SVC obstruction, myxedema, urinothorax (rupture of the ureter), protein-losing enteropathy, pulmonary embolism.
- **Exudative effusion:**
  - **Mechanism:** Inflammation resulting in leaky capillaries, leading to a protein-rich fluid.
  - **Causes:** Bacterial infection (pneumonia-associated ["parapneumonic"] effusion and empyema), neoplasm, pulmonary embolism with infarction, TB, viral infection, collagen vascular disease, pancreatitis, hemothorax, sarcoidosis, uremia, asbestosis, pericardial disease, chylothorax, iatrogenic (e.g., traumatic pleural tap).

 PLEURAL FLUID APPEARANCE

- **Bloody:** Neoplasm, TB, traumatic tap, pulmonary embolus, hemothorax.
- **Low glucose:** Neoplasm, TB, empyema, RA (extremely low glucose).
- **Lymphocytic:** Viral infection, TB, malignancy.
- **Milky (triglyceride rich):** Chylothorax.

RECOMMENDATIONS FOR PLEURAL FLUID ANALYSIS

- **CBC with differential:** Evaluate for signs of infection or trauma (e.g., ↑ RBCs).
- **Protein and LDH ratios** (Light's criteria): Pleural fluid protein/serum protein > 0.5 and pleural fluid LDH/serum LDH > 0.6 (or pleural fluid LDH > 2/3 upper limit of normal serum LDH) are suggestive of an exudate as opposed to a transudate.
- **Amylase:** High amylase supports esophageal rupture, pancreatic pleural effusion, or malignancy.
- **pH:** If < 7.30, suggests empyema, rheumatoid pleurisy, tuberculous pleurisy, or malignancy (normal pH is 7.60).
- **Glucose:** If < 60 mg/dL, suggests bacterial infection, rheumatoid pleuritis, or malignancy.
- **Gram stain:** To look for bacteria.
- **Cytology:** To reveal malignant cells.

Signs of "complicated" effusion include puslike appearance, a ⊕ Gram stain, low pH (< 7.3), low glucose (< 60 mg/dL), and high LDH (> 1000 IU/L).

WORKUP

- CXR may show blunting of the costophrenic angles. A decubitus CXR can determine whether the fluid is free-flowing or loculated.
- Thoracentesis ("pleural tap") or open biopsy is the definitive diagnostic test. A needle biopsy of pleura diagnoses tuberculous effusion. All parapneumonic effusions require a diagnostic tap.

TREATMENT

- Transudative effusion:
    - Address the underlying condition.
    - Perform a therapeutic lung tap when massive effusion leads to dyspnea.
- Exudative effusion:
    - **Malignant:** Consider pleurodesis (injection of an irritant such as talc into the pleural cavity to scar the two pleural layers together) in symptomatic patients who are unresponsive to chemotherapy and radiation therapy. Therapeutic thoracentesis, pleuroperitoneal shunting, and surgical pleurectomy are alternatives.
    - **Parapneumonic:** Consider drainage via a chest tube for a "complicated" parapneumonic effusion or an empyema.
    - **Hemothorax:** Place a chest tube to control bleeding by the apposition of pleural surfaces; determine the amount of blood loss; and assess the risk of infection and late fibrothorax.

Pneumonia

Pneumonia is defined by infection of the bronchoalveolar unit with an associated inflammatory exudate. Community-acquired pneumonia (CAP) causes the greatest number of deaths of any infectious disease in the United States. Causes include the following:

Streptococcus pneumoniae is the most common cause of CAP.

- **"Typical" infectious pneumonia:** Bacteria from the nasopharynx.
- **"Atypical" infectious pneumonia:** Organisms inhaled from the environment (e.g., bacteria, especially *Mycoplasma*; viruses, fungi); often difficult

to visualize on Gram stain and not susceptible to antibiotics that act on the cell wall (e.g., β-lactams).

- For persistent, recurrent infections, consider underlying lung injury, obstruction (e.g., bronchogenic carcinoma, lymphoma, Wegener's granulomatosis, TB, *Nocardia*, *Coxiella burnetii*, *Aspergillus*), or ↓ immune status.

SIGNS AND SYMPTOMS

- **Classic "typical" symptoms:** Productive cough (purulent yellow or green sputum), hemoptysis, tachypnea, dyspnea, fever/chills, night sweats, pleuritic chest pain.
- **Atypical pneumonia:** Classic symptoms may be the same as those above, or may present with a more gradual onset of symptoms, including dry cough, myalgias, headaches, sore throat, and pharyngitis.
- Physical exam reveals bronchial breath sounds, bronchophony, dullness to percussion, whispered pectoriloquy, egophony, ↑ tactile fremitus, and possible crackles or wheezes (see Table 4-8).

WORKUP

- **CBC:** Demonstrates leukocytosis and left shift (an immature form of WBCs are present) with bands.
- **CXR:** Shows lobar consolidation or patchy or diffuse infiltrates.
- **Sputum Gram stain and culture and blood culture:** Identify the pathogenic organism, the organism's susceptibility to antibiotics, and the presence of bacteremia. Evidence does not support routine sputum or blood culture in patients with CAP.
- **ABGs and pulse oximetry:** Poor O_2 saturation and acid-base disturbances may be seen in severe cases.
- Urine antigens for *Legionella* and pneumococcus can be helpful.

TREATMENT

- Initial treatment is empiric (fluoroquinolones or ceftriaxone/azithromycin) and is based on the suspected etiology, with revision of the medical regimen once Gram stain and culture and sensitivities are obtained (see Table 4-9).

TABLE 4-8. Pulmonary Diagnostic Tips

PHYSICAL FINDING	PLEURAL EFFUSION	PNEUMONIA	PNEUMOTHORAX
Breath sounds	↓	↓ vesicular but ↑ bronchial	↓
Adventitial sounds	Inspiratory crackles	Egophony ("E" →"A"), bronchophony, whispered pectoriloquy	None
Percussion	Dull	Dull	Hyperresonant
Tactile fremitus	↓	↑	↓

Elderly patients with CAP and patients with underlying COPD or DM may have minimal signs on exam. Your level of suspicion should remain high in these patients.

A good sputum sample has many PMNs and few epithelial cells. Otherwise, suspect contamination by oral flora.

Classic disease-specific clues to pneumonia:

- *Rust-colored sputum:* pneumococcus
- *"Currant-jelly" sputum:* Klebsiella
- *Cold agglutinins:* Mycoplasma
- *CD4 < 200 and/or ↑ LDH:* Pneumocystis carinii (now P. jiroveci) pneumonia

Azithromycin is often used for **Legionella** *coverage.*

Intermediate- to high-level penicillin resistance in S. pneumoniae ranges from 20% to 35%; fluoroquinolone resistance is 3–4%.

- The Patient Outcomes Research Team (PORT) score can be calculated to assess the need for hospitalization.
- Consider hospitalization for patients > 65 years of age or for those with co-morbidities, immunosuppression, altered mental status, aspiration, malnutrition, alcohol abuse, tachypnea, hypotension, sepsis, hypoxemia, or multilobar involvement.
- PORT score, age, and time to antibiotic administration (< 4 hours) all affect mortality.
- Any patient admitted to the hospital likely warrants IV antibiotics. However, a patient who has been afebrile for > 24 hours can switch to an oral antibiotic. Some physicians will discharge the patient once oral antibiotics are tolerated and have the patient finish the course of antibiotics (7–14 days total) on an outpatient basis. Others may elect to ensure that the patient remains afebrile on the oral antibiotic before discharge.
- While the patient is in the hospital, encourage incentive spirometry, chest physical therapy, hydration, and ambulation to loosen consolidation and improve aeration.

TABLE 4-9. Treatment of Pneumonia

DEMOGRAPHICS	SUSPECTED PATHOGENS	INITIAL COVERAGE (NONVIRAL)
Outpatient CAP, age < 60, otherwise healthy	*S. pneumoniae, Mycoplasma pneumoniae, Chlamydia pneumoniae, Haemophilus influenzae,* viruses.	Macrolide (clarithromycin or azithromycin), doxycycline, or β-lactam.
CAP with age > 60 or with comorbidity (e.g., COPD, heart failure, renal failure, diabetes, liver disease, EtOH abuse)	*S. pneumoniae, H. influenzae,* aerobic gram-⊖ rods (GNRs—*E. coli, Enterobacter, Klebsiella*), *S. aureus, Legionella,* viruses.	Second-generation cephalosporin (cefuroxime) or amoxicillin/ clavulanate (Augmentin). Add azithromycin if atypicals (*Legionella, Mycoplasma, Chlamydia*) are suspected. Alternatively, fluoroquinolone monotherapy.
CAP requiring hospitalization	*S. pneumoniae, H. influenzae,* anaerobes, aerobic GNRs, *Legionella, Chlamydia.*	Azithromycin with a second- or third-generation cephalosporin (cefotaxime or ceftriaxone) or a β-lactam with a β-lactamase inhibitor. Alternatively, fluoroquinolone monotherapy.
Severe CAP requiring hospitalization	*S. pneumoniae, H. influenzae,* anaerobes, aerobic GNRs, *Legionella, Mycoplasma, Pseudomonas.*	Macrolide, third-generation cephalosporin with antipseudomonal activity (ceftazidime). Consider vancomycin if MRSA is a possibility.
Nosocomial pneumonia (i.e., patient hospitalized > 48 hours or in a long-term care facility > 14 days)	GNRs, including *Pseudomonas, S. aureus, Legionella,* and mixed flora.	Aminoglycoside and third-generation antipseudomonal cephalosporin.

INDICATIONS FOR PNEUMOCOCCAL VACCINATION

Recommendations of the CDC National Immunization Program are that the following receive pneumococcal vaccination:

- Patients ≥ 65 years of age and children 2–23 months of age.
- Patients with chronic/systemic illness (e.g., heart disease, sickle cell disease, diabetes, cirrhosis, pulmonary fibrosis).
- Patients with ↓ immune function (e.g., AIDS, lymphoma, leukemia, asplenia, nephrotic syndrome).
- Alaskan natives and selected Native American populations.

COMPLICATIONS

- Some 30% of pneumococcal pneumonia patients exhibit bacteremia.
- There is an ↑ risk for MI and stroke (*NEJM* 351:2611–2618, 2004).

REFERENCES

- Fine MJ et al. A prediction rule to identify low-risk patients with community-acquired pneumonia. *NEJM* 336:243–250, 1997. Discusses the manner in which PORT scores can be used to risk-stratify patients.
- Niederman MS. Review of treatment guidelines for community-acquired pneumonia. *Am J Med* 117 Suppl 3A:51S–57S, 2004. A clinical review of pneumonia treatment strategies.

Acute Renal Failure (ARF)

Defined as an abrupt ↓ in renal function leading to the retention of creatinine and BUN, often accompanied by oliguria (urine output 100–400 mL/day) or anuria (urine output < 100 mL/day). Clinical manifestations are nonspecific and include malaise, fatigue, anorexia, oliguria, nausea/vomiting, and hypertension. ARF is categorized as prerenal, intrinsic, and postrenal. A summary of the etiologies, distinguishing features, and treatment of each of these three subtypes can be found in Figure 4-4. The fractional excretion of sodium (Fe_{Na}) is an important way to distinguish prerenal from intrinsic renal failure (see Figure 4-4):

$$Fe_{Na} = (\text{urine Na/plasma Na}) / (\text{urine creatinine/plasma creatinine}) \times 100\%$$

COMPLICATIONS

- **Volume overload** leads to CHF and hypertension. Pay careful attention to fluid balance and optimize hemodynamics (mean arterial pressure, cardiac output).
- **Metabolic acidosis:** Replace bicarbonate if HCO_3^- is ≤ 16 or serum pH is < 7.2.
- **Hyperkalemia and hyperphosphatemia** are common and can usually be treated with dietary restriction (K ≤ 40 mEq/day, PO_4 < 800 mg/day).
- After relief of obstruction, **postobstructive diuresis** can lead to inappropriate loss of fluid and electrolytes, which must often be replaced.

A small fluid challenge (0.5–1.0 L NS) can help distinguish prerenal from intrinsic ARF in oliguric patients who are not volume overloaded. In prerenal ARF, ↑ kidney perfusion leads to ↑ urine output and (usually) ↓ creatinine, and the Fe_{Na} is < 1% before rehydration.

HIGH-YIELD FACTS

INTERNAL MEDICINE

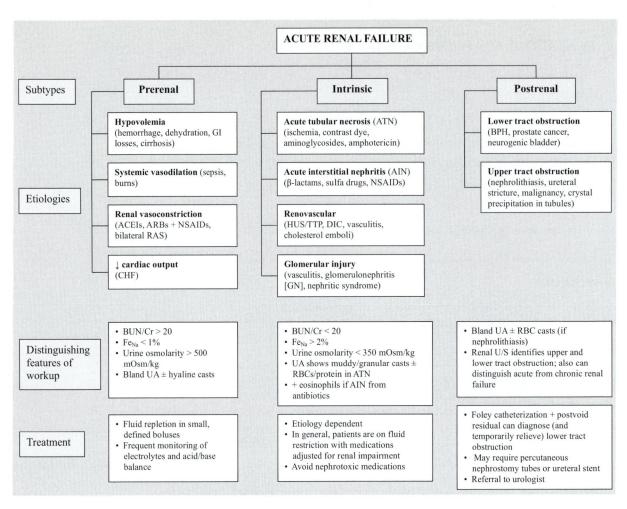

FIGURE 4-4. Summary of acute renal failure.

Indications for dialysis—

AEIOU

Acidosis unresponsive to medical therapy
Electrolyte abnormalities (K > 6.5 mEq/L)
Ingestions (methanol, ethylene glycol)
Overload (fluid)
Uremic symptoms (e.g., pericarditis, encephalopathy)

Chronic Kidney Disease (CKD)

Defined as three or more months of reduced GFR (< 60 mL/min/1.73 m^2) and/or kidney damage (abnormal pathology, blood/urine tests, or imaging). CKD is a growing problem, affecting 16.8% of the U.S. population and a disproportionately higher number of African-Americans. CKD is classified into five stages on the basis of GFR (see Table 4-10). In adults, a commonly used estimate of GFR is derived from the Modification of Diet in Renal Disease study equation:

$$\text{GFR (mL/min/1.73 m}^2) = 175 \times (S_{Cr})^{-1.154} \times (\text{age in years})^{-0.203} \times 0.742 \text{ (if female)} \times 1.12 \text{ (if black)}$$

SIGNS AND SYMPTOMS

CKD is initially asymptomatic and can be detected only by a rise in serum creatinine. As GFR declines, the following symptoms develop, usually around stage 3 or 4, as a result of the retention of solutes and nitrogenous waste (also indicated by ↑ BUN):

■ **General:** Anorexia, nausea/vomiting, fatigue, pruritus, a metallic taste in the mouth, fetor uremicus (breath smelling of urine/ammonia), uremic frost (white urea crystals on the skin).

TABLE 4-10. Stages and Management Goals of Chronic Kidney Disease

STAGE	GFR	GOALS
1 (normal or ↑ GFR)	≥ 90	Diagnose and treat underlying conditions (particularly if reversible); cardiovascular risk reduction.
2 (mild)	60–89	Estimate progression; determine if the patient is likely to need renal replacement therapy (RRT).
3 (moderate)	30–59	Monitor for and treat any complications.
4 (severe)	15–29	Continue to monitor and treat complications; prepare for RRT.
5 (end-stage renal disease)	< 15	RRT; dialysis (hemo- or peritoneal dialysis) is often used as a bridge to transplant if the patient is on a waiting list for cadaveric renal transplantation.

- **Cardiovascular:** Hypertension, often with resultant LVH; pericarditis, accelerated atherosclerosis, volume overload, CHF, hyperlipidemia.
- **Neurologic:** Peripheral neuropathy, encephalopathy (↓ attention and memory), seizures, stupor, coma.
- **Hematologic:** Anemia (due to ↓ production of erythropoietin by the kidneys), iron deficiency (anemia of chronic disease).
- **Metabolic:** Hyperkalemia, metabolic acidosis, ↑ PO_4, ↓ Ca^{++} (due to vitamin D_3 deficiency and binding with excess PO_4), $2°$ hyperparathyroidism leading to osteoporosis.

WORKUP

- Where possible, diagnose and treat the underlying etiology.
- Obtain frequent lab work to monitor for signs of uremia and worsening kidney function. Labs should include serum creatinine, BUN, PO_4, Ca^{++}, albumin, K^+, HCO_3^-, hemoglobin, PTH to assess for hyperparathyroidism, UA, and a first-morning urine spot protein/creatinine ratio to evaluate for proteinuria.

TREATMENT

- **General:**
  - Avoid nephrotoxic drugs (NSAIDs, aminoglycosides, contrast); early referral to a nephrologist.
  - Avoid blood draws on one arm and avoid subclavian lines to preserve vasculature for future access (e.g., AV fistula).
- **Cardiovascular:**
  - ACEIs/ARBs for hypertension with a BP goal of < 130/80 (have been shown to ↓ the progression of CKD).
  - Sodium restriction and/or loop diuretics to prevent volume overload; statins to lower LDL cholesterol (goal < 100 mg/dL).
- **Hematologic:** Administer weekly injections of an erythropoietin analog

HIGH-YIELD FACTS

INTERNAL MEDICINE

(epoetin or darbepoetin) only if hemoglobin is < 12 mg/dL in females or < 13.5 mg/dL in males (patients should be warned that new guidelines may soon change this trend due to ↑ mortality; see below). Give iron supplementation to maintain sufficient iron stores (% transferrin saturation > 20% and ferritin > 100 ng/mL).

- **Metabolic:** Dietary restriction (Na, K, PO_4, Mg); Kayexalate as needed for hyperkalemia; bicarbonate or citrate if HCO_3^- is < 22; oral PO_4 binders (calcium carbonate taken with meals) and calcitriol (1,25-OH vitamin D) for renal osteodystrophy.
- **Renal replacement therapy (preparation starts in stage 4 kidney disease):** Includes hemodialysis, peritoneal dialysis, and renal transplantation (either living-donor or cadaveric). If available, renal transplantation is the treatment of choice, as it has been shown to ↓ mortality and ↑ quality of life.

REFERENCES

- National Kidney Foundation Kidney Disease Outcomes Quality Initiatives (NKF-KDOQI) Clinical Practice Guidelines. Available online at www.kidney.org/professionals/kdoqi/guidelines.cfm. Commonly used guidelines for the management of complications of chronic kidney disease.
- Phrommintikul A et al. Mortality and target haemoglobin concentrations in anaemic patients with chronic kidney disease treated with erythropoietin: A meta-analysis. *Lancet* 369(9559):381–388, 2007. A recent study that found significantly higher all-cause mortality rates as well as higher rates of AV fistula access thrombosis in patients with CKD who had been treated with recombinant human erythropoietin. The study suggested that future guidelines might consider an upper limit for target hemoglobin concentrations.

Glomerular Disease

Glomerular disease encompasses a broad differential of diseases that all lead to injury to the glomerulus, impaired GFR, and the appearance of protein and/or blood cells in the urine. The two general categories are **nephrotic** and **nephritic syndromes** (see Table 4-11).

NEPHROTIC SYNDROME

Renal biopsy may be useful for histologic workup (e.g., rapidly progressive glomerulonephritis from Goodpasture's or Wegener's has characteristic crescents made of monocytes in Bowman's space).

- Characterized by severe proteinuria (> 3.5 g/day), generalized edema, hypoalbuminemia, and hyperlipidemia. Hypercoagulability may result from an imbalance of clotting factors in the coagulation cascade (due to an overall ↓ in anticoagulation proteins, especially antithrombin 3 [lost in urine], and to ↑ hepatic synthesis of precoagulant proteins such as fibrinogen).
- **Signs/Sx:** Presents with generalized edema (puffy eyes in the morning, pitting edema in the legs, pleural effusions, and/or ascites) and foamy urine. Also associated with an ↑ risk of thromboembolism and infection (especially from encapsulated organisms) due to loss of immunoglobulins.
- **Workup:** UA reveals proteinuria; a 24-hour urine collection is preferred. Serum studies reveal hyperlipidemia (↑ LDL cholesterol) and albumin < 3 g/dL. A renal biopsy may be useful.
- **Tx:** Etiology dependent, but protein and salt restriction, diuretics, anticoagulants, and antihyperlipidemics are indicated. Steroids may be necessary for severe disease.

TABLE 4-11. Summary of Renal Syndromes

SYNDROME	SOURCE	COMMON ETIOLOGIES	UNCOMMON ETIOLOGIES
Nephrotic syndrome	1° renal disease	Minimal change disease, focal segmental glomerulosclerosis (FSGS).	Membranous GN (75% idiopathic, but 2° causes include SLE, penicillamine, gold, NSAIDs, HBV, HCV, syphilis, and malignancy).
	Systemic disease	Diabetic nephropathy.	Renal amyloidosis, SLE WHO Class V.
Nephritic syndrome (with low serum complement levels)	1° renal disease	Postinfectious GN.	Membranoproliferative GN. HCV, cryoglobulinemia.
	Systemic disease	SLE WHO Class III/IV, infectious endocarditis.	
Nephritic syndrome (with normal serum complement levels)	1° renal disease	IgA nephropathy; rapidly progressive, ANCA-associated, pauci-immune GN.	Hereditary nephritis (Alport's syndrome).
	Systemic disease	SLE WHO Class II.	Anti–basement membrane disease (Goodpasture's syndrome), vasculitis (polyarteritis nodosa, microscopic polyarteritis, Wegener's granulomatosis, Henoch-Schönlein purpura), TTP, HUS.

NEPHRITIC SYNDROME

- An inflammatory disorder characterized by acute onset of oliguria (urine output < 400 mL/day) and ARF. Hematuria (smoky-colored urine due to RBCs and RBC casts), subnephrotic-range proteinuria, hypertension, and edema are also present. The signs and symptoms of nephritic syndrome can be remembered using the mnemonic **PHAROH**.
- **Signs/Sx:** Presents with tea-colored urine, ↓ urine output, hypertension, and edema in dependent areas (including the periorbital and scrotal regions), although edema is not as significant as in nephrotic syndrome.
- **Workup:** UA reveals hematuria and some degree of proteinuria; serum studies show ↓ GFR with elevated BUN and creatinine. Complement, ANA, ANCA, and anti-GBM antibodies should be measured. A ⊕ anti-streptolysin O (ASO) titer indicates postinfectious glomerulonephritis.
- **Tx:** Etiology dependent, but hypertension, fluid congestion, and uremia should generally be treated with salt and water restriction. Diuretics, dialysis, steroids, and stronger immunosuppressants may be administered as necessary.

> *Presentation of nephritic syndrome—*
>
> **PHAROH**
>
> **P**roteinuria (usually minimal compared to nephrotic syndrome)
> **H**ypertension
> **A**zotemia (↑ BUN)
> **R**BC casts
> **O**liguria
> **H**ypertension

Hyponatremia

Hyponatremia is, in general, an excess of body water in relation to serum sodium, with serum sodium < 135 mEq/L. It is believed to be the most common electrolyte disorder and has numerous etiologies, which may be categorized by osmolar and volume status (see Figure 4-5).

SIGNS AND SYMPTOMS

- Mild hyponatremia may be asymptomatic, especially if chronic. When hyponatremia is acute or of increasing severity, clinical manifestations are mostly neurologic; an acutely ↓ plasma osmolality gradient favors water movement into cells, leading to cerebral edema.
- **Plasma osmolality < 240 mOsm/kg:** Confusion, muscle cramps and twitching, nausea, lethargy, headache, seizures.
- **Serum sodium < 120 mEq/L:** Status epilepticus, stupor, and coma may ensue.

DIFFERENTIAL

Pseudohyponatremia (due to hyperlipidemia or hyperproteinemia).

WORKUP

Plasma and urine osmolality, plasma and urine electrolytes, and urine volume must be measured. These labs can then be used to categorize the type of hyponatremia (see Figure 4-5).

TREATMENT

- Address the underlying etiology, with specific treatment methods varying by volemic status:
    - **Hypovolemic:** Replete volume with NS.
    - **Euvolemic/hypervolemic:** Salt and water restriction.
- Symptomatic patients may initially need rapid correction of sodium levels (2 mEq/L/hr) for the first few hours until symptoms resolve. In general, however, hyponatremia should be treated at a measured pace, with no more than 10–12 mEq/L corrected for the first day and 18 mEq/L over the first two days.

Nephrolithiasis

Nephrolithiasis, commonly known as a kidney stone, most commonly occurs in men, with a peak age of onset in the 20s and 30s. Stones usually result from an imbalance of salts and minerals that are normally found in the urinary tract. Some 75–80% are composed of calcium (calcium oxalate or, less commonly, calcium phosphate; seen in high-oxalate diets, hyperparathyroidism, and sarcoidosis). Other stone types include struvite/magnesium ammonium phosphate (more common in females, and often due to UTIs with urease-producing *Proteus*), cystine (associated with hereditary cystinuria), uric acid (in patients with gout or those undergoing chemotherapy), and indinavir (in patients undergoing HIV treatment).

SIGNS AND SYMPTOMS

- **Classic symptoms:** Progressive, severe flank pain that radiates to the inguinal region. Patients often writhe in bed from colicky pain. Physical exam often reveals CVA tenderness.

Premenopausal women are at particularly high risk of cerebral edema (25-fold higher risk than men) during an acute hyponatremic episode.

What dreaded complication may result from overly rapid correction of hyponatremia?
Central pontine myelinolysis.

What are the most common elements found in stones?
Magnesium, phosphorus, calcium, and ammonia.

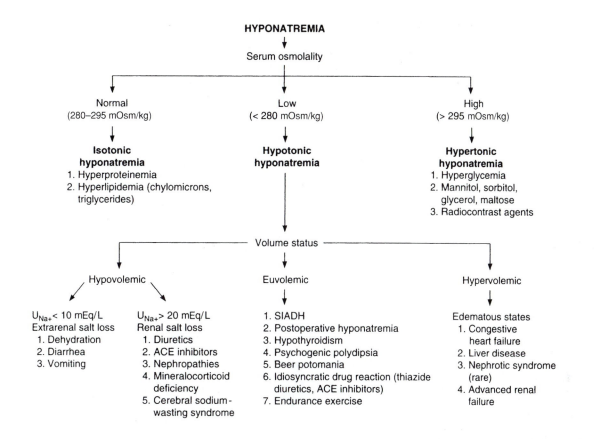

HYPONATREMIA
↓
Serum osmolality

| Normal (280–295 mOsm/kg) | Low (< 280 mOsm/kg) | High (> 295 mOsm/kg) |

Normal (280–295 mOsm/kg)
↓
Isotonic hyponatremia
1. Hyperproteinemia
2. Hyperlipidemia (chylomicrons, triglycerides)

Low (< 280 mOsm/kg)
↓
Hypotonic hyponatremia

High (> 295 mOsm/kg)
↓
Hypertonic hyponatremia
1. Hyperglycemia
2. Mannitol, sorbitol, glycerol, maltose
3. Radiocontrast agents

Volume status

Hypovolemic

$U_{Na+} < 10$ mEq/L
Extrarenal salt loss
1. Dehydration
2. Diarrhea
3. Vomiting

$U_{Na+} > 20$ mEq/L
Renal salt loss
1. Diuretics
2. ACE inhibitors
3. Nephropathies
4. Mineralocorticoid deficiency
5. Cerebral sodium-wasting syndrome

Euvolemic
1. SIADH
2. Postoperative hyponatremia
3. Hypothyroidism
4. Psychogenic polydipsia
5. Beer potomania
6. Idiosyncratic drug reaction (thiazide diuretics, ACE inhibitors)
7. Endurance exercise

Hypervolemic
Edematous states
1. Congestive heart failure
2. Liver disease
3. Nephrotic syndrome (rare)
4. Advanced renal failure

FIGURE 4-5. Workup of hyponatremia.

(Reproduced, with permission, from Tierney LM et al. *Current Medical Diagnosis & Treatment*, 41st ed. New York: McGraw-Hill, 2002: 893.)

■ **Associated symptoms:** Hematuria, nausea, vomiting, dysuria, tenesmus, and oliguria (in the setting of obstruction of the bladder or urethra or, less commonly, bilateral obstruction of the ureters); ↑ risk of UTIs proximal to the stone.

DIFFERENTIAL

Renal infarct, lumbar disk disease, aortic dissection, renal malignancy, pyelonephritis, trauma, glomerulonephritis.

WORKUP

■ UA with culture to evaluate pH and the presence of bacteria, blood, and crystals.
■ CT without contrast is often the first imaging choice, as it can identify all types of stones and can also help differentiate the various causes of the flank pain.
■ Renal ultrasound can identify hydronephrosis if obstruction is suspected; it is also a good choice for pregnant women to minimize radiation.
■ AXR will detect 90% of stones but will miss uric acid stones, which are radiolucent.

Risk factors for nephrolithiasis:

■ *Family history*

■ *Age 20–40*

■ *Diet (high protein, low fluids)*

■ *Medications*

■ *Immobility*

■ *Ileostomy*

■ *Liver disease*

■ *Renal disease (medullary sponge kidney, RTA, polycystic kidney disease)*

TREATMENT

- Treatment varies by stone type, but all patients should have adequate fluid intake to ↑ urine output to > 2.5 L/day.
- Analgesia is an important part of treatment and often requires IV medications (ketorolac is an effective IV NSAID that is often used to avoid narcotics).
- Some 80% of small stones (those < 4 mm) will pass spontaneously, although this may be painful.
- Stones > 5 mm require more invasive procedures, such as extracorporeal shock-wave lithotripsy, retrograde ureteroscopy (for midureteral stones), or percutaneous nephrolithotomy.
- Even with treatment, recurrence is common (10% per year). Preventive measures include ↑ fluid intake, dietary restriction (low protein, nitrogen, and sodium; minimizing oxalate-containing foods), maintaining adequate calcium intake, and administration of thiazides (which ↓ urinary calcium excretion). For uric acid stones, urine should be alkalinized with potassium citrate, and allopurinol should be considered.

GASTROENTEROLOGY

Approach to Abdominal Pain

Visceral pain and **parietal** pain present with different qualities and can help localize the source of abdominal pain to various anatomic locations. The location of the pain can also indicate not only the organs involved but the possible pathophysiologic processes that might be occurring.

- **Visceral pain** involves distention of a hollow organ or viscus and is dull and crampy, poorly localized, and vague.
- **Parietal pain** involves the parietal peritoneum, is sharp and stabbing, and is well localized (see Table 4-12).

WORKUP

- When evaluating abdominal pain, consider narrowing the differential by assessing the pain in terms of (1) pain quality, (2) pain location, and (3) physical exam findings.
- Key findings indicating an emergency include absent bowel sounds (e.g., pancreatitis, bowel ischemia, acute abdomen), high-pitched bowel sounds (e.g., obstruction), rebound tenderness, abdominal rigidity, involuntary guarding, and pulsatile masses. Attention should also be heightened when patients have point tenderness, a ⊕ Murphy's sign, or palpable masses.

TREATMENT

Treatment is etiology specific.

Cirrhosis

Defined as the irreversible destruction of normal hepatic architecture with characteristic diffuse fibrosis and regenerative nodules. The most common cause in the United States is alcohol abuse; the most common etiology worldwide is viral hepatitis. Other etiologies are as follows:

- **Metabolic diseases:** Wilson's disease, hemochromatosis, α_1-antitrypsin deficiency.

Albumin, PT, and bilirubin are tests of liver function. AST, ALT, and alkaline phosphatase are ↑ when there is hepatocellular injury or cholestasis.

TABLE 4-12. **Characterization of Abdominal Pain by Location**

LOCATION	ORGANS AFFECTED	POSSIBLE DISEASE ENTITIES
Right upper	Liver, gallbladder, kidney, small bowel	Hepatitis, cholelithiasis, choledocholithiasis, cholecystitis, biliary colic, 1° sclerosing cholangitis, 1° biliary cirrhosis, pyelonephritis, hepatic tumors/abscesses, right lower lobe pneumonia, MI, pericarditis (pain ↓ when sitting forward), perforated ulcer.
Epigastric	Stomach, abdominal aorta, pancreas	Cardiac disease, gastritis, PUD, pancreatitis, abdominal aortic aneurysm.
Left upper	Spleen, kidney, small bowel	Splenomegaly, splenic infarct, splenic rupture, pyelonephritis, pneumonia, MI, pericarditis, perforated ulcer.
Periumbilical	Abdominal aorta, small bowel, appendix	Abdominal aortic aneurysm or dissection, ischemic bowel (abrupt, episodic pain out of proportion to exam that worsens with food intake), small bowel obstruction (crampy, episodic pain that worsens with food and/or vomiting that ↑ with any PO intake), umbilical hernia, appendicitis, gastroenteritis.
Right lower	Appendix, ovary, fallopian tubes, kidney, ureter, intestines, testes	Nephrolithiasis (flank pain), pyelonephritis, appendicitis, Meckel's diverticulum, right-sided diverticulitis, IBD or other forms of colitis, ovarian cyst, PID, tubo-ovarian abscess (TOA), ectopic pregnancy, testicular or ovarian torsion, epididymitis.
Suprapubic	Bladder, uterus, ovaries, fallopian tubes	UTI, bladder or cervical cancer, PID, bladder outlet obstruction, endometriosis, mittelschmerz disease, ovarian cyst, ectopic pregnancy.
Left lower	Ovary, fallopian tubes, kidney, ureter, intestines, testes	Nephrolithiasis, pyelonephritis, left-sided diverticulitis, IBD or other forms of colitis, ovarian cyst, PID, TOA, ectopic pregnancy, testicular or ovarian torsion, epididymitis.

- **Drugs and toxins:** INH, methyldopa, acetaminophen, methotrexate, carbon tetrachloride.
- **Biliary diseases:** 1° biliary cirrhosis or chronic biliary obstruction.
- **Other:** Cardiac cirrhosis or impaired venous drainage of the liver (e.g., IVC or hepatic vein [Budd-Chiari] occlusion).

SIGNS AND SYMPTOMS

- Fatigue, malaise, and peripheral edema.
- Physical exam reveals stigmata of liver disease, summarized in Figure 4-6.
- **Hepatic encephalopathy:** The etiology remains unclear, although serum ammonia levels are ↑. With more severe forms, asterixis, confusion, and coma are evident.
- **Hepatorenal and hepatopulmonary syndromes:** Hepatorenal syndrome is marked by oliguria, low Fe_{Na}, and failure of the azotemia to respond to fluid bolus.

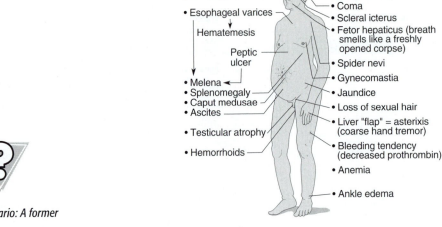

Effects of portal hypertension
- Esophageal varices
  ↓
  Hematemesis
  Peptic ulcer
- Melena ◄
- Splenomegaly
- Caput medusae
- Ascites
- Testicular atrophy
- Hemorrhoids

Effects of liver cell failure
- Coma
- Scleral icterus
- Fetor hepaticus (breath smells like a freshly opened corpse)
- Spider nevi
- Gynecomastia
- Jaundice
- Loss of sexual hair
- Liver "flap" = asterixis (coarse hand tremor)
- Bleeding tendency (decreased prothrombin)
- Anemia
- Ankle edema

FIGURE 4-6. Signs and symptoms of cirrhosis and portal hypertension.

(Adapted, with permission, from Chandrasoma P, Taylor CE. *Concise Pathology*, 3rd ed. Stamford, CT: Appleton & Lange, 1998: 654.)

Clinical scenario: A former alcoholic presents with confusion. On exam, he is found to have a flapping tremor of the wrists with extension. What are you thinking about? Hepatic encephalopathy (the tremor described is asterixis).

DIFFERENTIAL

Nephrotic syndrome, CHF, constrictive pericarditis, abdominal malignancy, peritoneal TB.

WORKUP

- Cirrhosis severity is defined by the Child-Pugh criteria (see Table 4-13) and the Model for End-Stage Liver Disease (MELD) score.
- Other laboratory studies include ammonia (↑), BUN (↓ due to a fall in protein production), sodium (hyponatremia), CBC (anemia, thrombocytopenia), and transaminases/alkaline phosphatase (↑).
- Additional tests are etiology dependent and include ANA, anti–smooth muscle antibody, anti-LKM (presence indicates autoimmune hepatitis), ceruloplasmin (↓ serum level indicates Wilson's disease), α-fetoprotein (↑ in hepatocellular carcinoma), iron studies (↑↑↑ ferritin and TIBC indicate hemochromatosis), and serum electrophoresis (absence of α-globulin indicates α₁-antitrypsin deficiency).
- RUQ ultrasound may show fatty infiltration of liver consistent with nonalcoholic fatty liver disease.
- The serum-ascites albumin gradient (SAAG), derived from paracentesis, is an excellent general test but is invasive.

In general, "decompensation" indicates cirrhosis with Child-Pugh class B, and this level is the accepted criterion for applying for liver transplantation. The timing of renal transplantation is generally based on the MELD score.

TREATMENT

- Lifestyle changes are critical in those with a substance abuse history.
- For ascites, recommend sodium restriction, potassium-sparing diuretics combined with a loop diuretic, and large-volume paracentesis. A transjugular intrahepatic portosystemic shunt that connects the portal vein to the IVC is effective for refractory ascites but can precipitate encephalopathy.
- Esophageal varices can be treated with nonselective β-blockers (to prevent initial bleeding). Bleeding varices are a medical emergency and can be treated with IV vasopressin (with nitroglycerin), IV somatostatin, endoscopic sclerotherapy or band ligation, and balloon tamponade.

FACTOR	POINTS: 1	POINTS: 2	POINTS: 3
Serum bilirubin (mmol/L) [mg/dL]	< 34 [< 2.0]	34–51 [2.0–3.0]	> 51 [> 3.0]
Serum albumin (g/L) [g/dL]	> 35 [> 3.5]	30–35 [3.0–3.5]	< 30 [< 3.0]
Ascites	None	Easily controlled	Poorly controlled
Neurologic changes	None	Minimal	Advanced coma
Prothrombin time	0–4	4–6	> 6
INR	< 1.7	1.7–2.3	> 2.3

[a] The Child-Pugh score is calculated by adding the scores of the five factors (range 5–15). The Child-Pugh class is A (a score of 5–6), B (7–9), or C (≥ 10).

Reproduced, with permission, from Braunwald E et al. *Harrison's Principles of Internal Medicine,* 15th ed. New York: McGraw-Hill, 2001: 1711.

DIAGNOSTIC TESTS

SERUM-ASCITES ALBUMIN GRADIENT (SAAG)

SAAG ≥ 1.1: Indicates the presence of portal hypertension, with etiologies including cirrhosis and congestive disease (CHF, Budd-Chiari syndrome).
SAAG < 1.1: Pancreatitis, bfxile duct leak, peritoneal TB, or metastases.

■ Management of hepatic encephalopathy includes protein restriction, lactulose (to promote ammonia excretion with three bowel movements a day), and neomycin (to inhibit ammonia-producing bacteria in the colon).
■ Consider liver transplantation for refractory disease.

Hepatitis

Acute or chronic inflammation of the liver is considered hepatitis. The most common causes include hepatitis viruses (see Table 4-14) and alcohol abuse. Autoimmune/granulomatous and drug-induced hepatitis are rarer entities.

SIGNS AND SYMPTOMS

■ **Acute hepatitis:** Often starts with a viral prodrome (malaise, fatigue, URI symptoms, nausea, vomiting, joint pain) followed by fever and diarrhea.
■ **Chronic hepatitis:** Presents with symptoms of chronic liver disease and cirrhosis.
■ Physical exam reveals jaundice, scleral icterus, hepatomegaly, splenomegaly, lymphadenopathy, and RUQ tenderness.

Name the major risk factors for viral hepatitis. IV drug use (HBV, HCV), unprotected sexual intercourse (HBV), overseas travel (HAV, HEV).

What percentage of alcoholics develop hepatitis? Roughly 15–20%.

TABLE 4-14. Hepatitis Viruses

VIRUS	TYPE	MODE OF TRANSMISSION	INCUBATION PERIOD	COMPLICATIONS
HAV	RNA; picornavirus	Fecal-oral—e.g., shellfish (a preventive vaccine is available).	Abrupt; 30 days.	None (no risk of chronic hepatitis or cancer).
HBV	DNA; hepadnavirus	Blood borne—percutaneous, sexual, possibly oral, perinatal (a vaccine is available).	Insidious; 8 days.	Chronic hepatitis (10% of those infected), cirrhosis (30%), hepatocellular carcinoma (3–5%).
HCV	RNA; flavivirus	Blood borne—percutaneous (especially IV drug users); possibly perinatal.	Insidious; 50 days.	Chronic hepatitis (80% of those infected), cirrhosis (30%), hepatocellular carcinoma.
HDV	Defective RNA virus; delta virus	Percutaneous, sexual (requires coinfection).	Insidious.	More severe HBV.
HEV	RNA; calicivirus-like	Fecal-oral (especially patients 15–40 years of age in developing countries).	Abrupt; 40 days.	Fulminant hepatitis with 20% mortality in pregnant women (no risk of chronic hepatitis or malignancy).

What transaminase finding indicates alcoholic hepatitis?

AST/ALT > 2:1.

Some 30% of HCV-infected patients have comorbid major depression, making interferon treatment more difficult.

DIFFERENTIAL

Systemic shock with liver hypoperfusion, neoplasm (hepatocellular carcinoma or metastatic lesions from colon cancer), abscess, toxoplasmosis, rickettsial diseases, biliary obstruction, systemic viral illnesses (e.g., mononucleosis).

WORKUP

- **Acute hepatitis:** CBC and LFTs; viral serology if HBV is suspected (see Figure 4-7).
- **Chronic hepatitis:** Hepatitis virus serology, liver biopsy, transaminases (must be ↑ for > 6 months). ↑ alkaline phosphatase and, in severe cases, ↑ PT may also be observed.

TREATMENT

- **Acute hepatitis:**
    - Supportive, including rest and assessment of sick contacts.
    - For HBV/HCV, consider α-interferon.
    - Steroids can be used for severe alcoholic hepatitis.
- **Chronic hepatitis:**
    - α_{2b}-interferon (or pegylated interferon) and lamivudine.
    - α-interferon and ribavirin for chronic HCV. Viral RNA is assayed to assess treatment response.

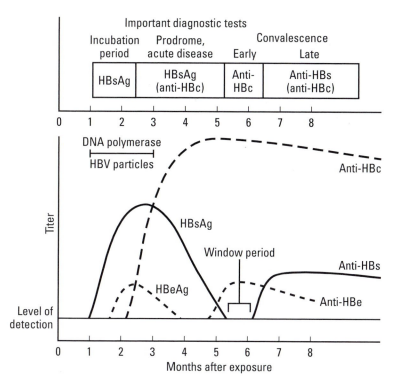

FIGURE 4-7. Serum antibody and antigen levels in HBV.

(Reproduced, with permission, from Bhushan V et al. *First Aid for the USMLE Step 1*. New York: McGraw-Hill, 2005: 197.)

Diarrhea

Diarrhea is the excretion of > 250 g of stool per day. **Acute diarrhea** is usually infectious, often has a sudden onset, and lasts < 3 weeks. **Chronic diarrhea** has a broader differential, often waxes and wanes, and generally persists for > 3 weeks. The basic mechanisms of diarrhea can include ↑ secretion of water and electrolytes, ↑ osmotic load in the colonic lumen, malabsorption, altered colonic motility, and exudative inflammation of colonic mucosa. The etiologies and presentations of major subtypes are outlined in the paragraphs that follow.

SIGNS AND SYMPTOMS

- **Secretory diarrhea:** Occurs when secretagogues such as endogenous endocrine products (VIPomas, serotonin), endotoxins/infection (cholera), and GI luminal substances (e.g., bile acids, fatty acids, laxatives) stimulate ↑ levels of fluid transport across the epithelial cells into the intestinal lumen.
- **Osmotic diarrhea:** Due to the presence of poorly absorbed substances that retain water in the intestinal lumen. This can be attributable to the ingestion of excess osmoles (e.g., mannitol or sorbitol ingestion), to the ingestion of substrate that is subsequently converted to excess osmoles, or to the presence of a genetic enzyme deficiency for a particular diet (e.g., lactase deficiency).
- **Malabsorptive diarrhea:** Due to the inability to digest or absorb a particular nutrient, which can in turn be attributable to bacterial overgrowth, pancreatic enzyme deficiency, or altered motility/anatomy (e.g., celiac disease).

Diarrhea is technically defined as the excretion of > 250 g of stool daily, although patients may consider the term to have different meanings. Obtain a clear history!

Clinical scenario: A woman who was recently treated with clindamycin presents with bloody diarrhea. What might you suspect is the reason? C. difficile colitis. How might you initiate treatment? Oral metronidazole or oral vancomycin.

In patients who have been traveling, don't forget to think about parasites. In patients who have eaten shellfish, think about Vibrio species and Norwalk virus. In patients who have eaten undercooked poultry, think about Campylobacter and Salmonella.

Not all vomiting is associated with preceding nausea. A sudden presentation is known as precipitate vomiting.

WORKUP

- Obtain a complete history, including recent sick contacts, recent travel, immune status, and antibiotic use.
- **Acute diarrhea:** Does not require laboratory investigation unless the patient has a high fever, bloody diarrhea, or diarrhea lasting > 4–5 days.
  - If studies are warranted, check for fecal leukocytes (Wright's stain), bacterial culture, *Clostridium difficile* toxin, and O&P.
  - Consider sigmoidoscopy or colonoscopy in patients with severe proctitis, bloody diarrhea, or possible *C. difficile* colitis.
- **Chronic diarrhea:** Differentiate osmotic from secretory forms (see also Figure 4-8):
  - Secretory diarrhea may be watery; osmotic diarrhea may be greasy or bulky.
  - Osmotic diarrhea will improve with fasting, but secretory diarrhea will not.
  - A stool osmotic gap > 50 mOsm/kg H_2O suggests an osmotic diarrhea.
  - The differential diagnosis for colitis includes ischemia as well as inflammatory or infectious causes.

TREATMENT

- **Acute diarrhea:**
  - Oral or IV fluids and electrolyte replacement.
  - Antidiarrheal agents (e.g., loperamide or bismuth salicylate) may improve symptoms but are contraindicated in patients with bloody diarrhea, high fever, or systemic toxicity (e.g., *E. coli* O157:H7, *Salmonella*).
  - Antibiotic use is controversial in that it is beneficial for treating certain organisms (e.g., *C. difficile*) but possibly harmful for others (*Salmonella* and *E. coli* O157:H7). Treat patients with antibiotics if there is a high likelihood of bacteremia (especially immunosuppressed patients).
- **Chronic diarrhea:**
  - Treat underlying causes and avoid dietary substances contributing to diarrhea. Consider antibiotics to treat bacterial overgrowth.
  - Loperamide, opioids, clonidine, octreotide, cholestyramine, and enzyme supplements can also be tried.

Gastritis

Gastritis, or inflammation of the gastric mucosa, can be divided into **acute** and **chronic** types. Causes include the following:

- **Acute "stress" gastritis (superficial lesions that evolve rapidly):** NSAID use, alcohol, and stress from severe illness (e.g., Curling's ulcers in burn patients).
- **Chronic "nonerosive" gastritis:** Has two subtypes:
  - **Type A gastritis:** Fundal gastritis 2° to autoantibodies to parietal cells. Accounts for 10% of chronic gastritis cases and is often comorbid with pernicious anemia, thyroiditis, and other autoimmune disorders.
  - **Type B gastritis:** Antral gastritis caused by NSAIDs (the most common cause), *H. pylori*, CMV, and HSV. Accounts for 90% of chronic gastritis cases.

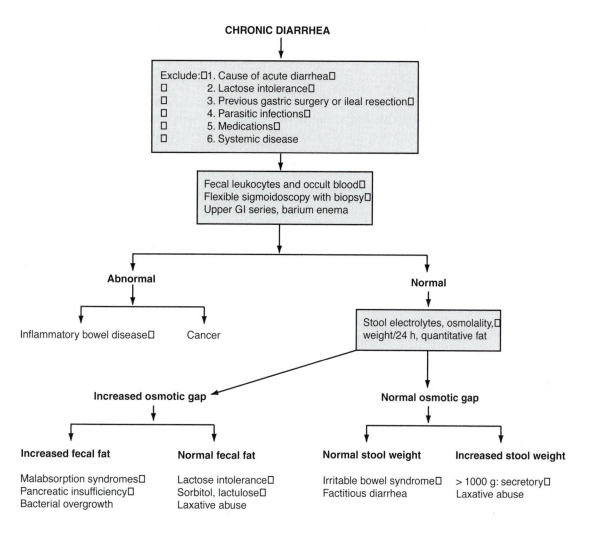

CHRONIC DIARRHEA

Exclude: 1. Cause of acute diarrhea
2. Lactose intolerance
3. Previous gastric surgery or ileal resection
4. Parasitic infections
5. Medications
6. Systemic disease

Fecal leukocytes and occult blood
Flexible sigmoidoscopy with biopsy
Upper GI series, barium enema

Abnormal

Inflammatory bowel disease   Cancer

Normal

Stool electrolytes, osmolality, weight/24 h, quantitative fat

Increased osmotic gap

Increased fecal fat

Malabsorption syndromes
Pancreatic insufficiency
Bacterial overgrowth

Normal fecal fat

Lactose intolerance
Sorbitol, lactulose
Laxative abuse

Normal osmotic gap

Normal stool weight

Irritable bowel syndrome
Factitious diarrhea

Increased stool weight

> 1000 g: secretory
Laxative abuse

FIGURE 4-8. Decision diagram for the diagnosis of causes of chronic diarrhea.

(Reproduced, with permission, from Tierney LM et al. *Current Medical Diagnosis & Treatment*, 41st ed. New York: McGraw-Hill, 2002: 585.)

SIGNS AND SYMPTOMS

■ Although usually asymptomatic, patients can present with indigestion, nausea, vomiting, anorexia, and GI bleeding (hematemesis, melena).
■ Type B gastritis may lead to an ↑ risk of PUD and gastric cancer.

WORKUP

Upper endoscopy and biopsy; testing for *H. pylori*.

TREATMENT

■ ↓ intake of offending agents (especially NSAIDs and alcohol).
■ Antacids, H₂ blockers, PPIs, and/or antibiotics for *H. pylori*.
■ Patients at risk for stress ulcers (e.g., ICU patients) should be given prophylactic H₂ blockers/PPIs on admission.

Alcohol, caffeine, nicotine, chocolate, and fatty foods can reduce LES tone and ↑ reflux.

What condition classically resembles a corkscrew on an upper GI radiographic series? Esophageal spasm.

Barrett's esophagus is columnar metaplasia of the distal esophagus 2° to chronic acid irritation. It is associated with an ↑ risk of esophageal adenocarcinoma.

BARRett's—

Becomes
Adenocarcinoma;
Results from
Reflux

Gastroesophageal Reflux Disease (GERD)

GERD is defined as symptomatic tissue irritation and damage resulting from the backflow of gastric contents into the esophagus. Its prevalence ranges from 36% to 44% in U.S. adults; risk factors include obesity, pregnancy, and scleroderma. Transient LES relaxation is the most common etiology, but GERD can also be due to an incompetent LES, abnormally acidic gastric contents, disordered gastric motility, delayed gastric emptying, and hiatal hernia.

SIGNS AND SYMPTOMS

- Presents as heartburn (substernal burning) that typically occurs 30–90 minutes after a meal, worsens with reclining, and improves with antacid use, standing, or sitting.
- Other symptoms include sour taste ("water brash"), regurgitation, dysphagia, epigastric pain, halitosis, morning cough, laryngitis, chronic cough, and wheezing/dyspnea (which can mimic or exacerbate asthma).

DIFFERENTIAL

- PUD, infectious (CMV/candidal) or chemical esophagitis, gallbladder disease, achalasia, esophageal spasm (most common in adults).
- CAD and pericarditis.

WORKUP

- Physical exam is typically normal unless GERD is 2° to systemic disease (e.g., scleroderma).
- Upper endoscopy should be performed if the patient has longstanding symptoms or to identify and grade esophagitis or Barrett's esophagus.
- Esophageal manometry and 24-hour pH monitoring.
- Obtain an AXR, a CXR, and a barium swallow (of limited use, but can help diagnose hiatal hernia and possibly motility problems).
- Can often be treated empirically, with further testing conducted only if treatment fails.

TREATMENT

- **Lifestyle modification:** Weight loss, head-of-bed elevation, avoidance of late meals.
- **Pharmacologic management:** H₂ blockers, PPIs, promotility agents.
- **Surgical intervention:** For severe hiatal hernia or congenital cases; Nissen fundoplication is the most common intervention (since the advent of PPIs, this is performed very infrequently).
- Upper endoscopy with biopsy is useful in monitoring for Barrett's esophagus and esophageal adenocarcinoma.

COMPLICATIONS

Esophageal ulceration, esophageal stricture, aspiration of gastric contents, upper GI bleeding, Barrett's esophagus.

Peptic Ulcer Disease (PUD)

Peptic ulcers are breaks that occur in the gastric or duodenal mucosa (and in some cases the submucosa). Duodenal ulcers are five times more common than gastric ulcers. The lifetime incidence of PUD is 5–10%. Duodenal ulcers are associated with excess gastric acid production; gastric ulcers are associated with impaired mucosal defenses without acid hypersecretion. The three major causes of PUD are as follows:

- NSAID use.
- Chronic *H. pylori* infection (plays a causative role in > 90% of duodenal ulcers as well as in 60–70% of gastric ulcers).
- Acid hypersecretory states such as Zollinger-Ellison syndrome.

SIGNS AND SYMPTOMS

- PUD usually presents with chronic or periodic burning/dull/aching epigastric pain.
- Pain from duodenal ulcers can be alleviated with food and antacids but usually recurs roughly three hours later.
- Pain from gastric ulcers can worsen with food intake, leading to weight loss.
- Less common symptoms of PUD include nausea, hematemesis with "coffee-ground" or bright red emesis, blood in the stool/melena, early satiety, or pain radiating to the back.

DIFFERENTIAL

- GERD, perforation, gastric cancer, gastritis, nonulcer dyspepsia, esophageal rupture, Zollinger-Ellison syndrome.
- Pancreatitis (acute or chronic), cholecystitis, choledocholithiasis, IBS.
- Ureteral colic.
- CAD, angina, MI, aortic aneurysm.

WORKUP

- Physical exam reveals epigastric tenderness and, if active bleeding is present, a ⊕ stool guaiac. A "succussion splash" (the sound of air and fluid in a distended stomach) can also be heard as a result of gastric outlet obstruction roughly three hours after eating.
- Upper endoscopy and concurrent biopsy of the lesion can be used to rule out active bleeding and determine the presence of malignancy.
- *H. pylori* can be detected by endoscopic biopsy with a direct rapid urease test (*Campylobacter*-like organism or CLO test), urease breath tests, or serum IgG (which is less expensive but less sensitive, indicating only exposure, not active infection); all have a sensitivity of > 90%.
- Barium contrast upper GI series.

TREATMENT

- Treatment has three major goals: protecting the mucosa, decreasing acid production, and eradicating *H. pylori* infection if present (see Table 4-15).
- All exacerbating agents (NSAIDs, nicotine, alcohol) should be discontinued.
- Antacids, H$_2$ blockers (e.g., cimetidine, ranitidine, famotidine), PPIs (e.g., omeprazole, lansoprazole), and sucralfate are used to promote healing.
- All patients with symptomatic gastric ulcers for > 2 months despite therapy must undergo endoscopy with biopsy to rule out gastric adenocarcinoma.
- Refractory cases (rare) may require a surgical procedure such as vagotomy (proximal gastric vagotomy is preferred) or a highly selective truncal vagotomy with antrectomy.

Rule out Zollinger-Ellison syndrome with serum gastrin levels in cases of GERD and PUD that are refractory to treatment. Serum gastrin is usually > 500 pg/mL. Patients with Zollinger-Ellison syndrome also have a paradoxical rise in serum gastrin with secretin stimulation.

What is the most common source of hemorrhage in PUD? Erosion into the gastroduodenal artery.

Some 10% of gastric ulcers are found to harbor adenocarcinoma on biopsy.

TABLE 4-15. Treatment of *H. pylori* Infection

TREATMENT	TYPE	AGENTS	DURATION	EFFECTIVENESS
1°/first-line treatment	Quadruple therapy	PPI + bismuth subsalicylate + amoxicillin + metronidazole	1 day	95% eradication
	Triple therapy	Tetracycline (or amoxicillin) + bismuth subsalicylate + metronidazole	14 days	84–90% eradication
		PPI + amoxicillin (or metronidazole) + clarithromycin	7–14 days	88–92% eradication
		Ranitidine or PPI + amoxicillin + metronidazole	12 days	89–90% eradication
	Double therapy	Ranitidine + clarithromycin	14 days	80–85% eradication
Second-line/ refractory cases	Quadruple therapy (extended)	PPI + bismuth subsalicylate + tetracycline + metronidazole	4–7 days	Variable

PUD
Perforates into the **P**eritoneal space and **P**enetrates into adjacent organs

COMPLICATIONS

Hemorrhage, gastric outlet obstruction, perforation (usually anterior ulcers), intractable disease.

Irritable Bowel Syndrome (IBS)

A functional disorder characterized by continuous or recurring symptoms of abdominal pain and irregular bowel habits. Patients most commonly present in their teens and 20s, but since the syndrome is chronic, they can present at any age. Some 22 million people in the United States are affected, with a two- to threefold ↑ prevalence in females. The etiology is unknown but may involve a disruption in normal colonic motility and altered neurologic perceptions. GI inflammation and alterations in natural GI flora may also play a role.

Some 50–94% of IBS patients who seek medical care suffer concurrently from psychiatric disorders such as major depression or generalized anxiety.

SIGNS AND SYMPTOMS

- Abdominal pain that is relieved by a bowel movement.
- Change in frequency.
- Change in consistency.
- Alternates between constipation and diarrhea. Generally one of those states predominates.

DIFFERENTIAL

IBD, mesenteric ischemia, diverticulitis, PUD, celiac disease, colonic neoplasia, infectious or pseudomembranous colitis, gynecologic disorders.

WORKUP

- Physical exam is often unremarkable except for mild abdominal tenderness.
- The Rome II system for IBS diagnosis is a clinical assessment (see below).
- Evaluate for red flags (see below).
- Obtain CBC, electrolytes, TSH, ESR, stool cultures, abdominal films, contrast CT, and barium contrast studies to rule out other conditions.
- Manometry may be used to assess sphincter function.

TREATMENT

- **Lifestyle changes:** ↑ fiber intake and ↓ consumption of gas-producing foods (e.g., legumes).
- Psychological assurance from physicians.
- Pharmacologic therapy may include antidiarrheals (e.g., loperamide), antispasmodics, anticholinergics (e.g., dicyclomine and hyoscyamine), and antidepressants.
- Other medications include cholestyramine (for diarrhea-type IBS) and alosetron (a 5-HT$_3$ antagonist for women with severe chronic or diarrhea-predominant IBS). The availability of alosetron is limited owing to reports of ischemic colitis.

DIAGNOSTIC TESTS

ROME II CRITERIA FOR THE DIAGNOSIS OF IBS

- At least 12 weeks (continuous or recurrent; need not be consecutive), in the preceding 12 months, of abdominal discomfort/pain with two of the following:
  - Relief with defecation
  - Change in frequency of stool
  - Change in form or appearance of stool
- The Rome criteria presume no identifiable structural or biochemical explanation for these symptoms. Symptoms that may exclude a diagnosis of IBS include the following:
  - Pain interfering with sleep
  - Hematochezia
  - Unintentional weight loss
  - Fever or chills

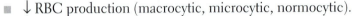

Anemia

Defined as a ↓ number of total RBCs, a ↓ in hemoglobin, or a ↓ in hematocrit. Etiologies are numerous (see Figure 4-9) but can be distinguished according to the following general mechanisms:

- ↓ RBC production (macrocytic, microcytic, normocytic).
- ↑ RBC destruction (e.g., hemolysis, which can be intracorpuscular or extracorpuscular and intravascular or extravascular).
- ↑ blood loss. Chronic loss can lead to a production problem through iron deficiency.

The first mechanism has a ↓ reticulocyte count, whereas the second and third mechanisms have an ↑ reticulocyte count.

SIGNS AND SYMPTOMS

- Usually asymptomatic, but may present with fatigue, dyspnea, dizziness, and/or exertional angina.
- Mildly anemic patients will have a normal physical exam, but those with moderate to severe anemia can have pallor of the skin and conjunctiva, a flattened jugular vein, tachycardia, and a systolic flow murmur.
- Depending on the cause, there may be other physical manifestations of disease. These include the following:

Be aware of folate deficiency 2° to medications (e.g., methotrexate, TMP-SMX, sulfa drugs).

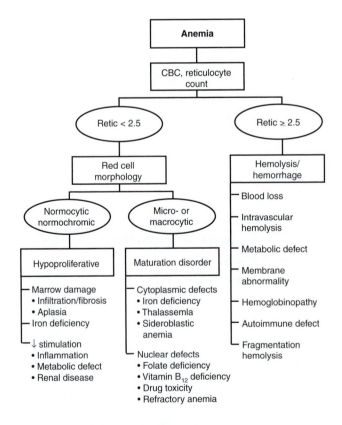

FIGURE 4-9. The physiologic classification of anemia.

(Reproduced, with permission, from Braunwald E et al. *Harrison's Principles of Internal Medicine*, 15th ed. New York: McGraw-Hill, 2001: 352.)

150

- **B$_{12}$ deficiency:** Peripheral neuropathy with loss of position and vibratory sense.
- **Blood loss** (e.g., malignancy).
- **Sickle cell disease:** Pain crisis, acute chest.
- **Hypothyroidism:** Menorrhagia, dry and coarse skin and hair, personality change, loss of lateral eyebrows, periorbital edema.
- **Severe iron deficiency:** Angular cheilitis, atrophic glossitis, ↑ bilirubin, ↑ platelet count, weak nails, koilonychia.

WORKUP

- CBC, iron studies (iron saturation and serum ferritin; see Table 4-16), serum B$_{12}$, serum folate, reticulocyte count, and peripheral blood smear.
- Coombs' test and PT/PTT to differentiate normocytic hemolytic anemias if hemolysis is found on the peripheral smear.
- Other lab tests are etiology specific and include TSH (for hypothyroidism), fecal occult blood (GI bleed), LFTs (liver disease), BUN and creatinine (renal disease), and SPEP or UPEP (multiple myeloma).
- Bone marrow biopsy is indicated if the patient presents with pancytopenia, macrocytic anemia with an unknown etiology, or a myelophthisic process (infiltration of the marrow space).

TREATMENT

Treatment depends on etiology.

ENDOCRINOLOGY

Diabetes Mellitus (DM)

Although DM is occasionally diagnosed on admission when it presents as diabetic ketoacidosis (DKA) or as hyperosmolar hyperglycemic nonketotic coma

A Schilling test can help differentiate whether the cause of B$_{12}$ deficiency is inadequate diet, lack of intrinsic factor (pernicious anemia), bacterial overgrowth, or a terminal ileal disease.

TABLE 4-16. Iron Studies in Microcytic Anemia

DISORDER	SERUM IRON	SERUM FERRITIN	TIBC	PERCENT SATURATION	HEMOGLOBIN ELECTROPHORESIS PATTERN
Iron deficiency anemia	↓	↓	↑	↓	Normal
Anemia of chronic disease	↓	↑	↓	↓	Normal
α-thalassemia	Normal	Normal	Normal	Normal	Normal for one- and two-gene deletions; abnormal for four-gene deletions.
β-thalassemia	Normal	Normal	Normal	Normal	↓ A1, ↑ A2, ↑ F
Sideroblastic anemia	↑	↑	↓	↑	Normal

(HHNK), it is most often seen as a chronic medical issue. DM is a metabolic syndrome of abnormal hyperglycemia 2° to ↓ insulin or abnormal insulin resistance coupled with inadequate levels of insulin secretion to compensate. It can be classified into two types:

- **Type 1 DM:** Formerly known as insulin-dependent diabetes mellitus (IDDM).
  - Caused by autoimmune destruction of pancreatic β-islet cells (anti-GAD and anti-insulin antibody), resulting in insulin deficiency.
  - Accounts for 10% of cases and is most commonly diagnosed in juveniles.
  - Not associated with obesity.
  - Strongly associated with HLA-DR3 and -DR4, but has a weak genetic predisposition.
  - Characterized by a lack of insulin, thus necessitating exogenous insulin.
- **Type 2 DM:** Formerly known as non-insulin-dependent diabetes mellitus (NIDDM).
  - Comprises > 85% of DM cases.
  - Usually occurs in patients > 40 years of age with abdominal obesity, but the prevalence in adolescent and young adults is increasing, presumably as a result of the epidemic of childhood obesity.
  - Has a strong genetic predisposition.
  - Results from ↑ insulin resistance in peripheral tissues, hyperinsulinemia to compensate for the resistance, and eventual burnout by the pancreatic islet cells, leading to ↓ insulin production. The mainstay of therapy is oral hypoglycemic medication, but many patients will ultimately require insulin therapy as the pancreatic islet cells burn out.

SIGNS AND SYMPTOMS

- Type 1 patients commonly present with polydipsia, polyuria (including nocturia), and polyphagia. Type 1 is also commonly associated with rapid or unexplained weight loss.
- Type 2 DM patients typically have a more insidious onset of symptoms, and at the time of diagnosis they may already have end-organ damage. Patients may complain of fatigue, candidal infections, poor wound healing, or blurred vision due to a change in the hydration status of the lens.

DIAGNOSTIC TESTS

DIAGNOSTIC CRITERIA FOR DIABETES

- **Prediabetes:** Blood glucose 100–125 mg/dL or 140–199 mg/dL after a two-hour glucose tolerance test with 75-g challenge.
- **DM:** Two of the following values met on two occasions (either the same test or two different tests):[a]
  - A two-hour glucose tolerance test > 200 mg/dL.[b]
  - A fasting (eight-hour) serum glucose > 126 mg/dL.
  - Classic symptoms (polyuria, polydipsia, or unexplained weight loss) **and** random glucose > 200 mg/dL.

[a] HbA_{1c} is not recommended for the diagnosis of diabetes but is useful for follow-up purposes.
[b] Diagnostic gold standard.

DIFFERENTIAL

- Other pancreatic disease (e.g., chronic pancreatitis, hemochromatosis, cystic fibrosis).
- Hormonal abnormalities (e.g., glucagonoma, Cushing's syndrome, acromegaly).
- Medications (e.g., corticosteroids, thiazide diuretics, phenytoin).
- Gestational DM, stress, diabetes insipidus (central or nephrogenic).

WORKUP

Laboratory testing is necessary to make a definitive diagnosis according to National Diabetes Data Group (NDDG) and World Health Organization (WHO) criteria. This includes the following:

- Urine glucose and urine ketones.
- ↑ hemoglobin A_{1c} (HbA_{1c}): Used to monitor the efficacy of and compliance with therapy over the preceding three months.

TREATMENT

- **Type 1 DM:**
  - A regular regimen of insulin injections (see Figure 4-10). Insulin may be delivered through daily subcutaneous injections or through an insulin pump, which delivers a continuous, predetermined dosage of insulin, supplemented by bolus insulin injections at mealtimes. Inhaled insulin was approved by the FDA in 2006, but its high cost has limited its use.
  - Vigilant monitoring of blood glucose at home, as tight glycemic control of glucose reduces end-organ damage.
  - Careful monitoring for end-organ damage.
- **Type 2 DM:** Lifestyle modification (weight loss, diet, and exercise) is first-line treatment to ↑ insulin sensitivity in target tissues. If glucose levels fail to normalize, start on oral hypoglycemic therapy (before resorting to insulin injections).

C-peptide is **low** in type 1 DM and **present** in type 2 DM. The C-peptide test measures endogenous insulin production.

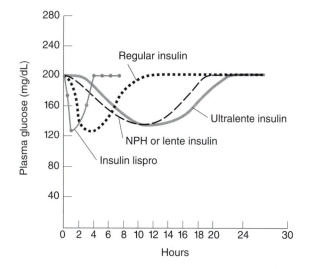

FIGURE 4-10. Effects of various insulins in a fasting diabetic patient.

(Reproduced, with permission, from Tierney LM et al. *Current Medical Diagnosis & Treatment*, 41st ed. New York: McGraw-Hill, 2002: 1220.)

- **Metformin:** First-line therapy; ↑ peripheral uptake of glucose and inhibits hepatic gluconeogenesis. Also results in weight loss. The most serious side effect is fatal lactic acidosis.
- **Sulfonylureas (e.g., glyburide, glipizide, tolbutamide):** ↑ pancreatic secretion of insulin. Side effects include weight gain and hypoglycemia.
- **Glitazones:** ↑ insulin sensitivity in the muscle and liver. Because troglitazone has been associated with hepatotoxicity, monitoring of LFTs is necessary.
- **Acarbose:** ↓ intestinal absorption of carbohydrates by inhibiting the breakdown of oligosaccharides. A major side effect is postprandial GI discomfort.

PREVENTION

- **Outpatient diabetes management** includes encouraging a regular diet and exercise; monitoring HbA_{1c} every 3–4 months (goal < 7%, although tighter control to < 6% or 6.5% is preferred and may be indicated in some individuals); a yearly spot microalbumin-to-creatinine ratio to monitor kidney function (goal < 30 μg/mg); regular BP monitoring (goal < 130/80); yearly lipid monitoring (goal LDL < 100, TG < 150, HDL > 40); low-dose aspirin for patients > 40 years of age with other cardiac risk factors; a yearly dilated retinal exam; and a podiatric exam yearly or as needed.
- Regardless of serum cholesterol level, statin therapy ↓ the risk of major vascular events.

COMPLICATIONS

Acute complications of DM are as follows:

- **Type 1 DM: DKA/hyperglycemia-induced crisis.** Lack of insulin causes the liver to turn fat into ketone bodies, a fuel used primarily by the brain.
    - Precipitated by the "five I's": Infections, Ischemia (MI), Iatrogenic (alcohol, corticosteroids, thiazide diuretics), Intra-abdominal processes (pancreatitis, cholecystitis), and Insulin deficiency (failure to take enough insulin).
    - Signs/Sx: Patients often present with abdominal pain, vomiting, Kussmaul respirations (a rhythmic, gasping, and very deep breathing pattern; "air hunger"), and a fruity/acetone breath odor. Patients are severely dehydrated with many electrolyte abnormalities (e.g., hypokalemia, hypophosphatemia, ↑ anion gap metabolic acidosis) and may also develop mental status changes such as somnolence, stupor, coma, and death if not rapidly treated.
    - Tx: Aggressive IV fluids, potassium, and insulin to correct electrolyte abnormalities; treatment of the initiating event.
- **Type 2 DM: HHNK coma.**
    - Precipitated by acute stress and dehydration.
    - Signs/Sx: Presents as profound dehydration, mental status changes, and an extremely high plasma glucose (> 600 mg/dL) without ketoacidosis. May be fatal.
    - Tx: IV fluids, insulin, and aggressive electrolyte replacement.

Both type 1 and type 2 DM lead to the following **chronic complications** as the disease progresses:

- **Retinopathy (proliferative or nonproliferative):** Appears when diabetes has been present for at least 3–5 years. Some 98% of type 1 and 80% of type 2 patients eventually have evidence of disease. Preventive measures

What is the Somogyi effect? Nocturnal hypoglycemia leads to ↑ morning glucose as a result of the release of counterregulatory hormones. Treat patients by decreasing rather than increasing nighttime insulin.

What is the dawn phenomenon? Early-morning hyperglycemia caused by ↓ effectiveness of insulin at that time.

include laser photocoagulation and tight control of blood glucose (HbA_{1c} < 7%) and BP.

- **Diabetic nephropathy:** Glomerular damage that initially manifests as microalbuminuria, which over time leads to compensatory hyperfiltration and ends with permanent loss of function. Diabetes is the most common cause of adult kidney failure (necessitating dialysis) in the developed world. Therapy with ACEIs prevents microalbuminuria.
- **Neuropathy:** Peripheral, symmetric, sensorimotor neuropathy resulting in foot trauma and diabetic ulcers. Treat with preventive foot care, analgesics, and TCAs.
- **Macrovascular damage:** Cardiovascular, cerebrovascular, and peripheral vascular disease. Cardiovascular disease is the most common cause of death in diabetic patients.

REFERENCE

The Diabetes Control and Complications Trial Research Group. The effect of intensive treatment of diabetes on the development and progression of long-term complications in insulin-dependent diabetes mellitus. *NEJM* 329:977–986, 1993. A landmark article in which type 1 DM patients with absent or mild retinopathy at baseline were randomized to intensive or conventional blood glucose management. A statistically significant ↓ in the appearance or progression of retinopathy, nephropathy, and neuropathy was demonstrated.

INFECTIOUS DISEASE

Fever of Unknown Origin (FUO)

FUO is one of the more vexing dilemmas in internal medicine. It is defined as a fever of at least 38.3°C (101°F) for at least three weeks, with an undetermined source after one week of workup in the hospital. In adults, infections and cancer account for > 60% of cases. Broadly, FUO can be divided into four etiologic categories:

In what percentage of FUO is no cause identified? In some 10–15% of cases.

- **Infectious:** TB and endocarditis (e.g., HACEK organisms) are the most common systemic infections causing FUO, whereas occult abscess is the most common cause of localized infections. *Acinetobacter*, MRSA, and coagulase-⊖ staphylococci cause many nosocomial infections.
- **Neoplastic:** Leukemias and lymphomas are the most common cancers that cause FUO; hepatic and renal cell carcinomas are the most common solid tumors.
- **Autoimmune:** Responsible for 15% of cases. Includes Still's disease, temporal arteritis, RA, SLE, and polyarteritis nodosa.
- **Miscellaneous:** Includes drug fever, cirrhosis, alcoholic hepatitis, granulomatous hepatitis, sarcoidosis, hyperthyroidism, Addison's disease, Whipple's disease, recurrent pulmonary embolism, factitious fever, and IBD.

WORKUP

- Obtain a complete history and physical; rule out sepsis.
- Obtain a CBC with differential, ESR, LFTs, and multiple blood cultures.
- Imaging studies may include CXR, CT, and MRI.
- Additional tests, depending on suspicion, include echocardiography (e.g., TEE), bone marrow biopsy, skin biopsy, lymph node biopsy, liver biopsy, and exploratory laparotomy.

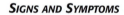

TREATMENT

- Start broad-spectrum antibiotics empirically in severely ill patients, but discontinue if the fever does not abate.
- Avoid empiric steroids except for vasculitis.

Human Immunodeficiency Virus (HIV)/Acquired Immunodeficiency Syndrome (AIDS)

Which virus is more infectious: HIV or hepatitis B? Hepatitis B by 50 to 100 times.

HIV affects five million new patients annually worldwide, with > 40 million people currently infected and 20 million fatalities attributed to AIDS since 1981. In the United States, symptomatic disease most commonly presents around age 30. HIV is more prevalent in males than in females, but as transmission via heterosexual contact ↑, the incidence in women is likewise rising. HIV is spread almost exclusively through the transmission of bodily fluids. Risk factors for HIV infection include the following:

- Unprotected anal, oral, and vaginal sex.
- Needle sharing and accidental sticks (or mucocutaneous exposure).
- Multiple transfusions of blood (and blood products).
- Infants of HIV-⊕ mothers are also at risk.

SIGNS AND SYMPTOMS

- Many HIV-infected individuals are initially asymptomatic.
- Some 50–60% of HIV-infected patients may present with flulike symptoms (fever, malaise, rash, headache, sore throat, generalized lymphadenopathy) during acute seroconversion.

WORKUP

- **Serum screening:** Both ELISA and the Western blot for HIV must be ⊕. Further testing involves HIV viral load (the number of viral RNA copies per milliliter of blood) and CD4 count.
- **Infectious screens:** PPD; VDRL; antibodies against CMV, toxoplasmosis, HBV, HAV, and HCV.
- Additional tests include CBC, electrolytes, LFTs, creatinine, CXR, Pap smear, and a pregnancy test for women (if indicated).

CRITERIA FOR THE DIAGNOSIS OF AIDS

AIDS is defined as either a CD4 count of < 200 cells/mm³ or the presence of an AIDS-defining illness.

- **AIDS-defining illnesses** include CMV infection, *Mycobacterium avium-intracellulare* infection, progressive multifocal leukoencephalopathy (PML), HSV esophagitis or recurrent oral/genital lesions, candidal esophagitis, AIDS wasting syndrome (cachexia), invasive fungal infection, toxoplasmosis, PCP, Kaposi's sarcoma, lymphoma (CNS), TB, and pneumococcal pneumonia.

- Additional opportunistic infections include candidal vaginitis, VZV reactivation, oral hairy leukoplakia, and chronic diarrhea from *Cryptosporidium, Microspora,* and *Isospora.*

TREATMENT

Treatment depends primarily on CD4 count and viral load.

- Begin highly active antiretroviral therapy (HAART) if the CD4 count is < 500 cells/mm^3 or if the patient has an AIDS-defining illness. The optimal timing of treatment initiation is still controversial.
- Treatment regimens usually include a protease inhibitor (e.g., saquinavir, ritonavir, indinavir) and two nucleoside analogs (e.g., AZT, ddI, 3TC, D4T).
- Once-daily and reduced-pill regimens are becoming available for patients for whom adherence is an issue. Patients should not be treated with HAART if adherence is an issue. Ninety percent adherence is probably more likely to induce new resistance patterns than 20% adherence.
- 1° prophylaxis of various opportunistic infections is indicated if CD4 counts fall below particular levels or if symptoms are present (see Table 4-17). Prophylaxis can be discontinued when the CD4 count ↑ adequately.

TABLE 4-17. Preventable Opportunistic Infections Associated with AIDS

ORGANISM	INDICATIONS FOR PROPHYLAXIS
PCP	CD4 < 200, oral candidiasis, or unexplained fever for > 2 weeks.
S. pneumoniae	CD4 ≤ 200.
Toxoplasma gondii	CD4 < 100 and IgG to Toxoplasma.
Mycobacterium avium–intracellulare	CD4 < 75.
Histoplasma capsulatum	CD4 < 100 in endemic areas.
Candida albicans	CD4 < 50.
Cryptococcus neoformans	CD4 < 50.
Mycobacterium tuberculosis (TB)	Skin test > 5 mm, active TB contact, or prior ⊕ skin test without treatment.
Influenza virus	All patients (yearly).
VZV	Significant exposure without a history of disease or vaccination.
HBV	Susceptible anti-HBcAg-⊖ patients.
HAV	Susceptible anti-HAV-⊖ patients.

HIV TESTING PROTOCOL

The **ELISA** test is a general HIV screening measure that detects the presence of anti-HIV antibodies in the bloodstream. The test has high sensitivity but moderate specificity, leading to numerous false ⊕s. Those with a ⊕ ELISA test must have a follow-up **Western blot** to confirm HIV infection.

COMPLICATIONS

Most patients recover from the initial retroviral syndrome and enter the latency phase, during which they are asymptomatic despite high levels of viral replication. Eventually the patient's immune system cannot control the infection, at which point CD4 counts fall, and AIDS and opportunistic infections ensue.

Tuberculosis (TB)

What is the most common extrapulmonary site of TB infection? The kidney, but TB can affect nearly every organ system.

After declining in the 1980s, infection with *Mycobacterium tuberculosis* is once again increasing in prevalence. TB primarily affects the lungs but may involve other organ systems, with presentations ranging from cough to meningismus. Worldwide, it is responsible for more infectious disease deaths than any other single agent, and two billion individuals are carriers. Spread is via infectious airborne droplets that lead to 1° and then 2° phases of infection. Risk factors include the following:

■ Immunosuppression (e.g., HIV, solid organ transplantation, TNF inhibitors, carcinoma), alcoholism, preexisting lung disease (e.g., silicosis), diabetes, CKD/dialysis, old age, homelessness, malnourishment/low body weight, and crowded living conditions with poor ventilation (e.g., military barracks).
■ Immigrants from Africa, Latin America, Asia, and Caribbean countries as well as persons with known exposure to infected patients are also at ↑ risk.

SIGNS AND SYMPTOMS

CXR findings in active pulmonary TB:

■ *Enlarged, calcified mediastinal lymph nodes and calcified pulmonary granulomas (Ghon complex) in the apical and posterior areas of the upper lobes of the lungs*
■ *Apical pleural scarring*
■ *Cavitary lesions*

■ Symptoms of active pulmonary TB include productive cough, hemoptysis, weakness, anorexia, weight loss, malaise, night sweats, and fever. Symptoms can resemble those of bacterial pneumonia.
■ Physical exam reveals dullness to percussion with ↓ tactile fremitus if effusions are present.
■ Extrapulmonary manifestations include scrofula (cervical lymphadenopathy) and Pott's disease (spinal spread).

DIFFERENTIAL

Pneumonia (bacterial, fungal, viral), other atypical mycobacterial infections, HIV infection, HIV-related opportunistic infections (e.g., PCP), lung abscess, lung cancer, sarcoidosis, UTI.

WORKUP

■ Presumptively diagnosed with CXR and a ⊕ acid-fast stain of the sputum. Culture of *M. tuberculosis* from sputum may take several weeks given its slow incubation period.
■ A ⊕ PPD test is indicative only of previous exposure to *M. tuberculosis* and may not be present in immunocompromised individuals (e.g., HIV-infected patients) who have TB.

TREATMENT

■ For active TB, antimycobacterial therapy should be instituted immediately and the patient should be isolated.
■ Vitamin B_6 (pyridoxine) is commonly given with INH to prevent the common side effect of peripheral neuritis.
■ For outpatients, directly observed therapy may be necessary to ensure adherence and prevent drug resistance.
■ Respiratory isolation should be instituted when TB is suspected.
■ Prophylactic treatment for HIV-⊕ and HIV-⊖ patients < 35 years of age who show conversion to a ⊕ PPD but who have no symptoms of active pulmonary TB on CXR include INH therapy for nine months. Many physicians forgo INH prophylaxis in patients > 35 years of age because the risk of INH-induced liver toxicity ↑ with age.

REFERENCE

Small PM, Fujiwara PA. Management of tuberculosis in the United States. *NEJM* 345:189–200, 2001. An excellent review article on the treatment of TB, including treatment in drug-resistant and HIV-associated cases. Also provides a summary of tuberculin skin reactions and patient compliance issues.

Urinary Tract Infection (UTI)

UTIs are most commonly caused by ascending infections and occur 30 times more frequently in women than in men (due to a short urethra). UTIs in men

TB is a reportable disease according to local and state health departments.

TB multidrug treatment regimens:

■ *Induction phase: INH + pyrazinamide + rifampin + ethambutol for eight weeks*
■ *Standard full course: INH + rifampin for nine months*

Depending on sensitivity, short-course regimens (postinduction) include:

■ *INH + rifampin (twice weekly) for six months*
■ *INH + rifapentine (once weekly) for six months*

HIGH-YIELD FACTS

INTERNAL MEDICINE

DIAGNOSTIC TESTS

PPD TESTING FOR TB

PPD is injected intradermally on the volar surface of the arm. The transverse length of induration is measured at 48–72 hours. BCG vaccination typically renders a patient PPD ⊕ for at least one year. The size of induration that indicates a ⊕ test for particular populations is as follows:

■ **> 5 mm**: HIV or risk factors, close TB contacts, CXR evidence of TB.

■ **> 10 mm**: Indigent/homeless, immigrants from developing nations, IV drug users, those with chronic illness, residents of health and correctional institutions.

■ **> 15 mm**: All others.

A ⊖ reaction with ⊖ controls implies anergy from immunosuppression, old age, or malnutrition and thus does not rule out TB.

Severe sepsis starting from a UTI must be considered in any elderly patient with altered mental status.

are usually due to congenital abnormalities or, in elderly men, to prostatic enlargement. Risk factors also include sexual intercourse, diaphragm and/or spermicide use, urinary tract instrumentation (e.g., Foley catheters), DM, and immunosuppression. Common microbial causes are listed in Table 4-18.

SIGNS AND SYMPTOMS

- Presents with dysuria, suprapubic pain, nocturia, and ↑ frequency and urgency.
- Patients with pyelonephritis can have fever, chills, flank pain, and CVA tenderness.

DIFFERENTIAL

- **Common:** Vaginitis, vulvar HSV lesions, allergic reactions, nephrolithiasis, TOA, infected ovarian cyst, appendicitis, epidural abscess, diskitis, vertebral osteomyelitis.
- **Rare:** Bladder cancer, mycobacterial infection.

WORKUP

- **UA:** ⊕ leukocyte esterase and nitrites, ↑ urine pH (if *Proteus* is present), and hematuria. Microscopic exam will show pyuria (> 2–5 WBCs/hpf) and possibly WBC casts (in pyelonephritis). Nitrites are the most specific test.
- **Culture:** The diagnostic gold standard is > 100,000 colony-forming units

UTI agents—

SEEKS PP

S. *saprophyticus*
E. *coli*
Enterobacter
Klebsiella
Serratia
Proteus
Pseudomonas

TABLE 4-18. GU Tract Infections

CONDITION	COMMON ORGANISMS	TREATMENT

Uncomplicated UTI/pyelonephritis	*E. coli* (50–80%), *Staphylococcus saprophyticus* (10–30%), *Klebsiella pneumoniae* (8–10%), *Proteus mirabilis*	**Acute, uncomplicated UTI:** Fluoroquinolone or TMP-SMX DS (× 3 days), cephalexin (× 5 days), or nitrofurantoin (× 7 days). Always treat men for seven days.
		Recurrent UTI:
		  ■ **Related to coitus:** TMP-SMX DS (× 1 dose, postcoital).
		  ■ **Unrelated to coitus:** TMP-SMX, cephalexin, or nitrofurantoin (× 3–7 days). May be continued for six months for prophylaxis.
		Acute, uncomplicated pyelonephritis (outpatient): Fluoroquinolone or amoxicillin/clavulanate (× 4 days).
		Acute, uncomplicated pyelonephritis (inpatient): IV fluoroquinolone or ampicillin/sulbactam until afebrile 24–48 hours; then PO ciprofloxacin (× 14 days).

Complicated UTI	*E. coli* (30–60%), *Proteus* (10%), *Klebsiella, Serratia* spp., *Pseudomonas aeruginosa, Enterococcus faecalis, Enterobacter* spp.	High-dose fluoroquinolone (ciprofloxacin 1000 mg QD, levofloxacin 300 mg QD, or ofloxacin 300 mg BID). Treat until asymptomatic and then continue for 2–14 days.

of bacteria per milliliter of clean-catch urine; however, urine cultures are reserved for recurrent UTIs, pyelonephritis, complicated UTIs, and those in men, pregnant women, and immunocompromised patients.

■ CT imaging may be helpful in delineating the extent of disease.

TREATMENT

Treatment is initially empiric (see Table 4-18).

Sepsis

Septic shock and multiorgan dysfunction are the most common causes of death in patients with sepsis, and rapid diagnosis is critical. Knowledge of relevant nomenclature is also necessary:

■ **Bacteremia:** Refers to the presence of bacteria in the blood.
■ **Systemic inflammatory response syndrome (SIRS):** Presents with fever/hypothermia, tachypnea, tachycardia, and leukocytosis/leukopenia.
■ **Sepsis:** Defined as suspected or proven infection plus SIRS.
■ **Severe sepsis:** Sepsis with organ dysfunction (hypotension, hypoxemia, oliguria, metabolic acidosis, thrombocytopenia, or mental status changes).
■ **Septic shock:** Severe sepsis with hypotension despite adequate fluid resuscitation (see the Emergency Medicine chapter for more details on septic shock).

SIGNS AND SYMPTOMS

With SIRS, expect (1) a body temperature > 38°C or < 36°C; (2) a heart rate > 90 bpm; (3) tachypnea as manifested by a respiratory rate > 20 breaths per minute or hyperventilation as indicated by a $PaCO_2$ of < 32 mmHg; and (4) an alteration in the WBC count, such as a count > 12,000/mm^3, a count < 4000/mm^3, or the presence of > 10% immature neutrophils ("bands").

WORKUP

Directed at finding a source of infection—blood and urine cultures, CXR, stool for *C. difficile*.

TREATMENT

■ Therapy should ideally be provided early and includes **aggressive fluid resuscitation, lung-protective ventilation, broad-spectrum antibiotics,** possibly **steroids, tight glucose control,** and possibly **activated protein C.**
■ Broad-spectrum antibiotics should be aimed at covering organisms such as MRSA, penicillin-resistant pneumococci, fungi, and gram-positive bacteria but should be adjusted once an organism and its drug sensitivities are determined.

REFERENCE

Russell JA. Management of sepsis. *NEJM* 355(16):1699–1713, 2006. An excellent overview of the pathophysiology and treatment of early and late sepsis.

Treat asymptomatic bacteriuria in patients with chronic pyelonephritis. Do not treat asymptomatic bacteriuria in patients with indwelling catheters.

Chronic complicated UTIs show ↓ responsiveness to antibiotics and may result from structural abnormalities/changes or functional disorders, pregnancy, DM, AIDS, indwelling catheters, or renal obstruction.

Systemic Lupus Erythematosus (SLE)

SLE is an inflammatory autoimmune disorder that primarily strikes young women, with a female-to-male ratio of 8:1. It is a multisystem disease that is characterized by recurrent exacerbations ("flares") and remissions due to autoantibody formation and immune complex deposition. There is a familial concordance and a correlation with HLA-DR2 and -DR3. African-American women are at especially high risk.

Some 90% of SLE patients are women of childbearing age.

The presence of antiphospholipid antibody (including lupus anticoagulant and anticardiolipin antibody) ↑ the risk of stillbirth and abortion in pregnancy.

SIGNS AND SYMPTOMS

SLE is one of the "great imitator" diseases, with famously protean manifestations as outlined in the mnemonic **SOAP BRAIN MD** and in Figure 4-11.

DIFFERENTIAL

■ Drug-induced lupus and mixed connective tissue disease (MCTD) can present with multisystem involvement and autoantibodies.
■ Discoid lupus presents with the characteristic skin manifestations without systemic involvement.
■ Also consider epilepsy, dermatitis, MS, psychiatric disorders, porphyria, and ITP.

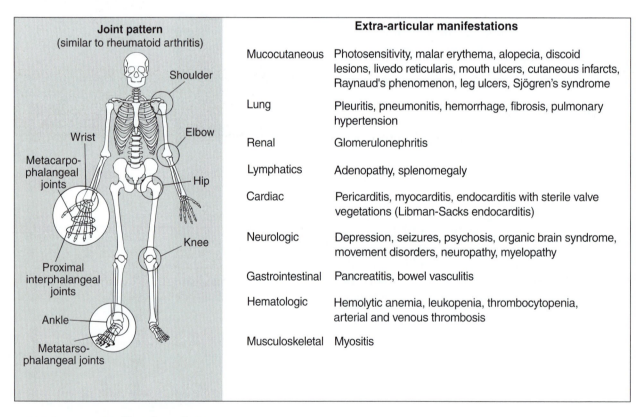

Joint pattern (similar to rheumatoid arthritis)	Extra-articular manifestations	
Shoulder, Elbow, Wrist, Metacarpophalangeal joints, Hip, Proximal interphalangeal joints, Knee, Ankle, Metatarsophalangeal joints	Mucocutaneous	Photosensitivity, malar erythema, alopecia, discoid lesions, livedo reticularis, mouth ulcers, cutaneous infarcts, Raynaud's phenomenon, leg ulcers, Sjögren's syndrome
	Lung	Pleuritis, pneumonitis, hemorrhage, fibrosis, pulmonary hypertension
	Renal	Glomerulonephritis
	Lymphatics	Adenopathy, splenomegaly
	Cardiac	Pericarditis, myocarditis, endocarditis with sterile valve vegetations (Libman-Sacks endocarditis)
	Neurologic	Depression, seizures, psychosis, organic brain syndrome, movement disorders, neuropathy, myelopathy
	Gastrointestinal	Pancreatitis, bowel vasculitis
	Hematologic	Hemolytic anemia, leukopenia, thrombocytopenia, arterial and venous thrombosis
	Musculoskeletal	Myositis

FIGURE 4-11. Manifestations of SLE.

- The American Rheumatism Association criteria for SLE (1997) require that patients fulfill at least four of the manifestations outlined in the **SOAP BRAIN MD** mnemonic.
- Because of the variable presentation of SLE, it may take several years before a formal diagnosis can be made. Recently revised criteria suggest the identification of three manifestations, with confirmatory antibody screening testing as a second step.
- Antibody tests are the best screening tool for this disease and other autoimmune disorders (see Table 4-19). Most patients with SLE will have a ⊕ ANA; however, many other disorders are ANA ⊕, including Sjögren's syndrome, scleroderma, RA, polymyositis, and dermatomyositis.
- Other tests routinely performed are complement system levels (↓ during flares), electrolytes, CBC, and renal function measures (serum creatinine, spot urine protein/creatinine ratios).

TREATMENT

There is no single treatment for SLE, as treatment depends largely on the systemic manifestations of the disease. Patients are initially treated with NSAIDs, which effectively treat serositis and arthritis.

- Steroids are used for flares.
- Disease-modifying antirheumatic drugs (DMARDs) are used preventively to ↓ the incidence of flares and ↓ the need for steroids. Hydroxychloroquine (Plaquenil), methotrexate, cyclophosphamide, and azathioprine are used in progressive or refractory cases. Hydroxychloroquine is especially effective in treating arthritis, skin disease, and fatigue.
- Cyclophosphamide (Cytoxan) and mycophenolate (CellCept) with steroids are effective for lupus nephritis.
- Pregnant women with prior fetal loss and the presence of antiphospholipid antibodies should receive low-dose heparin.
- Drug-induced lupus resolves when the offending medication is discontinued.

COMPLICATIONS

Survival with treatment ranges from 90% to 95% at two years and up to 75% at 20 years; mortality results from end-organ damage (especially renal failure) and opportunistic infections 2° to immunosuppression.

GENERAL MEDICINE

Outpatient Screening

Table 4-20 summarizes suggested outpatient screening measures in the United States.

Systemic manifestations of SLE—

SOAP BRAIN MD

Serositis (pleuritis, pericarditis, myocarditis)
Oral aphthous ulcers
Arthritis (especially small joints of hand/wrist)
Photosensitivity
Blood abnormalities (hemolytic anemia, thrombocytopenia, leukopenia, lymphopenia)
Renal disease (proteinuria or urinary cellular casts)
ANA ⊕
Immunologic abnormalities (⊕ anti-dsDNA, ⊕ anti-Sm, antiphospholipid)
Neurologic abnormalities (lupus cerebritis; seizures or psychosis)
Malar rash (photosensitive butterfly-shaped rash on face)
Discoid rash

HIGH-YIELD FACTS

INTERNAL MEDICINE

TABLE 4-19. Common Autoantibodies and Associated Conditions

SERUM TEST	RELATED CONDITIONS AND PREVALENCE OF FINDINGS
RF	RA (80%), SLE (15–35%), Sjögren's syndrome (75–95%), MCTD (50–60%). **RF may also be detected in the setting of viral infection, syphilis, TB, sarcoidosis, and malignancy.**
Anti–cyclic citrullinated peptide 2 (CCP2)	RA (often precedes diagnosis by several years).
ANA	Drug-induced lupus (100%), SLE (99%), scleroderma (97%), Sjögren's syndrome (96%), MCTD (93%), polymyositis/dermatomyositis (78%), RA (40%). **ANA may also be detected in 5% of healthy adults.**
Anti-dsDNA	Very specific for SLE (60%), and titers parallel disease activity (especially renal disease).
Antihistone	Drug-induced lupus (90%), SLE (50%).
Anti-Sm	Very specific for SLE (20–30%).
Anti-Ro (anti-SS-A)	Sjögren's syndrome (75%), SLE (40%; ↑ risk of neonatal SLE).
Anti-La (anti-SS-B)	Sjögren's syndrome (40%), SLE (10–15%; ↑ risk of neonatal SLE).
Antiphospholipid (anticardiolipin or anti-β2 glycoprotein 1 and antiprothrombin)	1° antiphospholipid syndrome or 2° disease (e.g., SLE).
Anticentromeric	Scleroderma (22–36%).
Anti-topo-I (anti-Scl-70)	Scleroderma (22–40%).
Anti-Jo1	Polymyositis/dermatomyositis (30%).
Anti–thyroid peroxidase	Hashimoto's thyroiditis.
Anti–smooth muscle	Autoimmune hepatitis.
Antimitochondrial	1° biliary cirrhosis.
c-ANCA/antiproteinase	Wegener's granulomatosis (90%).
p-ANCA/anti-MPO	Wegener's granulomatosis (10%). **Also detected in crescentic GN, microscopic polyangiitis, and Churg-Strauss syndrome.**
Anti-GBM	Goodpasture's syndrome.
Antitransglutaminase	Celiac disease.
Complement C3/C4 (↓ levels)	SLE, cryoglobulinemia. **Also detected in GN.**
HLA-B27	Ankylosing spondylitis (50–95%), reactive arthritis (Reiter's syndrome) (50–80%), psoriatic arthritis (50–80%), IBD-associated arthritis (50–80%).

TABLE 4-20. Outpatient Screening Measures

TARGET	METHOD	INTERVAL/AGE RANGE	RECOMMENDING ORGANIZATION[a]
Colon cancer	Flexible sigmoidoscopy	Every 3–5 years in patients > 50 years of age.	ACS
	Fecal occult blood testing	Yearly in patients > 50 years of age.	USPTF
	Digital rectal examination	Yearly in patients > 40 years of age.	ACS
	Colonoscopy	Every 10 years in patients > 50 years of age.	ACG
Prostate and breast cancer	Prostate examination	Yearly in patients > 50 years of age.	ACS
	Breast self-examination	Monthly after age 20 if desired by the patient (no consensus).	ACS
	Clinician breast exam	Every three years for patients 20–40 years of age; yearly for patients > 40 years of age.	USPTF
	Mammography	Every 12–33 months for patients $\geq$ 40 years of age.	NIH
Gynecologic cancer	Pap smear	Yearly for sexually active patients or those 18–65 years of age. Every three years after three normal smears.	USPTF
	Pelvic exam	Every 1–3 years in patients 20–40 years of age; yearly in patients $\geq$ 40 years of age.	USPTF
	Endometrial tissue biopsy	At menopause.	ACS
Lung cancer (smokers)	CXR (controversial)	Periodic.	
	High-resolution CT (under study)		
STDs (high-risk patients)	Gonorrhea culture	Periodic.	USPTF
	Chlamydia culture	Periodic.	USPTF
	Syphilis (RPR/VDRL)	Periodic.	USPTF
	HIV serology	Periodic.	USPTF
TB (high-risk immunosuppressed patients, immigrants)	PPD	Yearly.	USPTF
CAD	Total serum cholesterol	Every five years in patients $\geq$ 35 years of age.	USPTF

[a]ACS = American Cancer Society, ACG = American College of Gastroenterology (2000), USPTF = U.S. Preventive Services Task Force (1996).

Because internal medicine covers so many domains, you should set achievable goals in your bid to attain a solid fund of knowledge. The following is a list of core topics that you are likely to encounter in the course of your medicine rotation and on a shelf examination.

- **Cardiology:**
  - Acute coronary syndrome (e.g., angina pectoris, unstable angina, Prinzmetal's angina; see Emergency Medicine)
  - Acute myocardial infarction (see Emergency Medicine)
  - Arrhythmias (e.g., bradyarrhythmias, tachyarrhythmias, atrial fibrillation)
  - Cardiomyopathies
  - Congestive heart failure
  - Hypertension
  - Infective endocarditis, myocarditis, and pericarditis
  - Syncope
  - Valvular heart disease
- **Pulmonology:**
  - Acute respiratory failure
  - Asthma (see Emergency Medicine)
  - Chronic cough
  - Chronic obstructive pulmonary disease
  - Interstitial lung disease
  - Lung cancer
  - Pleural effusion
  - Pneumonia
  - Pneumothorax (see Emergency Medicine)
  - Pulmonary embolism (see Emergency Medicine)
  - Pulmonary nodules and masses
- **Nephrology:**
  - Acid-base disturbances
  - Acute renal failure
  - Chronic renal failure and uremia
  - Electrolyte disorders (e.g., hyponatremia and hypernatremia, hypo- and hyperkalemia)
  - Glomerular disease
  - Nephrolithiasis
- **Gastroenterology:**
  - Abdominal pain
  - Diarrhea
  - Disorders of swallowing (e.g., achalasia, esophageal cancer)
  - Gastritis
  - Gastroesophageal reflux disease
  - Gastrointestinal bleeding (see Surgery)
  - Gastrointestinal cancer
  - Hepatic disease (e.g., cirrhosis, hepatic encephalopathy, hepatitis, portal hypertension)
  - Inflammatory bowel disease (e.g., Crohn's disease, ulcerative colitis; see Surgery)
  - Irritable bowel syndrome
  - Malabsorption
  - Pancreatitis (see Surgery)
  - Peptic ulcer disease

- **Hematology:**
  - Anemia, including hemolytic anemias
  - Coagulation disorders (e.g., excessive bleeding and hypercoagulable states)
  - Neutropenic fever
- **Oncology:**
  - Breast cancer
  - Leukemias
  - Lymphadenopathy
  - Lymphomas
  - Paraneoplastic syndromes
  - Prostate cancer
- **Endocrinology:**
  - Adrenal disorders (e.g., hyperaldosteronism, hypoaldosteronism, Addison's disease, Cushing's disease), diabetes insipidus (central and nephrogenic)
  - Diabetes mellitus (types 1 and 2), including diabetic ketoacidosis
  - Hyper- and hypocalcemia
  - Hyperlipidemias (e.g., familial hypercholesterolemia)
  - Gonadal disorders (e.g., testicular feminization, 5α-reductase deficiency)
  - Nutritional disorders (e.g., osteomalacia, scurvy, pellagra, beriberi)
  - Pituitary disorders (e.g., acromegaly)
  - Thyroid disorders (e.g., Graves' disease, Hashimoto's thyroiditis)
- **Infectious disease:**
  - Animal-borne diseases (e.g., Lyme disease, rabies, malaria)
  - CNS infections (e.g., meningitis, encephalitis; see Neurology)
  - Fever of unknown origin
  - HIV and AIDS
  - Intra-abdominal infections (e.g., spontaneous bacterial peritonitis)
  - Respiratory tract infections (e.g., pneumonia, URI)
  - Sexually transmitted diseases (e.g., chlamydia, syphilis, gonorrhea, HSV)
  - Tuberculosis
  - Urinary tract infection
- **Rheumatology:**
  - Fibromyalgia
  - Gout and pseudogout
  - Osteoarthritis
  - Rheumatoid arthritis
  - Sarcoidosis
  - Septic arthritis
  - Seronegative spondyloarthropathies (e.g., ankylosing spondylitis)
  - Systemic lupus erythematosus
  - Vasculitis (e.g., polyarteritis nodosa, temporal arteritis)
- **General medicine:**
  - Health maintenance issues
  - Medical ethics issues
  - Outpatient management
  - Outpatient screening

CORE CLERKSHIPS IN

Neurology

Welcome to your neurology rotation! In this highly academic and scientific field, you will discover one of the things neurologists love most to do: talk, talk, and talk about neurology. So get ready for lengthy rounds in which you'll discuss detailed differentials, neuroscience, and the latest research while simultaneously attempting to answer the ever-present question, "Where's the lesion?" Of course, you won't be expected to learn all of neurology in a few weeks—so, as is the case in many other rotations, your questions will be more important than your answers.

"Where's the lesion?"

How Do I Excel in Neurology?

Neurology rotations differ notably from site to site, so the first thing you need to find out is how your responsibilities will be divided among inpatient wards, outpatient clinics, consult-liaison, and neurosurgery. Inpatient neurology tends to be like medicine: You get to manage patients with neurologic diseases who frequently have active medical issues as well. For this reason, you'll need to know your medicine while managing patients on the neurology wards. Day-to-day activities include following labs and neuro exams, writing notes, and playing a supportive role in management. The workload tends to depend on the number of students per team, the presence of interns, the number of admissions, and the inpatient census. To make the most out of this rotation, don't hesitate to ask your residents/attendings on the first day: Who evaluates me? What are my responsibilities? Whom can I ask for help? What is the call schedule, and is it home call or in house? For more details on how the day is often set up, refer to Chapter 1.

One of your primary goals during this rotation should be to learn how to conduct and present a complete screening neurologic exam. In addition, you should plan to read about your patients and understand the neuroanatomy, pathophysiology, and treatment involved in their care. **Always** try to trace the neuroanatomic pathways that might underlie your patient's symptoms so that you can better localize the lesion.

Patients on this rotation tend to be admitted for ischemic strokes and hemorrhages, status epilepticus, meningitis and encephalitis, Guillain-Barré syndrome (GBS), myasthenic crises, and acute changes in mental status of unknown etiology, with some variation from hospital to hospital. Trauma and tumor patients are often managed by neurosurgery. Outpatient clinics are a great place to see a spectrum of common and uncommon nonacute diseases, such as peripheral neuropathies, MS, migraine, and movement disorders. If you have a particular area of interest, such as neuromuscular disorders, you may want to find out if you can spend a few afternoons each week seeing patients in clinic and observing electrophysiologic testing. In general, you are encouraged to seek out the full range of interesting experiences neurology offers. Your residents and attending will likely be impressed by your initiative, and you will benefit from the experience.

Other ground rules, as always, are to be prompt and courteous, take good care of your patients, try to know them better than anyone else, read about their diseases, ask questions, give clear presentations, and demonstrate your interest in the subject. Focus on the basics by reviewing neuroanatomy and studying disease presentation, workup, and treatment. You shouldn't be expected to un-

HIGH-YIELD FACTS

NEUROLOGY

derstand obscure diseases or to track down remote articles (unless your patient happens to have a rare and interesting condition), but if you find yourself researching a case out of genuine interest, your residents and fellow students might appreciate seeing a report or an article that you have uncovered. At the very least, your residents will notice your effort and quite possibly learn from you. You may also want to develop a list of course objectives that fit your future aspirations—perhaps focusing on the execution of the neuro exam and on a basic understanding of the common neurologic diseases.

Finally, don't forget to bring your penlight, stethoscope, reflex hammer (three key tools), eye chart, tuning fork (512 Hz for testing hearing; 256 Hz for vibration testing), pins for pain sensation testing (don't reuse!), and cotton swabs for corneal reflex. You should also bring an ophthalmoscope if you have one.

Key Notes

Don't forget to report imaging studies and lumbar puncture (LP) results. If LP results are not available in the computer system in the morning, call the lab to see if they have been processed so that you can include them in your presentation. LP results often have a significant impact on decisions about the A&P.

Neurology admission notes are like medicine notes, with a few key distinctions:

- Indicate the handedness of the patient (e.g., "46-year-old RH [right-handed] male").
- Take a full medical history as well as a neurologic history, including a history of seizures, cerebrovascular accidents (CVAs, aka strokes), transient ischemic attacks (TIAs), diabetes mellitus (DM), myocardial infarctions (MIs, aka heart attacks), and other indicators of peripheral vascular disease.
- When you are documenting the neuro exam, remember that while the admission history and physical (H&P) is expected to include the full exam, progress notes can be more brief. An example of a brief physical/neuro exam with commonly used abbreviations is shown below. When presenting your examination of the patient, neurologists expect information to be presented in a certain order. Please refer to the example below for the suggested order.
- The assessment and plan (A&P) is a good place to organize and summarize. In it, you should include important symptoms and findings; localize the lesions to an anatomic location; and, finally, give an organized differential diagnosis by likelihood. This process, more than anything else, will make you shine as a student of neurology.

Key Procedures

Before attempting an LP, always rule out the possibility of herniation. Any patient who presents with altered mental status, immunosuppression, or focal neurologic deficits should have head imaging (a CT scan is fine).

The main procedure involved in inpatient neurology is the LP, known to your patients as the dreaded "spinal tap." Make sure your resident knows that you are interested in doing LPs. Check *Clinical Neurology, Clinician's Pocket Reference,* Ferri's *Care of the Medical Patient,* or similar guides for a description of the procedure. Contraindications to performing an LP include a suspected intracranial mass lesion, local infection, a spinal cord mass, and coagulopathy. Also remember that the patient must give informed consent for an LP (although this is not always possible in cases with altered mental status), and you must write a procedure note documenting the indication for the procedure and a summary (see Chapter 1 for a sample procedure note). You should also find a good and enthusiastic teacher and ask for plenty of supervision early on. Attempting a difficult LP alone can be a nightmare both for you and for the patient.

SAMPLE NEUROLOGY PHYSICAL EXAM

Gen: Well-developed, well-nourished, pleasant male in NAD.

VS: T 37.2, P 59, BP 167/89, RR 18, Sat 98% RA.

Skin: Anicteric, no rashes, no bruises.

HEENT: Head normocephalic. Ears symmetric with no gross deformity. Nose without deviation; no epistaxis. O/P normal with moist mucous membranes, no lesions, and no bleeding.

Neck: Stiff neck, ⊕ Brudzinski, ⊕ meningismus. No LAD or swollen glands.

Lungs: CTAB with no W/R/R.

Cardiac: RRR, S1S2 nl, no M/R/G.

Abd: Obese, soft, NTND, normal reactive bowel sounds × 4 quadrants, no masses.

Ext: No C/C/E.

MSE: The patient is A&O × 3. There is an adequate fund of recent and remote information.

Follows commands.

7-digit span; able to attend and concentrate.

Memory: 3/3 registration; 0/3 → 2/3 with prompts at 5 minutes.

Speech: Patient can name, repeat, and follow instructions and is fluent. No dysarthria.

CN:

I: Not tested.

II: Vision intact with no APD; visual fields are full to confrontation independently. Fundi normal; no papilledema, exudates, hemorrhages.

III, IV, and VI: PERRL directly and consensually and to accommodation. EOMI with smooth pursuits; no nystagmus noted on any aspect of gaze.

V: Facial sensation normal to touch in all three divisions. Masseter strength normal bilaterally. No pain with palpation of the temples.

VII: Facial appearance symmetric at rest. No asymmetry on grimace.

VIII: Hearing normal to finger bilaterally.

IX and X: Soft palate elevation symmetric and normal.

XI: Shoulder shrug performed with normal strength and is symmetric. No sternomastoid weakness.

XII: No tongue atrophy or fasciculations. Tongue midline.

Motor: Normal muscle tone and bulk of arms and legs.

No fasciculations or tremor at rest. LUE spasticity.

Strength 4/5 throughout LUE and LLE; 5/5 RUE and RLE.

⊖ drift; ⊖ orbit.

Key:

A&O × 3 = alert and oriented to person, place, and time

APD = afferent pupillary defect

BP = blood pressure

C/C/E = clubbing/cyanosis/edema

CN = cranial nerves

CTAB = clear to auscultation bilaterally

EOMI = extraocular movements intact

HEENT = head, eyes, ears, nose, and throat

LAD = lymphadenopathy

LE = lower extremities

LLE = left lower extremity

LUE = left upper extremity

M/R/G = murmurs/rubs/gallops

MSE = mental status examination

NAD = no acute distress

NTND = nontender, nondistended

O/P = oropharynx

P = pulse rate

PERRL = pupils equal, round, and reactive to light

RA = room air

RAM = rapid alternating movements

RLE = right lower extremity

RR = respiratory rate

RRR = regular rate and rhythm

RUE = right upper extremity

Sat = oxygen saturation

UE = upper extremities

VS = vital signs

W/R/R = wheezes/rhonchi/
rales

Sensory: Grossly intact to light touch, vibration, and pinprick throughout bilateral UE and LE. Proprioception normal in hands and feet. Romberg test ⊖.

Coordination: RAM: slow with LUE, normal with RUE.

Normal finger-to-nose and heel-to-shin.

No dysmetria.

Gait: Normal casual gait with normal station and arm movement, normal tandem, cannot walk on heels or tiptoes.

Reflexes: Biceps, brachioradialis, patellar, Achilles 2/4 bilaterally. 2+ reflexes on the LLE and LUE. 3+ reflexes on the RLE and RUE. Plantar responses are down-going bilaterally.

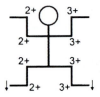

HIGH-YIELD CLINICAL TOPIC CHECKLIST

The most important things to learn on your neurology rotation are the screening and complete neurologic exams as well as the workup and management of common neurologic problems such as headache, seizure, meningitis, and stroke. Toward these goals, you should focus on the H&P, on the development of differentials, and on the recognition of emergency conditions. This is also a good time to learn about the indications for and interpretation of investigational studies, especially CT, MRI, LP, and, perhaps, EEG, EMG, and nerve conduction studies. The following is a list of 11 high-yield topics that are used extremely frequently on most neuro rotations.

❏ **The complete neurologic exam:** Mental status, cranial nerves, motor, sensory, gait and coordination, reflexes.
❏ **Imaging basics:** CT, MRI, contrast imaging.
❏ **LP:** Indications, procedural skills, interpreting results, when an LP is contraindicated.
❏ **Stroke:** Clinical features, risk factors, treatments, prevention.
❏ **Coma:** Assessing a comatose patient, use of the Glasgow Coma Scale, primitive brain stem reflexes, workup and treatment, etiologies.
❏ **Delirium and dementia.**
❏ **Headache:** Migraine, cluster, tension, 2° headaches.
❏ **Low back pain, spinal cord injuries:** Cord compression, cord lesions.
❏ **Movement disorders:** Parkinson's disease, Huntington's disease.
❏ **Seizures:** Partial (focal), generalized, absence, tonic-clonic, status epilepticus.
❏ **Weakness:** Upper motor neuron vs. lower motor neuron; anatomic localization and diagnosis.

Don't expect to master the neuro exam in just a few weeks. Instead, spend time creating a systematic approach toward the exam and learning to feel comfortable with its components. Perhaps the best approach is to carefully observe the exams (and notes) of your residents and attendings, taking note of how (and why) they choose to abbreviate or focus their exams. Also pay attention to which specific neurologic exams help them find subtle deficits. Tables 5-1 through 5-5 provide information on a complete exam; shown below is the abbreviated version.

Create a systematic approach!

Screening Exam for Mental Status

A mental status exam should include the following elements (see also Table 5-1):

- **Assess consciousness** and **orientation.** Assess each patient's orientation to person, place, date, and time. If a patient's level of consciousness and attention are abnormal, the other components of the exam will be more difficult to interpret.
- **Assess attention.** Can the patient follow commands? Can he or she concentrate on giving a history? If not, check an A-test or a digit span (a better test). In a digit span, the patient is asked to repeat a series of numbers, such as "201495" (the ability to repeat 5–7 numbers is normal). For the A-test, you recite a series of numbers and letters and ask the patient to raise his or her hand each time the letter A is heard.
- Pay attention to the patient's use of **language** as well as his or her **comprehension** of your requests during the exam. Ask patients if they know what is going on with their care and condition. Check repetition and naming (a sensitive test for aphasia).
- Finally, check **memory** and **higher cognitive function.** Ask the patient how he or she got to the hospital. What tests were done today? Ask the patient to recall three items after five minutes. Who is the president? Test abstraction. What does it mean when you say, "Two heads are better than one"?

Screening Exam for Cranial Nerves

A cranial nerve screening exam should include the following elements (see also Table 5-2):

- Focus on the eyes: check acuity, visual fields (by confrontation), pupillary size/shape/constriction to light and accommodation, and extraocular movements (EOM). Ask about diplopia. If diplopia is present, ask the patient if it is still present with one eye closed. If the diplopia is present with only one eye open, it is termed *monocular diplopia* (vs. binocular diplopia, in which the double vision is present only when both eyes are open). Don't leave out the funduscopic exam.
- Check light touch and temperature sensation in the face using the "cold" tuning fork. Check corneal reflexes if the patient has a depressed level of consciousness. Intact corneal reflexes will tell you that both CN V and CN VII are intact.
- Check the face for asymmetry. Check for symmetric movement of the facial muscles. Determine if any facial weakness detected is central (only the lower half of the face is affected) or peripheral (one entire half of the face is affected).

Cranial nerve testing:
- *The pupillary reflex tests CN II and III.*
- *The corneal reflex tests CN V and VII.*
- *The vestibulo-ocular reflex tests CN VI, IV, and III.*
- *The gag reflex tests CN IX and X.*

TABLE 5-1. Mental Status Exam

WHAT YOU'RE TESTING	WHAT YOU'RE LOOKING FOR	WHAT YOU'RE DOING
Level of consciousness	Alertness	Observe—are the eyes open? Does the patient appear drowsy?
	Orientation	Can the patient answer the following: ■ What's your name? ■ What is the day of the week/month/year? ■ Where are you? ■ What floor? Patients are "O × 3" if they know their name, the date, and their location.
	Response to voice	Call the patient's name; ask to open eyes.
	Response to pain	Try sternal rub or pinching extremities, and watch response for purposefulness.
Attention	Ability to focus on a task	Ask the patient to repeat digit spans (e.g., "02139") or use the A-test (see text).
Language	Comprehension of spoken word	Ask the patient to close his or her eyes, show three fingers, and touch the right ear with the left thumb.
	Comprehension of written word	Hold up a card reading, "Close your eyes."
	Repetition of phrases	Have the patient repeat sentences such as "No ifs, ands, or buts" or "Around the rugged rock the ragged rascal ran" and write, "Today is a sunny day."
	Fluency of speech	Is speech intelligible, fluent, and grammatical? Can the patient write a complete sentence?
	Naming	Try pointing to a watch and its parts to elicit "watch, band, crystal."
Concentration	Ability to maintain focus	Have the patient serially subtract 7 from 100 (or 3 from 20) or spell the word *world* backwards.
Mood, insight, thought process, and content	Look for signs of depression, other psychiatric disturbance, and denial	Ask the patient, "How are your spirits?" "Do you know why you are here in the hospital?"
Memory	Registration	List three words (e.g., *cat, pencil, banana*) and ask the patient to repeat them.
	Short term	Three minutes later, ask the patient to recall three items. Offer prompts if the patient is unable to do so (such as "a kind of animal," "used to write," "a kind of fruit"); can also try current events.
	Long term	Ask for birth date, Social Security number, and history.
Higher cognitive function	Fund of knowledge	Ask for names of current/past presidents.
	Calculations	Try simple addition and division (how many quarters in $2.50) and subtraction (making change from $5.00 for $1.39).
	Abstractions	Ask the patient to interpret a proverb such as "A rolling stone gathers no moss." Be aware of cultural differences.
	Constructions	Ask the patient to copy sketches (square, cube) and to draw a clock (analog).

TABLE 5-2. **Cranial Nerve Exam**

What You're Testing	What You're Looking For	What You're Doing
Optic nerve	Visual acuity	Use the Snellen eye chart.
	Visual fields	Test by confrontation if the patient cooperates; estimate by visual threat otherwise.
	Ocular fundi	Look for papilledema, retinal/subhyaloid hemorrhages, retinopathy, and/or optic atrophy.
Oculomotor nerve	Pupillary function	Check baseline size, shape, and symmetry; direct and consensual constriction (using penlight); and accommodation.
	Levator palpebrae function	Check for elevation of the eyelid and ptosis.
	Superior rectus, inferior rectus, inferior oblique function	EOM—elevate, depress, and elevate the adducted eye, respectively.
Trochlear nerve	Superior oblique function	EOM (depress the adducted eye).
Abducens nerve	Lateral rectus function	EOM (abduction).
	Assessment of EOM	Ask the patient to follow a target in the shape of the letter *H* and look for full movement and coordination.
Trigeminal nerve	**Motor:** Temporalis, masseter muscles	Palpate muscles as the patient clenches teeth.
	Sensory: V_1, V_2, V_3	Check sensation to the forehead, cheek, and jaw.
	Reflex: Corneal blink	Touch the cornea with cotton thread or tissue. (Not usually performed on conscious patients because of the safety risk.)
Facial nerve	Motor to facial muscles (also checked in motor response to corneal reflex)	Check raised eyebrows, tightly squinted eyes, smile, and puffed-out cheeks for asymmetry.
Vestibulocochlear nerve	Auditory function	Grossly test hearing by rubbing fingers together by each ear or scratching a pillow. Also consider doing Weber and Rinne tests.
	Vestibular function	Check for nystagmus and a history of vertigo.
Glossopharyngeal nerve	**Sensory:** Palate, pharynx, gag reflex	Stroke the back of the throat.
Vagus nerve	**Motor:** Palate, pharynx, vocal cords	Check the voice for hoarseness and articulation; check palatal elevation, uvular position, and gag reflex.
Spinal accessory nerve	**Motor:** Trapezius	Have the patient shrug the shoulder with resistance.
	Motor: Sternocleidomastoid	Have the patient turn the head to the side against resistance.
Hypoglossal nerve	**Motor:** Tongue	Examine the tongue in the mouth for position, atrophy, and fasciculations; have the patient protrude the tongue and move it side to side while checking for asymmetry.

What would cause ptosis? A lesion in the sympathetic nerves (above T1) that innervate the smooth muscle of the eyelid or a CN III palsy or dysfunction of the neuromuscular junction.

DTRs and nerve roots tested:

- *Biceps = C5, C6*
- *Brachioradialis = C5, C6*
- *Triceps = C6, C7*
- *Patella = L2–L4*
- *Achilles = S1*

Be familiar with dermatomal patterns:

- *T4 = nipple*
- *T7 = xiphoid process*
- *T10 = umbilicus*
- *L1 = inguinal ligament*
- *S2–S4 = penile/anal zones*

- Determine if there are gross differences in hearing between the ears. Check for vestibular dysfunction by inspecting gait and doing a Romberg test.
- Listen to the voice for hoarseness and dysarthria.
- Determine if the tongue and uvula are midline.

Screening Exam for Motor Nerves

A motor nerve screening exam should include the following components (see also Tables 5-3 through 5-5):

- Observe! Does the patient have atrophy, abnormal movements or postures, or a tendency to favor one side of the body? Are there localizing findings?
- Check tone in all four extremities. ↑ tone refers either to spasticity or to rigidity. *Spasticity* is a state in which the muscles are in a persistent state of ↑ involuntary reflex activity in response to a stretch. By contrast, the term *rigidity* is used to describe an involuntary ↑ in the resistance of a muscle to a passive stretch that is uniform throughout the range of motion of the muscles being stretched and is **not** velocity dependent. Rigidity and spasticity are often confused and can be difficult to distinguish, but they are two separate and distinct phenomena. In rigidity, DTRs are not hyperactive as they are in spasticity.
- Check strength throughout the major muscle groups in the upper and lower extremities using the standardized grading scale (see Table 5-4). Note asymmetries between the right and left extremities or between proximal and distal muscle groups.
- Check the strength of finger extension, index finger abduction, big toe dorsiflexion, and plantar flexion to look for subtle distal weakness.
- Check pronator drift by asking the patient to extend both arms with palms up and eyes closed. Weakness manifests as pronation or downward drift.
- Check for the **orbit sign** by asking the patient to make fists and revolve them around each other as if boxing a punching bag. Cortical spinal tract weakness leads the weak hand to "orbit" around the strong hand.
- Check rapid hand movements such as quickly tapping the index finger on the thumb for weakness or loss of coordination. Also check rapid foot tapping.
- Check DTRs (biceps, triceps, brachioradialis, patellar, ankle) and plantar responses (see Table 5-5 for a grading scale).
- Check for functional weakness of gait with heel and toe walking. Assess tandem and casual gait.

Screening Exam for Sensation

Consists of the following (see also Table 5-6):

- Check pain (or temperature) sensation in the hands and feet.
- Check vibration (or joint position sense) in the hands and feet.
- Check light touch on the arms and legs to look for asymmetry.

IMAGING BASICS

After you have conducted a complete neurologic exam, you should theoretically be able to localize a lesion in the nervous system. However, modern neurology increasingly relies on imaging for confirmation and diagnostic pur-

TABLE 5-3. Motor Nerve Exam

WHAT YOU'RE TESTING	WHAT YOU'RE LOOKING FOR	WHAT YOU'RE DOING
Appearance	Bulk (atrophy, hypertrophy), fasciculations, spasms, spontaneous motion.	Observing.
Tone		Passively move wrists, elbows, ankles, and knees; remind the patient to relax, shake gently, move evenly through range of motion, and then move abruptly (note pattern of resistance).
Rigidity	↑ tone in full range of motion, not dependent on rate or location; may be constant (lead-pipe rigidity) or cogwheel rigidity.	
Spasticity	↑ tone in most arm flexors and leg extensors that ↑ as rate of motion ↑; noted more at initiation of motion than at continuation.	
Flaccidity	↓ tone; joints tend to flop and hyperextend like a rag doll.	
Paratonia	Changes in tone over time/position caused by an inability to relax.	
Strength	Discover the pattern of weakness (or absence of weakness). Explore the extent of weakness and elucidate possible etiologies.	History (weakness, clumsiness); screening exam (see below). Focused motor exam based on information given in history and screen. Also use functional testing (see the entry on gait below). **Examination tips:** Give the patient mechanical advantage (start with the joint in midposition) and apply force to overcome the patient's strength, not to match it. Palpate the muscle belly during the exam.
Reflexes	DTRs (jaw, biceps, brachioradialis, triceps, finger flexors, patellar, thigh adductors, ankle jerk). Superficial reflexes (abdominal, cremasteric). Pathologic reflexes (Babinski, frontal release).	Ask the patient to relax and position the limbs and alternate from side to side for comparison. Watch for clonus, and record briskness (see Table 5-5 for grading). Pay attention to symmetry! For Babinski (plantar response), stroke the lateral plantar surface of the foot with a key and look for the direction of big toe motion (dorsiflexion = Babinski's sign).
Coordination	Point-to-point testing. Rapid movements (strength and coordination).	**Finger-to-nose test:** Have the patient touch his nose and then your finger; repeat. **Heel-to-shin test:** Have the patient run the heel up and down the opposite shin from knee to foot. Index finger tapping on the thumb; foot tapping on the ground.
Gait	Normal gait. Important for testing power of the lower extremities; functional testing is more sensitive than manual testing. Test for ataxia (tandem gait). Test for distal weakness. Test for proximal weakness.	Is gait balanced and coordinated with feet no wider than shoulders and arms swinging? Can the patient walk in a line heel to toe? Have the patient walk on toes (plantar flexion) and on heels (dorsiflexion of ankles). Have the patient hop on one foot or try a knee bend (standing on one foot). Can the patient get out of the chair without using arms?

HIGH-YIELD FACTS

NEUROLOGY

TABLE 5-4. Muscle Strength Grading

Score	Strength
0	No movement.
1	Flicker of contraction.
2	Full range of motion with gravity eliminated.
3	Full range of motion against gravity.
4	Full range of motion against gravity and some resistance.
5	Full power.

poses. You will thus be a step ahead if you familiarize yourself with the basic imaging modalities used in neurology before you start your rotation.

The two modalities used most in neurology are CT and MRI. Both modalities have their advantages and disadvantages, and each is indicated under different circumstances. Always identify what type of image you are looking at before trying to interpret it; otherwise, you may run into some trouble.

Computed Tomography (CT)

CT scans are basically three-dimensional x-rays. The images show high-attenuation (white) bony structures surrounding the brain and often show a darker (low-attenuation) cortical ribbon surrounding the white matter; CSF appears black. The image quality of CT scans is generally considered inferior to that of MRIs. Even so, there are specific circumstances in which CT is far more useful than MRI. These include the following:

■ **Suspected skull fracture:** Because CT uses x-rays for imaging, bone abnormalities are easily discerned. Bone cannot be imaged using MRI.
■ **Suspected intracranial bleeds:** Acute bleeds appear white on CT scans within 20 minutes of their onset. CT is especially useful in suspected intracerebral hemorrhages and subarachnoid bleeds (e.g., ruptured aneurysms),

CT:

Bone = white

CSF = black

TABLE 5-5. DTR Grading

Score	Strength
0	Absent.
1	Hypoactive.
2	Normal.
3	Hyperactive with spread across a joint.
4	Hyperactive with clonus.

TABLE 5-6. Sensory Exam

What You're Testing	What You're Looking For	What You're Doing
Sensory modalities	Pain	Pricking with a safety pin or a cotton swab stick broken in half.
	Temperature	Touching with a cool tuning fork.
	Vibration	Touching a buzzing tuning fork to bone and joint.
	Joint position sense	Moving the patient's finger or toe up or down.
		Romberg test: Have the patient stand with feet together and eyes closed for 10 seconds. If the patient is okay with the eyes open but not with the eyes closed, the test is ⊕.
	Light touch	Lightly touching the patient with finger or cotton.
Higher sensory function	**Graphesthesia:** The ability to recognize objects by touch.	Ask the patient to identify an object in the hand without seeing it, such as a paper clip, or to identify heads/tails of a coin.
	Point localization: The ability to localize sensory input.	Quickly touch the patient; then ask to identify location.
	Extinction: The ability to recognize dual, bilateral stimuli.	Touch the same areas bilaterally and ask the patient to identify the location of the stimulus.

allowing one to look for blood around the cerebral peduncles. By contrast, blood takes hours to appear on the MRI scanners used in most hospitals.

■ **Trauma:** CT is faster and safer than MRI when a patient may have metallic implants, fragments (e.g., trauma), or pacemakers in the body. Obviously, when time is of the essence, CT is preferable to MRI.

■ **Monitoring hydrocephalus:** The ventricles are relatively large structures. Therefore, the monitoring of ↑ ventricle size (hydrocephalus) does not require high-resolution imaging. The cheaper and faster imaging modality (CT) is thus preferred.

Magnetic Resonance Imaging (MRI)

MRI uses a combination of magnetic field and radio-frequency (RF) waves to produce images. Different timing sequences and RF waves can be used to produce different types of MRI images. You should know the two major types of MRI: T1 and T2. However, don't worry about what T1 and T2 mean from a physics perspective; instead, be able to recognize both types, and know what each can tell you about the brain.

T1:

Bone = no signal

CSF = black

T2:

Bone = no signal

CSF = white

DWI:

Ischemic areas = white

An LP is performed between which vertebrae? Between L4 and L5 (the level of the iliac crests).

In bacterial meningitis, think of bacteria as being made of protein and consuming glucose (high CSF protein, low CSF glucose), causing an acute inflammatory reaction (PMNs).

■ **T1:** T1 images look like what you expect the brain to look like—gray matter is darker, white matter is lighter, and CSF is black (i.e., it does not produce any signal). Remember, bone does not produce an MRI signal. In general, T1 images are used for studying the anatomy of the brain. Pathology may also be appreciated in these images as lighter or darker areas, but such areas will not be very pronounced. Classically, very bright areas on a T1 image will contain a high degree of protein, fat, subacute blood, or contrast agent. Note that the spatial extent of pathology is often underestimated by T1 imaging. Gadolinium enhancement can be used to ↑ the resolution of certain pathologic processes.

■ **T2:** T2 images are almost the inverse of T1—gray matter is lighter, white matter is darker, and CSF appears white. Unlike T1 images, pathology in T2 images will stand out (as bright white). Pathology appears white owing to edema and water accumulation in the area of pathology. Note that both edema and CSF have a large water component, and therefore both appear white. T2 is the study of choice for identifying pathology.

■ **Fluid attenuation inversion recovery (FLAIR) imaging:** A FLAIR image is similar to a T2 image except that the bright CSF has been subtracted away. Thus, one's eye is drawn to areas of abnormal signal, making the signal easier to recognize.

■ **Diffusion-weighted imaging (DWI):** A specific T2 sequence with which you should be familiar, DWI is used in suspected cases of acute stroke to determine if an ischemic event is occurring in the brain. As expected, the ischemic area appears white. DWI is especially useful because it reveals ischemic areas within minutes of onset.

Contrast

CT and MRI studies will often be ordered with contrast. Contrast material is designed to remain within blood vessels. Thus, adding contrast to a study will accomplish two tasks. First, the contrast can elucidate vascular anatomy and suggest the presence of any occlusions. Second, contrast seen outside of the vessels suggests compromise of the blood-brain barrier. If the blood-brain barrier is interrupted, contrast will "leak" into the brain and enhance the signal from that region. This tells the clinician about the severity of the condition and can also ↑ the resolution of a study. Iodinated contrast agents are used for CT contrast, and gadolinium is used for MRI contrast.

In a small subset of the population, severe contrast reactions may occur, so it is important to obtain a history of any prior reactions to contrast during CTs. In addition, it is now believed that gadolinium can on rare occasions cause a progressive, chronic syndrome known as nephrogenic fibrosing dermopathy, or nephrogenic systemic fibrosis. This syndrome clinically resembles scleroderma and eosinophilic fasciitis, and it affects patients with a history of renal insufficiency. Although relatively uncommon, the syndrome has caused some hospitals in the United States to pay closer attention to the routine use of gadolinium in MRI studies.

LUMBAR PUNCTURE (LP) RESULTS

As you read through this chapter, you will notice that in many cases an LP may be ordered to narrow the differential. Table 5-7 provides CSF profiles for the various neurologic diseases you may encounter.

TABLE 5-7. CSF Profiles

	RBCs (PER mm³)	WBCs (PER mm³)	GLUCOSE (mg/dL)	PROTEIN (mg/dL)	OPENING PRESSURE (cm H₂O)	APPEARANCE	GAMMA GLOBULIN (% PROTEIN)
Normal	< 10	< 5	~ 2/3 of serum	15–45	10–20	Clear	3–12
Bacterial meningitis	↔	↑ (PMN)	↓	↑	↑	Cloudy	↔ or ↑
Viral meningitis	↔	↑ (mono)	↔	↔ or ↑	↔ or ↑	Most often clear	↔ or ↑
SAH	↑↑	↑	↔	↑	↔ or ↑	Yellow/ red	↔ or ↑
GBS	↔	↔	↔ or ↑	↑↑	↔	Clear or yellow (high protein)	↔
MS	↔	↔ or ↑	↔	↔	↔	Clear	↑↑
Pseudo-tumor cerebri	↔	↔	↔	↔	↑↑↑	Clear	↔

REFERENCE

Negrini B et al. Cerebrospinal fluid findings in aseptic versus bacterial meningitis. *Pediatrics* 105:316–319, 2000. A retrospective chart review study challenging the notion that neutrophil predominance in CSF is indicative of bacterial meningitis. Although many may doubt the results, the study provides a good overview of factors to consider when evaluating CSF profiles.

STROKE

Stroke is a clinical syndrome defined by the acute onset of a focal neurologic deficit resulting from a disturbance in blood flow. This disturbance can be either ischemic (85%) or hemorrhagic (15%). A stroke that does not resolve symptomatically is referred to as a **cerebrovascular accident (CVA)**. If the deficit reverses within 24 hours, the event is redesignated a **TIA**. However, TIA symptoms generally reverse in roughly one hour. TIAs also significantly ↑ the risk of future stroke, especially within 48 hours of the TIA. The etiologies of **ischemic stroke** include the following:

■ **Cardiac:**
  ■ **Atrial fibrillation (AF):** The most common cause of cardioembolic stroke. Patients with AF have a five- to sixfold greater risk of stroke than the general population.

The treatment of meningitis is a time-sensitive matter—the earlier treatment is given, the better the outcome. So try to get CSF results as soon as possible! If you admit a patient overnight and the results are not in the computer by morning rounds, call the lab.

Risk factors for stroke include the following:

- *Nonmodifiable: Age, male gender, ethnicity (African-American, Hispanic, Asian), genetics.*
- *Modifiable: Hypertension, DM, smoking, heavy alcohol intake, cocaine use, obesity, hypercholesterolemia, carotid stenosis, AF.*

Ischemic strokes are much more common than hemorrhagic strokes.

Stroke sites and affected areas/deficits:

- *MCA: Contralateral trunk/arm/face, Broca's, Wernicke's (dominant), neglect (nondominant).*
- *ACA: Leg/foot, cognitive changes, bladder incontinence.*
- *PCA: Vision, reading, writing.*
- *Basilar: Coma, "locked-in" syndrome, cranial nerve palsies, drop attacks.*

- **Other cardiac causes:** Include embolism of mural thrombi, thrombi from diseased or prosthetic valves, other arrhythmias, endocarditis (septic, fungal, or marantic emboli), and paradoxic (venous) emboli in patients with right-to-left shunt in the heart (from ASD or patent foramen ovale).
- **Large vessel atherothrombosis** (internal and common carotids, basilar and vertebral arteries): Accounts for 35% of all strokes and roughly 40% of ischemic strokes. Symptoms are typically maximal at onset and may slowly improve.
- **Small vessel atherothrombosis:** Lacunar infarcts (the source of 20% of all strokes) occur in regions supplied by small perforating vessels and result from either atherosclerotic or hypertensive occlusion. They commonly occur in the basal ganglia, brain stem, and internal capsules (due to small vessel disease).
- **Other:** Less common causes of ischemic stroke include the following:
  - **Hematologic disorders,** including **hypercoagulable** states such as sickle cell disease, polycythemia, thrombocytosis, leukocytosis, malignancy, hereditary coagulopathies, and collagen vascular disease.
  - Fibromuscular dysplasia (young females), inflammatory diseases, arterial dissection, migraine, venous thrombosis.

Hemorrhagic strokes are most often caused by hypertensive rupture of small vessels, AVMs, hemorrhage conversion of ischemic strokes, amyloid angiopathy, cocaine use, and/or bleeding diatheses.

SIGNS AND SYMPTOMS

- Presentation depends on the location of the stroke; different **vascular** territories will have different presentations (see Table 5-8).
- The time course varies for thrombotic, embolic, and hemorrhagic strokes.
  - **Thrombotic strokes:** Evolve in minutes to hours and may follow a TIA.
  - **Embolic strokes:** Often present with the full deficit acutely and do not evolve.
  - **Hemorrhagic strokes:** Onset can include headache and/or altered mental status; deficits may not strictly follow vascular territories due to hematoma expansion and edema surrounding the bleed.
- Exam may reveal signs of arrhythmias (e.g., AF) and atherosclerotic disease (carotid and/or subclavian bruits). Remember, however, that the presence of bruits is not very sensitive for carotid stenosis.

DIFFERENTIAL

Todd's paralysis (postictal), subdural or epidural hematoma, brain abscess, brain tumor, MS, migraine headache, metabolic abnormalities, neurosyphilis, conversion disorder.

WORKUP

The goal of workup is twofold: (1) to urgently determine whether the stroke is ischemic or hemorrhagic, and (2) if the stroke is ischemic, to ascertain whether it can be reversed within a three-hour window using tPA both to salvage ischemic brain and to prevent further strokes. Concurrently, one must localize the lesion, rule out other lesions, and determine the etiology. Tests include the following:

TABLE 5-8. Stroke Sites and Resulting Neurologic Deficits

Vessel[a]	Region Supplied	Neurologic Deficit
Anterior circulation		
MCA	Lateral cerebral hemisphere; deep subcortical structures.	Combined deficits of superior/inferior divisions; may see coma and ↑ ICP.
Superior division	Motor/sensory cortex of face, arm, hand; Broca's area.	Contralateral hemiparesis of face, arm, and hand; expressive aphasia if dominant hemisphere.
Inferior division	Parietal lobe (visual radiations, Wernicke's area), macular visual cortex.	Homonymous hemianopia, receptive aphasia (dominant), impaired cortical sensory functions, gaze preference, apraxias, and neglect (nondominant).
ACA	Parasagittal cerebral cortex.	Contralateral leg paresis and sensory loss.
Ophthalmic artery	Retina.	Monocular blindness.
Posterior circulation		
PCA	Occipital lobe, thalamus, rostral midbrain, medial temporal lobes.	Contralateral homonymous hemianopia, memory or sensory disturbances.
Basilar	Ventral midbrain, brain stem, posterior limb of internal capsule, cerebellum, PCA distribution.	Coma, cranial nerve palsies, apnea, cardiovascular instability.
Deep circulation		
Lenticulostriate, paramedian, thalamoperforate, circumferential arteries	Basal ganglia, pons, thalamus, internal capsule, cerebellum.	"Lacunes." Pure motor or sensory deficits, ataxic hemiparesis, "dysarthria–clumsy hand" syndrome.

[a] MCA = middle cerebral artery; ACA = anterior cerebral artery; PCA = posterior cerebral artery.

- CT without contrast to distinguish ischemic from hemorrhagic stroke (see Figure 5-1). Note that ischemic strokes, which appear on CT scan as a loss of gray-white differentiation or as a hypodensity, are generally not visible for at least 3–6 hours after symptom onset.
- MRI to identify early ischemic changes (use DWI and the FLAIR sequence to differentiate new from old ischemic regions, respectively), to identify neoplasms, and to adequately image the brain stem and posterior fossa.
- CBC, coagulation panel, lipid panel, ESR, and CRP.
- TSH, RPR, B_{12}/folate, glucose, and HbA_{1c} to investigate other causes of acute neurologic symptoms.
- ECG, echocardiography (transesophageal echocardiography [TEE] is most sensitive for mural thrombi).
- Vascular studies for extracranial disease by carotid ultrasound; magnetic resonance angiography (MRA), CT angiography, or traditional angiography to look for intracranial disease.
- Blood cultures; screening for hypercoagulable states (if there is a history of bleeding, this is the first stroke, or the patient is < 50 years of age).

For stroke patients, especially those with new stroke or age < 50, consider B_{12}/folate, ESR, RPR, CRP, TSH, a lipid panel, HbA_{1c}, urine toxicology, and a hypercoagulable workup (INR, aPTT, antithrombin III, protein C/S, antiphospholipid/anticardiolipin antibody, sickle cell trait).

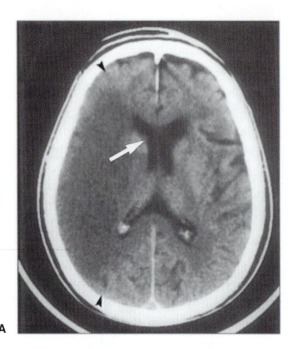

A

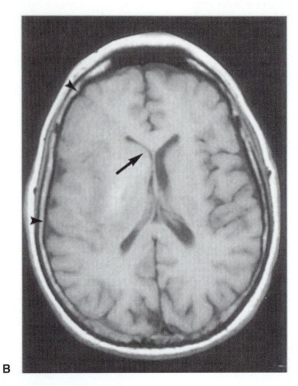

B

C

FIGURE 5-1. **CT/MRI findings in ischemic stroke in the right MCA territory.**

(A) CT shows low density and effacement of cortical sulci (between arrowheads) and compression of the anterior horn of the lateral ventricle (arrow). (B) T1-weighted MRI shows loss of sulcal markings (between arrowheads) and compression of the anterior horn of the lateral ventricle (arrow). (C) T2-weighted MRI scan shows ↑ signal intensity (between arrowheads) and ventricular compression (arrow). (Reproduced, with permission, from Aminoff MJ et al. *Clinical Neurology*, 3rd ed. Stamford, CT: Appleton & Lange, 1996: 275.)

CONTRAINDICATIONS TO tPA THERAPY

Major contraindications to tPA therapy are as follows:

1. SBP > 185 or DBP > 110 mmHg despite aggressive antihypertensive therapy.

2. Prior intracranial hemorrhage, stroke, or head trauma in the last three months.

3. Recent MI.

4. Current anticoagulant therapy with an INR > 1.7 or use of heparin in the last 48 hours with prolonged PTT.

5. A platelet count < 100,000/mm³.

6. Major surgery in the past 14 days or GI/urinary bleeding in the past 21 days.

7. Seizures present at the onset of stroke.

8. Blood glucose < 50 or > 400 mg/dL.

9. Age < 18.

TREATMENT

- **Acute:** Treatment consists of the following measures aimed at reperfusion, neuroprotection, and salvage:
    - Watch for symptoms or signs of brain swelling, ↑ ICP, or herniation.
    - Revascularize thrombotic disease using tPA within three hours of ischemic onset (measured from the last time the patient is confirmed to have been "well"). The three-hour time limit is an absolute. Some people who receive tPA undergo hemorrhagic conversion and may suffer a worse fate. Rule out hemorrhagic stroke, and screen for contraindications.
    - ASA is associated with ↓ morbidity and mortality in acute ischemic stroke presenting ≤ 48 hours from onset
- **Prevention and long-term treatment:**
    - For cardioembolic strokes, rule out hemorrhagic stroke before starting anticoagulation. Heparin and warfarin therapy can prevent further embolization; target an INR of 2–3 for warfarin therapy.
    - Antiplatelet agents such as aspirin, clopidogrel (Plavix), and dipyridamole/aspirin can be given for small-vessel (lacunar) strokes and when anticoagulation is either not indicated or contraindicated.
    - Carotid endarterectomy is appropriate in the setting of asymptomatic stenosis > 60% or symptomatic/asymptomatic stenosis > 70%. Do not use in 100% blockage.
    - Manage modifiable risk factors, especially hypertension, DM, and hypercholesterolemia.

*In treating stroke, avoid the "Hypos": **Hypo**tension, **Hypo**xemia, and **Hypo**glycemia. Maintain SBP approximately 20 mmHg above the patient's normal level to ensure adequate cerebral perfusion (permissive hypertension), and do not lower unless it is > 220/> 130.*

REFERENCE

Executive Committee for the Asymptomatic Carotid Atherosclerosis Study. Endarterectomy for asymptomatic carotid artery stenosis. *JAMA* 273:1421–1428, 1995. North American Symptomatic Carotid Endarterectomy Trial (NASCET) investigators. Clinical alert: Benefit of carotid endarterectomy for patients with high-grade stenosis of the internal carotid artery. *Stroke* 22: 816–817, 1991. The classic and original reports that established the criteria for surgical management of carotid disease for asymptomatic and symptomatic patients, respectively.

Aphasia is a general term used to describe language disorders. Aphasias generally result from insults (e.g., strokes, tumors, abscesses) to the language centers in the "dominant hemisphere." The left hemisphere is dominant in 90% of right-handed people and in 50% of left-handed people. Just as the job of the motor cortex is to move the body, the job of the language centers is to name. Therefore, a patient with a naming deficit of any kind is said to have an aphasia.

To characterize an aphasia, assess the patient's language abilities in three domains: **production, comprehension,** and **repetition.** Reading and writing are other aspects of language you may want to evaluate. There are eight main types of aphasias, six of which are described here (see Table 5-9). The two principal aphasias with which you should be familiar are Broca's and Wernicke's (see Figure 5-2).

Broca's Aphasia

Broca's aphasia is an expressive aphasia; it is a disorder of language production and repetition with intact comprehension. It is often 2° to a superior MCA stroke.

SIGNS AND SYMPTOMS

- Speech is nonfluent, with ↓ rate, short phrase length, and impaired articulation.
- Repetition is impaired, but comprehension is intact. Patients are noticeably frustrated with their speech because they are aware of their deficit.

*Aphasia is a problem with language and usually results from a **cortical** lesion. Dysarthria is a problem with articulation that usually involves a **subcortical** lesion such as an internal capsule or brain stem lesion.*

HIGH-YIELD FACTS

NEUROLOGY

TABLE 5-9. Summary of Aphasias

TYPE	FLUENCY	COMPRE-HENSION	REPETITION	NAMING	READING	WRITING	LESION LOCALIZATION
Broca's	↓	Normal	↓	↓	↓	↓	Posterior inferior frontal gyrus
Wernicke's	Normal	↓	↓	↓	↓	↓	Posterior superior temporal lobe
Conduction	Normal	Normal	↓	↓	Normal	↓	Arcuate fasciculus
Global	↓	↓	↓	↓	↓	↓	Large portion of left hemisphere
Transcortical motor	↓	Normal	Normal	Mildly ↓	Normal	↓	ACA/MCA border zone
Transcortical sensory	Normal	↓	Normal	↓	↓	↓	PCA/MCA border zone

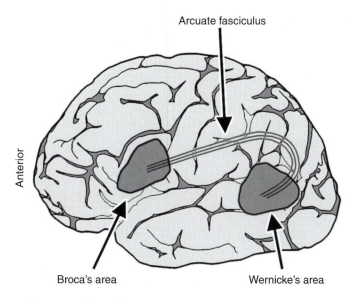

Arcuate fasciculus

Anterior

Broca's area

Wernicke's area

FIGURE 5-2. Broca's and Wernicke's areas.

Broca's and Wernicke's areas are the two major language centers in the brain. The arcuate fasciculus connects these two areas. Injury to the arcuate fasciculus results in language repetition errors.

- Associated features include arm and face hemiparesis, hemisensory loss, and apraxia of oral muscles due to the proximity of Broca's area (the posterior inferior frontal gyrus) to the motor and sensory strips (the pre- and postcentral gyri, respectively).

TREATMENT

Treat the underlying pathology; begin speech therapy (has varying outcomes with an intermediate prognosis).

Wernicke's Aphasia

Wernicke's aphasia is a receptive aphasia; it is a disorder of language comprehension and repetition without a deficit in language production. The lesion is often in the left posterior superior temporal lobe and is often 2° to a left inferior MCA stroke.

SIGNS AND SYMPTOMS

- Speech is fluent but empty of meaning.
- Comprehension, naming, and repetition are impaired, with frequent use of marked neologisms (made-up words) and paraphasic errors (word substitutions).
- No notable hemiparesis or dysarthria is present.
- Patients are often unaware of their deficit because they lack comprehension.

TREATMENT

Treat the underlying pathology; begin speech therapy (even though it is not as successful as in Broca's aphasia).

*Broca's is **B**roken speech.*

*Wernicke's is **W**ordy but makes no sense.*

Name another brain lesion characterized by Wernicke that is not to be confused with Wernicke's aphasia. Wernicke-Korsakoff's encephalopathy, resulting from thiamine deficiency, often 2° to alcoholism. A lesion in the mammillary bodies leads to confabulations and anterograde amnesia.

Transcortical Aphasias

Transcortical motor aphasia and transcortical sensory aphasia are marked by impaired language motor output (production deficit) and impaired language comprehension ("sensory"), respectively. Both are distinct from Broca's and Wernicke's in that repetition remains intact.

Conduction Aphasia

A conduction aphasia is a subtle aphasia that can be easily missed because both language production and comprehension remain intact, but language repetition is impaired. Conduction aphasias are said to result from damage to the arcuate fasciculus.

Global Aphasia

A global aphasia is, as the name implies, a global deficit of language production, comprehension, and repetition. It is the most serious and devastating of all the aphasias and is associated with the most widespread insult to the brain. It also carries the worst prognosis.

COMA

Defined as a profound suppression of responses to external and internal stimuli caused either by catastrophic structural injury to the CNS or by diffuse metabolic dysfunction. Coma etiology is the best predictor of coma outcomes; whereas coma 2° to drug overdose is associated with 5–10% mortality, coma 2° to anoxia carries a 90% mortality. In addition, the younger the patient, the better the prognosis.

The severity of coma is measured by the Glasgow Coma Scale (GCS), which consists of three parts: motor (6 points), verbal (5 points), and eye opening (4 points). A mnemonic often used in the ER as a general (not strict) rule is, "At GCS < 8, intubate."

The reticular activating system is necessary for consciousness. This structure extends from the brain stem, through the thalamus bilaterally, and to the cerebral hemispheres bilaterally. Bilateral hemispheric insults, bilateral thalamic insults, or brain stem insults lead to coma. Etiologies can be broken down as follows:

- **Supratentorial processes:** Hemorrhage (epidural, subdural, or intraparenchymal), infarction, abscesses, and tumors. Must be recognized in order to prevent potential herniation and compression of the midbrain and brain stem.
- **Infratentorial lesions:** Hemorrhage (pons, cerebellum, or posterior fossa), vertebrobasilar strokes, and tumors of the brain stem or cerebellum. Infratentorial masses require prompt evacuation due to impending compression/damage to the brain stem.
- **Metabolic causes:** Electrolyte or endocrine disturbances; ethanol, drugs, or toxins.
- **Miscellaneous:** Infectious or inflammatory disease; subarachnoid blood; generalized seizure activity or postictal states.

Patients with an initial GCS score of 3 or 4 have approximately 95% mortality at one month.

SIGNS AND SYMPTOMS

The physical exam should check for vital signs, trauma, nuchal rigidity, and funduscopic changes. However, the patient's presentation will vary with the etiology of the coma (see Table 5-10).

TABLE 5-10. Presentation of Coma Based on Etiology

INITIAL PRESENTATION	ETIOLOGY
Sudden onset	Brain stem infarctions, SAH.
Initially focal but rapidly progressive	Intracerebral hemorrhage.
Subacute	Tumor, abscess, subdural hematoma.
Focal neurologic deficits	Structural lesions.
No focal signs	Diffuse processes such as metabolic or drug intoxication.

DIFFERENTIAL

- Locked-in states (central pontine myelinolysis, brain stem stroke, advanced ALS).
- Persistent vegetative state.
- Trauma with diffuse cortical injury or hypoxic ischemic injury.
- Nonconvulsive status epilepticus.

WORKUP

- The absence or asymmetry of **primitive brain stem reflexes** can help localize the lesion and elucidate coma etiology.
    - **Pupil size:** Are pupils symmetric? A "blown pupil" may be a sign of ipsilateral uncal herniation.
    - **Pupillary light reflex:** A normal pupillary light reflex is said to occur when the pupils constrict symmetrically to light shone into either eye.
    - **Corneal reflex:** Normally, both eyes blink in response to corneal irritation (usually with a Q-tip or a cotton swab).
    - **Oculocephalic reflex (or "doll's eye" reflex):** The **vestibulo-ocular reflex (VOR)** or **oculovestibular reflex** is a reflex eye movement that stabilizes images on the retina during head movement by producing an eye movement in the direction opposite to head movement, thereby preserving the image on the center of the visual field. For example, when the head moves to the right, the eyes move to the left and vice versa. Because slight head movements are present all the time, the VOR is very important for stabilizing vision. The VOR does not depend on visual input and works even in total darkness or when the eyes are closed.
- Hot/cold-water calorics:
    - When active, the semicircular canals are responsible for moving the eyes opposite to the activated canal. Therefore, when a canal is inactive, the eyes will move slowly toward the inactive canal. The brain recognizes this discrepancy and initiates a corrective fast-phase jerk (called a saccade) back to the midline. Since infusion of cold water into an ear will inactivate that semicircular canal, the eyes will move toward the cold-water infusion followed by nystagmus in the opposite direction (fast-phase opposite).

GCS scoring: Think "Four-Eyes," the roman numeral V (Verbal) for Five, and the rest adds up to Fifteen.

Determining coma etiology is critical because it is the best predictor of outcomes.

HIGH-YIELD FACTS

NEUROLOGY

Reactive pupils in a patient with absent oculocephalic reflexes cannot be truly localized and point to a toxic/metabolic insult.

Normal eye deviations (fast phase) to caloric stimulation—

COWS

Cold
Opposite
Warm
Same

Why is dextrose administered? One common cause of coma is severe hypoglycemia.

- Note that nystagmus is always described in the direction of the fast phase. If the eyes look slowly toward the stimulus side with no fast-phase correction, the brain stem is intact and the lesion is in the cerebral hemispheres. If there is no movement of the eyes, then the lesion involves the brain stem. To help recall the normal caloric response, remember the mnemonic **COWS** (see below).
- Test passive muscle tone, DTRs, the Babinski reflex, and ankle clonus.
- Look for unusual **respiratory patterns:**
    - **Cheyne-Stokes:** A crescendo-decrescendo pattern due to bilateral hemisphere dysfunction.
    - **Central neurogenic hyperventilation:** Rapid deep breathing due to midbrain damage.
    - **Apneustic breathing:** Prolonged inspiration with subsequent apnea due to pontine dysfunction.
    - **Ataxic breathing:** Irregular breathing due to medullary dysfunction.
- **Localize the lesion:** This requires that structural and diffuse processes be differentiated.
- **Labs:** Check glucose and electrolytes, LFTs, BUN, creatinine, PT/PTT, CBC, ABGs, and blood cultures (if sepsis is suspected). In addition, a toxicology screen (for alcohol and drugs of abuse) and an LP (if CNS infection is suspected) should be ordered.
- **Imaging:**
    - A CT scan is indicated, particularly if a structural lesion, trauma, or SAH is suspected.
    - Remember **"stick, scan, and wave"**—include LP, MRI, and EEG in the coma workup, in addition to the evaluation of metabolic disturbances.

TREATMENT

- **Stabilize the patient:** Attend to **ABCs**—**A**irway, **B**reathing, and **C**irculation.
- **Reverse the reversible:** Administer **DON'T:** **D**extrose, **O**xygen, **N**aloxone, and **T**hiamine.
- **Prevent further damage:** This requires recognition of the progressive and/or treatable etiologies of coma. Some things to look for include the following:
    - Signs of herniation can be managed by decreasing ICP and/or by surgical decompression. It is important to detect supratentorial processes early on and to follow neurologic changes vigilantly.
    - Signs of meningitis include fever and nuchal rigidity; patients with possible meningitis should receive IV antibiotics immediately and an LP within four hours.
    - Signs of SAH warrant emergent CT and LP.
    - Seizure activity should be considered and treated if verified by clinical findings (shaking, gaze deviation, pupillary dilation) or EEG.
    - Trauma may suggest cervical spine injury and may warrant cervical x-rays and/or a CT.
- **Investigate further:** Management can shift to the treatment of metabolic disturbances and further investigation, if indicated, by ECG, CXR, and EEG.

REFERENCE

Teasdale G, Jennett B. Assessment of coma and impaired consciousness: A practical scale. *Lancet* 2:81–84, 1974. The classic paper that introduced the now-popular GCS.

Differentiating delirium and dementia can be challenging. Although both conditions reflect a so-called alteration of mental status and a global ↓ in cognition, delirium and dementia differ in terms of their etiologies, their time course, and the cognitive domains affected. Delirium and dementia are compared in the paragraphs that follow and in Table 5-11.

Delirium

A transient disturbance of consciousness with altered **attention**, concentration, orientation, and perception that is not attributable to dementia alone and develops over a short period of time (hours to days). All human beings, even medical students, are at risk for delirium; younger and healthier people have higher reserve, allowing them to sustain more insults before delirium sets in. The elderly are at particular risk for delirium 2° to medical illness, polypharmacy, and pre-existing dementia. The more common etiologies are provided in Table 5-12.

- UTI and pneumonia are among the most common causes of delirium in the elderly.
- Other predisposing factors include unfamiliar surroundings, sleep deprivation, sensory deprivation, and sensory overload.
- Iatrogenic delirium may result from medications.
- Any medical condition can cause delirium in a susceptible patient, including uremia, dehydration, and hypoxia.

SIGNS AND SYMPTOMS

- Waxing and waning consciousness and perceptual disturbances (hallucinations, delusions, agitation, persecutory thoughts) are common.
- Anxiety, paranoia, or combativeness may be present. Symptoms often worsen at night, a phenomenon known as "sundowning."
- Also characterized by ↓ attention span, ↓ short-term memory, and reversed sleep-wake cycles.

WORKUP

- Perform a thorough H&P, particularly for fevers, chills, nausea, vomiting, bowel movements, nutrition, medications (e.g., narcotics or benzodiaz-

> *Causes of delirium—*
> **MOVE, STUPID**
>
> **M**etabolic
> **O**xygen
> **V**ascular
> **E**ndocrine/**E**lectrolytes
> **S**eizures
> **T**umor/**T**rauma/
>   **T**emperature
> **U**remia
> **P**sychogenic
> **I**nfection/**I**ntoxication
> **D**rugs/**D**egenerative
>   diseases

TABLE 5-11. Dementia vs. Delirium

	DEMENTIA	**DELIRIUM**
Hallmark feature	Memory loss.	Fluctuating orientation.
Level of arousal	Normal.	Stupor or agitation.
Development	Slow and insidious.	Rapid.
Reversibility	Often irreversible.	Frequently reversible.
Other comments		Brain damage predisposes. Most common in children and the elderly. Course fluctuates; duration is brief.

TABLE 5-12. Common Causes of Delirium

TYPE OF INSULT	EXAMPLE
Metabolic	Hepatic encephalopathy, thiamine deficiency, hypoglycemia.
Oxygen	Hypoxia/hypercarbia.
Vascular	MI, anemia.
Endocrine/Electrolytes	Hyponatremia, hypercalcemia, fluid imbalance, hyper-/hypothyroidism.
Seizures	Ictal/postictal.
Tumor/**T**rauma/**T**emperature	
Uremia	Acute renal failure, dehydration.
Psychogenic	
Infection	UTI, pneumonia, meningitis, sepsis.
Intoxication	Alcohol, benzodiazepines, carbon monoxide, barbiturates, hallucinogens, opioids.
Drugs/**D**egenerative diseases	

epines), substance use (e.g., alcohol, illicit drugs), and recent illnesses. Pay particular attention to signs of infection or dehydration on physical exam. Check vital signs and perform a complete neurologic exam.
- Consider chronic medical conditions that may make the patient more susceptible to delirium (including dementia!).
- Obtain electrolytes (including calcium), a CBC with differential (to rule out infection), a UA (to rule out UTI), and a urine toxicology screen.
- Other labs include the following:
  - ABGs (to rule out hypoxia).
  - ECG (to rule out MI).
  - CXR (to rule out pneumonia, TB, CHF, and the like).
  - LFTs (to rule out hepatic encephalopathy).
  - Also consider TFTs, EEG (to rule out seizures), RPR or VDRL, LP (to rule out meningitis/encephalitis), and serum B_{12} and folate (to rule out vitamin deficiencies and malnutrition).
- CT and MRI should be performed if (1) head trauma or CNS pathology is suspected **after** lab work is done and is found to be noncontributory to a medical diagnosis, or (2) there is a high index of suspicion of CNS pathology.
- LP should be considered, especially if the patient is febrile with or without meningismus.

TREATMENT

- Treat the underlying cause of delirium.
- Normalize fluid and electrolyte status, and provide an appropriate sensory environment (windows and light).
- Use nonsedating antipsychotics (e.g., haloperidol) for agitation (except in alcohol withdrawal).
- Avoid benzodiazepines for sedation, as they will worsen most patients' symptoms (except in the setting of alcohol or benzodiazepine withdrawal, when benzodiazepines are clearly indicated).

Dementia

A chronic, progressive, global decline in multiple cognitive areas, especially memory loss. Other cognitive deficits include aphasia (language disturbance), apraxia (inability to execute commands), agnosia (disruption of recognition), and disturbances in executive function (e.g., abstraction). Alzheimer's disease accounts for 70–80% of all cases; other etiologies are outlined in the mnemonic **DEMENTIAS**:

- **D**egenerative diseases: Parkinson's, Huntington's, Pick's, Lewy body disease.
- **E**ndocrine: Thyroid, parathyroid, pituitary-adrenal axis.
- **M**etabolic: Alcohol, fluid electrolytes, vitamin B_{12}, glucose, hepatic/renal disease, Wilson's disease.
- **E**xogenous: Heavy metals, carbon monoxide, drugs.
- **N**eoplasm.
- **T**rauma: Subdural hematoma.
- **I**nfection: Meningitis, encephalitis, abscess, endocarditis, HIV, syphilis, prions, Lyme disease.
- **A**ffective disorders: Pseudodementia 2° to depression.
- **S**troke/Structure: Multi-infarct (vascular) dementia, ischemia, vasculitis, normal pressure hydrocephalus.

> **The 5 A's of dementia—**
>
> **A**mnesia
> **A**phasia
> **A**gnosia
> **A**praxia
> **A**bstract thought disturbances

Be careful not to mistake inattentiveness or depression for cognitive decline.

WORKUP

- **Conduct a thorough H&P:** Talk to family members about the time line of symptom progression. How long have there been problems? Are there other symptoms, such as tremor, rigidity, staring episodes, loss of consciousness, or excessive somnolence?
- **Labs/imaging:**
  - Obtain a CBC, electrolytes (including calcium), glucose, BUN/creatinine, LFTs, TFTs, B_{12} levels, and RPR or VDRL.
  - Neuroimaging (CT or MRI) is also indicated at some point to identify specific patterns of brain atrophy consistent with a particular etiology—e.g., frontotemporal vs. vascular dementia.
  - Consider an LP, ESR, folate, HIV, CXR, UA, 24-hour urine for heavy metals, and a urine toxicology screen.

TREATMENT

- Prevent further insult to the brain by avoiding toxic agents, normalizing diet, and treating any underlying disease that may be exacerbating the dementia.
- Avoid benzodiazepines, as they will often exacerbate disinhibition and confusion.

- Low-dose atypical antipsychotics (e.g., risperidone) may be used for agitation.
- Treat any associated depression.
- Support for the caregiver is essential.

Alzheimer's Disease (AD)

Risk factors for AD include **age,** female gender, family history, Down syndrome, ApoE4 homozygosity, and low educational level. Pathology includes neurofibrillary tangles, neuritic plaques with amyloid deposition, amyloid angiopathy, and neuronal loss. Survival is approximately 5–10 years from the onset of symptoms, and death is usually 2° to aspiration pneumonia or other infections.

SIGNS AND SYMPTOMS

- Anterograde amnesia is the first sign of AD.
- Subsequent cognitive deficits include aphasias, acalculia, depression, agitation, and apraxia.

WORKUP

Medicare now partially covers PET scans for AD.

- AD is a clinical diagnosis of exclusion that can be definitively diagnosed only on autopsy.
- Neurobehavioral and neuropsychological tests can be ordered to identify specific cognitive deficits.
- PET is increasingly being used to determine specific patterns of hypometabolism that may be highly sensitive and specific for diagnosing AD.

TREATMENT

Does AD affect life expectancy? Yes. Life expectancy from the time of diagnosis is approximately half that of age-matched controls.

- **Anticholinesterase inhibitors** (rivastigmine, galantamine, or donepezil) are first-line therapy. Tacrine can cause hepatotoxicity.
- Vitamin E (α-tocopherol) and selegiline, both of which are antioxidants, may slow cognitive decline.

REFERENCE

Larson EB et al. Survival after initial diagnosis of Alzheimer disease. *Ann Intern Med* 140(7):501–509, 2004. A study that found median survival from the time of diagnosis to be 4.2 and 5.7 years for men and women, respectively.

DYSEQUILIBRIUM

Equilibrium is maintained through the input of visual, vestibular, and proprioceptive sensory systems and through processing by the cerebellum and brain stem. **Dysequilibrium,** or "dizziness," is a vague term that may signify a number of phenomena, including the following:

- **Non-neurologic causes:**
  - **Presyncope:** A feeling of impending loss of consciousness. Common causes include hypotension, MI, vasovagal reaction, cardiac conduction abnormalities, and valvular disease.
  - **Psychogenic:** Anxiety, depression, psychosis, hyperventilation, hypochondriasis.

- Neurologic causes:
  - Dysfunction of the vestibular system leading to an **illusion of movement**. Examples include the following:
    - **Peripheral dysfunction** of the labyrinthine structure or the vestibular nerve.
      - **Benign paroxysmal positional vertigo (BPPV):** Responsible for 50% of cases of peripheral dysequilibrium. Marked by brief spells of vertigo triggered by changes in head position; caused by loose debris within the posterior canal of the inner ear.
      - **Ménière's disease:** Intermittent vertigo due to dilation and periodic rupture of the endolymphatic compartment of the inner ear. Hearing loss and tinnitus are also common. Symptoms can be controlled with a low-sodium diet.
      - **Other:** Acoustic neuroma (vestibular schwannoma), viral labyrinthitis.
    - **Central dysfunction** resulting from brain stem or cerebellar processes such as stroke, tumor, or MS.
  - Dysfunction leading to loss of balance **without an illusion of movement.** Examples include visual disturbances, peripheral neuropathies, and ataxias.

SIGNS AND SYMPTOMS

- Dysequilibrium manifests clinically as vertigo or ataxia (incoordination without weakness of voluntary movement of the eyes, speech, gait, trunk, or extremities).
- Peripheral and central vertigo are compared and further discussed in Tables 5-13 and 5-14. The **intrinsic brain stem signs** cited in Table 5-13 refer to signs such as ataxia, dysarthria, cranial nerve abnormalities, and motor system dysfunction.

WORKUP

- Through the history, determine what the patient actually means by "dizziness," paying particular attention to the duration of the "dizzy spells" (seconds vs. minutes or hours) and the precipitating events. Patients will often report dizziness after feeling faint, lightheaded, or ataxic, so it is important to carefully listen to the patient's description of symptoms and ask questions to elucidate differences between these symptoms.

Vertical nystagmus is pathognomonic for a central lesion.

TABLE 5-13. Central vs. Peripheral Dysequilibrium

	PERIPHERAL	CENTRAL
Vertigo	Often intermittent; severe.	Often constant; usually less severe.
Nystagmus	Always present; unidirectional, never vertical.	May be absent, unidirectional, or bidirectional; may be vertical.
Hearing loss or tinnitus	Often present.	Rarely present.
Instrinsic brain stem signs	Absent.	Often present.

TABLE 5-14. Etiologies of Peripheral and Central Dysequilibrium

PERIPHERAL VESTIBULAR DISORDERS	ACUTE CENTRAL ATAXIAS	CHRONIC CENTRAL ATAXIAS
BPPV	Drug intoxication	MS
Ménière's disease	Wernicke's encephalopathy	Cerebellar degeneration
Acute peripheral vestibulopathy	Vertebrobasilar ischemia/infarction	Hypothyroidism
Otosclerosis	Inflammatory disorders	Wilson's disease
Cerebellopontine-angle tumor	Cerebellar hemorrhage	Creutzfeldt-Jakob disease
Vestibulopathy/acoustic neuropathy		Posterior fossa masses
		Ataxia-telangiectasia

- Rule out other cranial nerve deficits, motor weakness, orthostasis, cardiac arrhythmia, and ear canal occlusions.
- Perform the Dix-Hallpike maneuver for BPPV (see below).
- Test for cerebellar dysfunction; perform the Romberg test and observe the patient's stance and gait. Test for dysmetria, checking finger-to-nose and heel-to-shin coordination; these should be unimpaired in peripheral processes.

THE DIX-HALLPIKE MANEUVER

In the Dix-Hallpike maneuver, vertigo is elicited with a change in the patient's head position. The patient is brought from a sitting to a supine position, with the head turned 45 degrees to one side and extended about 20 degrees backward. Once the patient is supine, his/her eyes are typically observed for about 30 seconds. If no nystagmus ensues, the patient is brought back to a sitting position. Following an additional delay of about 30 seconds, the other side is tested. A ⊕ Dix-Hallpike test consists of a burst of nystagmus and can provide clear evidence of a peripheral lesion.

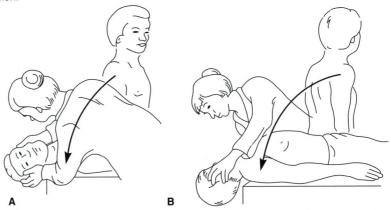

A   B

(Reproduced, with permission, from Lalwani AK. *Current Diagnosis & Treatment in Otolaryngology: Head and Neck Surgery*, 2nd ed. New York: McGraw-Hill, 2007, Figure 56-1.)

HIGH-YIELD FACTS

NEUROLOGY

- Test for nystagmus, paying close attention to direction and character. BPPV is usually torsional nystagmus toward the affected side.
- If necessary, obtain an audiogram, brain stem auditory evoked responses, and an electronystagmogram to distinguish peripheral from central dysequilibrium.
- Obtain an MRI if the patient shows signs of central involvement or if a peripheral disturbance cannot be explained by a benign etiology.

TREATMENT

- Use antihistamines (especially meclizine), anticholinergics such as scopolamine, benzodiazepines, or sympathomimetics to treat benign conditions such as BPPV and Ménière's disease.
- The reverse of the Dix-Hallpike maneuver can be used to treat BPPV, although the condition usually subsides spontaneously in weeks to months.
- Discontinue vestibulotoxic drugs such as quinidine, alcohol, and aspirin.
- Treat the underlying disorder if known (e.g., thiamine deficiency, hypothyroidism).

Other tests for dysequilibrium might include TFTs, B_{12} level, and CSF for cells and oligoclonal bands (WBCs in a CSF sample indicate infection, while oligoclonal bands can indicate MS).

HEADACHE

1° headache is generally classified into three categories: migraine, tension, and cluster. However, headache may also be the presenting symptom of serious neurologic disease and should therefore be taken seriously, as it is your job to differentiate between benign and life-threatening causes. Etiologies include the following:

- **Acute:** SAH, hemorrhagic stroke, seizure, meningitis, acutely elevated ICP, hypertensive encephalopathy, post-LP (spinal headache), ocular disease (glaucoma, iritis), new migraine headache.
- **Subacute:** Temporal arteritis, intracranial tumor, subdural hematoma, pseudotumor cerebri, trigeminal/glossopharyngeal neuralgia, postherpetic neuralgia, hypertension.
- **Chronic/episodic:** Migraine, cluster headache, tension headache, sinusitis, dental disease, neck pain.

WORKUP

There are four important questions that you should ask with regard to headache:

- **Is this a new or an old headache?** Is it qualitatively different from headaches the patient has had in the past? Is it the "worst headache of my life"? Any new, severe headache warrants an emergent workup and probably a CT (for "acute" causes of headaches listed above, especially SAH).
- **What are the characteristics of the pain?** Characterize onset, duration, quality, location, and alleviating and aggravating factors.
- **Are there any associated symptoms or relevant past medical history?** Ask about nausea, vomiting, fever, weight loss, neck pain, and jaw claudication. Also ask about a present and past history of cancer or immune compromise (e.g., HIV). Patients with migraines often have a family history of migraines.
- **Are there associated neurologic symptoms?** Look for ⊕ (paresthesias, visual stigmata) or ⊖ (weakness, numbness, ataxia) symptoms. Focal deficits and papilledema warrant immediate workup. Ask about photophobia, dizziness, neck stiffness, and a history of auras.

Recent-onset headaches require immediate workup! If associated with focal neurologic deficits or papilledema, do a CT or MRI to rule out more serious etiologies. Also rule out meningitis or SAH with an LP if symptoms are acute in onset.

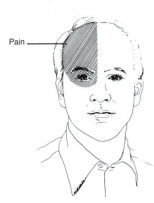

Pain ———

FIGURE 5-3. Distribution of pain in migraine headache.

Pain in migraine headache is most commonly hemicranial. Pain can also be holocephalic, bifrontal, or unilateral frontal. (Reproduced, with permission, from Aminoff MJ et al. *Clinical Neurology*, 3rd ed. Stamford, CT: Appleton & Lange, 1996: 91.)

Migraine Headache

Migraines afflict up to 18% of women (most commonly beginning before age 30) and 6% of men and tend to run in families. The etiology is not fully understood; vascular abnormalities (e.g., intracranial vasoconstriction and extracranial vasodilation) may be 2° to a disorder of serotonergic neurotransmission.

SIGNS AND SYMPTOMS

- A throbbing headache lasting between 2 and 20 hours. Headache is usually unilateral but may also be bilateral. In addition, it is generally frontal and retro-orbital but may also be occipital.
- Often precipitated by identifiable triggers, including the intake of certain foods (e.g., chocolate, caffeine), skipping meals, stress, menses, OCP use, and bright light.
- Associated with nausea and vomiting, photophobia, and noise sensitivity (see Figure 5-3).
- **"Classic migraines"** are preceded by a visual aura in the form of either scintillating scotomas (bright light or flashing lights, often in a zigzag pattern, moving across the visual field) or field cuts.
- **"Common migraines"** are not associated with these symptoms and can be bilateral and periorbital.

WORKUP

- Imaging may not be necessary in the absence of abnormal neurologic findings or fever. CT with contrast or MRI may be warranted if there are focal findings on exam (migraine itself can be associated with transient focal neurologic defects).
- Remember that subacute blood becomes isodense with brain after 2–14 days. MRI may therefore be the imaging modality of choice depending on the history and time course.

TREATMENT

- Counsel patients to avoid known triggers, regulate sleep and dietary patterns, and exercise regularly.
- **Pharmacotherapy** includes the following:
  - **Abortive therapy:** ASA/NSAIDs, sumatriptan and other triptans, ergots (partial 5-HT$_1$ agonists), and, rarely, opiates (although opiates should be avoided if possible). Triptans are contraindicated in patients with CAD or in those with complicated migraine headaches (e.g., basilar migraines) that include focal neurologic symptoms.
  - **Prophylactic therapy:** Propranolol (β-blockers), verapamil (calcium channel blockers), amitriptyline (TCAs), and valproic acid (anticonvulsants). Narcotics should not be used prophylactically.

Cluster Headache

Cluster headaches affect approximately 1% of the population and are seen more often in men than in women. They are much less common than migraines. The average age of onset is 25. Cluster headache may be precipitated by alcohol intake or vasodilator use.

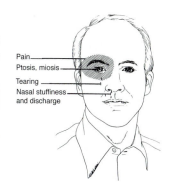

SIGNS AND SYMPTOMS

- A brief, severe, unilateral, periorbital headache lasting 30 minutes to three hours (see Figure 5-4). May present as "stabbing" eye pain that awakens the patient from sleep.
- Attacks tend to occur in clusters (hence the name), affecting the same part of the head and taking place at the same time of day (usually at night) and the same time of the year.
- Associated symptoms include ipsilateral tearing of the eye and conjunctival injection, Horner's syndrome, and nasal stuffiness.

WORKUP

No workup is necessary if the presentation is classic. However, imaging is often necessary to rule out a more catastrophic cause of this exceptionally painful syndrome (especially with initial presentation).

TREATMENT

- **Abortive therapy:** High-flow (100%) O_2, sumatriptan, ergots, intranasal lidocaine, corticosteroids.
- **Prophylactic therapy:** Calcium channel blockers, ergots, valproic acid, prednisone, topiramate, methysergide.

FIGURE 5-4. Distribution of pain in cluster headache.

Pain is commonly associated with ipsilateral conjunctival injection, tearing, nasal stuffiness, and Horner's syndrome. (Reproduced, with permission, from Aminoff MJ et al. *Clinical Neurology*, 3rd ed. Stamford, CT: Appleton & Lange, 1996: 92.)

Tension Headache

Tension headaches are chronic headaches that do not share the specific symptomatology of migraines. They are a diagnosis of exclusion and account for 75% of all headaches. If a history of nausea and vomiting, a history of photophobia, or a ⊕ family history is elicited, migraine headache is the more likely diagnosis. Many patients appear to have an overlap syndrome with components of both migraine and tension headaches.

SIGNS AND SYMPTOMS

- Presents as a tight, bandlike pain, especially posteriorly, that is exacerbated by noise, bright lights, fatigue, and stress. Associated with anxiety, poor concentration, and difficulty sleeping.
- Headaches are generalized but may be most intense in the occipital or neck region. The surrounding musculature may also be tightly contracted.
- Patients describe headache onset as occurring later in the workday—as distinguished from migraines, which can occur on awakening.
- No focal neurologic signs.

WORKUP

- A diagnosis of exclusion. Other causes of headache must first be considered.
- Headache diaries are helpful in isolating triggers and evaluating treatment trials.

TREATMENT

- Relaxation, massage, hot baths, regular diet, exercise, and avoidance of exacerbating factors may alleviate symptoms.
- Abortive medications are generally restricted to NSAIDs, although triptans and ergots may be considered.
- Prophylactic therapy is uncommon.

Differential diagnosis of headache:

Migraine: Often associated with an aura.

Cluster: Sharp, unilateral periorbital pain.

Tension: Bandlike pain.

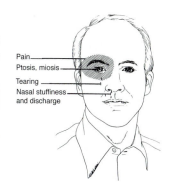

HIGH-YIELD FACTS

NEUROLOGY

- Analgesic overuse should be avoided, as it can precipitate an analgesic rebound headache syndrome. Analgesic rebound headaches are seen in 1% of the population, primarily in middle-aged women with underlying migraines.

Trigeminal Neuralgia (TN)

A neuropathic disorder causing episodes of intense pain in the distribution of the trigeminal nerve. Although its etiology is still not well defined, a possible framework involves compression of the trigeminal nerve near its connection with the pons causing injury to the myelin sheath, leading to erratic hyperfunctioning of the nerve. Aneurysms of the superior cerebellar artery, tumors, or arachnoid cysts may cause nerve compression. TN is sometimes associated with MS, especially in younger women.

SIGNS AND SYMPTOMS

- Presents with paroxysmal episodes of severe pain in the jaw, forehead, and scalp and around the eyes and lips. Episodes can occur up to hundreds of times a day.
- Symptoms are usually unilateral.
- Allodynia (an exaggerated response to otherwise non-noxious stimuli) of the face may also be noted.

TREATMENT

- Although there is no cure, medications can be of benefit.
    - Anticonvulsants (carbamazepine, phenytoin, topiramate) are first-line therapy.
    - Gabapentin, also an anticonvulsant, is often used in the treatment of neuropathic pain states (e.g., TN, postherpetic neuralgia). TCAs such as nortriptyline are also used for neuropathic pain.
    - Botox injections into the nerve may be of benefit.
- If medication fails, surgery may be attempted.

Pseudotumor Cerebri

Also known as idiopathic intracranial hypertension (IIH). Classically seen in obese women of childbearing age (those 20–45 years of age). Patients with pseudotumor cerebri have chronically elevated ICP, leading to papilledema. The main potentially permanent morbidity is vision loss resulting from decompensation of papilledema and progressive optic atrophy.

SIGNS AND SYMPTOMS

- Findings resulting from ↑ ICP are as follows:
    - **Headache** (the most common presenting complaint); nausea/vomiting.
    - **Pulse tinnitus:** A rhythmic or "rushing" sound heard in one or both ears that may be exacerbated by bending movements.
    - **Horizontal diplopia:** A falsely localizing "sixth nerve palsy." Other than this, patients should have no localizing signs.
- Findings resulting from papilledema include the following:
    - Transient visual dimming or blackouts, progressive peripheral vision loss, and blurring and distortion (i.e., metamorphopsia) of central vision.
    - Pain behind the eye or pain on eye movements.
    - Bilaterally swollen, edematous optic nerves consistent with papilledema on funduscopic exam.

- Acute and chronic papilledema can be clinically distinguished as follows:
  - **Acute:** Flame hemorrhages, venous engorgement, and hard exudates.
  - **Chronic:** Optic disk pallor.

WORKUP

- LP (preferably in lateral decubitus position) shows a high opening pressure (i.e., > 250 mm of water).
- CT/MRI reveals normal to small ventricles.

TREATMENT

- **Pharmacologic:**
  - **Diuretics:** Carbonic anhydrase inhibitors (e.g., acetazolamide).
  - **Corticosteroids:** In severe cases, a short course of high-dose steroids can be used to combat vision loss.
- **Procedural:**
  - Large-volume therapeutic LP.
  - Lumboperitoneal or ventriculoperitoneal CSF shunts and optic nerve sheath fenestration should be considered as last resorts.
- **Long term:** Weight loss; dietary changes (e.g., a low-sodium diet).

INTRACRANIAL NEOPLASMS

Intracranial neoplasms may be 1° (30%) or metastatic (70%).

- **1°:** Of all 1° brain tumors, 40% are benign and often affect those > 65 years of age. The most frequently reported 1° tumors include meningiomas and glioblastoma multiforme (GBM) in adults and medulloblastomas and astrocytomas in children. These rarely spread beyond the CNS.
- **Metastatic:** Metastatic tumors to the brain most commonly arise from breast, lung, kidney, and GI tract neoplasms or from melanoma. They most often appear at the gray-white junction and are characterized by rapid growth, invasiveness, necrosis, and neovascularization. One should suspect metastatic disease and seek a 1° source when multiple discrete neoplastic nodules appear in the brain simultaneously.

SIGNS AND SYMPTOMS

- Symptoms usually develop gradually and are due to local growth and resulting mass effect, cerebral edema, ventricular obstruction, and ↑ ICP.
- Patients often complain of persistent vomiting and headache or focal neurologic deficits.
- Other common symptoms include personality changes, lethargy, intellectual decline, aphasias, seizures, and mood swings.
- Only 30% of patients present with headache. When present, headache is typically dull and steady, worse in the morning, associated with nausea and vomiting, and exacerbated by coughing, changing position, or exertion.

WORKUP

- CT with contrast and MRI with gadolinium to localize and determine the extent of the lesion.
- Some brain tumors present as intracranial hemorrhages. These are typically located near the cortex, where blood vessels dramatically ↓ in size (as opposed to hypertension-related bleeds, which occur in deep gray matter such as the basal ganglia).

Two-thirds of 1° brain tumors in adults are supratentorial. Only one-third are supratentorial in children. Most CNS tumors are not 1° lesions but are metastases from the breast, lung, kidney, and other cancers.

- Certain metastatic brain tumors—e.g., those from thyroid cancer, melanoma, renal tumors, and choriocarcinoma—tend to bleed. Breast and lung metastases do not tend to bleed; however, 1° breast and lung tumors are often found in conjunction with brain hemorrhages due to these tumors' societal predominance.
- Histologic diagnosis may be obtained via CT-guided biopsy or during surgical tumor debulking, although the most likely diagnosis may be evident from tumor morphology and location on imaging studies.

TREATMENT

- Observation, radiation therapy, chemotherapy, or surgical resection, depending on tumor type (see Table 5-15).

TABLE 5-15. Common 1° Neoplasms

TUMOR	PRESENTATION	TREATMENT
Astrocytoma	Presents with headache and ↑ ICP. May cause unilateral paralysis in CN V–VII and CN X. Has a slow, protracted course. The prognosis is much better than that of GBM.	Resection if possible; radiation.
GBM (grade IV astrocytoma)	The most common 1° brain tumor. Often presents with headache and ↑ ICP. Progresses rapidly. Has a poor prognosis (< 1 year from the time of diagnosis).	Surgical removal and resection. Radiation and chemotherapy have variable results. Palliative care.
Meningioma	Originates from the dura mater or arachnoid. Has a good prognosis. Incidence ↑ with age.	Surgical resection; radiation for unresectable tumors.
Acoustic neuroma (schwannoma)	Presents with ipsilateral hearing loss, tinnitus, vertigo, and signs of cerebellar dysfunction. Derived from Schwann cells.	Surgical removal.
Medulloblastoma	Common in children. Arises from the fourth ventricle and leads to ↑ ICP. Highly malignant; may seed the subarachnoid space.	Surgical resection; radiation, chemotherapy.
Ependymoma	Common in children. May arise from the ependyma of a ventricle (commonly the fourth) or the spinal cord; may lead to hydrocephalus.	Surgical resection, radiation.

- GBM tumors are poorly responsive and require palliative care.
- Corticosteroids can be used to reduce vasogenic edema.

Parkinson's Disease

Parkinson's disease is a hypokinetic syndrome caused by the idiopathic depletion of dopamine in the substantia nigra and nigrostriatal tract. The usual age of onset is roughly 60 years, and life expectancy is approximately nine years from the time of diagnosis. Other insults that can cause a parkinsonian syndrome include neuroleptic and metoclopramide use, postencephalitis, toxic exposures (manganese, MPTP, carbon disulfide), bihemispheric ischemia, and trauma.

SIGNS AND SYMPTOMS

- The "**Parkinson's tetrad**" consists of the following (see also Figure 5-5):
  - **Resting tremor:** A coarse "pill-rolling" tremor that can affect the extremities, trunk, and head; one of the earliest signs.
  - **Rigidity:** Resistance to passive motion; "cogwheeling."
  - **Bradykinesia:** Includes difficulty initiating movement and slow execution. A festinating gait (a wide leg stance with short accelerating steps) without arm swing is also common.
  - **Postural instability:** Stooping, impaired righting reflex, freezing, falls.
- Other signs include masked facies, memory loss/mild dementia, micrographia, and a soft voice.

DIFFERENTIAL

- "**Parkinson's-plus**" syndromes (Parkinson's symptoms plus additional neurologic symptoms): Include progressive supranuclear palsy, corticobasal ganglionic degeneration, and Shy-Drager syndrome.
- **Other:** Essential tremor, depression, normal pressure hydrocephalus, and Wilson's disease can also present with tremors, psychomotor slowing, and instability.

TREATMENT

- Levodopa and carbidopa are dopamine analogs and are the mainstays of therapy. Catechol-O-methyltransferase (COMT) inhibitors such as entacapone ↑ the availability of levodopa to the brain and may ↓ motor fluctuation.
- Bromocriptine and pramipexole are dopamine agonists.
- Benztropine, an anticholinergic, and amantadine, a dopamine agonist, are useful for tremor symptoms.
- For intractable cases, surgical pallidotomy or chronic deep brain stimulation may be tried.

Huntington's Disease

Huntington's disease is a hyperkinetic autosomal-dominant disorder involving multiple abnormal CAG triplet repeats (< 29 is normal) in the huntingtin gene on chromosome 4p. The number of repeats expands in subsequent generations, leading to earlier expression and more severe disease. Life expectancy is 20 years from the time of diagnosis.

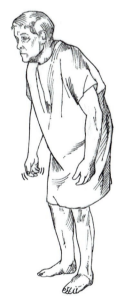

FIGURE 5-5. Patient with parkinsonism in typical flexed posture.

Note the masklike facies and resting hand tremor. (Reproduced, with permission, from Aminoff MJ et al. *Clinical Neurology*, 3rd ed. Stamford, CT: Appleton & Lange, 1996: 220.)

ESSENTIAL TREMOR VS. PARKINSON'S DISEASE

- **Essential tremor:**
  - Characterized by a postural/intention tremor. Fifty percent of patients have a ⊕ family history.
  - Alcohol reduces the tremor; tremor can affect the voice.
  - Treated with propranolol or primidone.
- **Parkinson's disease:**
  - Characterized by a **resting tremor.**
  - Other Parkinson's symptoms (e.g., bradykinesia, cogwheeling) are also present.
  - Treated with benztropine (effective only for tremor symptoms) or carbidopa/levodopa.

SIGNS AND SYMPTOMS

Presents at 30–50 years of age with gradual onset of symptoms:

- **Chorea:** Early motor symptoms of stiffness and rigidity give way to prominent choreiform activity. Patients are highly aware of their movements.
- **Altered behavior:** Irritability, moodiness, antisocial behavior, schizreniform illness, depression, suicidality.
- **Dementia.**

DIFFERENTIAL

Senile chorea, hemiballismus, Wilson's disease, Parkinson's disease.

WORKUP

- A clinical diagnosis.
- CT/MRI reveal cerebral atrophy, especially of the caudate and putamen.
- Genetic testing to determine the number of CAG repeats.

TREATMENT

- There is no cure, so treatment is symptomatic:
  - Reserpine to minimize unwanted movements.
  - Haloperidol for treatment of psychosis.
  - Antidepressants for depression; benzodiazepines for anxiety.
- Offer genetic counseling for offspring, with attention given to the social aspects of the disease.

SEIZURES

Cortical events characterized by excessive or hypersynchronous discharge by cortical neurons. The etiology is multifactorial, depending on a fine balance between (1) seizure threshold, (2) the presence of an epileptogenic focus, and (3) a precipitating factor or provocative event. A change in any of these factors can ↑ the frequency of seizures. For example, a 1° nervous system disorder may induce an epileptogenic focus that has a lower seizure threshold than "healthy tissue." Alternatively, systemic diseases or disturbances can lead to an altered seizure threshold. Some definitions related to seizures are essential:

- **Partial (focal) seizures** are seizures arising from a discrete region of one cerebral hemisphere; they can be categorized as simple or complex. Simple seizures do not involve a loss of consciousness; complex seizures cause a loss of consciousness.
- **Generalized seizures** are seizures involving both cerebral hemispheres, with loss of consciousness.

WORKUP/TREATMENT

The evaluation and treatment of a patient with a recent history of seizure should seek to answer the following questions:

- **Did the patient actually have a seizure?** A syncopal event with postsyncopal convulsion can easily be confused with a seizure.
    - Distinguish pseudoseizures (psychogenic) from true seizures (electrical). Serum prolactin levels are usually ↑ after true tonic-clonic seizures but are unaffected by pseudoseizures (they may also be unaffected by partial seizures). One should take care not to overinterpret prolactin levels, as they can also rise after a syncopal event.
    - In taking a history from the patient and from observers, ask about possible prodromes, onset, course, and postseizure period (see Table 5-16).
- **Was the seizure provoked by a systemic process?**
    - Non-neurologic etiologies include **hypoglycemia or hyperglycemia, hyponatremia, hypocalcemia, hyperosmolar states, hepatic encephalopathy,** uremia, porphyria, **drug overdose** (especially cocaine, antidepressants, neuroleptics, methylxanthines, and lidocaine), **drug withdrawal** (especially alcohol and other sedatives), eclampsia, hyperthermia, hypertensive encephalopathy, and cerebral hypoperfusion.
    - Workup should focus first on reversible causes and provocative factors.

Tonic-clonic movements do not exclude syncope.

Epilepsy is defined as a predisposition to recurrent, unprovoked seizures. Not everyone with seizures has epilepsy!

TABLE 5-16. Seizure vs. Syncope

	SEIZURE	**SYNCOPE**
Onset	Sudden onset with or without preceding aura. Focal sensory or motor phenomena. Sensation of fear, smell, memory.	Progressive lightheadedness; dimming of vision, faintness.
Course	Sudden loss of . with tonic-clonic activity. May last 1–2 minutes. Tongue laceration, head trauma, and bowel/urinary incontinence may be seen.	Gradual loss of consciousness, limp or with jerking. Rarely lasts > 14 seconds. Less commonly injured.
Postspell	Postictal confusion and disorientation.	Typically immediate return to lucidity.

Most seizures are self-limited and last < 2 minutes. Prolonged or repetitive seizures are called status epilepticus and constitute a medical emergency.

It is important to try to determine the etiology of seizures in order to guide treatment and elucidate the prognosis. In a patient with a known seizure disorder, consider subtherapeutic levels of medications or a new factor, such as infection or trauma.

Todd's paralysis is often confused with acute stroke and can be differentiated by MRI (DWI).

- **Was the seizure caused by an underlying neurologic disorder?** Seizures with focal onset (or focal postictal deficit) suggest focal CNS pathology. Seizures may be the presenting sign of a tumor, stroke, AVM, infection, or hemorrhage, or they may represent the delayed presentation of a developmental abnormality.
  - Patients without a known cause for their seizures should undergo neurologic evaluation, particularly for treatable causes (see Table 5-17).
  - The history should include past seizures; birth, childhood, and recent trauma; and developmental delays.
- **Is anticonvulsant therapy indicated?** Patients with a first seizure are frequently not treated when the underlying cause is unknown. However, one-third of idiopathic seizures will recur. Recurrence rates are higher in patients with abnormal EEGs or MRIs, with focal exams, or with irreversible predisposing factors (see Figure 5-6).

Partial (Focal) Seizures

Focal seizures arise from a discrete region in one cerebral hemisphere. Such seizures may, however, generalize to involve both hemispheres. Partial seizures are divided into simple and complex seizures.

SIGNS AND SYMPTOMS

- Presentation varies depending on the type of seizure.
  - **Simple partial seizures:** The clinical effects of focal seizures depend on the region of the cortex that is affected. Seizure foci in the motor or sensory areas (the frontal or parietal lobes, respectively) cause simple partial seizures and may lead to phenomena such as twitching of the face or tingling of the hand. Involvement of the insular cortex can lead to autonomic phenomena such as alterations in BP, changes in heart rate, and bronchoconstriction. There is **no alteration in consciousness.**
  - **Complex partial seizures:** These seizures can arise from any part of the cortex but classically involve the temporal lobe, frontal lobe, and occipital lobe, in descending order of frequency. Involvement of the temporal lobe or medial frontal lobe leads to complex partial seizures, with effects such as memories (déjà vu), feelings of fear, and "complex" actions such as lip smacking or walking. Involves an **impaired level of consciousness.**
- Postictally, Todd's paralysis may be seen, presenting with weakness or paralysis, often unilateral, that resolves over 24 hours. Often indicates a focal brain lesion.

DIFFERENTIAL

TIAs, panic attacks, pseudoseizures, syncope.

TABLE 5-17. Common Etiologies of Seizures by Age

INFANTS	CHILDREN (2–10)	ADOLESCENTS (11–17)	ADULTS (18–35)	ADULTS (35+)
Perinatal injury/ischemia	Idiopathic	Idiopathic	Trauma	Trauma
Infection	Infection	Trauma	Alcoholism	Stroke
Metabolic disturbance	Trauma	Drug withdrawal	Brain tumor	Metabolic disorders
Congenital/genetic disorders	Febrile seizure	AVM	Drug withdrawal	Alcoholism

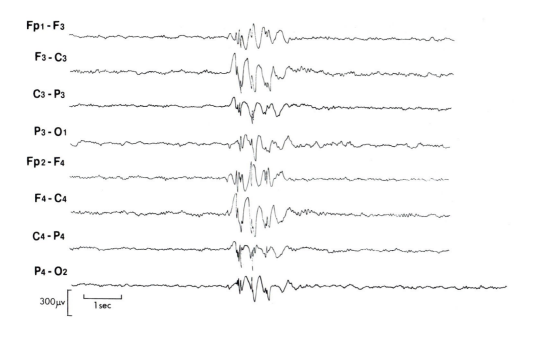

FIGURE 5-6. EEG in idiopathic seizures.

Note the burst of generalized epileptiform activity on a relatively normal background. (Reproduced, with permission, from Aminoff MJ et al. *Clinical Neurology*, 3rd ed. Stamford, CT: Appleton & Lange, 1996: 241.)

WORKUP

- Perform a detailed neurologic exam.
- Obtain a CBC, electrolytes, calcium, glucose, ABGs, LFTs, a renal panel, RPR, ESR, and a toxicology screen to rule out systemic causes.
- An EEG is often ordered to look for epileptiform waveforms and to confirm epileptiform seizures.
- Rule out a mass by MRI or CT with contrast. MRI is more sensitive and specific in seizure evaluations.

TREATMENT

- **Treat the underlying cause** if it is known.
  - For recurrent partial seizures, anticonvulsants such as phenytoin (Dilantin), carbamazepine (Tegretol), phenobarbital, valproate (Depakote), lamotrigine (Lamictal), gabapentin (Neurontin), and levetiracetam (Keppra) can be used.
  - In children, phenobarbital is the first-line anticonvulsant.
- For intractable temporal lobe seizures, surgical options include anterior temporal lobectomy.

Generalized Seizures

The two most common types of generalized seizures are absence (petit mal) and tonic-clonic (grand mal).

The side effects of phenytoin include gingival hyperplasia, hirsutism, and ↓ vitamin B_{12} levels.

ABSENCE (PETIT MAL) SEIZURES

Absence seizures begin in childhood, are often familial, and typically subside before adulthood.

SIGNS AND SYMPTOMS

- Characterized by brief, often unnoticeable episodes of impaired consciousness lasting only seconds and occurring up to hundreds of times per day.
- There is no loss of muscle tone, and patients have no memory of these events.
- Eye fluttering or lip smacking is common during absence seizures.

WORKUP

The EEG shows a classic **three-per-second spike-and-wave tracing** (see Figure 5-7).

TREATMENT

Ethosuximide is the first-line agent. Valproic acid or zonisamide may also be used.

TONIC-CLONIC (GRAND MAL) SEIZURES

SIGNS AND SYMPTOMS

- Tonic-clonic seizures begin suddenly with **loss of consciousness** and tonic extension of the back and extremities, continuing with 1–2 minutes of repetitive, symmetric clonic movements.
- Seizures are marked by **incontinence** and **tongue biting** (check for bite marks on the tongue).
- Patients may also appear cyanotic during the ictal period owing to poor respiratory function during the seizure.
- Consciousness is slowly regained in the postictal period.
- Postictally, the patient may complain of muscle aches and headaches.

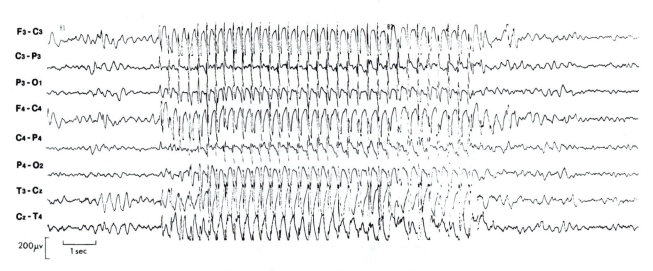

FIGURE 5-7. EEG of absence seizures with the classical three-spike-per-second pattern.

(Reproduced, with permission, from Aminoff MJ et al. *Clinical Neurology*, 3rd ed. Stamford, CT: Appleton & Lange, 1996: 240.)

DIFFERENTIAL

Syncope, cardiac dysrhythmias, brain stem ischemia, pseudoseizures.

TREATMENT

- Protect the airway.
- Manage the underlying cause.
- Otherwise, valproate, phenytoin, and carbamazepine are first-line anticonvulsant therapies. The choice of anticonvulsant depends on EEG, MRI data, and a careful history.

DEMYELINATING/DEGENERATIVE DISORDERS

Multiple Sclerosis (MS)

MS is an autoimmune demyelinating disorder of the CNS that is most likely T-cell mediated. Patients present with neurologic complaints that are separated in time and space and cannot be explained by a single lesion. MS has a female-to-male ratio of 2:1, shows a peak incidence at 20–40 years of age, and is thought to have a genetic component. MS grows more common with increasing distance from the equator, and these geographic differences have led to the hypothesis that it may be the result of a genetic predisposition coupled with a heretofore uncharacterized viral infection. The clinical course of MS is variable. The types of MS, in order of decreasing frequency, are relapsing-remitting, 2° progressive, 1° progressive, and progressive-relapsing.

> *The classic triad of MS—*
>
> **SIN**
>
> **S**canning speech
> **I**ntention tremor
> **N**ystagmus

SIGNS AND SYMPTOMS

Signs of MS are abundant, as the disease can affect any white-matter region of the CNS. They include the following:

- **Ocular symptoms:**
  - Optic pallor or atrophy.
  - Medial longitudinal fasciculus lesions leading to internuclear ophthalmoplegia and diplopia.
  - Optic neuropathy involving painful visual loss.
- **Bulbar symptoms:** Dysarthria; vertigo.
- **Spinal cord symptoms:**
  - Hyperreflexia; spasticity.
  - Limb weakness.
  - Paresthesias and pain. Patients will often present with a sensory level (e.g., numbness and tingling below a given dermatome) due to the organization of the spinal cord.
  - Urinary retention (leading to an ↑ risk of UTI).
  - **Lhermitte's sign** appears in some MS patients and presents as an electrical sensation running down the spine and into the lower extremities with neck flexion.

> *Factors exacerbating MS include infection, heat (referred to as **Uthoff's phenomenon**), trauma, the postpartum period, and vigorous activity. By contrast, pregnancy is often associated with a **decreased** frequency of exacerbations.*

DIFFERENTIAL

CNS tumors or trauma, multiple CVAs, vasculitis, vitamin B_{12} deficiency, CNS infections (Lyme disease, neurosyphilis), sarcoidosis, atypical presentations of other autoimmune diseases (e.g., SLE and Sjögren's syndrome).

WORKUP

- Diagnosed clinically by a history of multiple, separate neurologic attacks consisting of the following:

*Think MS with multiple
neurologic lesions separated
in time and space.*

> **MS treatment is as
> easy as ABC—**
>
> **A**vonex
> **B**etaseron
> **C**opaxone

*MS patients with the best
prognosis are those with a
relapsing-remitting course
with discrete exacerbations,
full recovery of function after
each episode, and an early
age of onset of the initial
attack.*

*Key distinctions between MS
and GBS:*

- *GBS produces no sensory
  level, whereas spinal cord
  demyelination does
  produce a sensory level.*
- *GBS produces hypo- or
  areflexia, whereas chronic
  MS often leads to
  hyperreflexia. Be careful,
  however, as an acute MS
  exacerbation can lead to
  areflexia for several days.*

- Two attacks and clinical evidence of two separate lesions, **or**
- Two attacks with clinical evidence of one lesion and laboratory evidence of another lesion.
- MRI shows multiple, asymmetric, often periventricular lesions in white matter, called plaques. Plaques extending as long spindles away from the ventricles are referred to as Dawson's fingers. Corpus callosum lesions are usually pathognomonic. Active lesions enhance with gadolinium on MRI.
- CSF analysis may show mononuclear pleocytosis (> 5 cells/μL) in 25% of cases, elevated free kappa light chains in 60% of cases, ↑ CSF IgG in 80% of cases, and oligoclonal bands in 90% of cases (nonspecific). Typically, there are no more than 50 WBCs in CSF.
- Other laboratory tests include visual, somatosensory, or brain stem evoked potentials.

TREATMENT

- There is no cure for MS.
- Immunomodulatory and immunosuppressive treatments can ↓ the number of relapses (by 30%) and can also reduce the severity of relapses in relapsing-remitting disease. Immunomodulators include **A**vonex (interferon-β1a), **B**etaseron (interferon-β1b), and **C**opaxone (copolymer 1).
- IV steroids should be given during acute exacerbations.
- Patients may also benefit greatly from physical therapy and symptomatic treatment of spasticity, pain, fatigue, and depression.

COMPLICATIONS

- The **Kurtzke five-year rule** states that the absence of significant motor or cerebellar dysfunction five years after diagnosis correlates with limited disability at 15 years. Fifteen years after diagnosis, approximately 20% of MS patients have no functional limitation; 70% are limited or are unable to perform major activities of daily living; and 75% are not employed.
- Morbidity and mortality are related to the accumulation of physical disabilities due to incomplete recovery from sequential attacks.

Guillain-Barré Syndrome (GBS)

An acute, rapidly progressive peripheral demyelinating disease, GBS is believed to be autoimmune in nature and is often associated with a viral URI prodrome or *Campylobacter jejuni* infection. Approximately 3500 cases are diagnosed each year in the United States, and some 85% of patients make a complete or near-complete recovery. The mortality rate is roughly 5%.

SIGNS AND SYMPTOMS

- Presents with rapidly progressive ascending paralysis. Classically, weakness and sensory symptoms begin distally (as with all peripheral nerve diseases) and ascend rapidly to involve the trunk, diaphragm, and cranial nerves.
- Reflexes are absent (this is a peripheral nerve disorder).
- Sensory symptoms such as numbness, tingling, and muscle aches are common, especially in the lower back.
- Autonomic deficits may be present.

WORKUP

- EMG and nerve conduction studies will show diffuse demyelination.
- LP reveals a CSF protein level > 55 mg/dL with little or no pleocytosis (**albuminocytologic dissociation**).
- MRI of the spinal cord to exclude cord compression.

TREATMENT

- Admit to the ICU for close monitoring. Be prepared to intubate patients if they develop impending respiratory failure (from paralysis of the diaphragm and accessory respiratory muscles).
- Watch for autonomic instability, including cardiac arrhythmias and gastroparesis. Autonomic instability is **a major cause of mortality.**
- Follow FVCs, not ABGs.
- Plasmapheresis and IVIG are first-line treatments. Steroids are **not** indicated in GBS.
- Aggressive rehabilitation is imperative. Most patients will regain premorbid function, but in severe cases this may take up to a year.

*Plasmapheresis and IVIG are first-line treatments for GBS. Steroids are **not** indicated in such patients.*

Amyotrophic Lateral Sclerosis (ALS)

A chronic, progressive degenerative disease of unknown etiology characterized by loss of upper and lower motor neurons (UMNs/LMNs). There are no associated sensory symptoms.

SIGNS AND SYMPTOMS

- Presents with asymmetric, slowly progressive weakness affecting the arms, legs, and cranial nerves. Some patients may present first with fasciculations.
- Also presents with UMN and/or LMN signs:
    - **UMN signs:** Spasticity, ↑ reflexes, upgoing toes.
    - **LMN signs:** Flaccidity, ↓ or absent reflexes, fasciculations, atrophy.
- Eye movements and sphincter tone are usually spared.

*UMN lesions—everything is **up** (tone, DTR, toe).*
*LMN lesions—everything is **lowered.***

WORKUP

- The clinical presentation is often diagnostic. Rule out systemic causes.
- EMG/nerve conduction studies show widespread denervation and fibrillation potentials.
- CT/MRI of the spine to exclude structural lesions that might account for UMN signs.

TREATMENT

- Supportive measures and patient education.
- Riluzole, a glutamate inhibitor, may prolong survival time.

UMN cell bodies are in the motor cortex and go to the spinal cord. LMN cell bodies are in the spinal cord and go to muscles.

DISORDERS OF THE NEUROMUSCULAR JUNCTION

Myasthenia Gravis

An autoimmune disease caused by circulating antibodies to postsynaptic acetylcholine receptors. It occurs at all ages, most often affecting young adult women. The disease can be associated with thymoma, thyrotoxicosis, and autoimmune disorders such as RA and SLE.

SIGNS AND SYMPTOMS

- Patients most often present with fluctuating ptosis or double vision due to weakness of the levator palpebrae and EOM.
- Weakness worsens with activity and throughout the day.
- Difficulty swallowing and proximal muscle weakness (e.g., difficulty climbing stairs, rising from a chair, or brushing hair) can also be present.
- Respiratory compromise and aspiration are rare but potentially lethal complications and are termed **myasthenic crises.**

WORKUP

- Often diagnosed on the basis of clinical findings. On exam, one can test how long patients can keep their eyes open.
- Carefully monitored testing with **edrophonium** (Tensilon, a short-acting cholinesterase inhibitor) is diagnostic; in a symptomatic patient, IV injection of edrophonium leads to rapid (and temporary) improvement of clinical symptoms.
- An abnormal EMG and a decremental response to repetitive nerve stimulation can yield additional confirmation.
- AChR antibodies are ⊕ in 85–90% of patients. Twenty percent of patients who are ⊖ for anti-AChR antibodies will have anti–muscle-specific kinase (anti-MuSK) antibodies.
- Antistriatal (striated muscle) antibodies are present in 85% of patients with thymoma. CT of the chest is used to evaluate for thymoma.

TREATMENT

- Long-acting anticholinesterase inhibitors prolong the action of acetylcholine in the synapse and overcome the antibodies by competition. These medications include neostigmine and pyridostigmine (Mestinon), which provide symptomatic relief.
- Prednisone and other immunosuppressive agents are the mainstays of treatment. Because symptoms can worsen with prednisone, however, patients must be closely monitored.
- In severe cases, known as myasthenic crises, plasmapheresis or IVIG may provide temporary relief (days to weeks).
- Thymectomy (regardless of the presence of thymoma) is associated with an ↑ rate of clinical remission and a better clinical outcome (especially in younger patients).

Lambert-Eaton Myasthenic Syndrome

A paraneoplastic disorder characterized by muscle weakness that often improves with repetitive contraction of the muscle (vs. myasthenia gravis, in which repetitive muscle contraction causes ↑ weakness).

SIGNS AND SYMPTOMS

- Often associated with small cell lung carcinoma (90% of cases).
- Weakness of the proximal muscles is seen, with the extraocular or bulbar muscles typically spared.
- DTRs are depressed or absent.

WORKUP

- Autoantibodies to presynaptic calcium channels.
- Chest CT for lung neoplasm.

MYASTHENIA GRAVIS VS. LAMBERT-EATON MYASTHENIC SYNDROME

- In **myasthenia gravis,** acetylcholine from the presynaptic nerve terminal cannot bind to the postsynaptic receptor because of antibodies attached to the ACh receptor.

- In **Lambert-Eaton myasthenic syndrome,** signal distortion is caused by an inadequate release of neurotransmitter, so with repeated contraction, the amount of neurotransmitter in the neuromuscular junction can build up in quantity and lead to transient ↑ strength.

TREATMENT

Guanidine hydrochloride is the mainstay of treatment. Anticholinesterases may also mitigate symptoms. Tumor resection can cure symptoms.

WEAKNESS

The key to working up a patient with complaints of weakness is to think anatomically. There are several locations in the chain of executing a movement where pathology can occur, and you should consider them all: the cortex, corticospinal tract (including brain stem pathology), spinal cord, anterior horn cells, nerve roots, plexus, peripheral nerves, neuromuscular junction, and muscle. True weakness involves a loss of motor power or strength and is exclusively a disorder of the motor system, localizing somewhere between the motor cortex and the muscles themselves.

You should first seek to differentiate UMN from LMN disease (see Table 5-18). Then try to pinpoint the location using your exam, thinking about what the affected muscles have in common (e.g., all are proximal; all are innervated by one nerve). As is always the case, the history, the physical, and the remainder of the neurologic examination are crucial in this process.

DIFFERENTIAL

The etiology of weakness is generally classified by anatomic localization. Although in most cases the physical exam and history will indicate a certain ana-

TABLE 5-18. Anatomic Localization: UMN vs. LMN Disease

CLINICAL FEATURES	UMN	LMN
Pattern of weakness	Pyramidal (arm extensors, leg flexors).	Variable.
Tone	Spastic (↑; initially flaccid).	Flaccid (↓).
DTRs	↑ (initially ↓).	Normal, ↓, absent.
Miscellaneous signs	Babinski's, other CNS signs.	Atrophy, fasciculations.

tomic level, don't get pigeonholed into a small differential; remember to consider all possible etiologies of weakness each time. Table 5-19 lists the location of lesions, the pattern of weakness expected, and associated etiologies.

WORKUP

The physical exam and history will largely shape the differential diagnosis and indicate which labs and tests to order. The patterns of laboratory and test results observed for the different etiologies of weakness are outlined in Table 5-20.

■ If a central lesion or UMN syndrome is suspected, CT or MRI of the brain (including the brain stem) and MRI of the spinal cord are often ordered.
■ If a peripheral neuropathy or a muscle-related weakness is suspected, tests should include CK, EMG, nerve conduction studies, and laboratory studies for treatable causes of peripheral neuropathy and myopathy. If there is a high index of suspicion for a demyelinating peripheral neuropathy, an LP may also be ordered.
■ In cases of high suspicion of myopathy, a muscle biopsy may be indicated.

Carpal Tunnel Syndrome

Results from compression of the median nerve at the wrist where it passes through the carpal tunnel. Most commonly seen in women 30–55 years of age. Risk factors include repetitive use injury, pregnancy, diabetes, hypothyroidism, acromegaly, RA, and obesity.

TABLE 5-19. Lesions in the Motor Pathways

LOCATION OF LESION	DISEASE TERM	WEAKNESS PATTERN	ETIOLOGIES
Intracranial		UMN, as described below.	Stroke, neoplasm, MS, hemorrhage, trauma, infection.
Spinal cord	Myelopathy	UMN at spinal level.	Compression, trauma, MS.
Anterior horn cell	Motor neuron disease	UMN/LMN; variable.	ALS, spinal muscular atrophy, poliomyelitis.
Nerve root	Radiculopathy	LMN at root level.	Compression, infection, meningeal mets, trauma.
Plexus	Plexopathy	LMN, mixed roots.	Trauma, neoplastic infiltration, idiopathic.
Peripheral nerve	Neuropathy	LMN, by nerve.	Metabolic, toxic, inflammatory, neoplastic.
Neuromuscular junction		Diffuse weakness.	Myasthenia gravis, Lambert-Eaton syndrome.
Muscle	Myopathy	Proximal weakness.	Muscular dystrophy, polymyositis, EtOH.

TABLE 5-20. Investigation of Patient with Weakness

TEST	SPINAL CORD	ANTERIOR HORN CELL DISORDERS	PERIPHERAL NERVE PLEXUS	NEUROMUSCULAR JUNCTION	MYOPATHY
Serum enzymes	Normal.	Normal.	Normal.	Normal.	Normal or ↑.
Electro-myography	With lesions causing axonal degeneration, there may be abnormal spontaneous activity (e.g., fasciculations, fibrillations) if sufficient time has elapsed after onset; with reinnervation, motor units may be large, long, and polyphasic.			Often normal, but individual motor units may show abnormal variability in size.	Small, short, abundant polyphasic motor unit potentials. Myositis—abnormal spontaneous activity.
Nerve conduction velocity	Normal.	Normal.	Slowed, especially in demyelinating neuropathies.	Normal.	Normal.
Muscle response to repetitive motor nerve stimulation	Normal.	Normal, except in the active stage of disease.	Normal.	Abnormal decrement or increment depending on stimulus frequency and disease.	Normal.
Muscle biopsy	May be normal in he acute stage but subsequently suggestive of denervation.			Normal.	Changes suggestive of myopathy (e.g., atrophy, fiber-type grouping).
Myelography or spinal MRI	May be helpful.	Helpful in excluding other disorders.	Not helpful.	Not helpful.	Not helpful.

SIGNS AND SYMPTOMS

- Wrist pain; numbness and tingling of the thumb, index finger, middle finger, and lateral half of the ring finger; weak grip; ↓ thumb opposition.
- Pain and symptoms are exacerbated by activities that require wrist flexion, such as typing, holding a cup of coffee, or opening a jar.
- Symptoms may awaken patients at night and are relieved by shaking out the wrists. Patients often complain of nocturnal pain and paresthesias.
- Thenar atrophy may occur in severe cases.

WORKUP

- Two clinical exams should be performed on suspected carpal tunnel patients:

What is the anatomic location of the carpal tunnel? Between the carpal bones and the flexor retinaculum.

- **Tinel's sign** (approximately 60% sensitivity and 65% specificity): Tapping on the palmaris longus tendon at the wrist over the median nerve to elicit a tingling sensation in the thumb and affected fingers.
- **Phalen's sign** (roughly 75% sensitivity and 35% specificity): Requires that the patient appose the dorsal aspects of the hands with the wrists flexed at 90 degrees for at least 30 seconds. The onset of paresthesias confirms the diagnosis.
- EMG and nerve conduction studies can be used to make a diagnosis, evaluate the degree of neural and motor compromise, and assess the severity of compression, especially in patients who exhibit persistent symptoms despite conservative management.
- Patients should also be evaluated for risk factors, including diabetes and hypothyroidism (myxedema).

TREATMENT

- Neutral wrist splints to wear both during the day and at night.
- Modification of repetitive activities and creation of a more ergonomic work environment.
- NSAIDs to control inflammation of the tendons.
- Direct injection of corticosteroid into the carpal space may also provide temporary relief.
- Surgical division of the transverse carpal ligament if symptoms persist.

SPINAL CORD COMPRESSION

A condition that develops when the spinal cord is compressed by any swelling or lesion, such as a tumor, an abscess, a ruptured or slipped intervertebral disk, or bone fragments from a vertebral fracture. Regardless of its cause, spinal cord compression is a medical emergency that requires swift diagnosis and treatment in order to prevent long-term disability from irreversible nerve damage.

SIGNS AND SYMPTOMS

- Presents with back pain and with ↓ sensation below the level of compression and/or with paralysis of the limbs below the level of compression.
- Urinary and fecal incontinence and/or urinary retention may also be seen.
- Hyperreflexia and Lhermitte's sign (an intermittent shooting electrical sensation) may be present.

WORKUP

- Conduct a thorough neurologic exam, and emergently obtain radiographs and an MRI of the spine (or CT myelography if the patient has a pacemaker).
- Investigate common causes, including tumors (especially metastatic non–small cell lung cancer, breast cancer, prostate cancer, renal cell carcinoma, lymphoma, and multiple myeloma) and infection leading to abscess. Look for track marks in patients with a history of IV drug use.

TREATMENT

- IV dexamethasone (a glucocorticoid) should be given to reduce edema around the lesion.

Cauda equina syndrome presents with saddle anesthesia (↓ perianal sensation), bowel/bladder dysfunction, low back pain, and lower extremity weakness. "Cauda equina" refers to the spinal nerve roots located below the sacral spinal cord (around L1).

- Urgent surgery is warranted if a localized lesion is identified and some hope of regaining function is predicted.
- In the setting of cancer-related compression, emergent radiation therapy may ↓ tumor bulk and help reduce compression.
- If complete paralysis is present for > 24 hours, the chances of recovery are significantly reduced.

OPHTHALMOLOGY

Although you may not encounter many ophthalmologic cases during your neuro rotation, it can be beneficial to have a grasp of at least some of the more common visual conditions seen in practice. A few of these are described briefly below.

Closed-Angle Glaucoma

SIGNS AND SYMPTOMS

- Characterized by extreme, sudden pain and blurred vision that may be accompanied by nausea and vomiting.
- Presents as a hard, red eye (from acute closure of the narrow anterior chamber angle) and is unilateral.
- The pupil is dilated and nonreactive to light.

Closed-angle glaucoma, but *open* pupil.

WORKUP/TREATMENT

- **This is a medical emergency!** Perform a slit-lamp exam and measure intraocular pressure by tonometry. It is important to emergently ↓ intraocular pressure with acetazolamide, mannitol, pilocarpine, and timolol to prevent damage that can lead to blindness.
- Peripheral laser iridotomy can be curative.

Open-Angle Glaucoma

SIGNS AND SYMPTOMS

- Can be asymptomatic, especially in the early stages.
- Suspect in patients > 40 years of age with frequent eyewear prescription changes, visual disturbances, and headaches.
- Visual defects start in the peripheral nasal fields.

WORKUP

Perform visual field testing, funduscopy, slit-lamp exam, and tonometry; look for cupping of the optic disk on slit lamp or funduscopy.

TREATMENT

- Treat with topical β-blockers (e.g., timolol) to ↓ aqueous humor production or with pilocarpine to ↑ aqueous humor outflow.
- Laser trabeculoplasty if medications fail.
- Patients > 40 years of age should have a yearly eye exam; those with a family history or diabetes should have more frequent exams.

Macular Degeneration

The leading cause of bilateral visual loss among the elderly in the United States.

SIGNS AND SYMPTOMS

Presents with painless loss of central vision.

WORKUP/TREATMENT

- On funduscopy or slit-lamp exam, look for pigment or hemorrhagic changes in the macular region.
- Laser photocoagulation may delay the loss of central vision, but the disease will often continue to progress.

Diabetic Retinopathy

Patients with DM should get regular eye exams for early detection of retinopathy. Good glucose control is key to minimizing the risk of developing retinopathy.

WORKUP

- **Nonproliferative retinopathy:** On slit-lamp exam, look for dot-blot hemorrhages, microaneurysms, exudates, and edema.
- **Proliferative retinopathy:** On slit-lamp exam, look for retinal neovascularization. The more advanced the disease, the more likely it is to progress to blindness.

TREATMENT

- **Nonproliferative retinopathy:** Focal laser photocoagulation to affected areas, especially when the process starts to affect the macula.
- **Proliferative retinopathy:** Treat with panretinal photocoagulation, in which laser burns are applied to the entire periphery of the retina to destroy ischemic areas (which release the vessel-growth signals).

COMMON CLERKSHIP TOPICS

The following is a list of topics that you should review during this rotation:

- **The complete neurologic exam:** Mental status, cranial nerves, motor, sensory.
- **Imaging basics:** CT, MRI.
- **Lumbar puncture:** Procedure and results.
- **Management of intracranial pressure.**
- **Aphasias:** Broca's, Wernicke's, transcortical, conduction, and global aphasias.
- **Coma:** Etiologies, assessing a comatose patient (Glasgow Coma Scale), primitive brain stem reflexes, workup and treatment, coma vs. persistent vegetative state vs. "locked-in" syndrome.
- **Cord compression/cord syndromes.**
- **Delirium and dementia,** Wernicke's encephalopathy, DTs, Alzheimer's disease.
- **Demyelinating/degenerative diseases:** MS, Guillain-Barré syndrome, ALS.
- **Dysequilibrium:** Central vs. peripheral, nystagmus.

- **Headache:** Migraine, cluster, tension, temporal arteritis.
- **Infections:** Meningitis, bacterial and viral (see Pediatrics), HIV infection (1° and opportunistic), TB and HSV infection, encephalitis, cerebral abscess, polio and postpolio syndrome.
- **Intracranial hemorrhages:** Subarachnoid, epidural, subdural, intraparenchymal (see Emergency Medicine for all).
- **Intracranial neoplasms:** 1°, metastatic, presentation, children vs. adults.
- **Low back pain, spinal cord injuries:** Cord lesions, cord compression, myelopathies, cervical spine injury.
- **Movement disorders:** Parkinson's, Huntington's, and Wilson's disease.
- **Seizures:** Partial, generalized, absence (petit mal), tonic-clonic (grand mal), status epilepticus (see Emergency Medicine).
- **Stroke:** Clinical features, risk factors, prevention, treatment/management.
- **Weakness:** UMN vs. LMN, differential based on anatomy, carpal tunnel syndrome.

CORE CLERKSHIPS IN

Obstetrics and Gynecology

Welcome to obstetrics and gynecology! This rotation is dedicated to acquainting future MDs with the basic principles of labor and delivery (L&D) and managing gynecologic issues, including medical, surgical, and social issues. You will be involved in prenatal care, annual well-woman examinations, contraceptive counseling, and numerous surgical procedures ranging from cesarean sections (C-sections) to a variety of gynecologic operations. Obstetrician/gynecologists are surgeons by nature who keep extremely demanding schedules and spend minimal time rounding and discussing differentials. For the next few weeks, you will thus be exposed to a whirlwind of activities covering a wide range of issues. Regardless of the field you ultimately enter, more than half of your patients will be women with potential gynecologic problems, so take advantage of this learning opportunity and have a good time!

What Is the Rotation Like?

OB/GYN rotations last approximately 6–8 weeks and differ vastly from school to school as well as from site to site. The basic setup consists of inpatient obstetrics, inpatient gynecology, and the outpatient clinic, where both obstetric and gynecologic patients are seen. Obstetrics can be one of the most rewarding and pleasant experiences in medical school, but it is not an easygoing discipline. The following outline summarizes the nature and duties of the rotation:

You should try to follow your patients from admission to delivery and postpartum care.

- **Obstetrics:** When you are in the obstetrics portion of your rotation, you will spend much of your time in the L&D suite.
    - **Responsibilities:**
        - Prerounding on antepartum **and** postpartum patients, and presenting those patients on ward rounds.
        - Evaluating patients in the triage area.
        - Writing the admission history and physical (H&P).
        - Monitoring the progress of laboring patients with residents and nurses. Patients in the L&D suite generally need an exam every 2–3 hours, so you can become a great resource by helping write progress notes.
        - Delivering babies, writing delivery notes, and checking labs.
    - **You should:**
        - Get to know the nursing staff very well, as much of L&D is in many instances handled by nurses or midwives.
        - Read about the basics of L&D (e.g., steps of labor, signs and symptoms of true labor, steps of delivery, and fetal heart tracing [FHT]), and learn about common complications that can arise (e.g., failure to progress, hypertension, fetal distress) and their appropriate management.
        - Always keep in mind that competence is only half the story. Knowing your patient well by periodically checking in on her to see if she needs anything—or just to comfort her—will impress not only your patient but your residents and attendings as well.
- **Inpatient gynecology:** As a surgically oriented specialty, inpatient gynecology is similar to general surgery. Rounding is early and fast; all the notes, rounding, and daily management planning for patients must be done prior to the surgeries that are planned for the day, which can start as early as 7:30 A.M.

- **Responsibilities:**
  - Prerounding on postoperative patients.
  - Presenting patients on ward rounds.
  - Writing notes (preoperative, operative, postoperative) on the patients whose surgeries you are involved with.
- **You should:**
  - **Try to plan out** which surgery you want to participate in the next day; read up on the surgery and on relevant anatomy; and learn something about the patient's history. Practice some basic suturing and knot-tying skills in the event that you are presented with a rare opportunity to help close an incision.
  - Learn some of the medical jargon common to surgeries, and be willing to **ask questions** pertaining to technique or to the prognosis of the surgery being performed.
  - Be ready to **answer questions** about the basic anatomy, surgical procedure, and prognosis of the surgery being performed.
- **Outpatient clinics:** The outpatient clinic is a great place to see both common and uncommon gynecologic and obstetric cases. The clinic experience is extremely helpful in that the skills and knowledge you will acquire there are likely to be applicable to most fields you may ultimately pursue, such as internal medicine, family practice, or surgery.
  - **Gynecology clinic:**
    - **Responsibilities:** Common gynecologic clinic issues are requests for birth control, routine health maintenance (breast exams, pelvic exams, Pap smears), abnormal vaginal bleeding, vaginal discharge, and lower abdominal pain.
    - **You should:** Perform a **focused H&P.** Like any other clinics at the hospital, this is a very fast-paced place, and your efficiency in taking a history and figuring out what the patient needs (e.g., prescriptions, results of diagnostic tests/labs, pelvic exam) will be greatly appreciated by residents and attendings alike.
  - **Obstetric clinic:**
    - **Responsibilities:** Patients are seen in the obstetric clinic to assess the adequacy of pregnancy progression, to screen for potential maternal-fetal complications, to help mothers adjust to their pregnancies, and to prepare mothers for childbirth. In addition, postpartum patients are seen for their regular six-week checkup or for any postpartum complications that may arise.
    - **You should:** Familiarize yourself with the **time course of prenatal labs** so that you are aware of which labs your clinic patients need at their visits.

Who Are the Players?

Team OB/GYN consists of a senior resident (R3 or R4), at least one junior resident (R2), and an intern (from OB/GYN, family practice, psychiatry, emergency medicine, or medicine). There may also be a fourth-year medical student doing his or her senior elective as well as one or two third-year medical students. Usually, there is one ward attending, although there may also be several private attendings, subspecialty attendings (maternal-fetal, gynecologic oncology), and fellows. Other important players on the team include the nursing staff and midwives (especially in L&D), who can teach you invaluable obstetric skills, and the anesthesiologists, who are needed for pain control both during labor and postoperatively.

Midwives can be your best allies in the L&D suite.

How Is the Day Set Up?

A typical day on an OB/GYN service may look like this:

	OB Service	GYN	Clinic
5:30–6:30 A.M.	Prerounds	Prerounds	
6:30–7:30 A.M.	Work rounds	Work rounds	
7:30 A.M.–4:00 P.M.	L&D	Operating room	Outpatient clinic (8:00 A.M.–5:00 P.M.)
4:00–6:00 P.M.	Wrap up work, do P.M. rounds if on GYN		

Call days are usually busy and are always in house. After you are done with your regular workday, you start call in L&D (usually at 5:00 P.M.) and see patients in triage while also following any laboring patients you might have. You and your resident will also see and potentially admit patients from the ER for acute obstetric or gynecologic care. You will usually be up all night—or, if you are lucky, get one or two hours of sleep. This is because there will often be someone delivering in the early hours of the morning or an emergency to keep you busy.

What Do I Do During Prerounds?

Depending on the size of your inpatient gynecologic service, prerounds should begin 30 minutes to one hour before work rounds. You should anticipate spending roughly 20–30 minutes on each patient you are following, depending on your stage in the year. As in surgery, most of your patients will be postoperative. The following outline lists prerounds activities by service.

- **Inpatient gynecologic service:**
  - Check vital signs overnight. Watch out for fever, hypotension, and ↓ O_2 saturation, which could indicate infection, loss of fluids, and pulmonary embolism/pulmonary edema/atelectasis, respectively.
  - Assess overnight fluid balance ("ins and outs"), including urine output. Since many gynecologic surgeries involve procedures that could potentially damage the ureters, it is imperative that you check for adequate urine output in order to rule out urinary obstruction.
  - Check labs, especially hematocrit if the patient lost a significant amount of blood during the operation.
  - Do a quick physical exam, and check the surgical wound to assess for drainage and possible infection. Review the chart for new notes, and write a concise progress note—all before work rounds.
- Obstetric service:
  - For **postpartum patients,** you should seek to accomplish the following:
    - Examine your patients' breasts.
    - Check fundus size and firmness, the extent of vaginal bleeding, and any wounds, such as sewn lacerations or cesarean incisions. A common complication of C-section is endometritis, and it is always good to let your residents know that you have considered that possibility during your exam.

- Make sure your notes are always cosigned by your residents; not only is this good medical practice, but you'll also get helpful feedback.
- For **antepartum patients,** you should ask the following questions during prerounds:
  - Do you feel the baby moving as much as usual?
  - Are you having any vaginal bleeding?
  - Are you having any abnormal vaginal discharge or gush of fluid?
  - Are you feeling contractions or pain?
  - Do you have any pain or discomfort with urination?

How Do I Excel in OB/GYN?

- **Be assertive.** Assertiveness is key to furthering your education and to scoring points with the people who evaluate you. So ask good questions (you should know something about the subject matter before doing so); get to know other patients on the service (for your own learning and in case you are asked to fill in); take the initiative to ask for demonstrations of procedures; volunteer for drawing blood (you need to practice anyway); do pelvic exams; participate in as many deliveries as you can; and try to dig up interesting and informative articles for your team.

Don't get shut out of learning the pelvic exam.

- **Be visible.** The L&D suite is a busy, crowded place, so unless you take the initiative, you may easily be forgotten. With this in mind, don't wait for your residents to call you for deliveries or interesting physical exam findings. Instead, know ahead of time which patients are likely to deliver during your shift, and anticipate that. Also bear in mind that most of the patients at the L&D suite need a progress note written every 2–3 hours, especially if they are on magnesium for tocolysis, so volunteer to write those notes before you are asked to do so.
- **Be the intern for your patients.** You will have patients assigned to you by your residents. Among other things, you will be responsible for obtaining each patient's H&P, writing progress notes, following up on diagnostic studies and pathology results, and presenting your patients to the team. In order to fulfill your responsibilities diligently, you will need to know and do everything you can for your patient. This means reading up on each case, carefully reviewing your patient's history, staying updated, and talking to your patient. These measures will allow you to actively participate in patient care and hence to act as your patient's strongest advocate.
- **Be knowledgeable in a general sense.** It is important to recognize that once residents become involved in a specialty, they tend to spend less time keeping up to date on everything else they learned in medical school. You can thus serve as a great asset to your team by providing new information about your patients' medical problems (e.g., diabetes, hepatitis, hypertension) and by recognizing psychiatric or social issues (e.g., postpartum depression, drug dependence, domestic violence).

*The key to success on the wards is to be a step ahead of your interns and residents. Write notes on triage patients **before** they ask you to do so!*

- **Work quickly, independently, and efficiently.** Residents appreciate students who can effectively contribute to the team—so order lab tests, make necessary phone calls, and write notes for patients. In addition, be focused, organized, and brief when presenting the patient. Remember, again, that in many ways this rotation is similar to surgery.
- **Know the expectations.** At the beginning of the rotation, be straightforward and ask the residents on your team exactly what they expect of you. You should also find out your attending's preferred format of patient presentation. Midway through the rotation, it is equally important to **get feedback** both from residents and from attendings with whom you have

worked. As part of this process, try to be assertive and ask for constructive feedback on what you should continue to do and areas in which you can improve. Be tactful, and communicate with the goal of maximizing your performance, education, and contribution to the team while on the clerkship.

While you are on this rotation, you may fall in love with OB/GYN and want to pursue it as a career. If this is the case, you should take additional steps. If you let your team know of your sincere interest in the field, they will be more than happy to lead you down the right track. Ask the interns and residents for advice on the politics of residency (e.g., which programs are good, which key people to get to know better, whom to ask for letters of recommendation, which senior electives to take). If possible, try to work with one of the key faculty members, who can write an influential letter of recommendation or serve as your adviser in your quest to match into the residency of your choice.

Survival Tips

In the course of your rotation, do not be discouraged if you encounter a patient who does not want a medical student to deliver her baby or even to be involved in her care. Many mothers want as little intrusion as possible into this sacred, personal moment in their lives, while others may be concerned about inexperienced students touching their newborn infant. Occasionally, male students may encounter some gynecologic patients who are uncomfortable with the notion of having a male in the examining room, much less a male student. On a rotation such as OB/GYN, in which you will be working very hard over long shifts, it can be easy to become frustrated when issues such as these arise. It is important, however, to respect a patient's wishes as well as to bear in mind that there may be specific reasons such requests may be made, such as a previous history of sexual abuse. So do not take it personally if a patient does not want you in the examination room. If this continues to happen frequently, you should discuss it with your resident. If you are a male medical student, being with an affable yet assertive female resident who cares about your educational experience may also be of great help in getting your foot in the door.

Here are a few additional tips for this rotation:

- Talk to OB patients early in labor and throughout the delivery. Establishing a rapport early on will increase the likelihood that you will be able to help with the delivery.
- Learn how to "count" and coach a patient through labor. A calm yet clear and assertive voice is usually appreciated.

Key Notes

Obstetrics admission note. The obstetric H&P is similar to a standard H&P but should include the following additional information:

- **Gravida:** The total number of times a patient has been pregnant, including the current pregnancy.
- **Para:** Four numbers that represent term deliveries, preterm deliveries, abortions (including elective, therapeutic, and spontaneous), and number of living children. This is often referred to as TPAL (term, preterm, abor-

tion, living). For example, a pregnant patient with one prior miscarriage and one prior term delivery would be a G3P1011.

- **Gestational age (GA):** Information on GA should be included along with information on the patient's last menstrual period (LMP) and estimated date of delivery, or EDD (which is the same as the due date and is often referred to as EDC, or estimated date of confinement).
- **Uterine contractions (UCs):** Information on the time of onset, frequency, and intensity of contractions should be noted.
- **Rupture of membranes (ROM):** The time of rupture and the color of the fluid should be described.
- **Vaginal bleeding:** This should include the duration of bleeding, its consistency (bright, red bleeding vs. old dark blood), and the number of pads.
- **Fetal movement:** Notation should be made as to whether fetal movement is normal, decreased, or absent.
- **Ultrasound history:** This should include GA at the time of the first ultrasound, whether anatomy was evaluated, and whether the size on ultrasound is equivalent to that expected based on the LMP, or "size equal to dates" (S = D).
- **Lab studies:** Include current lab results such as UA, CBC, and cultures.
- **Physical exam:** This should include a thorough physical, including a pelvic exam, which is commonly referred to as a sterile vaginal exam.
- **FHT:** Record baseline heart rate, variability, accelerations, and decelerations.
- **Tocometer:** Note the frequency of UCs and whether a regular or an irregular pattern is seen.
- **Ultrasound:** Describe findings such as vertex, breech, amniotic fluid index (AFI), and the location of the placenta.
- **Estimated fetal weight (EFW):** Specify whether the EFW was determined by Leopold's maneuver (feeling with hands) or measured by ultrasound.

Prenatal care. Key notes associated with prenatal care should include the following elements on the first visit:

- **Obstetric history:** Dates of pregnancies with GA at time of delivery, route (vaginal, C-section), and complications (including preeclampsia, abruption, previa, preterm labor, and unusually long labor).
- **Gynecologic history:** Menstrual history, STDs, OCP use.
- **Family history:** Congenital abnormalities, twins, bleeding disorders, hypertension, diabetes.
- **Social history:** Note any tobacco, alcohol, or drug use during pregnancy; occupational exposures (e.g., a nurse preparing chemotherapy agents); and the patient's involvement and/or relationship with the father of the baby. Also assess the patient's living situation.
- **Medical history:** Note any history of diabetes, hypertension, asthma, SLE, and the like.
- **Allergies.**
- **Medications:** List current medications and their dosages as well as medications used during pregnancy.
- **Prenatal labs:** Include blood type, Rh type, antibody screen, CBC, VDRL/RPR, rubella, HBsAg, UA and culture, Pap smear, gonorrhea culture (GC), chlamydia culture, PPD placement, VZV titer if there is no history of exposure, HIV if performed, maternal serum α-fetoprotein (MS-AFP) if performed, Down syndrome screening results if performed, and one-hour plasma glucose (PG) screening.

Always include the GA both by dates and by ultrasound when presenting a patient on L&D.

- **Diagnostic tests:** Ultrasound, amniocentesis if performed, chorionic villus sampling (CVS) if performed.
- **Physical exam:** A thorough exam is critical, particularly thyroid, heart, and lung evaluation and pelvic examination. It is important to evaluate the size of the uterus on pelvic exam in order to determine if it is consistent with gestational weeks. It is also vital to document the initial cervical exam so as to have a reference point in the event that there are future issues with preterm contractions or preterm labor.

Key notes for all subsequent visits should record the following:

- Fetal heart tones
- BP
- Urine dip
- Fundal height
- Weight gain
- Fetal movement
- Vaginal bleeding
- Contractions or cramping
- ROM
- Unusual vaginal discharge
- Dysuria
- Pelvic pressure

Delivery note. Some hospitals have preprinted delivery forms that allow you to simply fill in the blanks and check off appropriate boxes. If this is not the case, the following is a summary of the information that should be included in a delivery note:

- Age, gravida, para, therapeutic abortion (TAB), spontaneous abortion (SAB), GA.
- Onset of labor, ROM (with or without meconium).
- Indications for induction (if applicable).
- Obstetric, maternal, or fetal complications.
- Anesthesia/pain control (IV, epidural, general).
- Time of birth.
- Type of birth (NSVD, forceps assist, vacuum suction, C-section).
- Bulb suction, sex, weight, Apgar scores, presence of nuchal cord (tight or loose), number of cord vessels.
- Time of placental delivery, placenta expressed or delivered spontaneously, whether or not the placenta is intact.
- Episiotomy (how done, degree, how repaired) and/or lacerations (locations, degree, how repaired).
- Estimated blood loss (EBL).
- Disposition—e.g., mother to recovery room in stable condition; infant to newborn nursery in stable condition; future contraceptive plan (pills or condoms); breast-feeding vs. formula feed.

Postpartum note. The postpartum note is similar to the routine progress note that is written on most inpatients (subjective, objective—vitals, routine physical exam). Additional items that should be included in the postpartum note are as follows:

- Breast exam (soft, tender, engorged, signs of mastitis [erythema, warmth]).
- Fundus check (firmness, tenderness, location described relative to the umbilicus).
- Lochia (scant, minimal, heavy).

SAMPLE ADMISSION H&P

26 yo G3P1011 at 39 1/7 weeks by LMP 5/11/07 consistent with 10-week ultrasound presents c/o UCs 3–4 min, ⊕ FM, ⊖ ROM, ⊖ VB, ⊖ unusual vaginal discharge, ⊖ dysuria. Her due date is 2/15/08.

Prenatal care with Dr. Smith since 7 weeks for 11 visits.

Pregnancy complicated by:

UTI—treated with Keflex. TOC ⊖.

Pap smear c/w ASCUS—needs follow-up Pap smear 6 weeks postpartum.

PPD ⊕, CXR ⊖.

PNL: A+/−, RPR ⊖, rubella immune, HBsAg ⊖, HIV ⊖, Pap smear ASCUS, GC ⊖, chlamydia ⊖, 1-hour PG 121 (at 26 wks), PPD ⊕, CXR ⊖, declined screening for Down syndrome.

PMH: None.

PSH: Appendectomy age 9.

Meds: PNV, $FeSO_4$.

All: NKDA.

OB/GYN Hx:

Menarche age 13/menses q 28 days/lasts 3–5 days.

2000 NSVD, full term, uncomplicated 8-lb, 3-oz boy. No epidural.

1998 SAB in first trimester. No D&C needed.

H/o abnormal Pap smears—never had colposcopy or biopsy.

No h/o STDs.

Soc Hx:

Single, father of baby involved and supportive.

Denies T/E/D.

Fam Hx: Maternal grandmother with hypertension. No h/o birth defects or mental retardation.

Physical exam:

VS: T 37.2 BP 120/70 P 82 RR 18.

Gen: Uncomfortable with UCs.

Lungs: CTAB.

CV: RRR, II/VI SEM.

Abd: Soft, gravid, nontender.

Ext: 1+ edema, DTRs 2+ b.

SSE: No pooling. Nitrazine ⊖. Ferning ⊖.

SVE: 5 cm dilated/80% effaced/0 station.

Key:

ASCUS = atypical squamous cells of undetermined significance

b = bilateral

BP = blood pressure

c/o = complaining of

CTAB = clear to auscultation bilaterally

CV = cardiovascular

c/w = consistent with

CXR = chest x-ray

D&C = dilation and curettage

DTRs = deep tendon reflexes

$FeSO_4$ = ferrous sulfate

FM = fetal movement

h/o = history of

Hx = history

IUP = intrauterine pregnancy

NKDA = no known drug allergies

NSVD = normal spontaneous vaginal delivery

P = pulse rate

PMH = past medical history

PNL = prenatal labs

PNV = prenatal vitamins

PPD = purified protein derivative

PSH = past surgical history

RPR = rapid plasma reagin

RR = respiratory rate

RRR = regular rate and rhythm

SEM = systolic ejection murmur

SSE = sterile speculum exam

SVE = sterile vaginal exam

Key:

T/E/D = tobacco/alcohol (EtOH)/drugs

TOC = test of cure

Toco = tocometer

UTI = urinary tract infection

VB = vaginal bleeding

VS = vital signs

FHT: 130 sec, accels, reactive. No decelerations.

Toco: 4–5 min UCs.

Ultrasound: Vertex, AFI 11.4, placenta fundal.

EFW: 3650 g by Leopold's.

Assessment/Plan: 26 yo G3P1011 at 39 1/7 weeks with uncomplicated IUP in active labor.

1. Admit to L&D.

2. Obtain routine labs (type and screen, RPR, CBC).

3. Expectant management. Will start pitocin augmentation if UCs ↓ in frequency and there is insufficient cervical change

4. FHT reassuring. No signs of fetal distress.

5. Anticipate normal spontaneous vaginal delivery.

- Perineum (intact or separating).
- Breast-feeding status (problems with feeding; breast-feeding exclusively or supplementing with formula).
- Contraception desired (Depo-Provera injection, OCPs, condoms).

GYN operative note. The gynecology operative note contains the same information as the operative note for any other surgical service. This includes the following:

- Preoperative diagnosis (e.g., symptomatic uterine fibroids, cervical cancer, ovarian cyst).
- Postoperative diagnosis (usually "same").
- Procedure (e.g., total abdominal hysterectomy, ovarian cystectomy).
- Surgeons.
- Anesthesia (e.g., general endotracheal tube).
- EBL.
- IV fluids.
- Urinary output
- Findings.
- Complications (e.g., enterotomy).
- Pathology specimens (e.g., uterus, cervix, ovary).

Key Procedures

Delivering babies, cervical checks, Pap smears, cervical/vaginal cultures, external fetal monitoring, IV lines, basic suturing and knot tying, and retracting for visualization during procedures are the principal procedures on this rotation. Descriptions of most of these procedures can be found in major textbooks. However, the best way to learn is by observing and practicing, so let your residents know you are interested in these procedures.

SAMPLE POSTPARTUM PROGRESS NOTE

S—Eating solid foods. Breast-feeding without difficulty. No urinary complaints. Desires OCPs for contraception.

O—T$_{max}$ 37.2, T$_{current}$ 37.6, BP 120–127/70–76, P 82–85, RR 18–20, I/O 1200/1370.

Gen: NAD, awake and alert.

Lungs: CTAB.

CV: RRR, no murmurs.

Abd: Soft, nontender, minimally distended, BS.

Fundus: Firm, at umbilicus, not tender.

Perineum: 2nd-degree laceration repair intact.

Lochia: Minimal.

Extremities: No edema; no tenderness or evidence of DVT.

A/P—26 yo G3P2012 PPD#1 s/p NSVD at 39 1/7 weeks with uncomplicated labor course and delivery.

1. Ice packs to perineum.

2. Continue to encourage breast-feeding.

3. OCPs for contraception.

4. Anticipate d/c home tomorrow.

Key:

A/P = assessment and plan

BS = bowel sounds

d/c = discharge

DVT = deep venous thrombosis

I/O = intake/output

NAD = no acute distress

O = objective data

OCPs = oral contraceptive pills

PPD = postpartum day

S = subjective data

s/p = status post

What Do I Carry in My Pockets?

❑ Pregnancy wheel (to calculate and double-check EDC)
❑ OB/GYN handbook of your choice
❑ Penlight
❑ Stethoscope
❑ Index cards to keep track of your patients. Create cards with high-yield information, including the following:
  ❑ Steps of a vaginal delivery.
  ❑ Normal and abnormal labor patterns (e.g., duration, cervical dilation).
  ❑ Indications for C-section.
  ❑ Outlines of frequently written notes (preop, op, postop, delivery notes).
  ❑ The diagnosis and management of preeclampsia/eclampsia and other common maternal or obstetrical complications (e.g., abruptio placentae, placenta previa, preterm labor).

HIGH-YIELD CLINICAL TOPIC CHECKLIST

Read about these topics before you start the rotation. A full list of common clerkship topics can be found at the end of this chapter.

❑ Normal physiology of pregnancy
❑ Gestational diabetes

❏ Hypertension during pregnancy; preeclampsia/eclampsia
❏ First-trimester bleeding
❏ Third-trimester bleeding
❏ Normal labor and preterm labor
❏ Common vaginal infections
❏ PID
❏ Contraception
❏ Infertility

OBSTETRICS

Normal Physiology of Pregnancy

In pregnancy, multiple adaptations occur in each of the mother's organ systems to support the maternal-fetal unit (see Table 6-1).

TABLE 6-1. Maternal Changes During Pregnancy

SYSTEM	CHANGES	EFFECTS
Metabolic	↑ proteins, lipids.	↑ maternal fat deposition.
	↑ need for iron and folate.	Maternal anemia.
	↑ insulin sensitivity **early** in pregnancy; ↓ glucose tolerance later in pregnancy.	Narrow euglycemic range (normal 84 +/–10).
Blood	↑ plasma volume by 50%; ↑ RBC mass by 20–40%.	Physiologic anemia of pregnancy.
	↑ WBCs, fibrinogen, and coagulation factors 7, 8, 9, and 10.	Hypercoagulable stage of pregnancy.
Endocrine	↑ estrogen, progesterone, and aldosterone.	Water retention and mood changes.
	↑ prolactin.	Breast engorgement; preparation for milk production.
Skin, hair	↑ estrogen and progesterone.	Spider angiomata, palmar erythema.
	↑ testosterone.	Mild hirsutism, acne.
	↑ α-melanocyte-stimulating hormone.	↑ skin pigmentation (areolae, axillae, vulva).
Respiratory	↑ tidal volume; ↑ vital capacity.	Dyspnea; mild respiratory alkalosis.
	Slight ↑ in respiratory rate; upward displacement of diaphragm late in pregnancy.	
Cardiovascular	↑ cardiac output by 45% (primarily due to ↑ stroke volume).	Physiologic flow murmur; dependent edema.
	↓ peripheral vascular resistance.	↓ BP; supine hypotensive syndrome.
Renal	Dilation of the collecting system; ↑ GFR up to 60%.	↑ UTI frequency, hydroureter, pyelonephritis.
	↑ renal blood flow by 30–50%.	↑ urinary frequency, nocturia, glycosuria.
	↑ aldosterone, renin, and ADH.	Salt and water retention.
GI	↓ muscle tone leading to hypomotility.	Constipation, hemorrhoids.
	↓ LES tone; prolonged gastric emptying time.	Gastric reflux, hiatal hernia.
	Bile statis.	Gallstones.

Prenatal Care

Prenatal care is critical to the uneventful delivery of a healthy baby. Patients with little or no prenatal care can have complications arising from undiagnosed gestational diabetes, gestational hypertension, and intrauterine growth retardation (IUGR) as well as an inability to accurately estimate GA. The following subsections describe key aspects of prenatal care.

Accurate determination of the estimated due date is crucial to guiding management.

FREQUENCY OF VISITS

- **0–28 weeks' gestation:** Every month.
- **28–36 weeks' gestation:** Every 2–3 weeks.
- **36 weeks' gestation until delivery:** Every week until delivery.

ESTIMATED DATE OF CONFINEMENT

- **Nägele's rule:** LMP – 3 months + 7 days + 1 year.
- **Example:** If LMP is April 14, then EDC will be January 11 of the following year.

Nägele's rule for determining EDC: EDC = LMP – 3 months + 7 days. Exact dating uses EDC = LMP + 280 days.

DEFINITIONS

- **Embryo:** Fertilization to eight weeks.
- **Fetus:** Eight weeks to birth.
- **Previable:** < 24 weeks.
- **Preterm:** 24–37 weeks.
- **Term:** 37–42 weeks.

PRENATAL VISITS

At each prenatal visit, the following subjective and objective findings should be addressed and documented:

- **Subjective findings:**
  - Fetal movement.
  - Vaginal discharge and/or bleeding.
  - Abdominal cramps or UCs.
  - Leakage of fluid or signs of ROM.
  - Dysuria.
  - Blurred vision, headache, rapid weight gain, edema (after 24 weeks).
- **Objective findings:**
  - Weight, fundal height, BP, edema.
  - Dipstick urine protein and glucose.
  - Fetal heart tones (heard after 10–12 weeks).

FUNDAL HEIGHT

Fundal height is measured with a tape measure from the top of the pubic symphysis to the top of the fundus. Fundal height should correspond to GA as follows:

- **At 12 weeks:** At the pubic symphysis.
- **At 16 weeks:** Midway between the pubis and umbilicus.
- **At 20 weeks:** At the umbilicus.

■ **At 20–32 weeks:** Height above the pubic symphysis should equal GA in weeks.

See Figure 6-1 for a depiction of typical fundal height measurements.

Women planning a pregnancy should be advised to take supplemental folate (400 μg/day) beginning four weeks prior to conception to reduce the risk of neural tube defects.

NUTRITION

During pregnancy, the caloric requirement is ↑ by 300 kcal/day. Iron and folate supplementation is recommended. Guidelines are as follows:

■ **Normal weight gain:** 25–35 lbs for the entire pregnancy.
■ **First trimester:** 3–5 lbs total.
■ **Second trimester:** 0.5 lb/week.
■ **Third trimester:** 1 lb/week.

PRENATAL LABS

Table 6-2 outlines common prenatal laboratory studies.

What is the typical triple screen finding in Down syndrome? ↓ MSAFP, ↓ estradiol, ↑ hCG, and ↑ inhibin.

Medical Conditions in Pregnancy

GESTATIONAL DIABETES

Defined as glucose intolerance or diabetes mellitus (DM) that is first recognized during pregnancy. Affects 3–5% of all pregnancies and is the leading medical complication of pregnancy. During pregnancy, there is a tendency toward insulin resistance as the pregnancy progresses (2° to the effects of human placental lactogen, progesterone, cortisol, and prolactin). Risk factors include a previous or family history of gestational diabetes; obesity; and a previous history of a macrosomic baby (> 4500 g at birth), recurrent miscarriages, and stillbirths.

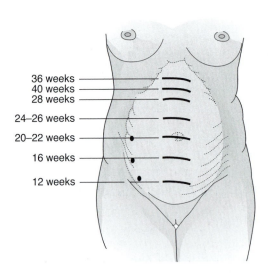

FIGURE 6-1. Height of the fundus at various times during pregnancy.

(Reproduced, with permission, from DeCherney AH et al. *Current Obstetric & Gynecologic Diagnosis & Treatment,* 8th ed. Stamford, CT: Appleton & Lange, 1994: 187.)

TABLE 6-2. Standard Prenatal Labs and Studies

GESTATION	LABS TO BE OBTAINED
Initial visit	Hematocrit/hemoglobin, type, Rh, and antibody screen.
	Infectious screen—rubella antibody titer, VDRL for syphilis screening, HBsAg, VZV titer in patients without a prior history of exposure, PPD, HIV.
	Cervical gonorrhea and chlamydia cultures.
	Cystic fibrosis screening if desired.
	Pap smear.
	UA and urine culture.
	Sickle prep in high-risk groups.
	Glucose test if the patient has risk factors for diabetes.
	Offer first-trimester screening for Down syndrome if desired.
	Ultrasound for dating purposes if LMP is unknown or discrepant with the exam.
	Offer CVS if indicated (e.g., for advanced maternal age, fetus at risk for genetic abnormality, or abnormal first-trimester screening).
16–20 weeks	Offer quad screen if desired.
	Offer MS-AFP if the patient previously had normal first-trimester screening or CVS.
	Amniocentesis if indicated.
	Ultrasound for anatomy evaluation at 18–20 weeks. If there is only one chance to conduct ultrasound, this is the best time during fetal development to assess the anatomy of the fetus.
26–28 weeks	Diabetes screening test for everyone (risk factors or not).
	Administer RhoGAM to patients initially determined to be Rh antibody ⊖; CXR if PPD ⊕.
34–38 weeks	CBC, VDRL, cervical chlamydia and gonorrhea (repeated if the patient is at high risk).
	Group B streptococcus (GBS) culture at 35–37 weeks.

SIGNS AND SYMPTOMS

- Largely asymptomatic in the mother.
- Presents with glycosuria, hyperglycemia, and/or an abnormal glucose tolerance test on routine prenatal screening at 26–28 weeks' gestation.
- Findings may include a fetus that is large for GA.

DIFFERENTIAL

Pregestational DM type 1 or 2, volume overload, simple sugar overload, urinary tract abnormalities.

WORKUP

- **Glucose challenge test at 26–28 weeks:**
  - Give a 50-g glucose load (a special sweet orange liquid).
  - Check blood glucose level one hour later.

What is the most common medical complication of pregnancy? Gestational diabetes.

- If > 140 mg/dL, follow up with a three-hour glucose tolerance test.
- If > 200 mg/dL, diagnose with gestational diabetes.
- **Glucose tolerance test if glucose challenge test is > 140 but < 200 mg/dL:**
  - Check blood glucose level at fasting (normal < 95).
  - Give a 100-g glucose load.
  - Check blood glucose level at one-, two-, and three-hour intervals.
  - Findings are abnormal if levels are > 180 mg/dL at one hour, > 155 mg/dL at two hours, and > 140 mg/dL at three hours. The patient has gestational diabetes if at least two levels are abnormal.
  - Repeat glucose tolerance test 2–4 months postpartum to diagnose those few women who will remain diabetic.

TREATMENT

Some 25–35% of women with gestational diabetes will develop diabetes in five years.

- Start with the American Diabetes Association (ADA) diet and monitor fasting blood glucose and one- or two-hour postprandial glucose levels.
- Facilitate patient education and diabetic clinic/dietitian consults.
- If studies reveal a persistent (one- to two-week) fasting blood glucose level > 95 mg/dL or a two-hour postprandial glucose level > 120 mg/dL, start glyburide or insulin.
- Although oral hypoglycemic agents were initially thought to be contraindicated in pregnancy, glyburide has recently been used in the third trimester with good success.

COMPLICATIONS

Complications from gestational diabetes can be divided into maternal and fetal (see Table 6-3).

HYPERTENSION IN PREGNANCY

What are the two most common causes of gestational hypertension? Preeclampsia and eclampsia.

Risk factors for hypertension in pregnancy include nulliparity or multiple gestations; extremes of age at pregnancy (< 15, > 35); vascular disease (e.g., hypertension 2° to lupus or diabetes); diabetes; and chronic hypertension. Subtypes are defined as follows:

- **Chronic hypertension:** Hypertension (BP > 140/90 mmHg measured two times at least six hours apart) prior to 20 weeks' gestation.
- **Gestational hypertension (formerly known as pregnancy-induced hypertension):** Hypertension after 20 weeks in a patient without a previous history of hypertension and without proteinuria.
- **Preeclampsia:** Gestational hypertension plus proteinuria (> 300 mg/24 hrs) +/– edema. Systemic endothelial damage leads to vascular spasm and

TABLE 6-3. Complications of Pregestational/Gestational Diabetes

MATERNAL	FETAL
Preterm labor	Macrosomia
Polyhydramnios	Shoulder dystocia
C-section for macrosomia	Perinatal mortality (2–5%)
Preeclampsia/eclampsia (fourfold)	Congenital defects (threefold)
Risk of future glucose intolerance or type 2 DM	Delayed organ maturity

capillary permeability, which in turn results in an ↑ ratio of thromboxane (a vasoconstrictor) to prostacyclin (a vasodilator). Because pathology is linked to the placenta, the only cure is delivery (i.e., removal of the placenta).

- ■ **Mild preeclampsia:** BP > 140/90 mmHg on two occasions at least six hours apart and proteinuria 300 mg – 5 g/24 hrs.
- ■ **Severe preeclampsia:** Any one of the following factors bumps up the diagnosis from mild to severe preeclampsia: BP > 160/110 mmHg on two occasions at least six hours apart; proteinuria > 5 g/24 hrs; platelets < 100; AST/ALT more than twice normal levels; oliguria; severe IUGR; pulmonary edema/cyanosis; CVA; severe headache; scotomata; RUQ pain; epigastric pain; nausea/vomiting.
- ■ **HELLP syndrome:** A variant of preeclampsia with a poor prognosis (see mnemonic). A patient with HELLP has severe preeclampsia even without other signs or symptoms of preeclampsia.
- ■ **Eclampsia:** Preeclampsia plus seizures (not due to neurologic disease). Endothelial damage leads to end-organ and CNS damage.

SIGNS AND SYMPTOMS

Table 6-4 lists the clinical presentation of hypertension in pregnancy.

DIFFERENTIAL

- ■ **Preeclampsia:** Renal disease, renovascular hypertension, 1° aldosteronism, Cushing's disease, pheochromocytoma, SLE.
- ■ **Eclampsia:** 1° seizure disorder, TTP.

WORKUP

- ■ **Blood tests:** CBC, platelet count, BUN/creatinine, LFTs.
- ■ **Coagulation tests:** Fibrinogen, fibrin split products (where indicated), PT/aPTT.
- ■ **Urine studies:** UA, serial urine protein, urine toxicology screen (an ↑ BP may be 2° to drugs).
- ■ **Fetal tests:** Ultrasound (to rule out oligohydramnios and IUGR), nonstress test (NST), biophysical profile (BPP).

> **HELLP syndrome:**
>
> **H**emolysis
> **E**levated **L**FTs
> **L**ow **P**latelets
> (thrombocytopenia)

The three most common symptoms preceding an eclamptic attack are headache, visual changes, and RUQ/epigastric pain.

If gestational hypertension occurs in the first trimester, suspect a molar pregnancy!

In eclampsia, 50% of seizures occur antepartum, 25% intrapartum, and 25% postpartum. Preeclamptic and eclamptic patients are at highest risk for seizure up to 24 hours postpartum; however, seizures have been reported up to six weeks after delivery.

TABLE 6-4. Signs and Symptoms of Preeclampsia and Eclampsia

MILD PREECLAMPSIA	SEVERE PREECLAMPSIA	ECLAMPSIA
Rapid weight gain, edema, JVD	Cerebral/visual changes (severe headaches, blurred vision, scotomata)	Seizures
Hyperactive reflexes, clonus	RUQ/epigastric pain	
	Pulmonary edema/cyanosis	
	↑ LFTs, ↓ platelet counts	
	↓ urine output	
	IUGR	

The presence of fetal cardiac activity on ultrasound is reassuring.

In a patient who presents with first-trimester bleeding, ask about past pregnancies, a history of abnormal Pap smears, and a history of PID.

In normal pregnancy, an intrauterine pregnancy can be visualized by transvaginal ultrasound when the β-hCG is > 1800–2000 and by transabdominal ultrasound when the β-hCG is > 3500–5000.

TREATMENT

The only cure for preeclampsia is delivery of the fetus and placenta (see Table 6-5).

Complications of Pregnancy

FIRST-TRIMESTER BLEEDING

Affects 20–30% of all pregnancies. Etiologies are as follows:

- SAB (complete, incomplete, missed, threatened, and septic abortion; intra-uterine fetal death), ectopic pregnancy (see the Emergency Medicine chapter for more details), cervical carcinoma, hydatidiform mole, genital tract trauma, or infections (e.g., cervicitis, genital tract trauma or infection). Can also be a normal part of pregnancy
- It is best to place SAB and ectopic pregnancy at the top of your list and rapidly rule out both of these common causes of first-trimester bleeding.

WORKUP

- Qualitative/quantitative β-hCG.
- Transvaginal ultrasound.
- Pelvic exam to assess cervical dilation and possible ectopic pregnancy (adnexal mass).
- Type and screen (for RhoGAM administration if Rh ⊖).

SPONTANEOUS ABORTION (SAB)

Abortion is the termination of pregnancy at < 20 weeks' GA or with an EFW of < 500 g. It occurs in 13–26% of all pregnancies. The various types of abortion are outlined and compared in Table 6-6. Etiologies are as follows:

TABLE 6-5. Management of Preeclampsia and Eclampsia

PREECLAMPSIA	ECLAMPSIA
If term or fetal lung is mature, deliver.	Monitor ABCs; give supplemental O₂.
If mild preeclampsia and immature fetus, hospitalize, observe, bed rest, and monitor mother and fetus closely.	Seizure control with MgSO₄.
Control BP (hydralazine, labetalol).	Limit fluids; insert Foley catheter to check I/Os; monitor magnesium levels and fetal status.
If severe preeclampsia, control BP with hydralazine or labetalol (goal BP < 140/110), prevent seizures with MgSO₄, and deliver when the patient is stable.	Deliver when stable.
Postpartum—continue MgSO₄ for the first 24 hours; monitor for magnesium toxicity (↓ reflex, respiratory paralysis, coma). Follow BP and heme, renal, and liver labs.	Postpartum—continue MgSO₄ for the first 24 hours, or at least for 24 hours after the last seizure. Follow BP and heme, liver, and renal labs.

TABLE 6-6. Types of Spontaneous Abortion

ABORTION	DEFINITION	CERVICAL OS	TREATMENT
Complete	All products of conception are expelled.	Closed.	RhoGAM if appropriate.
Threatened	No products of conception are expelled; membranes remain intact. Uterine bleeding is present; abdominal pain may be present; fetus is still viable.	Closed.	Avoid heavy activity; pelvic rest (e.g., no intercourse, no tampons); RhoGAM if appropriate.
Missed	No cardiac activity; no products of conception expelled; retained fetal tissue. No uterine bleeding.	Closed.	D&C; expectant management; RhoGAM if appropriate.
Incomplete	Some products of conception expelled.	Open.	D&C; RhoGAM if appropriate.
Inevitable	No products of conception expelled; uterine bleeding and cramps.	Open.	D&C or uterotonics to complete SAB; RhoGAM if appropriate. Patients are at risk for infection if managed expectantly.
Septic	Infection associated with abortion; endometritis leading to septicemia.	Varies.	Complete uterine evacuation, D&C, IV antibiotics, RhoGAM if appropriate. Maternal mortality is 10–50% if in septic shock.

- **Chromosomal abnormalities:** The most common etiology (roughly 60%).
- **Infections.**
- **Anatomic defects:** Septate/bicornuate uterus, cervical incompetence, adhesions.
- **Endocrine factors:** Progesterone deficiency, polycystic ovarian syndrome (PCOS).
- **Immunologic factors:** Lupus anticoagulant, antiphospholipid syndrome.

SIGNS AND SYMPTOMS

- Vaginal bleeding; passage of tissues.
- Abdominal pain.
- Hemodynamic instability in the presence of retained placental tissue or severe hemorrhage.

TREATMENT

- Establish hemodynamic stability.
- Administer RhoGAM to all Rh-⊖ patients (see Figure 6-2).
- Expectant management vs. uterine evacuation. If D&C is performed, chorionic villi should be identified.
- Antibiotics if infection present.

THIRD-TRIMESTER BLEEDING

Defined as any bleeding that occurs after 28 weeks' gestation. Complicates approximately 5% of all pregnancies.

Women with three or more consecutive SABs should be worked up for recurrent abortion (> 3 successive abortions).

Antiphospholipid antibody syndrome is present in 5–15% of women with recurrent abortions.

HIGH-YIELD FACTS

OBSTETRICS AND GYNECOLOGY

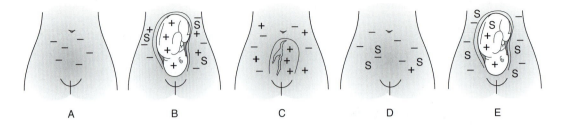

FIGURE 6-2. The significance of identifying Rh-⊖ mothers and giving them RhoGAM.

(A) Rh-⊖ woman before pregnancy. (B) Pregnancy occurs; the fetus is Rh ⊕. (C) Separation of the placenta. (D) Following delivery, Rh isoimmunization occurs in the mother, and she develops antibodies (S = antibodies). (E) The next pregnancy with an Rh-⊕ fetus. Maternal antibodies cross the placenta, enter the bloodstream, and attach to Rh-⊕ RBCs, leading to hemolysis. RhoGAM (Rh IgG) is given to the Rh-⊖ mother to prevent sensitization. (Reproduced, with permission, from DeCherney AH et al. *Current Obstetric & Gynecologic Diagnosis & Treatment*, 8th ed. Stamford, CT: Appleton & Lange, 1994: 339.)

What are the two most common causes of third-trimester bleeding? Abruptio placentae and placenta previa.

SIGNS AND SYMPTOMS

- Bleeding ranges from small amounts of spotting to passage of large clots.
- Abdominal pain and/or uterine tenderness suggests abruptio placentae.
- Profuse, painless bleeding is suggestive of placenta previa.

DIFFERENTIAL

- **Obstetric causes** (see Table 6-7): Abruptio placentae (30%), placenta previa (20%; see Figure 6-3), bloody show (loss of mucous plug with cervical dilation during the first stage of labor), uterine rupture.
- **Nonobstetric causes:** Genital tract lesions, cervical carcinoma.

WORKUP

Never do a vaginal exam prior to an ultrasound in a patient with third-trimester bleeding.

- CBC and PT/aPTT to rule out DIC; type and cross; UA and cervical cultures to rule out infection.
- If the location of the placenta is unknown, perform an ultrasound to rule out placenta previa before performing a vaginal exam.
- If no previa is found, perform a sterile speculum exam to evaluate the source of bleeding or ruptured membranes.
- Perform a vaginal exam to rule out labor.
- Fetal well-being tests:
  - Check for fetal heart tones and conduct an NST.
  - Consider amniocentesis for fetal lung maturity (FLM) for the assessment of delivery options.
  - Administer RhoGAM if Rh ⊖ and send a Kleihauer-Betke test to assess for extent of fetomaternal bleed.

TREATMENT

- Delivery for term patients.
- Bed rest and cautious tocolysis for stable preterm patients.
- In a mature fetus or in the presence of severe placental abruption, close fetal monitoring, amniotomy, and delivery are indicated (see Table 6-7).

TABLE 6-7. Abruptio Placentae vs. Placenta Previa

	ABRUPTIO PLACENTAE	PLACENTA PREVIA
Pathophysiology	Separation of normally implanted placenta from attachment to the uterus.	Abnormal implantation of the placenta near or at the cervical os. Classified as follows: ■ **Total:** The placenta covers the cervical os. ■ **Partial:** The placenta partially covers the os. ■ **Marginal:** The edge of the placenta extends to the margin of the os. ■ **Low lying:** The placenta is within reach of the examining finger, reached through the cervix.
Incidence	Incidence is 1 in 120, but accounts for 15% of perinatal deaths.	Incidence is 1 in 200.
Risk factors	Hypertension, abdominal or pelvic trauma, tobacco or cocaine use, previous abruption.	Prior C-sections, grand multiparity (> 5 previous deliveries).
Symptoms	**Painful** vaginal bleeding (although 10% of bleeding cases are concealed and there will be no overt bleeding); bleeding usually does not spontaneously cease. Abdominal pain, uterine hypertonicity, tenderness. **Fetal distress** is often present.	**Painless,** bright red bleeding (the bleeding source is usually the mother's except in cases of vasa previa); bleeding episode occurs at 29–30 weeks. Bleeding often ceases within 1–2 hours with or without UCs. Usually **no fetal distress.**
Workup	On transabdominal/transvaginal ultrasound, look for a retroplacental clot. One can rule in the diagnosis, but one cannot rule it out! Not highly sensitive. Abdominal exam may reveal tenderness. Clinical exam reveals signs of fetal distress, frequent UCs, and hypertonicity.	On transabdominal ultrasound, look for an abnormally positioned placenta; this test is very sensitive for ruling out this diagnosis.
Treatment	Stable patient with premature fetus— expectant management with continuous monitoring. Moderate to severe abruption—immediate delivery (vaginal delivery if fetal heart rate is stable; C-section if the mother or the fetus is in distress). Close fetal monitoring at all times. Amniocentesis to check fetal lung maturity if indicated.	No vaginal exam! Premature fetus (stable patient)—bed rest, tocolytics, serial ultrasound to check fetal growth; resolution of partial previa. If at or near term, amniocentesis to check fetal lung maturity; betamethasone to augment fetal lung maturity if indicated. Delivery by C-section (vaginal route if it resolves). Delivery in the presence of persistent labor, unstable bleeding requiring multiple transfusions, coagulation defects, or documented fetal lung maturity.
Complications	Hemorrhagic shock. Coagulopathy—DIC complicates 10% of all abruptions. Ischemic necrosis of distal organs. Recurrence rate is 5–16%; this risk ↑ to 25% after two previous abruptions. Fetal anemia.	Placenta accreta (up to 25% with one previous C-section and anterior placenta). Vasa previa. ↑ risk of congenital abnormalities. ↑ risk of postpartum hemorrhage. Fetal anemia.

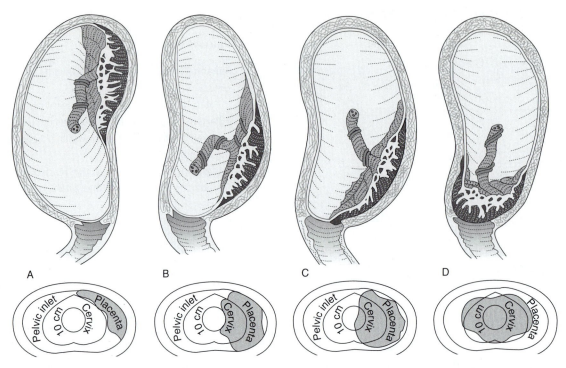

FIGURE 6-3. **(A) Normal placenta. (B) Low implantation. (C) Partial placenta previa. (D) Complete placenta previa.**

(Reproduced, with permission, from DeCherney AH et al. *Current Obstetric & Gynecologic Diagnosis & Treatment*, 8th ed. Stamford, CT: Appleton & Lange, 1994: 404.)

Labor and Delivery

NORMAL LABOR

Labor has two components: (1) UCs of sufficient frequency, duration, and intensity; and (2) cervical changes, including effacement (thinning) and dilation. Cervical dilation that occurs without UCs is not considered true labor. Similarly, UCs without cervical effacement and dilation are referred to as Braxton Hicks contractions, or false labor. The following are additional characteristics of normal labor:

What are the three signs of placental separation? Gush of blood; apparent umbilical cord lengthening; and the fundus of the uterus rises and firms.

- Onset of labor:
  - **Lightening:** A change in the shape of the abdomen with the sensation that the baby is less heavy. This event results from the descent of the fetal head into the pelvis.
  - **Bloody show:** Passage of blood-tinged mucus that is produced when the cervix begins to thin out (effacement). Cervical effacement commonly occurs before the onset of true labor, particularly in nulliparous patients.
- Assessment of labor:
  - Instruct the patient to report to the hospital for evaluation when:
    - Contractions occur every five minutes for at least one hour.
    - There is ROM (a large gush of fluid or continuous leakage).
    - There is significant bleeding.
    - There is a significant ↓ in fetal movement.
  - Cervical examination should evaluate the following:
    - **Effacement:** The length of the cervix as the cervix thins out and softens (%).

- **Dilation:** The size of the cervical opening at the external os (cm).
- **Position:** The location of the cervix with respect to the fetal presenting part.
- **Consistency:** From soft to firm, with soft indicating onset of labor.
- **Station:** The relationship of the fetal head to the level of the ischial spines. It ranges from –5 to +5 station (where 0 is defined to be the fetal head at the level of the ischial spines).
- **Stages of labor:** The stages of labor are as follows (see also Table 6-8 and Figure 6-4):
  - **First stage:** Onset of labor to complete (10-cm) cervical dilation.
    - **Latent phase:** From onset of labor to 4 cm of cervical dilation.
    - **Active phase:** From 4 to 10 cm of dilation; signifies a period of more rapid cervical dilation.
  - **Second stage:** From complete dilation to delivery of the infant.
  - **Third stage:** From delivery of the infant to delivery of the placenta.
- **Cardinal movements:** Babies undergo seven stereotypical cardinal movements for successful delivery. These movements, which constitute the second stage of labor, are as follows:

  1. Engagement
  2. Descent
  3. Flexion
  4. Internal rotation
  5. Extension
  6. External rotation
  7. Expulsion

- **Fetal lie, presentation, and position:** The orientation of the baby is described in relation to the maternal pelvis in the following manner:
  - **Fetal lie:** The long axis of the baby in relation to the long axis of the mother (longitudinal, transverse, oblique).
  - **Fetal presentation:** That part of the fetus which enters the pelvis first— e.g., vertex (head first), breech (buttocks or leg first), face, brow.

Leopold's maneuver is used to determine fetal lie and presentation.

The most common fetal orientation at delivery is longitudinal, vertex, occiput anterior (i.e., the baby's face emerges facing the mother's rectum).

TABLE 6-8. The Three Stages of Labor

STAGE	STARTS/END	EVENTS	AVERAGE DURATION (hrs)	
			NULLI[a]	MULTI[b]
First				
Latent	Regular UCs/cervix dilated up to 4 cm.	Highly variable duration; cervix effaces and slowly dilates.	6–20	4–14
Active	4-cm cervical dilation/complete cervical dilation (10 cm).	Regular and intense UCs; cervix effaces and dilates more quickly; fetal head progressively descends into the pelvis.	4–12	2–5
Second	Complete cervical dilation/delivery of the baby.	Baby undergoes all stages of cardinal movements.	1–3	0.5–1.0
Third	Delivery of the baby/delivery of the placenta.	Placenta separates and uterus contracts to establish hemostasis.	0–0.5	0–0.5

[a] Nulli = nulliparous (first-time mother).

[b] Multi = multiparous (delivered vaginally before).

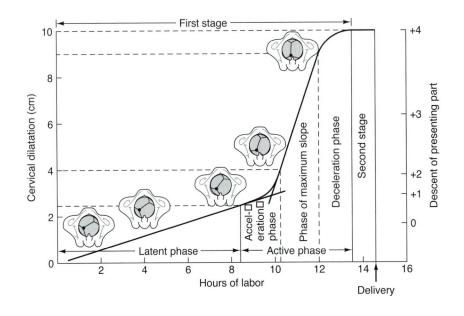

FIGURE 6-4. Cervical dilation, level of descent, and orientation of occipitoanterior presentation during various stages of labor.

(Reproduced, with permission, from DeCherney AH et al. *Current Obstetric & Gynecologic Diagnosis & Treatment*, 8th ed. Stamford, CT: Appleton & Lange, 1994: 211.)

> **Risk factors for preterm labor—**
>
> **MAPPS**
>
> **M**ultiple gestations
> **A**bdominal surgery during pregnancy
> **P**revious **P**reterm labor or delivery
> **S**urgery of the cervix

Premature ROM is rupture of membranes that occurs before the onset of labor, regardless of gestational age. Preterm ROM is rupture of membranes that occurs before 37 weeks' gestation. When both occur together, it is termed premature preterm rupture of membranes (PPROM).

■ **Fetal position:** The reference point of the fetal presenting part (for vertex presentation, the presenting part is the occiput; for breech presentation, the presenting part is the sacrum) to the maternal pelvis (right, left, anterior, posterior).

PRETERM LABOR

Preterm labor complicates 5–10% of all pregnancies. Risk factors for preterm labor can be described by the mnemonic **MAPPS**. However, half of all cases occur in patients without any risk factors. Diagnostic criteria are as follows:

■ **Preterm:** < 37 weeks' gestation.
■ **True labor:** UCs of sufficient duration and intensity to result in cervical dilation of > 2 cm or effacement of > 80%.

SIGNS AND SYMPTOMS

■ Abdominal, pelvic, or back pain.
■ Vaginal discharge; bloody show.
■ UCs; cervical dilation and/or effacement.
■ ROM.

DIFFERENTIAL

■ **False labor:** Contractions without cervical dilation or change.
■ **Appendicitis.**
■ **Local causes:** Cervicitis, genital tract infections, trauma, physiologic discharge.

WORKUP

- **Perform a cervical exam.**
- **Rule out infectious causes of preterm labor** with cervical cultures and a wet mount. Labs to send include CBC, urine tox screen, a UA and urine culture, and vaginal and cervical cultures for GBS, chlamydia, and gonorrhea.
- Perform a sterile speculum exam to evaluate for premature ROM. Tests to identify amniotic fluid vs. urinary leakage or excess vaginal discharge include the following:
    - **Vaginal pooling:** Gross visualization of amniotic fluid in the vagina.
    - **Nitrazine test:** Alkaline amniotic fluid turns the Nitrazine paper blue.
    - **Ferning test:** Amniotic fluid smeared on a slide forms "ferns" as it dries.
- Perform a serial exam and ultrasound to assess EFW, presentation, and amniotic fluid volume.

TREATMENT

- The course of management depends on the GA of the fetus. The main goal is to delay delivery until fetal lung maturity has been achieved.
- Consider tocolytics (e.g., indomethacin, nifedipine) if there is cervical change. Check for contraindications to tocolytics first (see the mnemonic **CHAMPS**). There is, however, no uncontested evidence that the use of tocolytics prolongs the length of gestation.
- Give betamethasone under the following conditions:
    - Estimated GA of 24–34 weeks with preterm labor; estimated GA of 24–32 weeks with PPROM.
    - Absence of uncontrolled maternal diabetes.
    - No need for immediate delivery (e.g., placental abruption with nonreassuring heart tracing).
- Amniocentesis may be considered, especially at 35–36 weeks' GA, to check for FLM. Amniotic fluid may also be collected from vaginal pooling and sent for testing in the setting of PPROM.
- Notify pediatrics on admission, not only for counseling of the patient as to the expected neonatal outcome but also to ensure that the pediatricians are aware of a potential preterm infant delivery.

ABNORMAL LABOR PATTERNS

A diagnosis of abnormal labor is considered in any case in which there is a variation in the normal pattern of cervical dilation or descent of the fetal presenting part. It occurs in 8–11% of all cephalic deliveries.

SIGNS AND SYMPTOMS

Table 6-9 describes patterns of abnormal labor. Also beware of false labor, which may be confused with arrest of dilation and has the following distinguishing characteristics:

- Irregular intervals and duration of UCs with no cervical dilation.
- Unchanged contraction intensity.
- Lower back and abdominal discomfort.
- Relief with sedation.

What could cause a false-⊕ Nitrazine test? Contamination from blood, semen, or vaginitis.

Tocolytics are ineffective if the patient is in active labor (cervical dilation ≥ 4 cm).

Contraindications to tocolytics–

CHAMPS

Chorioamnionitis
Hemorrhage
Abruption of placenta
Maturity of fetus
Preeclampsia/eclampsia
Severe IUGR

TABLE 6-9. Abnormal Labor Patterns

ABNORMAL PATTERN	THRESHOLD DURATION OF LABOR		POSSIBLE CAUSES
	NULLIPAROUS	MULTIPAROUS	
Precipitous	Completion of stages 1 and 2 in < 3 hours.		Unknown.
Protracted latent phase	> 20 hours	> 14 hours	Ineffective UCs; unripe cervix; abnormal fetal position; false labor.
Protracted active phase	> 12 hours or rate of cervical dilation < 1.2 cm/hr	> 6 hours < 1.5 cm/hr	Abnormal fetal position; fetopelvic disproportion; excess sedation; ineffective UCs.
Arrest of dilation in active contraction phase	Cervical dilation stops for > 2 hours		Ineffective UCs; fetopelvic disproportion; abnormal fetal lie, presentation, or position.
Arrest of fetal descent in second stage	> 2 hours without epidural > 3 hours with epidural	> 1 hour without epidural > 2 hours with epidural	Ineffective UCs; fetopelvic disproportion.

> **Causes of abnormal labor—**
>
> **The 3 P's**
>
> **P**owers (uterine contractions)
> **P**assenger (fetus)
> **P**assage (pelvic)

Shoulder dystocia is due to impaction of the fetal shoulder behind the pubic symphysis after delivery of the head.

DIFFERENTIAL

Normal or false labor; ineffective UCs; fetal malposition/fetopelvic disproportion.

WORKUP

- Obtain graphic demonstration of cervical dilation and effacement.
- Document on each vaginal exam the dilation of the cervix, the presence of the caput or molding of the fetal head, and the station and position of the fetal presenting part.
- The results of each examination should be assessed dynamically.
- Workup should then proceed with the systematic assessment of the "3 P's" of labor (see mnemonic):
  - **Powers (uterine forces):** Frequency and duration can be evaluated through manual palpation of the gravid abdomen during a contraction, by a tocodynamometer, and by an internal pressure catheter (this is the only way to measure the pressure generated by each UC).
  - **Passenger:** Estimation of fetal weight and clinical evaluation of fetal lie, presentation, and position.
  - **Passage:** Measurement of the bony pelvis is often a poor predictor of abnormal labor unless the pelvis is extremely contracted. Also assess for other physical obstacles (e.g., distended bladder or colon, uterine myoma, cervical mass).

TREATMENT

- **Precipitous labor:**
  - Stop any oxytocin use. Tocolytics are not proven to help.
  - Complications include uterine atony leading to postpartum hemorrhage and genital tract trauma.

- **Prolonged latent phase:**
  - Rest or augmentation of labor with oxytocin if "power" is the problem.
  - Amniotomy (i.e., artificial ROM [AROM]).
- **Protracted/arrested active phase:**
  - Intrauterine pressure catheter to measure the force of UCs.
  - AROM.
  - Augmentation with oxytocin if "power" is the problem.
  - C-section in the presence of fetopelvic disproportion or maternal/fetal distress.
- **Arrest in second stage:**
  - Attempt vaginal delivery if the mother and baby are doing well.
  - Augmentation with oxytocin.
  - Operative vaginal delivery (forceps, vacuum) if the vertex is low in the pelvis.
  - C-section in the presence of maternal/fetal distress, breech, or fetopelvic disproportion.

FETAL HEART RATE (FHR) MONITORING

The FHR is usually monitored continuously throughout labor to evaluate its effects on fetal intrapartum events. **External monitoring** is conducted with an ultrasound transducer affixed to the maternal abdomen. **Internal monitoring** is done through an electrode attached to the fetal scalp and requires that the membranes have been ruptured. Relevant variables are as follows:

- **Baseline FHR:** The normal range of the human FHR is 110–160 bpm. Abnormal patterns are as follows:
  - **Baseline tachycardia:** A baseline heart rate > 160 bpm for > 10 minutes. Etiologies include fetal hypoxia, maternal fever, fetal infection, maternal thyrotoxicosis, fetal anemia, fetal arrhythmias, and the use of β-sympathomimetic drugs such as terbutaline (see the mnemonic **FFAAST Heart**).
  - **Baseline bradycardia:** A baseline heart rate < 110 bpm for > 10 minutes. Etiologies include fetal hypoxia, damage to the conduction system of the fetal heart, maternal autoimmune disease, and treatment with drugs such as β-blockers.
- **Heart rate variability:** Represents the interplay between cardioinhibitory and cardioacceleratory centers in the fetal brain stem.
  - **Beat-to-beat variability is the most reliable indicator of fetal well-being** and is one of the best indicators of intact integration between the CNS and heart of the fetus.
  - **Short-term variability:** Variation on a "beat-to-beat basis" usually ranges from 3 to 5 bpm.
  - **Long-term variability:** Fluctuations with amplitudes of 5–20 bpm occurring at 3–5 cycles per minute.
- **Periodic changes:** Table 6-10 and Figure 6-5 outline patterns in FHR. Relevant definitions are as follows:
  - **Accelerations:** Transient increases in FHR above the determined baseline. Accelerations are reassuring and usually indicate fetal well-being.
  - **Early decelerations:** Decreases in FHR that begin with a contraction, reach a nadir at the peak of the contraction, and end with the completion of the contraction. Early decelerations result from pressure on the fetal head through a reflex response mediated by the vagus nerve with release of acetylcholine at the sinoatrial node. Early decelerations are

Early decelerations mirror the contraction as it happens and are innocuous. Repetitive late decelerations are a delayed mirror image and may be a sign of uteroplacental insufficiency.

TABLE 6-10. Fetal Heart Rate Patterns

	EARLY DECELERATION	LATE DECELERATION	VARIABLE DECELERATION
Significance	Benign	Abnormal	Benign/abnormal
Onset	Gradual	Gradual	Abrupt
When	End with UC	End after UC	Variable
Etiology	Head compression	Uteroplacental insufficiency	Umbilical cord compression/head compression
Initial treatment	None required	O_2, lateral decubitus position, oxytocin off	Amnioinfusion

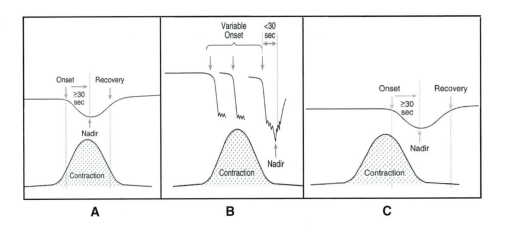

FIGURE 6-5. Features of early (A), variable (B), and late (C) decelerations on fetal heart monitoring.

(Reproduced, with permission, from Cunningham FG et al. *Williams Obstetrics*, 22nd ed. New York: McGraw-Hill, 2005: 452, 453, 454.)

innocuous and can be observed throughout labor without alteration in fetal condition or acid-base status.

- **Variable decelerations:** Slowing of the heart rate that may start before, during, or after the UC and is characterized by a rapid fall in FHR, often below 100 bpm, with a rapid return to baseline.
  - Decelerations are associated with umbilical cord compression and are mediated through the vagus nerve with sudden and often erratic release of acetylcholine at the fetal sinoatrial node.
  - This pattern is often seen with oligohydramnios or after ROM 2° to "decreased cushioning" of the umbilical cord. If the variable decelerations are severe and repetitive, hypoxia and metabolic acidosis may result.
- **Late decelerations:** Begin after the UC starts, reach their nadir after the peak of the contraction, and end after the contraction ceases.
  - Late decelerations are a sign of uteroplacental insufficiency resulting from ↓ uterine perfusion or ↓ placental function.
  - Associated with progressive fetal hypoxia and acidemia. May occur with any process that would predispose to insufficient blood flow and oxygenation of the fetus, such as placental abruption, excessive uterine activity, maternal hypotension, anemia, and IUGR.
  - Although repetitive late decelerations are considered nonreassuring, they have very poor positive predictive value. Ninety percent of the time, a fetus with repetitive late decelerations actually has a normal acid-base status.

A reactive tracing is a sign of fetal well-being. A reactive tracing has at least two accelerations in which the heart rate peaks 15 beats above the baseline for at least 15 seconds during a 20-minute period.

A fetus < 28 weeks' GA is neurologically immature and thus is not expected to have a "reactive" FHR.

Postpartum Complications

POSTPARTUM HEMORRHAGE

Defined as blood loss of > 500 mL within the first 24 hours of vaginal delivery or > 1000 mL following cesarean delivery. Hemorrhage can be sudden and profuse, or blood loss can occur more slowly but persistently. In either case, excessive bleeding is a serious and potentially fatal complication.

What is the most common cause of postpartum hemorrhage? Uterine atony.

DIFFERENTIAL

Uterine atony, genital tract trauma, retained placental tissue, uterine inversion, uterine rupture, cervical carcinoma (see also Table 6-11).

WORKUP/TREATMENT

The diagnosis and treatment of the three major causes of postpartum hemorrhage are discussed in Table 6-11.

Remember serial hematocrits in postpartum hemorrhage.

"POSTPARTUM BLUES"/POSTPARTUM DEPRESSION

"Postpartum blues" is a common disorder affecting new mothers, many of whom experience mild, short-lived crying, irritability, anxiety, and emotional lability. However, when symptoms are of at least two weeks' duration and include anhedonia, insomnia, changes in appetite, feelings of guilt, suicidality, or feelings of wanting to hurt the baby, the diagnosis is likely to be postpartum depression.

TABLE 6-11. Common Causes of Postpartum Hemorrhage

	UTERINE ATONY	GENITAL TRACT TRAUMA	RETAINED PLACENTAL TISSUE
Risk factors	Overdistention of the uterus (multiple gestations, macrosomia). Abnormal labor (prolonged labor, precipitous labor). Conditions interfering with UCs (uterine myomas, $MgSO_4$, general anesthesia). Uterine infection.	Precipitous labor. Operative vaginal delivery (forceps, vacuum extraction). Large infant. Inadequate laceration repair. Unrecognized cervical laceration.	Placenta accreta/increta/percreta. Preterm delivery. Placenta previa. Previous C-section/curettage. Uterine leiomyomas.
Workup	Palpation of a softer, flaccid, "boggy" uterus without a firm fundus.	Careful visualization of the lower genital tract to look for any laceration > 2 cm in length or bleeding.	Careful inspection of the placenta for missing cotyledons. Ultrasound may also be used to examine the uterus.
Treatment	The most common cause of postpartum hemorrhage (90%). Bimanual uterine massage. Oxytocin infusion. Empty bladder (overdistended bladder can prevent UCs). Methylergonovine maleate (Methergine) if the patient is not hypertensive and/or prostaglandin F2-alpha. (Hemabate) if the patient is not asthmatic. Rectal misoprostol may also be used.	Surgical repair of the physical defect.	Manual removal of the remaining placental tissue. Curettage with suctioning may also be used, with care taken to avoid perforating the uterine fundus. In cases of true placenta accreta/increta/percreta where the placental villi invade into the uterine tissue, hysterectomy may be required as a life-preserving therapy.

TREATMENT

Includes support groups, psychotherapy, and pharmacologic treatments such as antidepressants.

REFERENCE

Beck CT. Postpartum depression: It isn't just the blues. *Am J Nursing* 106(5): 40–50, 2006. A good description of postpartum blues vs. postpartum depression.

GYNECOLOGY

Abnormal Uterine Bleeding

Subtypes of abnormal uterine bleeding are distinguished as follows:

- **Polymenorrhea:** Menses with intervals that are too short (< 21 days).
- **Menorrhagia:** Menses that are too long (> 7 days) and/or excessive blood loss (> 80 mL) at **normal** intervals.

HIGH-YIELD FACTS

OBSTETRICS AND GYNECOLOGY

- **Hypermenorrhea:** Menses that are too long (> 7 days) and/or excessive blood loss (> 80 mL) at **regular but not necessarily normal intervals.**
- **Oligomenorrhea:** Menses with intervals that are too long (> 35 days).
- **Metrorrhagia:** Menses occurring at irregular intervals with intermenstrual bleeding.
- **Menometrorrhagia:** A combination of menorrhagia and metrorrhagia.

DIFFERENTIAL

- **Premenopause:**
    - **Pregnancy:** The most common cause. Keep in mind abnormal pregnancies such as ectopic pregnancy, threatened abortion, and incomplete abortion.
    - **Organic causes:** Blood dyscrasias, hypersplenism, hypothyroidism, sepsis, ITP, leukemia.
    - **Anatomic causes:** Malignancies, infections, endometriosis, ruptured corpus luteum cyst, fibroids, endometrial polyp, trauma.
    - **Dysfunctional uterine bleeding (DUB):** Bleeding without any other recognizable cause.
- **Postmenopause:**
    - **Atrophic vaginitis:** Most common.
    - **Endometrial cancer:** Must be ruled out with endometrial biopsy.
    - **Other:** Cervical cancer, vulvar cancer, hormone replacement therapy (HRT).

WORKUP

- Obtain an H&P, including a thorough menstrual and reproductive history.
- Assess the rate of bleeding, hemodynamic status, and orthostatic vitals; obtain a CBC.
- Conduct a pregnancy test.
- Determine whether the patient is having ovulatory or anovulatory cycles. The patient is ovulating if she has menstrual cycles at regular intervals.
    - If the patient **is not ovulating,** suspect DUB, most likely 2° to hormonal irregularities.
    - If the patient **is ovulating,** conduct further workup to rule out pathology:
        - Order a PT/aPTT to rule out coagulopathy, particularly if the patient is an adolescent and has just begun menstruating.
        - Evaluate for skin and hair changes, thyroid enlargement, galactorrhea, obesity, hirsutism, cervical motion tenderness (CMT), uterine size, cervical lesions, and adnexal tenderness.
        - Obtain an endometrial biopsy for women > 35 years of age.
        - Consider transvaginal ultrasound to check for uterine and ovarian masses/endometrial thickening (normally < 5 mm in postmenopausal women).

TREATMENT

- **Anovulatory bleeding:** After ruling out pathologies (uterine polyps, endometrial cancer), place patients on medroxyprogesterone acetate (Provera) or OCPs. Also consider HRT if the patient is perimenopausal (see Table 6-12).
- **DUB:**
    - For mild cases (hemoglobin > 11), treat with iron supplements, NSAIDs, and OCPs. Alternatively, high-dose progestins (norethindrone) can be used to normalize menses.

TABLE 6-12. General Management of Abnormal Uterine Bleeding

ACUTE UTERINE BLEEDING	RECURRENT UTERINE BLEEDING
High-dose estrogen (oral or IV)	GnRH agonists (Lupron)
High-dose OCPs	Danazol (multiple side effects)
D&C	D&C/endometrial biopsy to aid in diagnosis
	Endometrial ablation

- For severe cases (hemoglobin < 7), stabilize the patient first (blood transfusion, saline) and then start on IV estrogen or OCPs.
- For recurrent, severe cases, start on OCPs, Provera, or Depo-Provera with or without an estrogen supplement.
- If medical therapy fails, consider surgical options for DUB, which include hysteroscopy with D&C, endometrial ablation with laser or electrocautery, and hysterectomy.

Endometriosis

Defined as the presence of endometrial glands and stroma outside the uterine cavity. Affects 5–15% of premenopausal women, accounting for 40–50% of all surgeries for infertility. Evidence exists, however, for a genetic disposition in first-degree relatives. Sites affected (see also Figure 6-6) include the ovaries, the broad ligament, and the cul-de-sac. Etiologies include direct implantation of endometrial cells by retrograde menstruation; vascular and lymphatic dissemination of endometrial cells; and coelomic metaplasia of multipotential cells in the peritoneal cavity.

Fibroids are benign uterine tumors that may cause excessive menstrual bleeding, pelvic pain, and frequent urination.

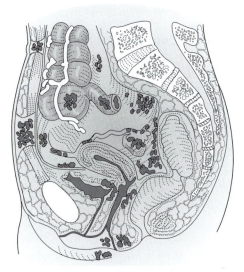

FIGURE 6-6. Common sites of endometriosis (dark ovals).

(Reproduced, with permission, from Doherty GM, Way LW. *Current Surgical Diagnosis & Treatment*, 12th ed. New York: McGraw-Hill, 2006: 1075.)

- Presents with pelvic pain (dysmenorrhea, dyspareunia, dyschezia), abnormal bleeding, and infertility.
- The disease is hormone dependent and usually improves after menopause.
- Physical exam reveals nodular thickening along the uterosacral ligament; a fixed, retroverted uterus; and tender, fixed adnexal masses (endometriomas).

DIFFERENTIAL

Most women with endometriosis are asymptomatic. However, patients can present with a wide range of symptoms, and the differential depends on the patient's specific complaints.

- **Chronic abdominal pain:** Chronic PID and pelvic adhesions.
- **Amenorrhea:** Causes of 1° and/or 2° amenorrhea.
- **Sudden-onset lower abdominal pain:** Ectopic pregnancy, appendicitis, PID, adnexal torsion, rupture of the corpus luteum, endometrioma.

WORKUP

- **Laparoscopy:** Offers a definitive diagnosis.
- **Biopsy:** Biopsy of "endometriosis-appearing lesions" reveals functional endometrial glands and stroma together with hemosiderin-laden macrophages.
- **Labs/imaging:** Pregnancy test, UA, ultrasound.

TREATMENT

Treatment should be individualized according to age, reproductive plans, and extent of disease.

- **Medical:** Aimed at inducing inactivity/atrophy of endometrial tissue.
  - **Hormonal manipulation:** OCPs, progestin, danazol, GnRH agonists.
  - All medical treatments are for symptomatic relief, not for cure, as they have no effect on the adhesions and fibrosis caused by endometriosis.
- **Surgical:**
  - **Conservative:** Laparoscopic removal of implants (excision, electrocauterization, laser ablation) that allows for future pregnancy.
  - **Definitive:** Total abdominal hysterectomy (TAH), bilateral salpingo-oophorectomy (BSO), lysis of adhesions, and removal of all implants. In premenopausal patients, some ovarian tissue may be left intact to prevent early menopause, although there may be a recurrence of endometriosis. In patients without endogenous estrogen production (e.g., patients who have no ovaries), HRT should be instituted. Some experts advocate waiting before starting HRT.

Amenorrhea

1° **amenorrhea** is defined as the absence of menses by age 16. 2° **amenorrhea** is defined as the absence of menses for three cycles or for six months with normal prior menses. Etiologies are as follows:

- 1° **amenorrhea:** Constitutional delay (physiologic), pituitary failure, gonadal failure/agenesis, androgen insensitivity syndrome, müllerian abnormality, genital tract outflow obstruction, pregnancy.
- 2° **amenorrhea:**
  - **Pregnancy:** The most common cause of amenorrhea.

Classically, endometriosis lesions are described as having the appearance of mulberries, raspberries, powder burns, and "chocolate cysts" (cysts on the ovaries filled with old blood).

For endometriosis, disease severity does not necessarily correlate with symptoms.

Medical treatment of endometriosis is symptomatic and will not improve a patient's ability to conceive.

Always check a pregnancy test. Pregnancy is a common cause of amenorrhea.

HIGH-YIELD FACTS

OBSTETRICS AND GYNECOLOGY

The workup for a patient with 1° amenorrhea is the same as that for 2° amenorrhea if the patient has both a uterus and breasts. If not, do a karyotype.

Do not start a patient on OCPs for amenorrhea until you are satisfied that you have determined an etiology. It may interfere with your workup.

- **Hypothalamic causes:** Hypothyroidism, hyperprolactinemia, anorexia.
- **Pituitary causes:** Tumor, hemosiderosis.
- **Ovarian causes:** PCOS, premature menopause (premature ovarian failure).

WORKUP/TREATMENT

The workup of amenorrhea should follow a logical progression:

- Determine if it is 1° or 2° amenorrhea. If 1°, refer to the workup described in Figure 6-7.
- 2° amenorrhea is divided into two groups: without galactorrhea and with galactorrhea. Workup should proceed as follows:
    - First, rule out pregnancy.
    - **With galactorrhea** (see Figure 6-8):
        - Check TSH. If abnormal, evaluate for thyroid disease.
        - If TSH is normal, check prolactin. If high, evaluate for pituitary tumor and drugs affecting pituitary function.
    - **Without galactorrhea** (see Figure 6-9):
        - Do a progestin challenge.
        - If ⊕ (withdrawal bleeding), there is adequate estrogen production, indicating anovulation.
        - If ⊖, check LH and FSH levels.
            - Low LH/FSH indicates that the main problem lies in the hypothalamic-pituitary axis (e.g., stress, nutritional imbalance, tumors) or is attributable to constitutional delay in a patient with 1° amenorrhea.

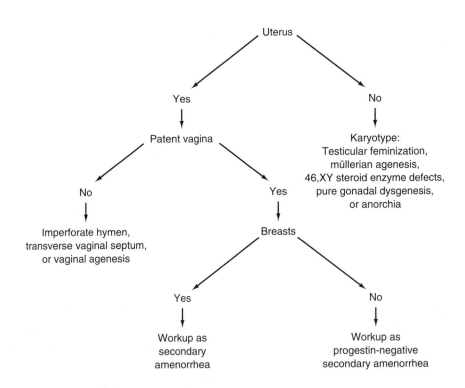

FIGURE 6-7. Workup for 1° amenorrhea.

(Reproduced, with permission, from DeCherney AH et al. *Current Obstetric & Gynecologic Diagnosis &Treatment*, 8th ed. Stamford, CT: Appleton & Lange, 1994: 1010.)

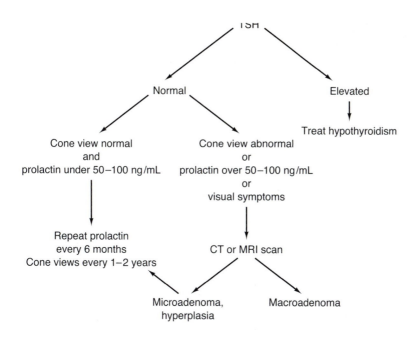

FIGURE 6-8. Workup for patients with 2° amenorrhea with galactorrhea and hyperprolactinemia.

(Reproduced, with permission, from DeCherney AH et al. *Current Obstetric & Gynecologic Diagnosis & Treatment*, 8th ed. Stamford, CT: Appleton & Lange, 1994: 1011.)

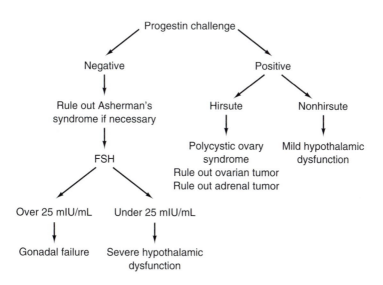

FIGURE 6-9. Workup for patients with 2° amenorrhea without galactorrhea and hyperprolactinemia.

(Reproduced, with permission, from DeCherney AH et al. *Current Obstetric & Gynecologic Diagnosis & Treatment*, 8th ed. Stamford, CT: Appleton & Lange, 1994: 1012.)

Contraception

Table 6-13 summarizes the various forms of contraception available and their failure rates during the first year of use (both "lowest expected" and "typical,"

TABLE 6-13. Forms of Contraception and Their Failure Rates

METHOD	HOW USED	PERCENTAGE OF WOMEN WITH PREGNANCY (%)[a]	
		LOWEST EXPECTED	TYPICAL
No method	No form of contraception	85.0	85.0
Hormonal agents			
Combination pill	Once-daily pill	0.3	8.0
Progestin-only pill	Once-daily pill	0.3	8.0
Depo-Provera	IM injection every 12 weeks	0.3	3.0
Barrier methods			
Male condom	With each intercourse	2.0	15.0
Female condom	With each intercourse	5.0	21.0
Diaphragm/ spermicide	With each intercourse	6.0	16.0
Spermicides	With each intercourse	18.0	29.0
Cervical cap	Parous with each intercourse	26.0	32.0
	Nulliparous with each intercourse	9.0	16.0
IUD (Copper T)	Inserted every 10 years	0.6	0.8
IUD (levonorgestrel-releasing)	Inserted every 5 years	0.1	0.1
Sterilization			
Female	One-time operation	0.5	0.5
Male	One-time operation	0.10	0.15
Behavioral methods			
Periodic abstinence	Calendar method	9.0	25.0
	Ovulation method	3.0	25.0
	Symptothermal	2.0	25.0
	Postovulation	1.0	25.0
Withdrawal	With each intercourse	4.0	27.0

[a]Data apply to the first year of use.

meaning the rate actually seen in the population). Common contraindications for combination estrogen/progesterone OCPs include the following:

- Women > 35 years of age who smoke.
- Those with a history of the following conditions:
  - Blood clots
  - CVA or CAD
  - Migraines with auras
  - Estrogen-dependent carcinoma
  - Jaundice with pill use
  - Diabetes with vascular involvement
  - Active liver disease
  - Known or suspected breast cancer
  - Known or suspected pregnancy
  - Thromboembolic disorders
  - Uncontrolled hypertension
  - Undiagnosed abnormal genital bleeding

Menopause

Defined as the permanent cessation of natural menses that marks the end of a woman's reproductive life. The average age at onset ranges from 45 to 55 years, with the median age 51 years. The climacteric period is the extended period of ↓ ovarian function beginning several years before and lasting years after menopause itself.

SIGNS AND SYMPTOMS

- **Perimenopausal symptoms:**
  - Irregular and infrequent menses.
  - Hot flashes, sleep disturbances, vaginal dryness, volatility of affect, sexual dysfunction, hair and nail brittleness.
- **Postmenopausal symptoms:** Genital tract atrophy (e.g., urinary incontinence), osteoporosis, cardiovascular diseases.

DIFFERENTIAL

Premature ovarian failure (menopause occurring prior to 42 years of age), which may be due to alkylating chemotherapy, smoking, autoimmune diseases, hysterectomy, or genetic predisposition.

WORKUP

- FSH, LFTs, cholesterol panel, CBC, UA.
- Obtain a mammogram, a Pap smear, and a bone density study (to screen for osteoporosis).
- Definitive diagnosis is made when serum FSH is > 25 mIU/mL at two separate times or when the LH/FSH ratio is > 2.

TREATMENT

- **HRT:** Estrogen plus progestin.
  - In light of recent reports of ↑ cardiovascular morbidity and breast cancer with prolonged HRT use, it is generally advised that hormone replacement be used only in symptomatic patients for short durations, and only after patients have been thoroughly informed about relevant risks and benefits. However, there has been substantial debate among

What form of contraceptive is recommended in nursing mothers? Progestin-only pills. What is the only contraceptive effective against STDs? Condoms.

Overall, the risk of any pregnancy, including ectopic pregnancy, is decreased with IUD use. In the event that a woman with an IUD does become pregnant, a greater proportion of the pregnancies will be ectopic.

↑ serum FSH levels in postmenopausal women are due to feedback from fewer oocytes and ↑ FSH requirements from resistant oocytes.

If a woman still has her uterus, a combined estrogen-progestin regimen should be used for HRT to prevent endometrial hyperplasia.

OB/GYNs about the NIH trial that prompted these recommendations, since the majority of patients studied had been postmenopausal years before starting HRT, and it remains unclear how well the results apply to perimenopausal women.

- **Side effects** include irregular bleeding (especially in the first six months), weight gain, fluid retention, and endometrial hyperplasia (rare if the patient is also taking progesterone).
- **Contraindications** include a history of breast cancer, endometrial cancer, liver disease, thromboembolic disease, or MI.

■ Patients should be advised to take calcium supplements, stop smoking, and exercise to prevent or minimize osteoporotic changes. An annual pelvic exam should be performed and a Pap smear and mammogram obtained. However, women > 30 years of age who have had three consecutive ⊖ Pap smears, have no history of CIN 2/3 or immune compromise (including HIV infection), and were not exposed to DES in utero can have Pap smears every 2–3 years.

REFERENCE

Rossouw JE et al. Risks and benefits of estrogen plus progestin in healthy postmenopausal women: Principal results from the Women's Health Initiative randomized controlled trial. *JAMA* 288(3):321–333, 2002. This is the well-known and widely cited Women's Health Initiative HRT study, which evaluated the major health benefits and risks of the most commonly used combined hormone preparation in the United States. The study concluded that overall health risks exceeded the benefits that would be obtained from the use of combined estrogen plus progestin. This critical study has significantly influenced the practice of HRT prescription in the United States.

Infertility

Defined as the inability to get pregnant after trying for one year. The most important determinant of infertility in a couple is the woman's age, as conception rates are more than halved by age 35 and over. However, infertility is just as often attributed to the male as to the female. Specific etiologies are as follows:

- **Males:** Often due to a ↓ sperm count, dysfunctional sperm, or impaired sperm delivery.
- **Females:** Often due to structural damage (e.g., damage to the fallopian tubes resulting from STDs or from endometriosis or fibroids), hormonal imbalances that can affect ovulation (including PCOS), or ovarian failure. **Both males and females:** Obesity, EtOH, smoking, improper nutrition, and age may all affect fertility.

WORKUP

- **Females:**
  - Workup should include measurement of body mass index (BMI); FSH and LH levels to assess ovarian function; evaluation of midluteal progesterone levels to confirm ovulation; cervical cytology and testing for STDs; ultrasound to image the ovaries and uterus; and/or hysterosalpingography to assess tubal patency.
    - If the woman has a history of irregular menses, prolactin and thyroid levels may be tested, and androgen levels may be evaluated if hyperandrogenism is suspected.
- **Males:** Workup involves a semen analysis, possible hormone testing, and ultrasound imaging to visualize structural abnormalities.

TREATMENT

- Often begins with lifestyle modification (e.g., smoking cessation and weight loss) and, if possible, treating underlying issues such as repair of a varicocele in the male.
- The next step often involves stimulation of ovulation with drugs such as clomiphene citrate or metformin in women with PCOS.
- Assisted reproductive technology includes in vitro fertilization and intracytoplasmic sperm injection. Some couples choose donor insemination.

REFERENCE

Balen AH, Rutherford AJ. Management of infertility. *BMJ* 335:608–611, 2007. Explores the factors involved in infertility, such as women's age, guidelines for assessment of infertility, and the principles of treatment, including assisted reproductive technology.

Polycystic Ovarian Syndrome (PCOS)

Affects 5–7% of females of reproductive age. Characterized by oligo- or amenorrhea, evidence of hyperandrogenism (e.g., hirsutism, acne, male-pattern hair loss), and a polycystic appearance to the ovaries on ultrasound. May also be associated with insulin resistance, fertility problems due to anovulation, and metabolic syndrome.

In PCOS, the ovaries have a characteristic "string of pearls" appearance due to multiple follicles lined up in the ovary. There is usually no dominant follicle, and ovulation does not occur.

DIFFERENTIAL

Includes other hormonal imbalances, such as Cushing's syndrome, hyperprolactinemia, and thyroid abnormalities.

WORKUP

- Obtain prolactin and TSH levels to rule out other causes of the characteristic signs and symptoms.
- Measure testosterone and DHEAS levels, both of which may be elevated (if excessively elevated, consider an androgen-secreting tumor).
- Transvaginal/pelvic ultrasound to visualize the ovaries.
- A fasting blood glucose or glucose tolerance test is often performed to screen for insulin resistance.

TREATMENT

- Weight loss in obese patients; treatment of insulin resistance; OCPs to normalize menstrual cycles and inhibit androgens.
- Women with PCOS who experience infertility may respond to weight loss, metformin, clomiphene citrate, and/or gonadotropin therapy.

REFERENCE

Norman RJ et al. Polycystic ovary syndrome. *Lancet* 370(9588):685–697, 2007. A review article detailing the endocrine disruptions, health complications, and management of PCOS.

Common Vaginal Infections (Vaginitis)

The normal vaginal flora consists of approximately 25 bacterial species. The vaginal environment is normally acidic (pH 3.3–4.2) 2° to colonizing lactobacillus-producing lactic acid. This acidic environment inhibits the growth of

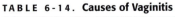

pathologic organisms. A less acidic environment can lead to bacterial proliferation and result in possible clinical infection. Table 6-14 outlines common etiologies of vaginitis.

SIGNS AND SYMPTOMS

- Vulvovaginal itch with or without a burning sensation.
- An abnormal odor.
- ↑ vaginal discharge.
- In examining the patient, always check the quantity, odor, and color of vaginal discharge.

DIFFERENTIAL

The differential diagnosis for ↑ vaginal discharge includes STDs and UTIs.

WORKUP

- **Wet prep:** Slide smears with saline and KOH.
- **Labs:**
  - Obtain a Gram stain of the vaginal discharge and a gonorrhea and chlamydia antigen test to rule out STDs.
  - UA of a clean-catch urine specimen to rule out UTIs.

TREATMENT

Treatments for the specific types of vaginitis are discussed in Table 6-14.

TABLE 6-14. Causes of Vaginitis

	BACTERIAL VAGINOSIS (USUALLY *GARDNERELLA*)	*TRICHOMONAS*	YEAST (USUALLY *CANDIDA*)
Relative frequency (%)	50	25	25
Discharge	Homogenous, grayish-white, watery; **fishy and stale odor.**	Profuse, malodorous, grayish, frothy; **"strawberry spots"** on cervix and vaginal wall.	Thick, white, **cottage-cheese** texture.
Vaginal pH	> 4.5	> 4.5	Normal
Saline smear[a]	**Clue cells** (epithelial cells coated with bacteria).	Motile trichomonads.	Pseudohyphae; budding yeast.
KOH smear	Fishy odor.	Nothing.	Pseudohyphae; budding yeast.
Treatment	Metronidazole.[b]	Metronidazole 2 g PO. Treat the partner, as this is considered an STD.	Miconazole (Monistat) or nystatin.

[a] If you see lots of WBCs and no organism on saline smear, suspect chlamydia.

[b] Patients taking metronidazole should not drink alcohol, as this can result in an Antabuse-like effect.

Sexually Transmitted Diseases (STDs)

Taken together, STDs are one of the most common gynecologic problems encountered in the outpatient setting. All sexually active patients must thus be examined with an awareness of a possible STD. Patients often have a past history of STDs, which can be elicited through careful and tactful history taking.

GENITAL HERPES

Herpes simplex is the **most common** STD and is highly infectious (75% rate). Etiologies are HSV type 2 (90%) and type 1 (10%).

SIGNS AND SYMPTOMS

- **1° infection:** Characterized by malaise, low-grade fever, and adenopathy.
  - **Prodromal phase:** Presents with mild paresthesia and burning.
  - Painful vesicular lesions arise 3–7 days after exposure.
- **Physical findings:** Physical exam reveals multiple clear vesicles that may have lysed, progressing to painful ulcers with red borders that coalesce and become secondarily infected. Lesions can be found on the vulva, vagina, cervix, perineum, and perianal area.

WORKUP

- Obtain a thorough sexual history and look for the physical findings outlined above.
- Tzanck smear of lesions and viral cultures.

TREATMENT

- **Expectant management:** Keep lesions clean and dry.
- **Acyclovir:** If diagnosed early in the outbreak, oral administration of acyclovir may ↓ the duration of symptoms. Prophylactic acyclovir may also be used for decreasing the frequency and severity of recurrence; IV acyclovir can be used for hospitalized cases or severe outbreaks, particularly in pregnancy or HIV infection.

CHLAMYDIA

Chlamydia is the **second most common** STD and is 10 times more common than gonorrhea. It can manifest as cervicitis, PID, or lymphogranuloma venereum (rare) and often coexists with gonorrhea. *Chlamydia trachomatis*, the etiologic agent, is an obligate intracellular parasite.

SIGNS AND SYMPTOMS

- Mild cases may be asymptomatic. More severe cases present with dysuria, an abnormal vaginal discharge, ectopic pregnancy, or infertility.
- Physical findings are subtle and nonspecific. A mucopurulent cervical discharge is often a clue, but many patients may not have any symptoms or discharge. Findings may be masked by coexisting gonorrheal infection.

WORKUP

- Monoclonal antibody test (faster).
- Enzyme immunoassay of the cervical secretion (has 95% specificity).
- Always check for **concomitant gonorrheal infection** (cultures, smear).

Some 20–50% of patients with an STD have coexisting infections, creating a low threshold for detecting other infectious diseases. All contacts of the patient must be treated.

What do you expect to see on Tzanck smear in patients with genital herpes? Multinucleated giant cells.

Gonorrhea and chlamydia travel together. When gram-⊖ diplococci are seen, add doxycycline to cover for chlamydia.

Lymphogranuloma venereum is an STD caused by Chlamydia that is usually seen outside of the United States. It is characterized by painless ulcers and large draining lymph nodes.

A one-time dose of azithromycin will cover both chlamydia and gonorrhea but may cause GI upset.

Roughly 15% of women infected with gonorrhea will progress to PID if untreated.

Which serotypes of HPV are highly associated with cervical cancer? Serotypes 16, 18, and 31.

TREATMENT

Azithromycin, tetracycline, or doxycycline (erythromycin may be substituted in allergic or pregnant patients). Treatment is associated with a 95% cure rate.

COMPLICATIONS

Insidious tubal damage leading to infertility.

GONORRHEA

Gonorrhea remains a very common infection. An ↑ frequency has also been observed with penicillin-resistant strains in asymptomatic infections. *Neisseria gonorrhoeae*, the etiologic agent, is a gram-⊖ intracellular diplococcus.

SIGNS AND SYMPTOMS

- Presents with a malodorous, purulent, yellow-green discharge from the cervix, vagina, Skene's ducts, urethra, or anus.
- Some 10–20% of affected heterosexual women also have gonorrhea infection in the pharynx.

WORKUP

- Gram stain of discharge.
- Cultures from the discharge on Thayer-Martin medium (80–95% sensitivity).
- Enzyme immunoassay for gonorrhea antigen.

TREATMENT

Maintain a low threshold for treating patients for gonorrhea; it is valid to treat on clinical grounds alone. The choice of antibiotics depends on the site of infection.

- For urethral, cervical, or rectal infection, use ceftriaxone, ciprofloxacin, or ampicillin.
- For pharyngeal infection, give ceftriaxone, ciprofloxacin, aqueous penicillin with probenecid, or tetracycline.

CONDYLOMATA ACUMINATA (VENEREAL WARTS)

Condylomata acuminata are almost as common as gonorrhea infection. Unlike other STDs, however, the sequelae may take years to manifest. The etiologic agent is HPV. Condylomata acuminata are commonly associated with serotypes 6 and 11; cervical neoplasia is associated with serotypes 16, 18, and 31.

SIGNS AND SYMPTOMS

- Presents with painless bumps, discharge, and pruritus.
- Physical findings include soft, fleshy, exophytic, papular, verrucous, flat, or macular growths on the cervix, vagina, vulva, urethral meatus, perineum, or perianal area. Lesions are often symmetrical.
- Coinfection with *Trichomonas* or *Gardnerella* is common.

The presumptive diagnosis is made with physical findings. The diagnosis can be confirmed with a biopsy of warts following 5% acetic acid staining.

TREATMENT

- **External and vaginal lesions:** Condylox, cryotherapy, CO_2 laser, or trichloro-acetic acid.
- **Cervical lesions:** Colposcopy and potential biopsy of the cervix; cryotherapy, laser, or loop electrosurgical excision procedure (LEEP).
- Lesions are often more resistant to therapy in pregnant, diabetic, and immunosuppressed patients.

Venereal warts and cervical dysplasia are associated with different serotypes of HPV.

SYPHILIS

The incidence of syphilis has been rising over the past few years owing to penicillin-resistant gonorrhea strains. *Treponema pallidum*, a motile spirochete, is the etiologic agent.

Pap smear of the cervix diagnoses only about 5% of patients infected with HPV.

SIGNS AND SYMPTOMS

Presentation depends on disease stage:

- **1° (10–60 days after infection):** Presents with a **painless ulcer** (chancre) of the vulva, vagina, cervix, anus, rectum, pharynx, lips, or fingers. The chancre heals spontaneously in 3–9 weeks.
- **2° (4–8 weeks after the appearance of the chancre):**
  - Low-grade fever, headache, malaise, generalized lymphadenopathy.
  - A diffuse, symmetric, asymptomatic maculopapular rash on the soles and palms.
  - Condyloma latum, which heals spontaneously in 2–6 weeks.
- **3° (1–20 years after the initial infection):** Destructive, granulomatous **gummas** can be seen that cause systemic damage to the CNS, heart, or great vessels. Complicated by aortitis, meningovascular disease, and tabes dorsalis.

What is a pathognomonic finding for 3° syphilis? The Argyll Robertson pupil, which refers to pupils that accommodate but do not react.

WORKUP

- **Screening test:** VDRL or RPR (rapid but nonspecific).
- **FTA-ABS/MHA-TP:** Very specific; perform if RPR is ⊕.
- Dark-field microscopy (motile spirochetes) of 1° or 2° lesions.

TREATMENT

- **Penicillin** is the treatment of choice for 1°, 2°, and 3° syphilis.
- Tetracycline or penicillin desensitization for allergic patients. In light of the risk of congenital syphilis, patients must be treated with penicillin during pregnancy.
- Transplacental spread can occur at any stage of syphilis and can lead to congenital syphilis.

What could cause a false RPR? Pregnancy, lupus, and antiphospholipid antibodies.

Pelvic Inflammatory Disease (PID)

Upper genital tract infection that usually results from an ascending infection from the cervix. The lifetime risk is 1–3%. Causative organisms include *Neisseria gonorrhoeae* (one-third of cases), *Chlamydia trachomatis*, and anaerobes/aerobes (e.g., *E. coli*, *Bacteroides*). Risk factors include multiple sexual partners, unprotected intercourse, new partners within 30 days of becoming symp-

The insertion of IUDs carry an ↑ risk of PID. They are indicated in monogamous women at low risk for STDs.

tomatic, cigarette smoking, and recent placement of an IUD or surgical instrumentation.

SIGNS AND SYMPTOMS

- Presents with a one- to three-day history of lower abdominal pain with or without fever; a vaginal discharge, recent menses, a history of sexual exposure, and a past history of PID may also be seen.
- Other findings include the following:
    - Lower abdominal tenderness.
    - CMT.
    - An adnexal mass and/or tenderness.

DIFFERENTIAL

Ectopic pregnancy, endometriosis, ovarian torsion, hemorrhagic ovarian cyst, appendicitis, diverticulitis, UTI.

What is a chandelier sign? Severe CMT on exam that makes the patient "jump for the chandelier."

WORKUP

- **Diagnostic criteria** are as follows:
    - A history of abdominal pain and findings of abdominal tenderness with or without rebound (90%).
    - CMT.
    - Adnexal tenderness (should be bilateral).
- **Additional criteria,** one of which is required to establish the diagnosis, are as follows:
    - A temperature > 38°C.
    - A WBC count > 10,000.
    - An inflammatory mass (tubo-ovarian abscess) on exam/sonography.
    - Culdocentesis that yields peritoneal fluid with bacteria and WBCs.
    - The presence of N. gonorrhoeae and/or C. trachomatis on the endocervix.
- **Labs:**
    - CBC (WBC > 10,000), ESR (> 15 mm/hr), β-hCG.
    - Gram stain of cervical discharge.
    - RPR/VDRL (to rule out syphilis); HIV and hepatitis screen.
- **Imaging:**
    - Ultrasound to detect an inflammatory mass.
    - Laparoscopy for the definitive diagnosis of edema and erythema of the fallopian tubes and purulent exudate. Note that laparoscopy has been shown to confirm the clinical diagnosis in approximately 60% of cases.

What is Fitz-Hugh–Curtis syndrome? Perihepatitis from ascending infection, generally from gonorrhea or chlamydia. It results in RUQ pain and LFT elevations.

TREATMENT

- **Outpatient treatment:** Oral cefoxitin or ceftriaxone and doxycycline.
- **Inpatient treatment:** IV cefotetan and doxycycline (orally or IV).
- Admit patients for IV antibiotics in the presence of the following:
    - A temperature > 38°C.
    - Suspected pelvic or tubo-ovarian abscess.
    - Nausea and vomiting that would prevent compliance with the administration of oral medications.
    - Signs of peritonitis.
    - Pregnancy.
    - A possible surgical emergency such as appendicitis.
    - Lack of clinical response to an oral regimen.
- **Surgery:** Warranted if the diagnosis is uncertain or if the patient has a tubo-ovarian abscess that is unresponsive to parenteral antibiotics.

COMPLICATIONS

- ↑ (tenfold) risk of an ectopic pregnancy.
- ↑ (fourfold) risk of chronic pelvic pain.
- Infertility (15% after a single episode and 75% after three episodes).
- Recurrent PID.
- Fitz-Hugh–Curtis syndrome (found in 15–30% of PID cases).

Urinary Incontinence

Affects almost half of women at least occasionally. Many women will not volunteer that this is an issue unless the subject is broached specifically by their care provider. As women age, they experience greater degrees of pelvic relaxation and a greater incidence of urinary incontinence, especially daily incontinence. Table 6-15 summarizes the main types of urinary incontinence as well as their risk factors, diagnosis, and treatment.

Ask your patients about urinary incontinence. Much of the time, they will not volunteer this information.

All patients complaining about urinary incontinence should have a UA and urine culture.

TABLE 6-15. Types of Urinary Incontinence

	STRESS	URGE	OVERFLOW	TOTAL
Symptoms	Urine loss with coughing, laughing, or straining.	Dribbling/leaking regardless of whether bladder is full. Sense of not being able to reach the bathroom in time.	Urinary retention, poor stream, straining to void.	Continuous urine leakage.
Risk factors	Menopause, pelvic relaxation, chronically ↑ intra-abdominal pressure (e.g., cough, ascites).	Neurologic disease (e.g., Alzheimer's, diabetes, Parkinson's). Most cases are idiopathic. UTIs. Bladder foreign bodies or irritants.	Epidural anesthesia (95% of cases). Neurologic disease (e.g., MS, spinal cord injury).	Pelvic surgery, pelvic radiation, PID.
Diagnostic tests	Standing stress test, cotton swab test, urethroscopy. Cystometrogram (distinguishes stress from urge incontinence). Normal residual volume.	Cystometrogram; normal/↓ residual volume.	Uroflowmetry; ↑ residual volume.	Localize the fistula with indigo carmine, methylene blue, or cystourethroscopy.
Treatment	Kegel exercises, estrogen replacement, α-agonists, pessaries, surgery to restore hypermobile bladder neck to anatomic position.	Anticholinergics, β-adrenergic agonists, smooth muscle relaxants, TCAs, Kegel exercises, behavior modification.	α-adrenergic agonists, striated muscle relaxants, cholinergic agents, self-catheterization, surgical removal of obstruction if present.	Surgery to repair fistula.

267

The most common cancers in
women are as follows:

1. Breast

2. Lung

3. Colorectal

4. Uterine

Annual Pap smears should
begin approximately three
years after the initiation of
sexual intercourse but no later
than 21 years of age.

Some 5% of ovarian tumors
are Krukenberg tumors, which
are tumors usually of GI origin
that are metastatic to the
ovary.

Gynecologic Oncology

Table 6-16 summarizes the essentials of the three important gynecologic cancers.

COMMON CLERKSHIP TOPICS

In OB/GYN, you should be able to generate a differential diagnosis for common problems; perfect a systematic way of working up a patient; gain experience in performing a thorough pelvic examination with a Pap smear; and, it is hoped, find an appreciation of the process of birth. You can also learn about commonly used modalities such as ultrasonography, cervical biopsies, and fetal monitoring. The following list outlines common disease entities, conditions, and topics that you are likely to encounter during your OB/GYN rotation and on a shelf examination.

- **Obstetrics:**
  - Normal physiology of pregnancy
  - Prenatal care
  - Medical conditions in pregnancy
    - Gestational diabetes
    - Hypertension in pregnancy
  - Complications of pregnancy
    - First-trimester bleeding
    - Spontaneous abortion
    - Ectopic pregnancy (see Emergency Medicine)
    - Hydatidiform mole
    - Third-trimester bleeding
- **Labor and delivery**
  - Normal labor
  - Preterm labor
  - Abnormal labor patterns
  - Fetal heart rate monitoring
  - Postpartum hemorrhage
- **Gynecology:**
  - Abnormal uterine bleeding
  - Amenorrhea
  - Common vaginal infections (vaginitis)
  - Contraception
  - Endometriosis
  - Gynecologic oncology
  - Infertility
  - Menopause
  - Pelvic inflammatory disease
  - Premenstrual syndrome
  - Sexually transmitted diseases
    - Genital herpes
    - Chlamydia
    - Gonorrhea
    - Condylomata acuminata
    - Syphilis
    - Urinary incontinence

TABLE 6-16. Common Gynecologic Cancers

	CERVICAL CANCER	ENDOMETRIAL CANCER	OVARIAN CANCER
Symptoms	Postcoital bleeding; foul discharge. May be asymptomatic.	Postmenopausal uterine bleeding; palpable abdominal and pelvic masses.	↑ abdominal girth (ascites). Often asymptomatic until late stages. GI and GU complaints; thrombophlebitis; lower abdominal pain/pressure.
Risk factors	Anything that ↑ the risk of or indication of human papillomavirus (**HPV**) infection, including venereal warts, early sexual activity, multiple sexual partners, and smoking.	Chronic, unopposed estrogen stimulation (e.g., PCOS). Obesity, nulliparity, endometrial hyperplasia, DM, hypertension, early menarche, late menopause, anovulation, family history.	Nulliparity, breast cancer, family history. OCPs may have a protective role in ↓ the risk of ovarian cancer.
Screening	Pap smear (performed at least once a year for sexually active women).	None (Pap smear is only 50% effective in detecting uterine cancer).	None (routine ultrasound and CA-125 are not cost-efficient).
Diagnosis	Punch and/or cone biopsy.	Endometrial biopsy; D&C.	Ultrasound, abdominal CT, CA-125 for epithelial cancers; AFP and β-hCG for germ cell cancers.
Treatment	**Early stage:** Cervical conization, hysterectomy, radiotherapy, radical lymphadenectomy. **Advanced stage:** Irradiation/chemotherapy only (surgery would harm the bladder and rectum without being effective).	TAH-BSO, and peritoneal washing for cytology +/− pelvic and aortic node sampling. Radiotherapy, chemotherapy, progesterone.	TAH-BSO, omentectomy, and peritoneal washing for cytology with or without pelvic and aortic node sampling. Tumor debulking, chemotherapy.
Prevention	Safe sex (condoms) to ↓ the risk of HPV infection. Smoking cessation; routine Pap smears.	Progesterone to oppose estrogen; low-fat diet, weight control.	OCPs. Oophorectomy in patients with a strong family history of ovarian cancer.
Notes	Some 85% are squamous cell carcinoma and 15% adenocarcinoma. Unless nephrostomy tubes are placed, renal failure is the most common cause of death in patients with end-stage cervical cancer.	The **most common gynecologic cancer.** The fourth most common cancer in women (after breast, colorectal, lung). Most are adenocarcinoma. Endometrial hyperplasia is the precursor lesion and is treated with progesterone.	The **most lethal** gynecologic cancer. Complications of ovarian cancer include ovarian rupture, torsion, hemorrhage, infection, and infarction. The most common cause of death in end-stage ovarian cancer is bowel obstruction.

HIGH-YIELD FACTS

OBSTETRICS AND GYNECOLOGY

Pediatrics

Welcome to pediatrics! The pediatric rotation is a six- to eight-week block at most medical schools. This time is split between the inpatient ward and the outpatient setting. Traditionally, more time has been devoted to the inpatient service, but this may change with the current emphasis on outpatient primary care. The outpatient portion of the rotation may be completed in a community pediatrician's office or in the hospital's outpatient clinic or emergency department. In addition, usually a week or less is devoted to the newborn service.

Who Are the Players?

The ward team typically consists of an attending, 1–2 upper-level residents, 2–4 interns, and 1–4 medical students.

Attendings. The attending may be a member of the general pediatric faculty or a member of one of the pediatric subspecialties. The attending is ultimately responsible for patients and generally rounds on a daily basis. During attending rounds, you will have an opportunity to formally present patients to someone who will be responsible for a large portion of your evaluation. Also note that because some time is usually devoted to didactics, it is advisable that you become familiar with your attending's areas of interest, as he or she is likely to focus on those topics during rounds. It would also be helpful for medical students to clarify expectations with their attendings at the start of the rotation so that attendings and students alike will have clear goals for the rotation.

Residents. The role of residents is to supervise the interns and medical students. Residents are responsible for most of the day-to-day teaching you will get on the service, so ask them to give you informal lectures and to show you interesting findings on the ward. You should also demonstrate an interest in doing procedures. Note that residents are a good source of articles as well. Finally, remember that residents play a critical role in your clinical evaluations.

Interns. Interns are responsible for monitoring patients' daily progress and for doing the "grunt work." Needless to say, these people are busy—but you can help them by following patients with them and writing a daily progress note. Discuss each patient's assessment and plan (A&P) with your intern, and make sure you understand the rationale behind all the orders you have written and tests you have requested; by doing so, you will be more informed when you present to the residents and attending. Interns may also play an important role in your evaluations. If you are asked to consult a specialist, make sure you know the specific questions being asked of them by the team.

Nurses, social workers, child life specialist. As on other services, these specialists are invaluable sources of information about your patients.

How Is the Day Set Up?

The schedule of a typical day on the ward is as follows:

7:00–8:00 A.M.	Prerounds: get signout from the person who cared for your patient overnight; check with the nurses caring for your patient; check chart, labs, and vitals; examine the patient; speak with parents
8:00–9:00 A.M.	Team rounds
9:00–10:00 A.M.	Attending rounds
10:00 A.M.–12:00 noon	Write progress notes, order labs, etc.
Noon–1:00 P.M.	Lunch or lunch conference
1:00–5:00 P.M.	Check afternoon labs, sign out to the team members, etc.

What Do I Do During Prerounds?

In pediatrics, most numbers (I's and O's, medication dosages) are reported on a per-kilogram basis.

Prerounding in pediatrics is similar to prerounding in internal medicine, but with a few variations. In general, children should be examined during prerounds even if they are still sleeping. However, you should ask your resident if there are patients who should not be examined prior to rounds in the morning. You may also awaken a patient's parents to ask how their child is doing. Allow yourself some extra time, as there are often calculations that need to be done prior to rounds. Also note that most numbers are reported on a per-kilogram basis. For example, input (fluids and formula) is reported as cc/kg/day and kcal/kg/day, and urine output is reported as cc/kg/hr. Medication dosages are also reported on a per-kilogram basis. You may need to allow 20 minutes per patient at the beginning of this rotation until you become more efficient.

How Do I Excel in Pediatrics?

As you have realized or will soon realize, your grades during the clinical years are more subjective than they were during the preclinical period. Nevertheless, there are some basic rules you can follow to help improve your evaluations:

■ **Know your patient.** You've probably heard this advice at least a thousand times, but it nonetheless remains a constant. You have the time to investigate patients thoroughly so that your busy interns, residents, and attendings can turn to you for the detailed information they may not have obtained during their workups. Important but often not thoroughly investigated aspects of the admission history and physical (H&P) are diet, immunization history, developmental milestones, and social history.

■ **Communicate with your patient.** Although earning the trust of your pediatric patient and parents is no small task, it is a necessity in effectively caring for your patient. You must therefore take every step you can to ensure that patients know why they are there and what you are doing for them. So take your time when explaining concepts and procedures, and do so at a level that is appropriate to the patient's age and developmental level. Because this may mean using very concrete terms and humor, try practicing on yourself or on a fellow student—and remember to be very, very patient.

- **Communicate with parents.** This rotation is unique in that you will need to interact with concerned (and, unfortunately, sometimes unconcerned) parents who will be in the room with you. You will likely have the most time to speak with a child's family, so you may enjoy a closer relationship with them than anyone else on the team. It is thus critical that you maintain an open line of communication regarding a child's condition, prognosis, and planned procedures. No one knows the patient better than the primary caregiver, so listen carefully. At times, parents may ask you questions that lie beyond your medical knowledge. An incorrect answer could undermine their trust in you, so you should never give an answer if you are unsure of its validity. It is okay to say, "I do not know, but I will find out from the resident for you." In this way, you will help alleviate the family's worries while showing your genuine concern for the child. You will not lose face for not having all the answers; to the contrary, parents will trust and respect you for being honest and keeping them well informed.
- **Show genuine interest in patients.** Make sure any interest you show is genuine, as nothing is worse than insincerity. Remember how frightened you were of doctors as a child? Try to alleviate some of your patients' fears.
- **Read about the patients you admitted on a given day as soon as you get the chance.** The sooner you read about a patient's problem, the more likely it will be that you will remember the topic—and the more knowledgeable you will be when you present to your team. During your reading, you will discover questions that you should have asked, new labs to order, and so on. If you want to be a superstar, do a quick PubMed search and learn about a hot topic of ongoing research to discuss with the team on rounds the following morning. This will allow you to make valuable contributions to the workup and to ask intelligent questions.
- **Practice your presentation.** Typically, the only time your attending has the chance to see you at work is during rounds, so use this time to your advantage. Try not to stutter and mumble your presentations; instead, make sure they are organized, precise, accurate, and, whenever possible, done from memory. Also make sure that the A&P sections are well thought out; discuss them with the intern or resident beforehand. Handing out a review article about the topic may not hurt either.
- **Ask for feedback.** The attendings and residents will usually schedule a time for feedback halfway through the rotation. If they don't schedule such time, ask for it. Then, ask them to give you a detailed evaluation of your performance, emphasizing areas in which you can improve. Never accept the answer that you are "doing fine," as "fine" may mean average or better—who knows? Ask for feedback on your written work (H&P and progress notes) as well.
- **Act professionally and respect your colleagues.** Nothing looks worse than a scenario in which team members are criticizing one another, especially in front of a patient. This undermines a patient's trust and can also compromise care. So if you need to say something to a colleague, save it until you leave the patient's room, and then express your thoughts tactfully. It is crucial to maintain team morale so that you can work together as a cohesive unit. Derogatory remarks are never appropriate on the wards (or anywhere else, for that matter). They're also a surefire way for you to trash your own evaluation.

Key Notes

The H&P and daily progress notes for pediatrics are similar to those of medicine, but there are a few variations:

- **Source:** You may obtain the history from the parent, patient, other caregiver, or any combination of the above. In any case, however, it is important to include the source of your information as well as your judgment on the reliability of that source (e.g., reliable, vague). This will enable your reader to place the information in context.

- **History of present illness (HPI):** Key pediatric questions include recent eating history (changes in appetite, poor feeding), number of wet diapers per day (fewer than three may indicate dehydration in an infant), bowel movements, a change in energy or irritability, ill contacts, recent travel, and other environmental changes. Try to present the history chronologically.

- **Past medical history (PMH):** This should include maternal history (mother's age, gravida, para, abortions, pregnancy course); details of the pregnancy (onset of prenatal care, weight gain, complications such as diabetes or hypertension, blood type, Coombs' test, rubella immunity status, RPR/VDRL); group B strep, chlamydia, HIV, PPD, and HBV status; drug/alcohol/tobacco use; details on labor and delivery (spontaneous or induced, duration, complications, presentation, method of delivery, presence of meconium); neonatal history (birth weight, gestational age [GA], complications in the nursery, length of stay); and a history of other hospitalizations, surgeries, or injuries. Note that the pregnancy and neonatal history may not be relevant to all admissions (e.g., adolescents admitted for pneumonia).

- **Nutrition:** For infants, include information on breast milk or formula type, frequency, and amount; for toddlers, include the introduction of cereal and baby foods as well as milk intake. For older children, discuss appetite and type of food eaten.

- **Growth:** For infants, plot length, weight, and head circumference on the growth chart and assess for trends. For children > 2 years of age, plot height, weight, and body mass index (BMI) on the growth chart.

- **Immunization:** This is an often-overlooked section that should not be missed in pediatrics. Ask to see the immunization record. During the winter season, ask about influenza status.

- **Developmental history:** Ask the parents when the child first began to sit, walk, and talk and when he or she completed toilet training. For children < 6 years of age, the Denver Developmental Assessment is a useful tool with which to gauge a child's language acquisition, gross and fine motor development, and social interactions. For older children, be sure to ask about school performance.

- **Family history (FH):** Focus on inherited diseases, consanguinity (i.e., inbreeding), sudden infant death syndrome (SIDS), miscarriages, early deaths, congenital anomalies, developmental delay, mental retardation, sickle cell disease, asthma, seizure disorders, atopy, and cardiovascular diseases. It is also helpful to include a pedigree chart.

- **Social history (SH):** This is an important section in pediatrics and should include information about the home environment (who lives there, smoking in the home, and the like), the child's interaction with the family, the primary caregiver, and parental contact information. A psychosocial assessment should be tailored to the age of the child; the basic components for adolescent patients are outlined in the mnemonic **HEADDSS.**

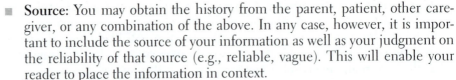

*Don't forget to plot **all** children on growth charts and assess trends! This may require obtaining information from the child's pediatrician.*

The psychosocial history—

HEADDSS

Home life
Education, **E**mployment
Activities (sports, school, friends)
Drugs (alcohol, tobacco, illicits)
Depression, suicide
Safety (seat belts, guns in the home, abuse)
Sexual activity

Tips for Examining Children

Infants from the age of six months on often have anxiety toward strangers. It is thus very common for a child to cry during the exam—but don't take it personally. Here are some more useful tips:

- Anxious children will search your eyes for good intentions. Kind eyes will get you far!
- Take off your white coat before entering the examination room (unless your attending prefers otherwise). Consider wearing a tie with cartoon characters on it, or perhaps wearing a sticker on your shirt. A stethoscope is much less threatening if you have a plush animal stethoscope cover. Observe the child's interactions with the parents, primary caregiver, and the like.
- For infants and toddlers, do as much of the exam as possible with the child in the parent's lap. If the patient is in respiratory distress (which may worsen with agitation, as would be the case with epiglottitis), the child should be left in the parent's arms.
- Distraction with a toy or even your name badge works well for young children (i.e., those < 2 years of age). Babies love mirrors, which can help you gauge how well they visually track objects. Giving older children a "task" to perform during your exam will also help ensure their cooperation.
- Let the child touch and play with the instruments. Demonstrate what you are about to do on yourself or on a parent to let the child know that the procedure is not painful. Save the invasive and painful parts of the exam for the end.
- It is best to perform the cardiac and pulmonary portion of the exam first, when the child is still quiet. Once you have accomplished this often-difficult task, move on to the other portions of the physical. Once you look in a child's mouth and ears, it is often the end of the line for the physical exam.
- With newborns, infants, and toddlers, observe, auscultate, and then palpate.
- Use age-appropriate terms.
- Smile and speak in a soft tone. Tell the child how well he or she is doing. Be funny whenever possible.

Take time to play with the young patient before attempting a physical exam.

Check the tympanic membranes last.

Variations in the physical exam are as follows:

- **Vital signs:** Information on temperature should include the method by which it was obtained: axillary, rectal, oral (only in children > 3 years of age), or tympanic. Rectal temperatures are the gold standard in pediatrics; axillary and tympanic temperatures, though often used, are inaccurate and unreliable. Oral temperatures are 1°F below rectal. Include weight (in kilograms and percentile range), height (in centimeters and percentile range), and head circumference (in centimeters and percentile range). Head circumference is routinely measured in children up to two years of age. Plot these values on graphs along with old values if available.
- **General appearance:** Be descriptive. Comment on alertness, playfulness, consolability, hydration status (tearing, drooling), respiratory status, development, social interactions, responsiveness (smiling, laughing), and nutritional status.
- **Skin:** Check for jaundice, acrocyanosis, mottling, birthmarks, cradle cap, rashes, and capillary refill.
- **Hair:** Note lanugo and Tanner stage.
- **Head:** Note circumference, sutures, shape, and fontanelles.
- **Eyes:** Note red reflex in the newborn, strabismus (cover test in preschoolers and corneal light reflex in infants), and scleral icterus.
- **Ears:** Use the largest speculum you can. One option to facilitate examining the ear is to have the parent hold the child facing you. Ask the parent to cross his or her leg over both of the child's legs. Also ask the parent to wrap one arm around the child's arm and body and to use the other arm to

Report vital signs as ranges with a maximum value.

Key:

AFOSF = anterior fontanelle open, soft, and flat

A/P = assessment and plan

AXR = abdominal x-ray, also known as a KUB, or kidney, ureter, bladder

BMP = basic metabolic panel

BP = blood pressure

BS ⊕ = bowel sounds present

CBC = complete blood count

CC = chief complaint

C/C/E = clubbing/cyanosis/edema

CN = cranial nerve

CTAB = clear to auscultation bilaterally

c/w = consistent with

d/c = discharge

DOA = day of admission

DTRs = deep tendon reflexes

EOMI = extraocular movements intact

F/C = fever/chills

FM = fine motor

G1P1 = gravida 1, para 1

GM = gross motor

GU = genitourinary

HBV = hepatitis B vaccine

HC = head circumference

HEENT = head, eyes, ears, nose, and throat

h/o = history of

HR = heart rate

HSM = hepatosplenomegaly

ID = identification

IUTD = immunizations up to date

SAMPLE PEDIATRIC ADMIT NOTE

CC: "Throwing up."

ID: 7-week-old previously healthy Caucasian male presents with progressive emesis × 1 week.

Source: Parents, reliable.

Referring physician: Dr. Paul Smith, pediatrician, (310) 555-8798.

HPI: This is the first hospital admission for this 7-week-old Caucasian male, who was in his USGH until 1 week PTA, when parents describe onset of emesis after feedings. Emesis occurred 1–2 times/day, looked like formula, and was NBNB. In the 3 days PTA, emesis ↑ in frequency, occurring within 10 minutes of every feeding, and became projectile in nature. On the DOA the mother noted projectile emesis to 2–3 feet of a dark brown color and decided to bring him to the ER. Patient has no prior history of similar symptoms. He feeds avidly and appears hungry after vomiting. Patient had 4 wet diapers in the past 24 hours. Parents deny F/C, diarrhea or constipation, weight loss, irritability, rashes, cough, rhinorrhea, or other URI symptoms. No h/o recent travel or ill contacts. In the ER, patient was given a 20 cc NS bolus × 1 and was admitted to pediatrics for further evaluation.

PMH:

1. **Past illnesses:** None.
2. **Surgical history:** None.
3. **Medications:** None.
4. **Allergies:** NKDA.
5. **Immunizations:** IUTD. Received HBV at birth. Well-child visit next week for 2-month vaccines.
6. **Birth history:** 3000-g 38-week-GA term male born via C-section for failure to progress to a 25 y/o G1P1 Caucasian female at Mercy Hospital. Apgar scores of 7 at 1 min and 9 at 5 min. Home in 2 days without complications. Pregnancy had been uneventful. Mother denies infections, exposures, tobacco, medication, or drug use.
7. **Diet:** Initial breast-feeding × 4 weeks. Now Enfamil with iron q 4 h at 2–4 oz per feed.
8. **Developmental history:** Has met developmental milestones. GM: Raises head and chest when prone. FM: Follows objects to midline. Language: Alerts to sound, social smile. Social: Recognizes parents.

FH: Father with pyloric stenosis at age 8 weeks. No other family history of congenital illness, developmental delay, or GI disease.

SH: Pt lives with his mother and father in an apartment. There are no siblings (patient is first-born). Parents are college educated. Father works as an accountant, and mother works part time as a lawyer. Paternal grandmother baby-sits. No smoking, pets, or firearms in the home.

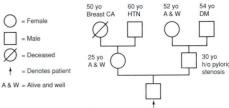

ROS: Unremarkable except as above.

PE: VS: T 98.4°F (rectal), HR 144, RR 48, BP 95/60 (right arm).

Growth: Wt 4.8 kg (50%), length 57 cm (50%), HC 38.7 cm (50–75%).

General: WD/WN 7-week-old male resting quietly in NAD.

Skin: Dry, warm, pink with good turgor. No jaundice, ecchymoses, or rashes.

HEENT:

    Head: NC/AT, AFOSF 1 × 1 cm, head shape symmetric.

    Eyes: PERRL, EOMI, RR intact bilaterally, anicteric, conjunctivae clear and moist.

    Ears: TMs nonerythematous, mobile; normal landmarks bilaterally.

    Nose: Patent nares, no nasal flaring or d/c.

    Mouth: Palate intact, no thrush, MMM, O/P clear without erythema or exudates.

    Neck: No LAD, no thyromegaly.

Chest: No respiratory distress, symmetric excursion, CTAB, no W/R/R.

Cardiac: RRR, nl S1S2, no M/R/G, femoral pulses 2+ bilaterally.

Abdomen: Soft, NTND, occasional peristaltic waves visible, BS ⊕, no masses or palpable "olive," no HSM.

GU: Nl circumcised male, both testes descended without masses or tenderness, no hernias present.

Back: No dimples or tufts.

Extremities: Brisk cap refill < 2 seconds, no C/C/E. No Barlow's/Ortolani's sign or hip clicks, skin folds symmetric.

Neuro: MS: Alert and active. CNs: Pupillary light reflex/face/palate symmetric, tongue midline. Motor: MAE, normal tone and bulk, strong suck; no sensory abnormalities noted. Reflexes: Moro present and symmetric, DTRs 2 bilaterally, palmar and plantar grasp intact, both toes upgoing.

Labs: CBC and BMP pending.

Studies: AXR: Nonspecific bowel gas pattern. No masses seen.

Abdominal US: Hypoechoic mass > 1.5 cm, c/w pyloric stenosis.

A/P: 7-week-old previously healthy Caucasian male with 1-week h/o progressive projectile emesis with confirmed pyloric stenosis on US.

1. **Emesis:** The clinical picture of progressive, projectile, nonbilious emesis in a first-born term male is consistent with the diagnosis of pyloric stenosis, which was confirmed on US. Patient does not appear dehydrated. However, prior to surgical intervention must r/o electrolyte abnormalities such as hypokalemic hypochloremic metabolic alkalosis 2° to persistent vomiting.
   - Check BMP results for electrolyte abnormalities.
   - Surgery consult to evaluate for pyloromyotomy.
   - NPO until surgery.
   - IV fluids at 1 × maintenance for hydration.

2. **Routine health maintenance:** Pt is up to date on his vaccinations.
   - Well-child visit for 2-month vaccines is scheduled.

hold the child's head. In an infant, pull the auricle backward and downward. In an older child, pull the external ear backward and upward to straighten the ear canal. Use an insufflator bulb to assess tympanic membrane mobility.

- **Nose:** Look for patent nares, nasal polyps, and nasal flaring (respiratory distress).
- **Mouth:** Note dentition, palate (cleft), and thrush. Use a gloved finger to evaluate the infant's palate and suck reflex.
- **Heart:** The average heart rate in a newborn is 140–160 bpm; in an older child, it is < 120 bpm. Always check for femoral pulses in infants to exclude coarctation. Innocent murmurs are found in up to 50% of normal children and are characterized by low intensity (I–II/VI), occurrence in systole, variation with position and respiration, and a musical quality.
- **Chest:** The average respiratory rate in a newborn is 40–60; in an older child it is 15–25. Expiration is more prolonged in infants than in adults; in young infants, respiratory movements are produced by abdominal movements. Look for any skin retraction between the rib or above the clavicles (a sign of respiratory distress).
- **Abdomen:** Deep palpation should be performed on every infant. Check the umbilicus (or stump), and check for hepatosplenomegaly and masses.
- **Back:** Check for scoliosis, tufts of hair, and deep sacral dimples.
- **Genitalia:** Circumcision, testes (descended bilaterally), hernias, labia (adhesions), hymenal opening, and Tanner stage should be noted.
- **Musculoskeletal:** Check for developmental hip dysplasia. With the infant supine, stabilize the pelvis with one hand, and then flex and adduct the opposite hip and apply gentle posterior pressure on the thigh. Feel for hip dislocation, which will usually relocate spontaneously upon release of pressure (Barlow maneuver). To reduce a dislocated hip, place one finger on the greater trochanter and one on the inner thigh, flex and abduct the hip, and lift the femoral head anteriorly, feeling for a clunk as it relocates into the acetabulum (Ortolani maneuver). Check range of motion, leg length, and symmetry of skin creases.
- **Neurologic:** Check tone, strength, neonatal reflexes (e.g., root, suck, grasp, Moro, stepping), Babinski, DTRs, and development.

The Nursery Rotation

Most students will spend a week or less on the nursery service, attending deliveries and working in the newborn nursery. As part of the nursery team, you will be paged to attend deliveries in which newborns may be at risk. The pediatric team is called for factors such as multiple gestations, preterm deliveries, cesarean sections, possible meconium aspiration, and known fetal anomalies. On arrival, the team obtains a brief history, sets up the infant warmer, and prepares resuscitation equipment such as O_2, suction, and intubation apparatus. The newborn is then shuttled from the obstetrician to the warmer, where the team goes to work. The baby is immediately dried off, the nose and mouth are suctioned, and the baby is rubbed and stimulated. The team provides ventilatory support, CPR, and/or advanced life support measures if necessary. Apgar scores are assessed at one and five minutes, and the baby receives an initial head-to-toe examination. If the baby appears vigorous and healthy, a brief delivery note is written, and the team's role may end there. If there are potential problems, the baby may be taken to the nursery for observation or admitted to the neonatal ICU (NICU).

The team will also take care of newborns in the nursery, write daily progress notes, and talk with new mothers. This portion of the pediatric rotation gives you a great opportunity to interact with neonatologists and newborns and to practice physical exams (before the onset of stranger anxiety). The nursery can have a fair amount of downtime, so this is a great time to get lectures or bedside teaching from your residents.

Key Procedures

The key procedures in pediatrics are lumbar puncture (LP), urine catheterization, IV line placement, and blood drawing. If the patient needs a painful procedure, parents are sometimes asked to leave the room, depending on the preference of the doctor. Drawing blood in newborns < 1 month of age is often accomplished with a heel or arterial stick. Ask a nurse or a resident to demonstrate the technique for you.

What Do I Carry in My Pockets?

The white coat is generally not used in pediatrics, so don't rely on those handy oversized pockets to store your peripheral brain and instruments of the trade.

- ❑ Toy for distraction
- ❑ Stethoscope
- ❑ Ophthalmoscope
- ❑ Otoscope with tips of different sizes and an insufflator bulb
- ❑ Penlight
- ❑ Tongue blades
- ❑ Calculator (to determine dosages for meds)
- ❑ Optional: stickers for a reward, cartoon Band-Aids

HIGH-YIELD CLINICAL TOPIC CHECKLIST

Read about these topics before you start the rotation. Most are discussed in this chapter. A full list of common clerkship topics can be found at the end of this chapter.

- ❑ Acute otitis media
- ❑ Asthma
- ❑ Bronchiolitis
- ❑ Congenital heart disease
- ❑ Fever management
- ❑ Immunizations
- ❑ Infant nutrition
- ❑ Lead poisoning
- ❑ Neonatal hyperbilirubinemia
- ❑ Sickle cell disease

WELL-CHILD CARE

Developmental Milestones

Pediatricians use a sequence of milestones to monitor children for normal developmental progress and to identify developmental delays. Assessments are typically divided into gross motor, fine motor, language, and social development. Table 7-1 summarizes the key developmental milestones. Obtain a copy of the Denver Developmental Screening Test II for more extensive guidelines. Table 7-2 describes classical neonatal reflexes. Most neonatal reflexes disappear by the sixth month of life. Infants with persistent primitive reflexes are at greater risk for developmental disability.

Failure to Thrive (FTT)

Refers to an inadequate growth rate in an infant or a child. Definitions include weight below the third percentile for age, weight < 80% of the ideal for age, or falling off the growth curve. Traditionally, FTT has been defined as either medical (**organic**) or psychosocial (**nonorganic**) in etiology, but the current teaching is that there is considerable overlap between the two. Nonorganic causes of FTT generally include neglect, abuse, or inadequate food intake (inadequate calories, improper formula preparation, or food refusal). Risk factors include low SES, low maternal age, maternal depression, caretaker neglect, chronic illness, genetic disease, and HIV infection. Although the differential is broad, the etiologies of organic FTT include the following:

- **GI dysfunction:** Pyloric stenosis, duodenal atresia, malabsorption, celiac disease.
- **Infection:** HIV, TB, intestinal parasites.

TABLE 7-1. **Key Developmental Milestones**

	TIME FRAME	MILESTONE
Gross motor	1 month	Lifts head when prone
	4 months	Rolls front to back
	5 months	Rolls back to front
	6 months	Sits upright
	12 months	Walks
Fine motor	Birth	Visually fixes
	1 month	Tracks to midline
	2 months	Tracks past midline
	6 months	Transfers objects
	12 months	Two-finger pincer grasp
Language	1 month	Alerts to sound
	3 months	Coos
	4 months	Orients to voice
	6 months	Babbles
	9 months	Mama, dada—nonspecific
	12 months	Mama, dada—specific
	15 months	Uses 4–6 words
Social	2 months	Social smile
	4 months	Laughs
	6 months	Stranger anxiety
	12 months	Imitates actions; comes when called
	18 months	May start toilet training

TABLE 7-2. Selected Neonatal Reflexes

REFLEX	TIMING	DESCRIPTION
Moro startle	Present at birth; disappears by 3–6 months.	Head extension leads to extension, adduction, and then abduction of the upper extremities.
Palmar grasp		Infants grasp a finger placed in the palm.
Rooting		Infants pursue an object placed around the mouth.
Stepping	Present at birth; disappears by 2–4 months.	Infants move their legs in a walking movement when they are held upright and leaning forward.
Asymmetric tonic neck	Present at birth; disappears by 4–9 months.	Turning the head while supine leads to ipsilateral extremity extension and contralateral flexion (fencer position).
Parachute		Infants extend the ipsilateral arm to support the body when tilted to one side while sitting.
Galant	Present at birth; disappears by 6–9 months.	Stroking the paravertebral region while the infant is prone causes the pelvis to move toward the stimulated side.
Babinski		Stroking the lateral plantar surface causes fanning and upgoing motion of toes.

- **Chronic disease:** CF, bronchopulmonary dysplasia, CHD.
- **Reduced growth potential:** Congenital syndromes, skeletal dysplasias.

SIGNS AND SYMPTOMS

- Weight below the third percentile for age.
- Weight < 80% of the ideal for age.
- Falling off the growth curve by crossing down two major percentile lines on a growth chart.
- Other signs and symptoms specific to the cause of FTT may include GI complaints, odd eating behavior, or lethargy.

Nonorganic causes of FTT are more common in developed countries.

283

WORKUP

- Observe caregiver-child interaction for potential underlying psychosocial issues.
- If labs are necessary, standard screening tests include a CBC, electrolytes, creatinine, albumin, protein, UA, and urine culture.
- With GI symptoms, order stool guaiac, culture, and O&P.
- Other tests include a sweat chloride test (for CF) and assessment of bone age. Tests for malabsorption (stool pH and reducing substances) may also be appropriate.

TREATMENT

- Varies according to etiology.
- Keeping a food diary that includes calorie count may be helpful.
- Encourage nutritional supplementation if breast-feeding is inadequate.
- Hospitalize for feeding, calorie counts, and observation if there is evidence of neglect or severe malnourishment or if no growth results from dietary modification.

REFERENCE

Schwartz ID. Failure to thrive: An old nemesis in the new millennium. *Pediatr Rev* 21:257–264, 2000. A well-organized discussion of a complicated topic.

Growth Parameters

At each pediatric visit, the weight, height, and head circumference of the patient are plotted on growth charts specific for gender and age. Over time, the clinician uses these growth charts to recognize potential growth abnormalities. Some helpful rules of thumb are summarized in Table 7-3.

How does FTT manifest on growth charts? Children fall off the weight curve first, then the height curve, and then the head circumference curve.

It is crucial to ask caretakers detailed information about formula preparation (i.e., powder, concentrate, or ready-to-feed formula, and how they are preparing the formulas).

As a general rule of thumb, babies triple in weight and double in length during the first year.

TABLE 7-3.   Growth Pearls

VARIABLE	GUIDELINES
Weight	**Average birth weight (BW):** 3.5 kg (7.7 lbs). ■ Some 5–10% of BW may be lost over the first few days. Formula-fed babies return to BW by the second week of life, whereas breast-fed babies should return to BW by the thrid week of life. ■ BW should double by 4–5 months, triple by one year, and quadruple by two years. **Average weight gain:** 30 g/day for 3–4 months; 10–20 g/day for 4–12 months; 5 lbs/year from age two to puberty.
Height	**Average birth length:** 50 cm (20 inches). **Average height:** 30 inches at one year; 3 feet at three years; 40 inches at four years (two times birth length); three times birth length at 13 years. **Average growth:** 2–3 inches per year from age four to puberty.
Head circumference	**Average birth head circumference:** 35 cm. **Average head circumference ↑:** 1 cm/month for one year. Some 90% of head growth occurs by age two.

REFERENCES

- American Academy of Pediatrics. Identifying infants and young children with developmental disorders in the medical home: An algorithm for developmental surveillance and screening. *Pediatrics* 118(1): 405–420, 2006. Updated guidelines from the AAP that provide an algorithm for developmental surveillance and, if warranted, developmental screening tests and well-child visits from birth to age three.
- Hagan J et al. *Bright Futures: Guidelines for Health Supervision of Infants, Children, and Adolescents,* 3rd ed. Arlington, VA: National Center for Education in Maternal and Child Health, 2007. A great resource for information on well-child care with updated guidelines from 2007. Bright Futures has a helpful Web site at www.brightfutures.org that offers a host of useful resources for health care providers and patients alike.
- National Center for Health Statistics. *2000 CDC Growth Charts: United States.* Available online at www.cdc.gov/growthcharts/. This site contains CDC growth charts for different age groups and both genders.

Immunizations

Tables 7-4 and 7-5 summarize recommended childhood immunization schedules. Listed below are contraindications and precautions related to vaccination.

CONTRAINDICATIONS

Contraindications to vaccination are as follows:

- Current moderate to severe acute illness.
- Severe allergy to a vaccine component or to a prior dose of vaccine.
- Anaphylactic reaction to eggs (influenza vaccine), gelatin (MMR), neomycin (MMR, IPV), polymyxin B (IPV), or streptomycin (IPV). Perform prior skin testing.
- Encephalopathy within seven days of prior pertussis vaccination (use DT instead of DTaP).
- Pregnancy, immune compromise, or use of high-dose steroids (oral polio, MMR, varicella).
- Recent administration of antibody-containing blood products (live injected vaccines).

PRECAUTIONS

Prior reactions to pertussis vaccine—e.g., fever > 40.5°C (> 105°F), shocklike state, persistent crying for > 3 hours within 48 hours of vaccination, or seizure within three days of vaccination.

REFERENCES

- American Academy of Pediatrics, Committee on Practice and Ambulatory Medicine. Recommendations for preventive pediatric health care. *Pediatrics* 120(6):1376, 2007. An updated guideline of all the necessary preventive health measures for children.
- Centers for Disease Control and Prevention. *2007 Immunization Schedules.* Available online at www.cdc.gov/vaccines/recs/schedules/. As of 2007, immunization schedules have been divided into childhood schedules (birth through 6 years), adolescent (7–18 years), and catch-up (for those children whose immunizations have been delayed by > 1 month).

*Prematurity, malnutrition, current antibiotic therapy, and the presence of mild acute illness and/or low-grade fever are **not** contraindications to immunization.*

Who might need a meningitis vaccine from a pediatrician? A high school senior about to enter a college dormitory, as well as children with sickle cell disease or functional asplenia.

TABLE 7-4. 2007 CDC Immunization Schedule (0–6 years)

VACCINE[a]	BIRTH	2 MONTHS	4 MONTHS	6 MONTHS	12–15 MONTHS	15–18 MONTHS	2 YEARS	4–6 YEARS
HBV	x	x		x				
DTaP		x	x	x		x		x
Hib		x	x	x	x			
IPV		x	x	x				x
Influenza[b]			x	x	x	x	x	x
PCV[c]		x	x	x	x			
MMR					x			x
Varicella					x			x
HAV[d]					x		x	
Meningococcal[e]							x	

[a] HBV = hepatitis B vaccine; DTaP = diphtheria, tetanus, acellular pertussis; Hib = *Haemophilus influenzae* type b; IPV = inactivated polio vaccine; PCV = pneumococcal conjugate vaccine; MMR = measles, mumps, rubella; HAV = hepatitis A vaccine.

[b] Influenza vaccine is recommended yearly for all children 6–59 months of age. The minimum age is six months for trivalent inactivated influenza vaccine and five years for the live attenuated influenza vaccine. Children who are < 9 years of age who are receiving influenza vaccine for the first time should receive two doses, separated by > 4 weeks for inactivated and > 6 weeks for live attenuated vaccine.

[c] PCV is recommended for all children 2–23 months of age; it is also recommended for certain high-risk groups > 24 months of age, but fewer doses are needed in older children.

[d] HAV is recommended for all children one year of age. The two doses in the series should be administered at least six months apart.

[e] Meningococcal vaccine is recommended for children 2–10 years of age with terminal complement deficiencies or anatomic/functional asplenia (e.g., sickle cell) as well as for certain other high-risk groups. Use of meningococcal conjugate vaccine (MCV4) is also an accepted alternative.

Infant Nutrition

BREAST MILK

- The American Academy of Pediatrics recommends exclusive breast-feeding for the first six months of life and continuation of breast-feeding through 12 months of age for optimal infant nutrition. After six months of age, breast-fed infants may require fluoride and iron supplementation, as maternal stores of iron are often depleted by that time.
- It is important for health care professionals to encourage breast-feeding to new mothers, preferably prior to delivery, as well as to provide support if they experience frustration with breast-feeding. Lactation consultants, who are available at many birthing centers and hospitals, can serve as excellent educational and support resources for new mothers.
- Advantages to breast-feeding include the following:
  - **Infant benefits:** Faster mother-infant bonding; ↓ risk of eczema and cow's-milk protein allergy; ↓ risk of serious infections due to the presence of maternal IgA antibodies.

TABLE 7-5. 2007 CDC Immunization Schedule (7–18 years)

Vaccine[a]	7–10 Years	11–12 Years	13–14 Years	15 Years	16–18 Years
DTaP		x			
HPV[b]		x			
MCV4[c]		x	x	x	x
PPV[d]		x	x	x	
Influenza	x	x	x	x	x
HAV[e]					x

[a] HPV = human papillomavirus; PPV = pneumococcal polysaccharide vaccine.

[b] Administer the first dose of the HPV vaccine series to females at 11–12 years of age. Administer the second dose two months after the first dose and the third dose six months after the first dose.

[c] Administer meningococcal conjugate vaccine at 11–12 years of age as well as to previously unvaccinated adolescents at high school entry (approximately 15 years of age). Also administer to previously unvaccinated college freshmen living in dormitories.

[d] PPV is recommended for certain high-risk groups.

[e] HAV is recommended for certain other groups of children, including those in areas where vaccination programs target older children.

- ■ **Maternal benefits**: ↓ risk of breast and ovarian cancer and earlier returns to prepregnancy weight.
- ■ **Economic benefits**: ↓ cost in comparison to formula and convenience (correct temperature, no preparation, no risk of mixing errors).
- ■ Health professionals almost universally agree that human breast milk provides the most complete form of nutrition for infants. However, human breast milk is **not** recommended when:
  - ■ The mother has been infected with HIV or is taking antiretroviral medications.
  - ■ The mother has active, untreated TB.
  - ■ The mother is infected with human T-cell lymphotrophic virus (HTLV) type I or II.
  - ■ The mother is using or is dependent on an illicit drug.
  - ■ The mother is taking chemotherapeutic drugs or is undergoing radiation therapy.

"Breast is best": For the vast majority of infants, breast-feeding is preferred over commercially available infant formulas.

REFERENCE

American Academy of Pediatrics. Policy statement on breastfeeding: Breast-feeding and the use of human milk. *Pediatrics* 115(2):496–506, 2005. This paper reviews the latest science on breast-feeding.

FORMULAS

If a mother chooses to use formula, many different types are available to her. However, formulas with iron are recommended. Formulas may be based in

All breast-fed infants should receive vitamin D supplementation (200 IU) to prevent rickets.

cow's milk or soy. Recently, formula manufacturers have added long-chain polyunsaturated fatty acids, which have been implicated in the promotion of growth, neurodevelopment, and visual acuity. Table 7-6 discusses recommended foods for the first year of life. Remember the following when guiding parents on infant nutrition:

- In the first two months of life, babies will eat 2–3 ounces (or approximately 10–20 minutes per breast) every 2–3 hours.
- New foods should be introduced after six months of age at a rate of one per week to allow for the identification of potential allergies.
- Avoid honey in children < 1 year of age in light of the risk of infant botulism.
- Avoid foods that may lead to choking, including nuts, raisins, and hot dogs.
- Currently, recommendations are to avoid cow's milk until 1 year of age; eggs until 2 years of age; and peanuts, tree nuts, and fish until 3 years of age. However, prevention of food allergies is a dynamic area of research, and these guidelines may change in the future.

Tanner Staging

Puberty follows a predictable sequence in all adolescents, but with variations in timing and the rate of change. The Tanner staging system is outlined in Table 7-7. Normal progression is as follows:

Menarche: Onset of menses.
Pubarche: Pubic hair development.
Thelarche: Breast development.

- **Males:** Testicular enlargement → penile enlargement → growth spurt → pubic hair.
- **Females:** Thelarche → growth spurt → pubic hair → menarche.
- **Precocious puberty** is defined in boys as 2° sexual characteristics presenting before nine years of age. These definitions have recently changed for girls in light of recent evidence that black girls mature earlier than do white girls. For girls, precocious puberty is now defined as the development of 2° sexual characteristics before age six for black females and before age seven for white females.

TABLE 7-6. Infant Nutrition

AGE	RECOMMENDED FOODS
Birth	Breast milk or formula with iron.
4–6 months	Iron-fortified single-grain cereal; supplemental water.
6–7 months	Strained fruit; consider fluoride supplementation (depends on local water supply).
7–8 months	Strained vegetables.
8–9 months	Well-chopped meats.
9–10 months	Cheese, egg yolk, protein-rich foods.
10–12 months	Soft finger foods: cookies, fruits, vegetables, meats.
12 months	Soft table foods; may start whole cow's milk.

TABLE 7-7. Tanner Stages

STAGE	MALE GENITALIA	FEMALE BREASTS	PUBIC HAIR
I	Childhood-size penis, testes, scrotum.	Preadolescent—elevation of papilla only.	None.
II	Enlargement of testes, scrotum.	Breast buds—elevation of breast and papilla.	Sparse, straight; downy hair on labia/penile base.
III	Enlargement of the penis, mainly in length.	Enlargement of the breast and areola, single contour.	Darker, coarse, curled hair.
IV	Continued penile enlargement, especially in breadth. Scrotal skin darkens; rugations are present.	Projection of the areola and papilla; separate contour (the 2° mound).	Adult-type hair limited to the genital area.
V	Adult size and shape.	Mature breast.	Adult quantity and pattern; spreads to thighs.

REFERENCE

Sun SS et al. National estimates of the timing of sexual maturation and racial differences among U.S. children. *Pediatrics* 110:911–919, 2002. This study demonstrated that blacks enter puberty earlier than do whites and Hispanics. It also provides gender- and race-specific reference norms.

CARDIOLOGY

Congenital Heart Disease (CHD)

CHD is present in approximately 0.8% of U.S. children and is generally divided into acyanotic disease ("pink babies") and cyanotic disease ("blue babies"). Cardiac defects with right-to-left shunts are categorized as cyanotic and those with left-to-right shunts as acyanotic. Workup includes CXR, ECG, an echocardiogram, and, in some cases, angiography. Further distinctions are as follows:

- **Acyanotic congenital heart conditions:**
  - Include PDA, ASDs, VSDs, and coarctation of the aorta.
  - Many septal lesions close spontaneously, but persistent or large lesions may require surgical intervention.
  - Lesions are often asymptomatic in early childhood, but as fetal circulation transitions into adult circulation over the first several weeks of life, left-to-right shunting ↑ and symptoms of CHF develop, usually between one and three months.
  - Large ASD or VSD lesions may lead to Eisenmenger's syndrome, in which a left-to-right shunt causes pulmonary hypertension and shunt reversal.

True central (gonadotropin-dependent) precocious puberty is much more common in females and is usually idiopathic. Despite this, order a CT or MRI to rule out CNS pathology as a potentially treatable cause.

Left-to-right shunts–

The 3 D's

AS**D**
VS**D**
P**DA**

- Cyanotic congenital heart conditions:
  - Include tetralogy of Fallot, transposition of the great vessels, truncus arteriosus, tricuspid atresia, hypoplastic left heart syndrome, and total anomalous pulmonary venous return (in which the pulmonary veins drain into the right heart).
  - Cyanotic lesions typically present in the first week of life because they have been dependent on the ductus arteriosus, which typically closes within the first week of life.
  - Nonoxygenated blood bypasses the lungs into the systemic circulation, and infants may present with cyanosis, respiratory distress, or shock either at birth or in the first weeks to months of life.
  - Transposition of the great vessels requires immediate surgical repair to sustain life.
  - Tetralogy of Fallot varies in presentation depending on the severity of the pulmonic stenosis component.
  - In many of these conditions, PGE_1 is used to maintain a PDA for collateral flow.
  - The definitive treatment in all cases is surgical repair.

REFERENCES

- Rosenthal A. How to distinguish between innocent and pathological murmurs in childhood. *Pediatr Clin North Am* 31:1229–1240, 1984. A highly useful, concise discussion of the features of childhood murmurs. An "oldie but goodie."
- Saenz RB et al. Caring for infants with congenital heart disease and their families. *Am Fam Physician* 59:1857–1868, 1999. A basic overview of CHD along with a discussion of medical and psychosocial treatment issues.
- www.pted.org. An interactive Web site of child and adult congenital heart disease, with helpful diagrams of each structural defect.

DERMATOLOGY

Diaper Rash

Diaper rash can be caused by irritant dermatitis from prolonged skin contact with urine and feces. 2° fungal infection of the skin with *Candida albicans* is common; 80% of diaper rashes lasting > 4 days are colonized with *Candida*.

SIGNS AND SYMPTOMS

- **Irritant dermatitis:** Ill-defined erythematous patches or plaques, often with scaling. Usually spare the inguinal folds.
- **Candidal infection:** Well-demarcated, beefy-red erythematous patches surrounded by satellite erythematous papules or pustules. Can be found within the inguinal folds.

WORKUP

- For **candidal infection,** the diagnosis is generally made by clinical appearance and distribution of lesions.
- To confirm the diagnosis, scrape a satellite lesion, stain with 10% KOH, and observe pseudohyphae under the microscope.

TREATMENT

- The diaper area should be kept clean and dry.
- Use barrier cream in moist areas.
- Treat candidal infections with topical antifungal agents (nystatin is first-line treatment for infants, but clotrimazole is an alternative for older children).
- Severe candidal infections can be treated with a low-potency topical steroid (e.g., 1% hydrocortisone cream) in conjunction with topical antifungal agents.

REFERENCE

Kazaks EL, Lane AT. Diaper dermatitis. *Pediatr Clin North Am* 47:909–919, 2000. A top-to-bottom review of a common outpatient topic.

Viral Exanthems

There are many causes of rash in children. The clinical history is often the key tool used to make the diagnosis. Common rashes caused by viruses are discussed in Table 7-8. Note that treatment consists mainly of supportive measures (e.g., fluids, treatment of discomfort from fever with acetaminophen) along with isolation while patients are contagious.

REFERENCES

- Crocetti M et al. Fever phobia revisited: Have parental misconceptions about fever changed in 20 years? *Pediatrics* 107(6): 1241–1246, 2001. A discussion of the important myth that pediatricians do not aim to treat fevers, but rather the discomfort associated with them.
- Gable EK et al. Pediatric exanthems. *Prim Care* 27:353–369, 2000. A good discussion of 12 major causes of viral exanthems in children.
- http://dermatlas.med.jhmi.edu/derm/. A thorough compilation of images that is constantly being updated by a widely respected pediatric dermatologist. It features many advanced search features that can facilitate the diagnosis of enigmatic rashes.
- Nguyen HQ et al. Decline in mortality due to varicella after implementations of varicella vaccination in the United States. *NEJM* 352(5):450–458, 2005.

*Avoid aspirin when treating fever in the setting of a viral infection, as it is associated with **Reye's syndrome,** a rare mitochondrial disorder characterized by acute and severe encephalopathy along with degenerative liver disease.*

GASTROENTEROLOGY

Intussusception

Occurs when one portion of the bowel telescopes into an adjacent portion, usually proximal to the ileocecal valve (see Figure 7-1). Intussusception is the most common cause of bowel obstruction in the first two years of life and affects males more often than females. Risk factors include polyps, Meckel's diverticulum, adenovirus or rotavirus infection, Henoch-Schönlein purpura, intestinal lymphoma, celiac disease, and CF.

SIGNS AND SYMPTOMS

- Presents with sudden onset of violent episodes of colicky abdominal pain interspersed with relatively normal periods.

TABLE 7-8. Viral Exanthems

DISEASE	CHARACTERISTICS
Rubeola (measles)	**Agent:** Paramyxovirus. **Prodrome:** Cough, Coryza, Conjunctivitis **(the 3 C's)** for 2–3 days. **Koplik's spots:** White-gray spots on the buccal mucosa; resolve before appearance of the rash. **Rash:** An erythematous maculopapular rash that begins on the head and spreads to the body; fades in the same pattern. **Fever:** High fever is present. **Complications:** Otitis media (common), encephalitis, pneumonia, subacute sclerosing panencephalitis (rare).
Rubella (German or three-day measles)	**Agent:** RNA/togavirus. **Prodrome:** Malaise followed by posterior cervical and suboccipital lymphadenopathy (often so mild that it may be missed or forgotten). Adolescents may develop transient polyarthralgias. **Rash:** A maculopapular rash that begins on the face and then generalizes, resolving in 3–5 days. **Fever:** On the first day of rash only. **Viral exanthem:** Petechiae on the palate (Forschheimer spots). **Complications:** Devastating results if a fetus is infected during gestation. Rarely, encephalitis and thrombocytopenia.
Roseola infantum (exanthem subitum)	**Agent:** HHV-6 and HHV-7. **Fever:** Abrupt onset of high temperature (> 40°C [> 104°F]) for 3–5 days; the child does not feel ill. **Rash:** As the fever drops, a maculopapular rash appears on the trunk, spreads peripherally, and resolves in 24 hours. **Complications:** Rapid temperature ↑ associated with febrile seizures.
Varicella (chickenpox)	**Agent:** VZV. **Transmission:** Highly contagious via respiratory droplets and contact with lesions until crusted over. **Prodrome:** Fever and malaise for one day. **Rash:** Pruritic teardrop vesicles on an erythematous base that start on the face and trunk and spread peripherally. Lesions break and crust over in one week. The classic finding consists of "crops" of lesions in different stages of healing. **Complications:** 2° skin infection is most common, but in immunocompromised children or neonates, fatal disseminated disease may occur (meningoencephalitis, hepatitis, pneumonitis). **Zoster (shingles):** Reactivation of varicella infection with painful skin lesions in a dermatomal distribution.
Erythema infectiosum (fifth disease)	**Agent:** Parvovirus B19. **Transmission:** Epidemics occur in the spring; contagious via respiratory secretions. **Prodrome:** Often absent; mild flulike illness for 7–10 days. **Rash:** "Slapped cheek" rash and circumoral pallor; then an erythematous, maculopapular rash spreads to the trunk and legs in a lacy, reticular pattern. Usually lasts 2–3 weeks. **Fever:** Low-grade or no fever. **Complications:** Aplastic crisis (sickle cell disease and other anemias), fetal anemia/hydrops fetalis (in utero infection), arthritis, encephalopathy.
Hand, foot, and mouth disease	**Agent:** Coxsackie A virus. **Transmission:** Contagious by direct contact. **Prodrome:** Fever, anorexia, and oral pain. **Rash:** "Football-shaped" vesicles with surrounding erythema on the hands and feet and oral ulcerations; resolves in one week. **Fever:** Present.

- The classic triad of intermittent colicky abdominal pain, vomiting, and bloody mucous stools is found in only one-third of patients; however, most will have at least one of these signs.
- Red "currant jelly" stools (rare), lethargy, and fever are more ominous signs.
- A "sausage-shaped" abdominal mass is felt on palpation.
- Abdominal tenderness; stool occult blood.

DIFFERENTIAL

Constipation, GI infection, Meckel's diverticulum, lymphoma (in children > 6 years of age), meconium ileus (neonates).

WORKUP/TREATMENT

- Assess and correct any volume or electrolyte abnormalities.
- AXRs may reveal a mass, an obstruction, or visible intussusception. Ultrasound can be used to establish the diagnosis in equivocal cases.
- Air-contrast or barium enema confirms the diagnosis and is also curative in 75% of cases. Peritoneal signs are an absolute contraindication to this procedure.
- If enema reduction is unsuccessful or the child has peritoneal signs, proceed to surgical reduction and resection of gangrenous bowel if present.

REFERENCES

- Harrington L et al. Ultrasonographic and clinical predictors of intussusception. *J Pediatr* 132:836–839, 1998. A concise discussion of how to diagnose intussusception.
- McCollough M, Sharieff GQ. Abdominal pain in children. *Pediatr Clin North Am* 53:107–137, 2006. An excellent overview of common causes of abdominal pain in children.

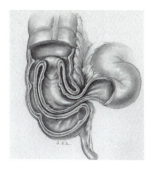

FIGURE 7-1. Intussusception.

(Reproduced, with permission, from Way LW, Doherty GM. *Current Surgical Diagnosis & Treatment*, 11th ed. New York: McGraw-Hill, 2003: 1323.)

Pyloric Stenosis

A gastric outlet obstruction caused by hypertrophy of the pyloric sphincter. It is more common in first-born males, exhibiting a male-to-female ratio of 4:1. The incidence is approximately 1 in 500 births.

Pyloric stenosis is more often seen in first-born males.

SIGNS AND SYMPTOMS

- The classic sign is projectile nonbilious emesis after feedings that gradually ↑ in intensity and frequency in the first 2–8 weeks of life.
- Infants appear hungry and initially feed well but later suffer from malnourishment and dehydration. They may reach a plateau in their growth curves or even lose weight.
- An olive-shaped mass may be palpable in the epigastric area.
- Gastric peristaltic waves may be visible.
- Hypochloremic hypokalemic metabolic alkalosis with dehydration is seen 2° to persistent emesis.

DIFFERENTIAL

Pylorospasm, overfeeding, gastroenteritis, hiatal hernia, duodenal atresia ("double bubble" sign on x-ray), esophageal stenosis, malrotation/volvulus, incarcerated hernias, meconium ileus, milk protein allergy, gastroesophageal reflux.

Which antibiotic is associated with pyloric stenosis?

Erythromycin.

WORKUP

■ Basic metabolic panel.
■ Ultrasound is highly sensitive and specific for hypertrophic pyloric stenosis.
■ AXR may show a dilated, air-filled stomach.

TREATMENT

■ NG tube placement; correction of dehydration and electrolyte abnormalities.
■ Surgical pyloromyotomy.

REFERENCE

Papadakis K et al. The changing presentation of pyloric stenosis. *Am J Emerg Med* 17:67–69, 1999. An interesting comparison of the presentations of pyloric stenosis over the past three decades.

GENETIC DISORDERS

Autosomal Trisomies (21, 18, 13)

There are many important chromosomal abnormalities in pediatrics. Table 7-9 outlines the three major autosomal trisomies with which you should be familiar.

TABLE 7-9. Autosomal Trisomies

DISORDER	CLINICAL FEATURES	FACTS AND PROGNOSIS
Trisomy 21 (Down syndrome)	Mental retardation, flat facial profile, Brushfield spots (speckled irises), transverse palmar crease (simian crease), flat nasal bridge with epicanthal folds, short stature. Cardiac defects (endocardial cushion/septal defects). ↑ incidence of ALL. Alzheimer's disease is seen in adulthood. Associated with GI anomalies (duodenal atresia, Hirschsprung's disease).	Incidence of 1 in 600 (↑ with advanced maternal age). Some 95% of cases are due to meiotic nondisjunction; 4% are due to a balanced translocation. Life expectancy is 30s–40s.
Trisomy 18 (Edwards' syndrome)	Severe mental/growth retardation, prominent occiput, rocker-bottom feet, low-set ears, horseshoe kidney.	Incidence of 1 in 3000; male-to-female ratio of 1:3. Some 90% die in the first year of life.
Trisomy 13 (Patau's syndrome)	Severe mental/growth retardation, scalp defects, microencephaly, polydactyly, agenesis of corpus callosum.	Incidence of 1 in 5000; 60% of those affected are female. Some 90% die in the first year of life.

REFERENCES

- American Academy of Pediatrics, Committee on Genetics. Health supervision for children with Down syndrome. *Pediatrics* 107:442–449, 2001. Health maintenance guidelines written for general pediatricians.
- Johns Hopkins University. *Online Mendelian Inheritance in Man (OMIM™)*. Available online at www.nslij-genetics.org/search_omim. html. A highly useful database that can help answer even the most obscure genetics questions that may arise during the pediatrics rotation.

HEMATOLOGY AND ONCOLOGY

Sickle Cell Disease

An autosomal-recessive disorder resulting from a mutation in the β-globin chain. Patients endure a chronic hemolytic anemia with intermittent acute events or "crises." These acute crises generally require hospital admission and include the following:

- **Vaso-occlusive crisis or "pain crisis"**: The most common cause of hospital admissions. Microvascular infarcts occurring in any tissue in the body lead to pain and organ dysfunction. Hand-foot syndrome (dactylitis), priapism, and avascular necrosis of the femoral head are forms of vaso-occlusive crisis. Pain crises typically occur in bones.
- **Acute chest syndrome**: The second leading cause of hospital admissions. Defined by the radiologic appearance of a new pulmonary infiltrate and fever; hypoxia may be present but is not required for diagnosis. The etiology is in many cases unknown, but infection and fat emboli (from bone marrow infarcts) are known causes.
- **Aplastic anemia**: Suppression of RBC precursors in bone marrow, often due to parvovirus B19 infection; leads to an acute and reversible reticulocytopenia. Most patients need transfusions for 1–2 weeks.
- **Hemolytic crisis**: An acute ↓ in hemoglobin resulting from exposure to oxidative stress, typically in patients with G6PD deficiency.
- **Acute splenic sequestration**: An acute ↓ in hemoglobin 2° to splenic pooling of RBCs with splenomegaly and hypovolemic shock. Typically occurs between six months and two years of age. Splenectomy should be considered if patients have had two or more events.
- **Serious infection**: By 2–4 years of age, sickle cell patients are also susceptible to life-threatening infections with encapsulated organisms (*Streptococcus pneumoniae, Haemophilus influenzae, Salmonella, Neisseria meningitidis*) due to functional asplenia.
- **Cerebrovascular disease**: Overt stroke (ischemic or thrombotic, involving large cerebral arteries) affects 11% of patients by age 20, and silent infarcts (involving sickling in microcirculation) are detected by neuroimaging studies in an additional 22%.
- **Other**: Pulmonary artery hypertension, renal papillary necrosis, hematuria, cholelithiasis (pigment stones), retinopathy. Heterozygotes with "sickle cell trait" generally have no manifestations of disease but may show painless hematuria or inability to concentrate urine.

SIGNS AND SYMPTOM

- A progressive hemolytic anemia develops after four months of age as fetal hemoglobin ↓. Patients may exhibit pallor, splenomegaly, jaundice, a systolic ejection murmur, and growth retardation. Dactylitis is common at initial presentation.

What is the most commonly isolated pathogen in osteomyelitis of a sickle cell patient? **Salmonella,** *followed by* S. aureus.

295

All sickle cell patients with fever need a workup for sepsis.

■ Any sickle cell patient with a temperature > 38°C must be evaluated for bacterial sepsis, septic joints, or osteomyelitis.
■ Sickle cell patients are frequently admitted for vaso-occlusive crises. Patients are at ↑ risk for acute decompensation when exposed to "triggers," which include hypoxia, changes in temperature, and dehydration.

WORKUP

■ Newborn screening at birth (mandated in 44 states and the District of Columbia).
■ Diagnose through the use of Sickledex preparations or by hemoglobin electrophoresis to determine the type and amount of hemoglobin present. Sickledex is inappropriate for use in newborns because large amounts of fetal hemoglobin can lead to a false-⊖ result.
■ During an acute crisis, appropriate tests may include blood culture and sensitivity, CBC, reticulocyte count, UA/urine culture and sensitivity, CXR, serum electrolytes, and type and cross.

TREATMENT

Sickle cell crisis pain can be severe and subjective, so don't be judgmental with pain medication.

■ **Pain crisis:** Treat with NSAIDs and/or opioids (morphine or hydromorphone, often using age-appropriate patient-controlled analgesia), hydration (1.5–2.0 times maintenance), and O_2 for hypoxia.
■ **Acute chest:** Broad-spectrum antibiotics (cephalosporin plus a macrolide), O_2, fluids, analgesics, incentive spirometry, and exchange transfusion in the presence of hypoxia or if hematocrit is < 18%.
■ **Stroke, priapism, and other complications:** Chronic exchange transfusions to keep HbS below 30%.
■ **Aplastic anemia, sequestration, hemolytic crisis:** Simple transfusion.

PREVENTION

The median life expectancy of sickle cell patients is 42 years for men and 48 years for women. The following are routine maintenance recommendations for patients with sickle cell disease:

■ Start prophylactic oral penicillin VK BID at diagnosis and continue until the child is at least five years of age.
■ Vaccinate against S. *pneumoniae*, H. *influenzae*, HBV, influenza, and N. *meningitidis*.
■ Give folic acid QD (this is somewhat controversial and is not a strict recommendation for children).
■ Screening should include **retinal exams** for sickle retinopathy (yearly starting at age eight), **hip radiographs** for avascular necrosis (yearly starting at age 10), and **echocardiography** for pulmonary artery pressures (every other year starting at age 10).
■ Hydroxyurea is used in children > 5 years of age with severe complications to ↑ the proportion of HbF and ↓ the incidence of vaso-occlusive events.
■ Bone marrow transplantation has been curative in some children.
■ Children with a history of stroke are placed on chronic exchange transfusion protocols to prevent future events.
■ Deferoxamine (Desferal) or the new oral iron chelator deferasirox (Exjade) is used with transfusion to prevent hemochromatosis.

REFERENCES

- Driscoll MC. Sickle cell disease. *Pediatr Rev* 28:259–268, 2007. An excellent overview of the pathogenesis, diagnosis, and management of sickle cell disease.
- Wethers DL. Sickle cell disease in childhood. *Am Fam Physician* 62:1013–1020, 1309–1314, 2000. A comprehensive, easy-to-read, two-part series on sickle cell disease.

Childhood Cancers

The most common childhood cancers are acute leukemias, CNS tumors (primarily posterior fossa or cerebellar tumors), and lymphomas. Other common pediatric tumors include Wilms' tumor, neuroblastoma, soft tissue sarcomas, and bone tumors. Although there are many important pediatric cancers, the key features of selected malignancies are discussed below.

The most common cancers in children:

1. Leukemia

2. CNS tumors

3. Lymphoma

4. Neuroblastoma

REFERENCE

Young G et al. Recognition of common childhood malignancies. *Am Fam Physician* 61:2144–2154, 2000. A primary care–oriented discussion of the most common childhood cancers.

ACUTE LYMPHOCYTIC LEUKEMIA (ALL)

ALL is the most common childhood cancer, exhibiting a peak onset at four years of age.

SIGNS AND SYMPTOMS

- Patients often present with lethargy, fever, bone pain, limp or refusal to bear weight, and CNS manifestations (including headache).
- Signs include petechiae, purpura and bleeding (from thrombocytopenia), pallor (from anemia), lymphadenopathy, hepatosplenomegaly, and testicular swelling.

DIFFERENTIAL

Aplastic anemia, immune thrombocytopenic purpura, rheumatic diseases (SLE, JIA), other malignancies, mononucleosis or other viral infections.

WORKUP

- Peripheral smear reveals large immature lymphoblasts, most of which express the common ALL antigen (CALLA).
- Bone marrow biopsy is critical to diagnosis, as the morphology of peripheral blasts may not reflect the true bone marrow morphology.
- Obtain a baseline CMP along with calcium, magnesium, and phosphorus levels to define baseline values prior to chemotherapy (to monitor for tumor lysis syndrome).
- LDH and uric acid levels are often ↑.
- Flow cytometry identifies the predominant cell type.
- Obtain a CXR, an LP, and a CT to screen for metastases.

TREATMENT

- **Chemotherapy** involves induction, consolidation, and maintenance phases of treatment. The total length of therapy is approximately two years for girls and three years for boys.

What are typical WBC counts in children with ALL? Although ALL is a lymphocyte-proliferative disorder, WBC counts can be low, normal, or high.

HIGH-YIELD FACTS

PEDIATRICS

- **Induction:** Commonly prednisone, vincristine, and L-asparaginase.
- **Consolidation:** Intrathecal methotrexate with or without cranial irradiation.
- **Maintenance:** 6-MP, methotrexate, vincristine.
- **Tumor lysis syndrome:**
  - The induction phase of chemotherapy induces rapid killing of tumor cells, releasing cytosol directly into the blood. Cells contain high concentrations of potassium, phosphate, and DNA, and thus hyperkalemia, hyperphosphatemia, and ↑ uric acid (a purine degradation product) result in acute renal failure.
  - Treat tumor lysis with fluids, diuretics, allopurinol, alkalinization of urine, and reduction of phosphate.

WILMS' TUMOR (NEPHROBLASTOMA)

Wilms' tumor is a renal tumor of embryonal origin and is the most common renal tumor in children. It is usually seen between one and four years of age and is associated with a family history of Wilms' tumor, Beckwith-Wiedemann syndrome (hemihypertrophy, macroglossia, visceromegaly, and embryonal tumors), Denys-Drash syndrome (nephropathy and genital abnormalities), **WAGR** syndrome (**W**ilms' tumor, **A**niridia, **G**enitourinary abnormalities, and mental **R**etardation), and neurofibromatosis. A small number of tumors are bilateral.

Wilms' tumor is one of the successes of pediatric oncology, with an overall cure rate > 85%.

SIGNS AND SYMPTOMS

- Most patients (85%) are diagnosed after the incidental discovery of a painless abdominal mass either by the parents or by the primary care physician during routine physical examination.
- Patients may complain of nausea, emesis, bone pain, weight loss, dysuria, and polyuria.
- Common findings include fever, hematuria, hypertension (due to renin secretion by tumor cells or by compression of renal vasculature), and, in boys, varicocele (due to spermatic vein compression).

DIFFERENTIAL

Neuroblastoma, polycystic kidneys, hydronephrosis, and other abdominal neoplasms must be excluded.

WORKUP

- Abdominal ultrasound reveals a solid intrarenal mass and is also used to examine the renal vasculature and the contralateral kidney.
- CT reveals hematogenous metastases (present at diagnosis in 10–15% of patients).
- CBC, LFTs, BUN/creatinine, UA.
- Chest CT or CXR to screen for metastases.

TREATMENT

- Abdominal exploration with tumor excision and nephrectomy.
- Postsurgical chemotherapy with vincristine and dactinomycin.
- Chest CT to screen for metastases.

REFERENCE

Kalapurakal JA et al. Management of Wilms' tumour: Current practice and future goals. *The Lancet Oncology* 5:37–46, 2004. A concise review article of the diagnosis and management of Wilms' tumor.

NEUROBLASTOMA

A tumor of the neural crest cells that make up the adrenal medulla and sympathetic nervous system. It is the most common malignant tumor of infants and most often presents in children < 5 years of age. There are familial cases in addition to associations with neurofibromatosis, Hirschsprung's disease, Beckwith-Wiedemann syndrome, and fetal hydantoin syndrome.

SIGNS AND SYMPTOMS

- Abdominal distention, anorexia, weight loss, malaise, and muscular symptoms may be seen, depending on the location of the tumor.
- Presents with a firm, smooth, nontender abdominal or flank mass.
- Hypertension (from compression of renal vasculature), fever, pallor, and periorbital bruising ("raccoon eyes") are also seen.
- Metastases to the liver, bone, and lymph nodes can lead to hepatosplenomegaly, leg swelling, bone pain, or lymphadenopathy. A skin rash, watery diarrhea (from secretion of VIP), and opsoclonus/myoclonus ("dancing eyes/dancing feet") may also be present.

Neuroblastoma is the most common malignant tumor of infancy.

DIFFERENTIAL

Wilms' tumor, Ewing's sarcoma, rhabdomyosarcoma, lymphoma, hepatoblastoma.

WORKUP

- CT of the abdomen, chest, and pelvis; bone scan and bone marrow aspirate; LP.
- Obtain a 24-hour urine collection for catecholamines (VMA and HVA are ↑ in 95% of patients).
- CBC, LFTs, coagulation panel, BUN/creatinine.

TREATMENT

- At diagnosis, 50% of children have distant metastases.
- Treat via excision of localized tumors. For intermediate- to high-risk stages, combination chemotherapy and/or adjunctive radiation may be used.

REFERENCE

Alexander F. Neuroblastoma. *Urol Clin North Am* 27:383–392, 2000. An excellent review paper on neuroblastoma.

IMMUNOLOGY

Juvenile Idiopathic Arthritis (JIA)

Formerly known as juvenile rheumatoid arthritis, JIA is a collagen vascular disease that is defined by persistent inflammation in > 1 joint for > 6 weeks in a patient < 16 years of age. Onset most commonly occurs at 1–3 years of age;

Roughly 5–8% of children with systemic JIA develop **macrophage activation syndrome,** *a life-threatening condition characterized by sudden-onset fever, pancytopenia, hepatosplenomegaly, liver dysfunction, DIC, hypofibrinogenemia, hyperferritinemia, and hypertriglyceridemia.*

girls are affected more often than boys (as with most rheumatic diseases). JIA is divided into three subtypes on the basis of clinical symptomatology: pauciarticular, polyarticular, and systemic.

SIGNS AND SYMPTOMS

- **Pauciarticular:**
  - Affects four or fewer joints, usually large joints (knees, ankles).
  - The most common form of JIA; the prognosis is good (~70% of patients go into remission after several years).
  - Chronic asymptomatic uveitis (more likely in ANA-⊕ patients) can lead to blindness in young children if not diagnosed by slit-lamp examination. Acute-onset uveitis is more common in older children.
- **Polyarticular:**
  - Affects five or more joints, usually large (knees, ankles) and small joints (hands, feet), as well as the temporomandibular joint and cervical vertebrae.
  - The second most common form of JIA.
  - RF seropositivity is associated with older age of onset, ⊕ ANA, and more severe disease.
- **Systemic (Still's disease):**
  - Clinical features include high, spiking fevers to > 39.4°C; a "salmon-colored" rash that comes and goes with fever; and unremitting and severe arthritis.
  - The least common form of JIA; associated with the worst prognosis (complete resolution is rare, and ~50% develop destructive arthritis).
  - RF and ANA are ⊖.
  - Boys and girls are equally affected.
  - Other symptoms include myalgias, pericarditis, pleuritis, lymphadenopathy, hepatosplenomegaly, and growth retardation.
  - Labs may show anemia of chronic disease, an ↑ WBC count, and ↑ acute-phase reactants (ESR, CRP, platelets).
- **All types:** Symptoms may include morning stiffness, easy fatigability (particularly later in the day), joint pain, and swelling. Involved joints are often warm with limited range of motion but are rarely erythematous.

DIFFERENTIAL

Lyme disease, seronegative spondyloarthropathies (for the pauciarticular type), rheumatic fever, SLE, occult infection, sarcoidosis, juvenile dermatomyositis, malignancy (for the systemic type).

WORKUP

- CBC and ESR.
- RF/ANA serologies.
- Radiographs can show soft-tissue swelling, osteopenia, joint space narrowing, or bony erosions.
- MRI is more sensitive for early joint changes.
- Synovial fluid analysis reveals leukocytosis (5000–30,000 WBCs/mm³) and elevated protein.

TREATMENT

- Most cases respond to NSAIDs. Aspirin is contraindicated because of the risk of Reye's syndrome.

- Give methotrexate for severe disease.
- Anti-TNF therapy (etanercept or infliximab) is appropriate for refractory polyarticular disease.
- Intra-articular steroids are helpful for joint pain and swelling. Administer systemic steroids for severe systemic disease or severe uveitis. Steroid eye drops and dilating agents are administered for most cases of uveitis.
- Stretching and morning baths are helpful for morning stiffness.
- Calcium supplements and weight-bearing exercises to prevent osteoporosis; physical therapy may prevent disability.

REFERENCES

- Goldmuntz E, White P. Juvenile idiopathic arthritis: A review for the pediatrician. *Pediatr Rev* 27:e24–e32, 2006. A nice discussion of the new classification system.
- Ravelli A, Martini A. Juvenile idiopathic arthritis. *Lancet* 369:767–778, 2007. A recent review of the diagnosis and management of JIA.

INFECTIOUS DISEASE

Fever Management

The management of a young child with fever depends on the age group of the child. Children are divided into three age groups for this purpose: < 28 days, 28–90 days, and 3–36 months. During your weeks on the pediatric ward, you will be admitting many febrile children. Be thankful that new management guidelines have diminished the number of hospitalizations for fever. To further your understanding of these new guidelines, a few definitions follow.

- Fever is defined as a rectal temperature > 38°C (> 100.4°F).
- To diagnose fever without a source, the etiology of the fever must not be evident after a careful H&P. Acute otitis media is usually not considered a sufficient source.
- "Toxic appearing" describes a clinical picture that includes lethargy, signs of poor perfusion, marked hypoventilation or hyperventilation, or cyanosis.
- "Lethargy" describes an altered level of consciousness characterized by poor or absent eye contact or failure of the child to recognize the parents or to interact with the environment.
- Low-risk criteria include a previously healthy term infant who is non–toxic appearing, has no sign of focal bacterial infection (other than otitis media), has a reliable home environment and follow-up care, and has a ⊖ lab evaluation, including a WBC count of 5000–15,000/mm³, a total band count < 1500/mm³, a normal UA (⊖ dipstick or < 10 WBCs/hpf), a CSF WBC count of < 10/mm³, and, if diarrhea is present, < 5 WBCs/hpf in the stool.
- A full sepsis workup includes the following:
  - LP and CSF culture, Gram stain, cells, glucose, and protein, and possibly HSV PCR.
  - Urine culture and UA.
  - CBC with differential, blood culture, and BMP (electrolytes, glucose, BUN/creatinine).

All toxic-appearing children must be hospitalized for antibiotics and must receive a full workup for sepsis.

MANAGEMENT OF A FEBRILE INFANT < 28 DAYS OLD

All febrile infants < 28 days old should be hospitalized for a full sepsis workup. Treatment includes the following:

In neonates, group B streptococci (GBS), enteric gram-⊖ bacilli, and Listeria are the most common bugs.

- Ampicillin and gentamicin ("amp and gent") or ampicillin and cefotaxime while awaiting culture results. Antibiotics should be administered before the LP if any delay in the LP is anticipated.
- HSV infection should also be considered and should be investigated in the history. Acyclovir may be started empirically pending the results of HSV PCR from CSF.

MANAGEMENT OF A FEBRILE INFANT 28–90 DAYS OLD WITHOUT A SOURCE

Most infants at this age who appear toxic need to be hospitalized, given a full workup for sepsis, and started on IV antibiotics. For non-toxic-appearing low-risk infants, outpatient management is adequate. There are two options that can be used to approach this problem:

- **Option 1:** CBC/blood culture; UA/urine culture; LP/CSF culture; ceftriaxone 50–75 mg/kg IM; reevaluate in 24 hours.
- **Option 2:** No blood or CSF culture; UA/urine culture only; no antibiotics if evaluation is normal and the patient is low risk; reevaluate in 24 hours.

MANAGEMENT OF A FEBRILE CHILD 3–36 MONTHS OLD WITHOUT A SOURCE

The risk of bacteremia (mainly S. *pneumoniae*) in this age group is small (1–3%). Again, however, all infants who appear toxic need to be hospitalized, given a complete workup for sepsis, and started on IV antibiotics empirically until cultures return ⊖ at 48 hours. If the child does not appear toxic and the temperature is < 39°C, no diagnostic tests or antibiotics may be necessary. The parents should be instructed to give the child acetaminophen 15 mg/kg q 4 h and to return to the office if the fever persists for > 48 hours or if the clinical condition deteriorates. A non-toxic-appearing child with a temperature > 39°C may need the following:

- CBC with manual differential.
- For an absolute band count > 1500/mm^3, a neutrophil count > 10,000/mm^3, or a WBC count > 15,000/mm^3, a blood culture and empiric ceftriaxone 50 mg/kg IM.
- A catheterized urine culture for circumcised males < 6 months of age, uncircumcised males < 12 months, or females < 2 years of age.
- A stool culture if there is evidence of blood or mucus in the stool or > 5 WBCs/hpf.
- A CXR in children with dyspnea, tachypnea, crackles, O$_2$ saturation < 95%, or ↓ breath sounds.
- Acetaminophen 15 mg/kg q 4 h for discomfort associated with fever.
- Reevaluation in 24 hours.
- An LP if blood cultures are ⊕ and the child is still febrile on reevaluation.

REFERENCES

- Baraff LJ. Management of fever without source in infants and children. *Ann Emerg Med* 36:602–614, 2000. An update of the classic 1993 guidelines for management of fever without a source in children 0–36 months of age.
- Pickering LK. 2006 *Red Book: Report of the Committee on Infectious Diseases*, 25th ed. Elk Grove Village, IL: American Academy of Pediatrics, 2006. The classic resource for information on pediatric infectious disease. The full text of the book, along with a visual library of more than 2000 images, is available online at http://aapredbook.aappublications.org/current.shtml.

Meningitis

An inflammation of the leptomeninges. Viruses causing meningoencephalitis include enteroviruses, mumps, measles, HSV, VZV, arboviruses, EBV, rabies virus, and adenovirus. The most common bacterial pathogens vary with age group (see Table 7-10). The Hib vaccine has nearly eliminated *H. influenzae* type b meningitis in the United States.

SIGNS AND SYMPTOMS

- **Kernig's sign:** Flexion of the hip to 90 degrees with subsequent pain on extension of the leg.
- **Brudzinski's sign:** Involuntary flexion of the knees and hips following flexion of the neck while supine.
- **Age-specific signs and symptoms:** See Table 7-11.

DIFFERENTIAL

Encephalitis, brain abscess, epidural or subdural empyema, mastoiditis, tumors, cysts, trauma, vasculitis, intracranial hemorrhage, bacterial endocarditis with septic embolism, demyelinating disorders, drug intoxication or side effects.

WORKUP

- **CT:** If there are signs of ↑ ICP such as focal neurologic findings or papilledema, obtain a CT before the LP to prevent potential brain stem herniation.
- **LP:** Obtain a CSF cell count with differential, glucose, protein, Gram stain, and culture (see Table 7-12). HSV PCR may be appropriate in certain situations. An opening pressure > 180 mmHg may indicate bacterial meningitis.

*Having a hard time keeping Kernig's and Brudzinski's signs straight? Think "Knee" for **K**ernig's sign and "**Br**ain" for **Br**udzinski's sign.*

In meningococcal meningitis (N. meningitidis), a rapidly spreading petechial rash is typical and may precede other symptoms.

TABLE 7-10. Common Bacterial Causes and Empiric Treatment of Meningitis

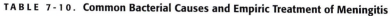

AGE	POTENTIAL BACTERIAL PATHOGENS	TREATMENT
Neonates (< 1 month)	Group B streptococcus (GBS), *E. coli, Listeria monocytogenes,* HSV.	Ampicillin (200 mg/kg) × 14–21 days for GBS and *Listeria.* Cefotaxime (100–150 mg/kg) for > 2 weeks after CSF sterilization for gram-⊖ organisms. Add acyclovir for suspected HSV.
Infants (1–3 months)	*S. pneumoniae, N. meningitidis,* GBS.	Cefotaxime (200 mg/kg) or ceftriaxone (100 mg/kg) and ampicillin (200 mg/kg) × 7–10 days for uncomplicated Hib or *N. meningitidis.* Cefotaxime (200 mg/kg) and vancomycin (40–60 mg/kg) × 10–14 days for *S. pneumoniae.*
Children (3 months – 18 years)	*N. meningitidis, S. pneumoniae, H. influenzae.*	Same as for infants.

TABLE 7-11. Age-Related Signs and Symptoms of Meningitis

AGE	SYMPTOMS	SIGNS
0–3 months	Paradoxical irritation (irritable when held and less irritable when not held), altered sleep pattern, respiratory distress, vomiting, poor feeding, diarrhea, seizures.	**Early:** Lethargy, irritability, temperature instability. **Late:** Bulging fontanelle, shock.
4–24 months	Altered sleep pattern, lethargy, seizures.	**Early:** Fever, irritability. **Late:** Nuchal rigidity (after 18 months), coma, shock.
> 24 months	Headache, stiff neck, lethargy, photophobia, myalgia, seizures.	**Early:** Fever, nuchal rigidity, irritability, papilledema, Kernig's sign, Brudzinski's sign. **Late:** Seizures, coma, shock.

- **Other labs/studies:**
  - CBC, electrolytes, glucose, blood culture.
  - The WBC count is usually ↑ in bacterial meningitis but is often unremarkable in aseptic meningitis.
  - EEG may be helpful in patients who present with seizures. Changes are usually nonspecific and are characterized by generalized slowing. Focal slowing in the temporal area is characteristic of HSV infections.

In aseptic meningitis, many patients feel better after the LP.

TREATMENT

The initial choice of antimicrobial is based on the most likely organisms involved given the patient's age group (see Table 7-10). Empiric antibiotics should be started immediately, even before the results of the LP and CSF analyses are known. Supportive care includes the following:

TABLE 7-12. CSF Findings in Meningitis

COMPONENT	NORMAL	BACTERIAL	HSV	OTHER VIRAL	TUBERCULOUS
Glucose (mg/dL)	40–80	< 30	> 30	> 30	20–40
Protein (mg/dL)	20–50	> 100	> 75	50–100	100–500
WBCs/µL	0–6	> 1000	10–1000	100–500	10–500
Neutrophils (%)	0	> 50	< 50	< 20	< 20
RBCs/µL	0–2	0–10	10–500	0–2	0–2

- Strict fluid balance in light of the risk of SIADH. Rehydrate with isotonic solution until the patient is euvolemic; then switch to two-thirds maintenance fluids.
- Frequent urine specific gravity assessment.
- Daily weights and daily measurement of head circumference in babies.
- Neurologic assessment; seizure precautions.
- Isolation may be necessary until the causative organism has been identified.

COMPLICATIONS

- **Acute:** Shock, seizures, subdural effusions (common with Hib infection), SIADH, subdural empyema, cerebral edema, ventriculitis, abscess.
- **Long term:** Deafness, epilepsy, learning disabilities, blindness, paresis, ataxia, hydrocephalus.
- Acute treatment with dexamethasone before or at the time of antibiotic administration may improve neurologic outcome in Hib meningitis but is not indicated in other causes of meningitis.

Pneumonia

Pneumonia is defined as inflammation of the lung parenchyma that may be infectious or noninfectious. It can be classified according to etiologic agent, patient age, host reaction, and anatomic distribution (e.g., lobar, interstitial, bronchopneumonia). Risk factors include anatomic malformations, immunodeficiencies, chronic lung disease 2° to prematurity, and exposure to cigarette smoke. The most common cause of pediatric pneumonia is viral infection (RSV, influenza, PIV, adenovirus); *S. pneumoniae* is the most common bacterial agent. In neonates, GBS and *Listeria* are potential agents. Infants 1–3 months of age may present with *Chlamydia trachomatis* pneumonia, while older children and teenagers are susceptible to *Mycoplasma* and *Chlamydia pneumoniae* infections.

Viruses are the leading cause of pneumonia in children.

SIGNS AND SYMPTOMS

Presents with tachypnea, tachycardia, cough, shortness of breath, malaise, fever, chest pain, and retractions. However, overall patterns of presentation may vary with the etiologic agent (see Table 7-13). Presenting symptoms also differ with age group:

The majority of large pleural effusions are caused by S. aureus pneumonia.

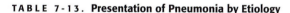

TABLE 7-13. Presentation of Pneumonia by Etiology

	SYMPTOMS	LUNG EXAM	CXR	WBC
Viral pneumonia	Cough, low-grade fever.	Diffuse crackles and wheezes.	Diffuse and streaky infiltrates.	Normal or ↑ with a lymphocyte predominance.
Bacterial pneumonia	High fever, cough, chills, dyspnea.	Focal crackles, ↓ breath sounds, dullness to percussion, egophony.	Lobar consolidation.	Leukocytosis with left shift.

- **Newborns:**
  - Usually show signs of respiratory distress, including tachypnea, cyanosis, nasal flaring, grunting, and retractions.
  - Sometimes exhibit signs of systemic infection, including poor perfusion, hypotension, acidosis, and leukopenia or leukocytosis, as well as nonspecific signs such as poor feeding, irritability, and lethargy.
  - Infants with *C. trachomatis* pneumonia are afebrile and may have conjunctivitis and a staccato cough.
- **Young children:**
  - Nonspecific complaints include abdominal pain, fever, malaise, GI symptoms, restlessness, apprehension, and chills.
  - Respiratory signs include tachypnea, cough, grunting, and nasal flaring. Children rarely expectorate, even with a productive cough.
- **Older children:**
  - Present with mild upper respiratory tract symptoms such as cough and rhinitis followed by abrupt fever, chills, tachypnea, chest pain, and productive cough.
  - Adolescents with *Mycoplasma* infections may present with prolonged cough in the absence of fever.

DIFFERENTIAL

Gastric aspiration, foreign body aspiration, atelectasis, congenital malformation, bronchopulmonary dysplasia, CHF, neoplasm, chronic interstitial lung disease, collagen vascular disease, pulmonary infarct.

What would aspiration pneumonia look like on CXR? Right middle or upper lobe infiltrates.

WORKUP

- Viral nasal wash or nasal swab for respiratory pathogens such as RSV, influenza, and parainfluenza.
- Obtain a CXR in ill-appearing infants and children, those who need hospitalization, and those who worsen clinically on antibiotics.
- The WBC count is often > 15,000/mL in bacterial pneumonia. A WBC count < 5000/mL in the newborn period may indicate sepsis.

TREATMENT

- Treatment should be based on age, clinical and CXR findings, immune status, and Gram stain of sputum, tracheobronchial secretions, or pleural fluid if available. See Table 7-14 for empiric antibiotic therapy by age group.
- Criteria for hospitalization include the following:
  - All children < 2 months of age.
  - Children > 2 months of age with respiratory distress, hypoxia, inability to take oral medications, failure to respond to oral antibiotics, immunosuppression, underlying cardiopulmonary disease, or evidence of empyema on CXR.
- Hospitalized children should be treated with IV antibiotics until afebrile and then given oral antibiotics to complete a total of 7–10 days of treatment.

REFERENCE

McIntosh K. Community-acquired pneumonia in children. *NEJM* 346: 429–437, 2002. An excellent review article on a common topic.

TABLE 7-14. Common Etiologies and Empiric Treatment of Pneumonia

AGE	ORGANISMS	EMPIRIC COVERAGE
Infants < 6 weeks	GBS, *C. trachomatis, S. aureus*, gram-⊖ enterics, RSV, CMV, HSV, enterovirus.	Ampicillin and gentamicin **or** ampicillin and cefotaxime. Add PO erythromycin for suspected *C. trachomatis.* Add IV acyclovir for suspected HSV.
6 weeks – 6 months	RSV, *S. pneumoniae*, Hib, group A streptococcus, *C. trachomatis* (until three months of age), *S. aureus.*	Supportive care for suspected viral pneumonia. **Mild to moderate illness:** PO amoxicillin or cefuroxime. **Severe illness:** IV cefuroxime or ceftriaxone.
6 months – school age	RSV (until two years of age), PIV, influenza virus, adenovirus, *S. pneumoniae.*	Supportive care for suspected viral pneumonia. **Mild to moderate illness:** PO amoxicillin, amoxicillin/clavulanic acid, or cefuroxime. **Severe illness:** IV cefuroxime or ceftriaxone.
School age	*M. pneumoniae, S. pneumoniae*, adenovirus.	**Mild to moderate illness:** PO azithromycin if *Mycoplasma* is suspected. **Severe illness:** IV cefuroxime or ceftriaxone with PO azithromycin. Vancomycin may be added after 24–48 hours if the child has not improved and there is suspicion of drug-resistant *S. pneumoniae.*

Acute Otitis Media

Acute otitis media (AOM) is a suppurative infection of the middle ear cavity. Children are more susceptible to infection owing to the angle of entry, short length, and ↓ tone of the eustachian tube. Up to 75% of children will have at least three episodes by the age of two. Bacteria such as *S. pneumoniae*, nontypeable *H. influenzae*, and *Moraxella catarrhalis* are responsible for roughly 80% of cases; viruses such as influenza A, RSV, and parainfluenza virus (PIV) account for approximately 20%. Conditions that predispose children to AOM include viral URIs, bottle feeding, pacifier use, passive exposure to tobacco smoke, day care, immunodeficiency, trisomy 21, hypothyroidism, and cleft palate. Breast-feeding ↓ the risk of AOM.

SIGNS AND SYMPTOMS

- Presents with ear pain, fever, crying, irritability, difficulty sleeping, difficulty feeding, vomiting, and diarrhea. Young children may tug on their ears. Often preceded by URI symptoms (cough, congestion, rhinorrhea).
- Otoscopic exam reveals abnormal color, opacification, ↓ mobility (tested with an insufflator bulb), or air-fluid levels in addition to signs of acute inflammation, including erythema and bulging of the affected tympanic membrane. Erythema alone is not sufficient for diagnosis, as it may result from vigorous crying.

What are the three most common bacterial pathogens that cause acute otitis media?
S. pneumoniae, *nontypeable* **H. influenzae,** *and* **M. catarrhalis.**

A diagnosis of acute otitis media requires:

1. *A history of acute onset of signs and symptoms.*
2. *The presence of middle ear effusions.*
3. *Signs and symptoms of middle ear inflammation.*

Don't rush to antibiotics when evaluating AOM; instead, consider your patient and whether an observational period of 2–3 days may be appropriate.

DIFFERENTIAL

Otitis media with effusion (fluid behind the tympanic membrane without evidence of inflammation), myringitis (inflammation of the eardrum with normal tympanic membrane mobility), otitis externa, mastoiditis, foreign body in the ear, ear trauma, a hard cerumen, mumps, toothache, pharyngitis, nasal congestion, temporomandibular joint dysfunction.

WORKUP

Diagnosed clinically according to the following three requirements:

- Acute onset of signs and symptoms.
- Middle ear effusions.
- Signs and symptoms of middle ear inflammation.

TREATMENT

- The treatment of AOM with antibiotics is controversial, as roughly 75% of all outpatient antibiotic prescriptions are for URIs, which many fear have led to the growing antibiotic resistance of respiratory pathogens.
- The American Academy of Pediatrics' clinical practice guidelines advocate an observational period of 48–72 hours with symptomatic treatment after 72 hours for children > 2 years of age with nonsevere illness, as well as for those six months to two years of age with an uncertain diagnosis (missing at least one of three requirements above) and mild symptoms.
- Given these caveats, recommended antibiotic usage is as follows:
  - Amoxicillin 80–90 mg/kg/day × 7–10 days is appropriate initial antibiotic therapy for most children.
  - High-dose amoxicillin/clavulanate (Augmentin) may be administered to cover for β-lactamase-⊕ pathogens and may also be given to patients who fail to improve on amoxicillin alone in 2–3 days or to those with severe illness. IM ceftriaxone is appropriate if patients fail to respond to amoxicillin/clavulanate.
- Children with > 3 infections in six months or four infections in one year should be considered for referral to an ENT specialist for tympanostomy tube placement or myringotomy.

COMPLICATIONS

Hearing loss with risk of language delay (for chronic otitis media with effusion), tympanic membrane perforation, scarring (tympanosclerosis), cholesteatoma (growth of desquamated stratified squamous epithelium in the inner ear), chronic otitis media, mastoiditis.

REFERENCES

- Rovers MM et al. Antibiotics for acute otitis media: A meta-analysis with individual patient data. *Lancet* 368:1429–1435, 2006. A meta-analysis that found antibiotic use to be beneficial in children < 2 years of age with bilateral AOM as well as in those with AOM and otorrhea. For most other children with milder disease, a observational period of 48 hours was found to be acceptable.
- Subcommittee on Management of Acute Otitis Media. American Academy of Pediatrics and American Academy of Family Physicians clinical practice guideline: Diagnosis and management of acute otitis media. *Pediatrics* 113:1451–1465, 2004. Detailed recommendations regarding the use of the observational "wait and see" approach for selected patients with AOM, along with guidelines on appropriate antibiotic usage.

Streptococcal Pharyngitis

Bacterial pharyngitis in a pediatric population is most commonly caused by group A β-hemolytic streptococcal infection (*Streptococcus pyogenes*). Streptococcal pharyngitis is important to identify and treat because of its potential complications, which are categorized as suppurative (peritonsillar and retropharyngeal abscesses) and nonsuppurative (acute rheumatic fever, postinfectious glomerulonephritis). Treatment can prevent most complications except for postinfectious glomerulonephritis.

SIGNS AND SYMPTOMS

- Sore throat, high fever, headache, malaise, and occasional abdominal pain.
- Absence of upper respiratory symptoms (no cough, rhinorrhea, or itchy, watery eyes).
- Tender anterior cervical lymphadenopathy.
- Enlarged, hyperemic tonsils with exudates.
- An erythematous pharynx.
- Palatal petechiae may be present.
- If fever and pharyngitis are accompanied by a characteristic erythematous "sandpaper-like" rash on the neck or trunk that later spreads to the extremities, the diagnosis is **scarlet fever.**

WORKUP

A ⊕ throat culture or streptococcal antigen detection test ("rapid strep test") distinguishes bacterial streptococcal pharyngitis from viral pharyngitis.

TREATMENT

- Penicillin VK PO × 10 days or azithromycin (for penicillin-allergic patients) × 5 days to prevent rheumatic fever.
- Empiric therapy is sometimes initiated after a culture has been sent if there is a high index of suspicion for streptococcal infection.

COMPLICATIONS

- **Postinfectious glomerulonephritis:**
  - May follow streptococcal pharyngitis or streptococcal skin infections within 1–2 weeks. (Note that this complication is **not** prevented by timely antibiotic administration.)
  - Signs include hematuria, proteinuria, ↓ urination, hypertension, pulmonary edema, and peripheral edema.
  - Complement levels (C3) may be low.
  - Typically self-limited and does not recur.
- **Acute rheumatic fever:**
  - An immune reaction that may arise 2–6 weeks after untreated streptococcal pharyngitis.
  - The diagnosis is made using the Jones criteria (see the mnemonic **JONES**).
  - Treatment involves penicillin, anti-inflammatory medications, and supportive therapy.
  - Given the high rate of recurrence, indefinite daily prophylactic penicillin should be started.

Streptococcal pharyngitis is very rare in children < 3 years of age.

The sensitivity of rapid strep tests ranges from 80% to 90%, but their specificity is > 95%. This means that false-⊖ results occasionally do occur, and you must base your treatment decisions on the entire clinical picture.

Jones criteria (major criteria) for acute rheumatic fever—

JONES

Joints—migratory polyarthritis involving > 2 joints
♥ pancarditis—new murmur (mitral or aortic insufficiency or Carey Coombs murmur) or symptoms of CHF
Nodules—over the joints, scalp, or spine
Erythema marginatum—a circinate, erythematous, maculopapular rash on the trunk and extremities
Sydenham's chorea—emotional instability, involuntary movements

UTI pathogens—

SEEKS PP

S. saprophyticus
E. coli
Enterobacter
Klebsiella
Serratia
Proteus
Pseudomonas

Which key tests should be ordered for a child with flank pain and a fever? CXR, UA, and urine culture. Flank pain can result from pyelonephritis or lower lobe pneumonia.

Urinary Tract Infection (UTI)

The simple definition of a UTI is growth of an abnormal number of bacterial colonies from the urine. UTIs can be classified as lower (cystitis, involving the bladder) or upper (pyelonephritis, involving the kidney). In infants, the source of bacteria is more often from hematogenous seeding of the kidneys, whereas in older children UTIs more often result from ascending infections of fecal flora. During the newborn period, the incidence of UTI is slightly higher in males; during childhood, it becomes 10 times more common in females. The predominant organisms responsible for UTI are *E. coli, Proteus, Klebsiella, Staphylococcus saprophyticus* (especially in adolescent females), and the enteric streptococci. Risk factors include vesicoureteral reflux, obstructive uropathy, renal calculi, bladder dysfunction, and intermittent catheterization. Infection in a small child should make you consider the possibility of abnormal anatomy.

SIGNS AND SYMPTOMS

- Vary by age (see Table 7-15).
- Cystitis presents with ↑ frequency and urgency, dysuria, incontinence, and suprapubic tenderness; hematuria and a low-grade fever may also be seen.
- Pyelonephritis is more likely to produce high fevers, chills, flank pain, nausea, vomiting, CVA tenderness (related to flank pain), and dehydration.

WORKUP

- Pyuria, hematuria, and bacteriuria on UA can suggest a UTI, but diagnosis requires a urine culture. A culture is ⊕ if:
  - More than 10^5 colonies/mL are obtained from a midstream clean-catch sample.
  - More than 10^4 colonies/mL are obtained from an intermittent ("in and out") catheterization sample.
  - Any colonies are obtained from a suprapubic tap sample.
- If the culture contains diphtheroid bacilli, *Staphylococcus*, or multiple organisms, suspect contamination and repeat the urine culture.
- Any toxic-appearing child should have blood cultures, a CBC with differential, electrolytes, and BUN/creatinine to rule out pyelonephritis and sepsis.

TABLE 7-15. Signs and Symptoms of UTI

NEWBORNS	INFANTS	PRESCHOOL	SCHOOL AGE
Fever	Fever	Fever	Fever/chills
Hypothermia	Irritability	Enuresis	Enuresis
Poor feeding	Poor feeding	Dysuria	Dysuria
Vomiting	FTT	Urgency	Urgency
Jaundice	Diarrhea	Urinary frequency	Urinary frequency
FTT		Abdominal pain	CVA tenderness
Sepsis		Vomiting	Hematuria
Apnea			
Diarrhea			

TREATMENT

- Empiric antibiotic treatment while awaiting sensitivity results.
- Give a five- to ten-day course of TMP-SMX or cephalexin for uncomplicated cystitis.
- Give "amp and gent" or cefuroxime for neonates, toxic-appearing patients, or children with suspected pyelonephritis.
- All patients can switch to oral antibiotics once clinically improved.
- Prophylactic antibiotic therapy (TMP-SMX or nitrofurantoin) is indicated in the following situations:
  - Prior to undergoing a VCUG.
  - Reflux of any grade in infancy and early childhood (see Figure 7-2).
  - Reflux of grades III–V in children > 5 years of age.
  - Patients with > 3 UTIs per year.

REFERENCE

American Academy of Pediatrics. Practice Parameter: The diagnosis, treatment, and evaluation of the initial urinary tract infection in febrile infants and young children. Available online at http://aappolicy.aappublications.org/practice_guidelines/index.dtl#T.

NEONATOLOGY

Apgar Score

The Apgar score is an objective tool that is used for evaluating the need to resuscitate a newborn and is determined at one minute and five minutes after birth. Assessment of the infant should begin immediately at birth, and the Apgar score alone should not be used to determine when to initiate resuscitation. In general,

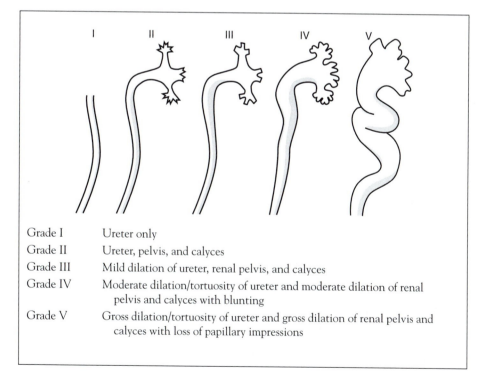

Grade I	Ureter only
Grade II	Ureter, pelvis, and calyces
Grade III	Mild dilation of ureter, renal pelvis, and calyces
Grade IV	Moderate dilation/tortuosity of ureter and moderate dilation of renal pelvis and calyces with blunting
Grade V	Gross dilation/tortuosity of ureter and gross dilation of renal pelvis and calyces with loss of papillary impressions

FIGURE 7-2. International classification of vesicoureteral reflux.

What the Apgar score measures—

APGAR

Appearance (color)
Pulse (heart rate)
Grimace (reflex
irritability)
Activity (muscle tone)
Respiratory effort

Which two TORCHeS
infections lead to intracranial
calcifications? CMV and
toxoplasmosis. CMV leads to
peri**V**entricular calcifications,
whereas to**X**oplasmosis leads
to diffuse calcifications in the
corte**X**.

scores of 8–10 indicate no need for resuscitation. Scores of 4–7 indicate a potential need for resuscitation, and infants should be carefully observed, stimulated, and given ventilatory support as needed. Scores of 0–3 indicate severe distress and the need for immediate resuscitation (see Table 7-16).

REFERENCE

Moster D et al. The association of Apgar score with subsequent death and cerebral palsy: A population-based study in term infants. *J Pediatr* 138:798–803, 2001. A population-based cohort study on the prognosis of infants with low Apgar scores.

Congenital Infections

Infections acquired in utero or in the perinatal period are commonly referred to by the acronym **TORCHeS**. These include **T**oxoplasmosis, **O**ther (parvovirus, *Borrelia*, VZV), **R**ubella, **C**ytomegalovirus, **H**SV/HIV/HBV, and **S**yphilis. Clinical findings common to many of these infections are intrauterine growth restriction, anemia and thrombocytopenia, hepatosplenomegaly, hydrops fetalis, jaundice, and chorioretinitis. Table 7-17 summarizes the distinctive clinical signs and symptoms of each.

Neonatal Hyperbilirubinemia

In the first week of life, most babies present with "physiologic jaundice," a benign condition with a peak bilirubin concentration up to 15 mg/dL. Bilirubin is primarily unconjugated and results from (1) ↑ RBC destruction as fetal hemoglobin is replaced with adult hemoglobin, and (2) ↓ clearance due to immature hepatocytes' inability to conjugate and thus excrete bilirubin as quickly as in adults. A total bilirubin > 15 mg/dL is considered pathologic. Subtypes are as follows:

- **Indirect (unconjugated) hyperbilirubinemia:** In addition to physiologic jaundice of the newborn, pathologic etiologies include hemolysis of any cause, including blood group incompatibility, internal bleeding, polycythemia, infants of diabetic mothers, congenital defects in bilirubin metabolism (e.g., Gilbert's syndrome, Crigler-Najjar syndrome), cephalohematoma, and breast-milk jaundice.

TABLE 7-16. Interpretation of the Apgar Score

	0	1	2
Color	Blue, pale	Body pink, extremities blue	Body and extremities pink
Heart rate	Absent	< 100/min	> 100/min
Reflex irritability	No response	Grimace	Cough or sneeze
Muscle tone	Limp	Some extremity flexion	Full extremity flexion
Respiratory effort	Absent	Weak cry	Strong cry

TABLE 7-17. TORCHeS Infections

INFECTION	EPIDEMIOLOGY	CLINICAL FEATURES	TREATMENT
Toxoplasma gondii	Maternal exposure to cat feces or poorly cooked meat. Fetal disease with 1° infection only. Highest risk of exposure is at 10–24 weeks' gestation.	Hydrocephalus, microcephaly, severe mental retardation, epilepsy, diffuse intracranial calcifications. Infants may be asymptomatic at birth.	Pyrimethamine + sulfadiazine.
HIV	Most mothers are asymptomatic with a high-risk history (prostitution, drug abuse, hemophilia).	Recurrent infections, hepatosplenomegaly, neurologic abnormalities, FTT. Some 10–25% develop AIDS symptoms between three and six months, depending on the use of perinatal antiretrovirals.	AZT, TMP-SMX (PCP prophylaxis), and other agents. Prevent with maternal pre-, intra-, and postpartum AZT; avoid breast-feeding.
VZV	First-trimester maternal chickenpox infection. Infections that develop within one week before or after delivery are associated with severe disseminated disease.	Microphthalmia, cataracts, cutaneous and bony abnormalities. Risk of zoster as an older child.	Acyclovir. Prevent with varicella-zoster immune globulin (VZIG) after exposure to VZV.
Rubella virus	Non-rubella-immune mother. Fever and rash in mother. The highest transmission risk is in the first trimester (80%). Virus may persist in infant's oropharynx for one year.	Microcephaly, cataracts, glaucoma, microphthalmia, "salt-and-pepper" chorioretinitis, "blueberry muffin" rash, B- and T-cell deficiencies, deafness, PDA, ASD, VSD. Infants may be asymptomatic at birth.	No treatment; vaccine preventable.
CMV	The most common congenital infection; sexually transmitted. 1° infection has the worst outcome, but reinfection can also produce disease. Infants may shed virus in urine for 1–6 years.	Sepsis, periventricular calcifications, microcephaly, pneumonia, deafness, severe mental retardation, hepatosplenomegaly. Infants may be asymptomatic at birth with late neurologic sequelae.	Ganciclovir may be effective. Prevent with CMV-⊖ blood products.

■ **Direct (conjugated) hyperbilirubinemia:** Causes include TORCHeS infections, metabolic disorders (galactosemia, α_1-antitrypsin deficiency, CF), bacterial sepsis, obstructive jaundice (biliary atresia), prolonged administration of TPN, and neonatal hepatitis. Direct hyperbilirubinemia is always of pathologic origin (see Table 7-18).

TABLE 7-18. Physiologic vs. Pathologic Jaundice

PHYSIOLOGIC JAUNDICE	PATHOLOGIC JAUNDICE
Not present until 72 hours after birth.	Present in the first 24 hours.
Total bilirubin ↑ < 5 mg/dL/day.	Total bilirubin ↑ > 0.5 mg/dL/hr.
Total bilirubin peaks at < 14–15 mg/dL.	Total bilirubin rises to > 15 mg/dL in formula-fed term and preterm infants. Total bilirubin can rise to > 17 mg/dL in breast-fed or full-term infants.
Direct bilirubin < 10% of total.	Direct bilirubin > 10% of total.
Jaundice resolves by one week in term infants and two weeks in preterm infants.	Jaundice persists beyond one week in term infants and two weeks in preterm infants.

Conjugated hyperbilirubinemia is always pathologic.

SIGNS AND SYMPTOMS

Jaundice starts in the head and progresses to the feet as bilirubin levels rise.

WORKUP

- **Indirect hyperbilirubinemia:** Blood typing, Coombs' test, CBC, blood smear, reticulocyte count.
- **Direct hyperbilirubinemia:** LFTs, bacterial and viral cultures, metabolic screening tests, hepatic ultrasound, sweat chloride test.

TREATMENT

- Phototherapy for term infants with bilirubin levels of approximately 15–20 mg/dL, depending on the infant's age and the cause of the hyperbilirubinemia. Skin bronzing may be seen after phototherapy in infants with direct hyperbilirubinemia.
- Exchange transfusions for bilirubin levels > 20 mg/dL if phototherapy fails.

COMPLICATIONS

Premature infants are more susceptible to kernicterus.

- The main concern with indirect hyperbilirubinemia is the development of kernicterus (bilirubin encephalopathy).
- Unconjugated bilirubin is lipid soluble and can cross the blood-brain barrier and precipitate in the brain, especially in the basal ganglia. Kernicterus typically occurs at levels > 20–25 mg/dL but can occur at lower levels in the presence of factors such as prematurity, asphyxia, hemolysis, and sepsis.
- Infants who survive the initial insult often develop a neurologic syndrome characterized by hypotonia, seizures, mental retardation, choreoathetoid movements, deafness (manifested by delayed language acquisition), impairment of eye movements (especially upward gaze), and dental enamel hypoplasia. Cognitive function is relatively spared.

BREAST-MILK VS. BREAST-FEEDING JAUNDICE

- **Breast-milk jaundice:** A syndrome of prolonged unconjugated hyperbilirubinemia that is thought to be due to an inhibition of bilirubin conjugation in the breast milk of some mothers. It is an extension of physiologic jaundice, peaks at 10–15 days of age, and declines slowly by 3–12 weeks of age.
- **Breast-feeding jaundice:** Attributable to poor feeding or inadequate breast-milk supply and ↑ enterohepatic circulation of bilirubin. It usually occurs during the first week of life and resolves when enteral intake improves. Treatment involves evaluating the breast-feeding pair and encouraging more feeding.

REFERENCES

- American Academy of Pediatrics Clinical Practice Guideline, Subcommittee on Hyperbilirubinemia. Management of hyperbilirubinemia in the newborn infant 35 or more weeks of gestation. *Pediatrics* 114(1):297–316, 2004.
- Dennery PA et al. Neonatal hyperbilirubinemia. *NEJM* 344:581–590, 2001. A good review of a key neonatology topic.

Respiratory Distress Syndrome (RDS)

The most common form of respiratory failure in preterm infants, RDS results from a deficiency of surfactant that leads to poor lung compliance, atelectasis, and hyaline membrane formation in the alveoli. Risk factors include maternal diabetes, hypothermia, asphyxia, and prematurity. RDS is seen in 65% of infants born at 29–30 weeks' gestation.

SIGNS AND SYMPTOMS

Presents with tachypnea (respiratory rate > 60), progressive hypoxemia, cyanosis, nasal flaring, intercostal retractions, and grunting in the first 72 hours of life.

DIFFERENTIAL

Transient tachypnea of the newborn, meconium aspiration syndrome, congenital pneumonia, spontaneous pneumothorax, diaphragmatic hernia, cyanotic heart disease.

WORKUP

CXR shows bilateral atelectasis with a "ground-glass" appearance and air bronchograms.

TREATMENT

- Intubation and ventilation (conventional, high frequency, or oscillator) may be required to maintain oxygenation.
- It is becoming increasingly recognized, however, that mechanical ventilation is associated with barotrauma and that high concentrations of supplemental O_2 may lead to oxygen toxicity. For this reason, it is recommended

Treatment with surfactant ↓
mortality from neonatal RDS.

Why does pretreatment of at-
risk mothers with
betamethasone ↓ the
incidence of RDS?
Corticosteroids ↑ the
production of surfactant by
type II pneumocytes.

that infants be extubated as quickly as can be tolerated and stabilized on CPAP.
- Surfactant replacement therapy ↓ mortality.
- Supportive care in a NICU (thermoregulation, close monitoring of fluids and acid-base balance, and maintaining adequate BP and perfusion) is required.

PREVENTION

- RDS can be avoided by preventing premature birth or by pretreating at-risk mothers with corticosteroids (betamethasone).
- Fetal lung maturity can be monitored in utero with the amniotic fluid lecithin-to-sphingomyelin (L/S) ratio and the presence of phosphatidylglycerol. An L/S ratio < 2 indicates a possible surfactant deficiency and the need for steroids.

COMPLICATIONS

Persistent PDA; bronchopulmonary dysplasia; pneumothorax/interstitial emphysema; retinopathy of prematurity.

REFERENCE

Gnanaratnem J, Finer NN. Neonatal acute respiratory failure. *Curr Opin Pediatr* 12:227–232, 2000. A practical review of neonatal RDS and its treatment.

NEUROLOGY

Febrile Seizures

Defined as seizures that arise in association with fever. Generally occur in children between six months and six years of age with an incidence of 3–4%. The risk of febrile seizures is slightly higher following the administration of some vaccines (e.g., MMR), but there are no associated long-term consequences, so patients should not forgo vaccination for this reason.

SIGNS AND SYMPTOMS

- Generally associated with a maximum temperature of 39°C or higher, and may be due to a rapid ↑ in temperature.
- Classified as simple or complex (see Table 7-19). Complex febrile seizures are characterized by episodes that last > 15 minutes, have focal features or postictal paralysis, or occur in a series with a total duration of > 30 minutes.

TABLE 7-19. Simple vs. Complex Febrile Seizures

SIMPLE FEBRILE SEIZURE	COMPLEX FEBRILE SEIZURE
Short duration (< 15 minutes)	Long duration (> 15 minutes)
Generalized	Focal
One seizure in a 24-hour period	More than one seizure in a 24-hour period ("cluster")

WORKUP

- **History:** Ask the parents to describe the nature of the seizure (focal vs. generalized), its duration (keep in mind that parents often overestimate duration), the number of seizures, the postictal state, and events preceding the seizure. Also ask about a history of previous seizure, a family history of febrile seizure, a history of trauma or ingestions, and the child's neurologic development and medication exposure.
- **Exam:** Check rectal temperature, vital signs, mental status, nuchal rigidity (note that this is valid only for children > 18 months of age), fullness of the fontanelle, and abnormalities or focal differences in muscle strength and tone.
- **Labs:** The following laboratory tests and imaging studies are helpful:
    - In younger children (< 12 months of age), a workup for sepsis should be performed, including CBC, blood culture, CSF for cell count, glucose, protein, and culture, and UA/urine culture.
    - An LP is necessary if CNS infection is suspected in children > 1 year of age.
    - A serum glucose determination is indicated in all seizure patients.
    - A head CT is indicated only if CNS disease is suspected (e.g., in the setting of macrocephaly, an abnormal neurologic exam, or signs and symptoms of ↑ ICP).
    - An EEG should be considered for complex febrile seizures.

Simple febrile seizures carry a better prognosis.

TREATMENT

- Antipyretics (e.g., acetaminophen) may be helpful in overall management but do not ↓ the recurrence rate.
- Appropriate treatment of any underlying illness.
- Diazepam per rectum may be used to stop prolonged seizures (> 5 minutes).
- In rare cases, daily prophylactic phenobarbital or valproic acid may be necessary for children with complex febrile seizures.

COMPLICATIONS

- Some 70% of children will never have another febrile seizure. The majority of recurrent seizures take place within one year of the initial episode.
- For simple febrile seizures, there is no ↑ risk of developmental, intellectual, or growth abnormalities, and the risk of developing epilepsy (2.4%) is not much higher than that of the general population (1.4%). Thus, the initiation of chronic antiepileptic medication is not recommended after one or more simple febrile seizures.
- Risk factors for developing epilepsy include complex febrile seizures, abnormal neurologic exams, neurologic or developmental abnormalities, and a family history of epilepsy.

REFERENCE

Sadleir LG, Scheffer IE. Febrile seizures. *BMJ* 334:307–311, 2007. A concise review article of febrile seizures.

What is the most common etiology of pediatric limp? Trauma.

Limp

Disturbances in gait are common in children and may present with a limp or with refusal to bear weight. A painful limp is typically acute in onset and may be accompanied by fever and irritability. A painless limp is usually slow in onset and may be associated with weakness or limb deformity. The causes of limp can be remembered with the mnemonic **STARTS HOTT** (see Table 7-20).

TABLE 7-20. Causes of Pediatric Limp

CONDITION	DIAGNOSIS/TREATMENT
Septic arthritis	The most common cause of painful limp in children 1–3 years of age; usually monoarticular. Agents include *S. aureus,* group A streptococcus, and *Neisseria gonorrhoeae* in sexually active teenagers. Presents with acute onset of pain, fever, warmth, swelling, reduced joint mobility, leukocytosis, and ↑ ESR. X-rays reveal joint space widening; joint aspiration shows turbid fluid with low glucose; WBC count is > 10,000 with neutrophilia. Treat with drainage and antibiotics.
Transient synovitis	Most common in males 3–8 years of age; may follow a viral URI. Presents with acute onset of pain, limp, and ↓ joint mobility in the hip. Afebrile or low-grade fever; no tenderness, warmth, or joint swelling; normal WBC count and ESR. Can be difficult to differentiate from septic arthritis. X-rays are normal; ultrasound may show effusion. Treat with bed rest and NSAIDs.
Aseptic vascular necrosis	Legg-Calvé-Perthes disease (LCPD)—femoral head; Köhler's disease—navicular bone; Sever's disease—calcaneus. LCPD occurs in males 4–9 years of age after interrupted blood supply to the femoral head; may be bilateral. Presents with painless limp or pain in the inner thigh, restricted motion, short stature, and muscle spasm. Afebrile; normal WBC count and ESR. X-rays reveal sclerosis of the femoral head and widened femoral neck. Treat with surgical or cast containment of the femoral head to prevent deformity and osteoarthritis.
Rheumatoid arthritis	See discussion of JIA.
Trauma	Obtain from history.
Slipped capital femoral epiphysis (SCFE)	Often seen in obese male adolescents or children in their growth spurts. May be bilateral; mostly gradual onset and progressive. Presents with dull pain referred to the thigh or knee that worsens with activity. X-rays (taken in frog-leg lateral position) reveal widened physis with posterior and medial displacement of the femoral head relative to the femoral neck (Klein's line). Treat with pinning and cast immobilization.

TABLE 7-20. **Causes of Pediatric Limp** *(continued)*

CONDITION	DIAGNOSIS/TREATMENT
Henoch-Schönlein purpura	Vasculitis in children 4–10 years of age. Presents with asymmetric migratory periarticular swelling, palpable purpura on the buttocks and legs, and abdominal pain. Complications include GI bleeding, intussusception (monitor for stool occult blood), and glomerulonephritis (monitor for hematuria/proteinuria). The disease is self-limiting; treat symptoms (NSAIDs for arthralgias) and complications (steroids for intestinal and CNS complications).
Osteomyelitis	Most common in boys 3–12 years of age; results from hematogenous (younger children) or direct spread. The most common etiologic agent is *S. aureus.* Neonates are at risk for GBS, *E. coli,* and anaerobic organisms; children are at risk for *Streptococcus, Pseudomonas* (foot puncture wounds in tennis shoes), *Pasteurella multocida* (dog and cat bites), and *Salmonella* (sickle cell patients). Young infants may have fever only; children may have fever, localized pain, ↓ mobility, erythema, and edema. X-rays are normal for 1–2 weeks. Labs show neutrophilic leukocytosis, ↑ ESR, and a ⊕ blood culture (approximately 50% are ⊕). Imaging includes bone scan and MRI (gold standard). Treat with IV and PO antibiotics for 4–6 weeks.
Tumor	Malignant pediatric bone tumors must be ruled out. **Ewing's sarcoma:** A small, round blue-cell tumor found in the femur and pelvis with early metastases. X-rays reveal an "onion-skin" appearance. Treat with chemotherapy; highly sensitive to radiation. **Osteogenic sarcoma:** Seen in adolescent boys more frequently than in girls; often metastasizes to the lung. Located in the distal femur, proximal tibia, and proximal humerus; presents with pain and a palpable mass. X-rays reveal Codman's triangle (periosteal elevation) and "sunburst sign" (calcification in soft tissues). Treat with surgery and adjuvant chemotherapy.
Tuberculosis	Skeletal TB results from hematogenous or direct spread from lymph nodes. Affects the vertebrae (Pott's disease), hips, fingers, and toes. Diagnose with biopsy and culture of affected bone. X-rays show destruction of the cortex. Treat with a four-drug regimen for two months; then use a two-drug regimen for 7–10 months (depending on local sensitivities).

REFERENCES

■ Kocher MS et al. Differentiating between septic arthritis and transient synovitis of the hip in children: An evidence-based clinical prediction algorithm. *J Bone Joint Surg Am* 81:1662–1670, 1999. Addresses the difficulty in differentiating these two conditions; examines the evidence and provides a clinical algorithm.

■ Lawrence LL. The limping child. *Emerg Med Clin North Am* 16:911–929, 1998. Outlines a thorough approach toward limp, including summaries of major causes and references for further reading.

Pediatric Fractures

A number of fracture types are specific to pediatrics. These include the following:

- **Torus fractures:** Involve "buckling" of the cortex with compression of the bone.
- **Greenstick fractures:** Incomplete fractures that break one side of a bone and bend the other.
- **Epiphyseal fractures:** Involve the growth plate (the weakest portion of a child's skeletal system) and are classified into five groups by the Salter-Harris system, which predicts the prognosis for a given fracture (see Figure 7-3).

PULMONOLOGY

Asthma (Reactive Airway Disease)

Ask about the allergic triad: asthma, atopic dermatitis, and allergic rhinitis.

A bronchial disorder characterized by inflammation, reversible smooth muscle constriction, and mucus production. Asthma is the most common chronic condition of childhood, affecting roughly 6% of children (and as many as 40% of children in urban settings), and will almost certainly be part of the inpatient pediatrics experience. Numerous research studies have shown that the prevalence of asthma has been increasing over the past several decades. 1° triggers include irritants such as cigarette smoke, air pollution, and ozone as well as allergens such as pollens, dust mites, pets, and cockroaches. Other triggers include exercise, cold weather, respiratory infections, drugs (aspirin, β-blockers), stress, foods, and food additives. Be sure to elicit a history of past severity, frequency of attacks, ER visits, hospitalizations, ICU admissions, intubations, courses of steroids per year, number of school days missed, and family history of asthma, allergies, and atopic disease. GERD and sinusitis can make asthma worse.

SIGNS AND SYMPTOMS

- Patients or parents may report chest congestion, persistent or nighttime cough, exercise intolerance, dyspnea, pneumonia, irritability, or feeding difficulties in younger children.

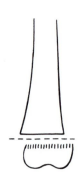 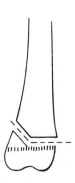 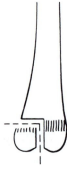 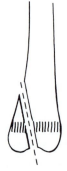 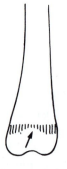

| I. Through growth plate | II. Through metaphysis and growth plate | III. Through growth plate and epiphysis into joint | IV. Through metaphysis growth plate, and epiphysis into joint | V. Crush of growth plate. May not be seen on x-ray |

FIGURE 7-3. Salter-Harris classification of epiphyseal fractures.

- Wheezing, coughing, tachypnea, tachycardia, prolonged expiration, hyperresonance, intercostal and subcostal retraction, and nasal flaring may be present on exam.
- Asthma can occur without overt wheezing (e.g., cough-variant asthma produces a chronic cough).
- Red flags include cyanosis, diminished breath sounds (due to poor air exchange), absence of wheezing, use of accessory muscles, increasingly labored breathing, and mental status changes (indicative of hypercarbia and/or significant hypoxemia with impending respiratory failure).
- **Status asthmaticus** refers to severe asthma attacks that may not be responsive to standard treatments. This is a life-threatening condition that may lead to respiratory acidosis and respiratory arrest. Patients must usually be hospitalized (often in an intensive-care setting) and mechanically ventilated.

Key indicators of asthma severity:
- *Frequent ER visits*
- *A history of intubation*
- *Hospitalizations*
- *Steroid use*

BEWARE OF ASTHMA WITHOUT WHEEZING

- During an asthma exacerbation, wheezes may actually be absent on lung exam.
- For wheezes to be produced, air must be moving through the lungs. In patients with a severe exacerbation, air movement may be so limited that wheezes are not heard.
- Once bronchodilator treatment is initiated and air movement ↑, wheezes may appear, indicating clinical improvement.
- Conversely, the disappearance of wheezes is important to note. While this may signal resolution of an exacerbation, it can also be an ominous sign that the patient's ability to move air through the lungs is decreasing. This exam finding indicates the need for more aggressive treatment.

DIFFERENTIAL

- Aspiration, foreign body.
- Bronchiolitis, pneumonia, bronchopulmonary dysplasia, CF, allergic bronchopulmonary aspergillosis (ABPA).
- GERD.
- Vascular slings, tracheoesophageal fistula.

WORKUP

The diagnosis is based on clinical findings. However, the following may be helpful:

- **PFTs:** ↓ vital capacity, ↑ functional residual capacity, ↑ residual volume, ↓ FEV_1, ↓ peak expiratory flow (PEF), and reversal of pulmonary abnormalities by inhalation of aerosolized albuterol.
- **Peak flow (PF) monitoring:** Measures how fast a patient can forcibly expire air after a maximal inhalation; reductions of 50–80% of predicted values indicate a mild to moderate obstruction, and readings < 30% of predicted indicate severe obstruction. PFs are also helpful in monitoring treatment efficacy.
- **CXR:** Nonspecific findings, but may find hyperinflation, depressed diaphragm, and atelectasis.

- **WBC count:** Eosinophilia.
- **ABGs:** Hypoxia, hypercarbia, respiratory acidosis during acute exacerbations. It is important to recognize increasing $PaCO_2$ as a sign of impending respiratory failure; with tachypnea, values should usually be well below 40.

TREATMENT

- Children < 1 year of age often require nebulized medication. Children 1–4 years of age may use a spacer with a face mask, and children > 4 years of age can use a metered-dose inhaler (MDI) with a spacer.
  - **Acute therapy:** Bronchodilators (nebulized albuterol 0.15 mg/kg in 2–3 cc NS or MDI two puffs q 1–6 h PRN) are immediately effective and are the mainstay of acute treatment. A five-day "pulse" of PO prednisone or IV methylprednisolone (Solu-Medrol) is highly effective but takes 4–6 hours to have an effect.
  - **Chronic therapy:** Avoid triggers; give inhaled corticosteroids for prevention. Leukotriene receptor antagonists are indicated for moderate to severe persistent asthma and may allow some patients to reduce their dependence on β_2-agonists and inhaled steroids. Cromolyn sodium and theophylline are rarely used in asthma management since the advent of inhaled steroids.
- Asthma is often classified by severity for the purpose of determining appropriate treatment (see Table 7-21). It is recommended that one begin with more aggressive therapy and then use a "step-down" approach to treatment. In addition to the maintenance medications listed in Table 7-21, all

TABLE 7-21. Classification of Asthma Severity

	SYMPTOMS	NIGHTS WITH SYMPTOMS	PEF OR FEV$_1$ (% OF PREDICTED)	MAINTENANCE MEDICATIONS
Step 4: severe persistent	Continual symptoms; limited physical activity; frequent exacerbations.	Frequent.	< 60%	Daily inhaled high-dose corticosteroids **and** long-acting bronchodilator **and** PO steroids 2 mg/kg/day.
Step 3: moderate persistent	Daily symptoms; two or more exacerbations per week. Exacerbations limit activity.	> 1 time per week.	60–80%	Medium-dose inhaled corticosteroids **or** low- to medium-dose inhaled steroid and long-acting bronchodilator; if needed, medium- to high-dose inhaled steroid and long-acting bronchodilator.
Step 2: mild persistent	Symptoms occur > 2 times per week but < 1 time per day. Exacerbations may affect activity.	> 2 times per month.	> 80%	Low-dose inhaled steroid.
Step 1: mild intermittent	Symptoms occur < 2 times per week. Asymptomatic between exacerbations.	< 2 times per month.	> 80%	No daily medication needed.

patients should have short-acting bronchodilators (albuterol) as needed during an acute attack.

REFERENCE

National Asthma Education and Prevention Program (United States Department of Health and Human Services). Expert Panel Report 3: Guidelines for the diagnosis and management of asthma, 2007. Available online at www.nhlbi.nih.gov/guidelines/asthma/asthgdln.htm. A comprehensive literature review and final report on the diagnosis and management of asthma.

Bronchiolitis

An acute inflammatory illness of the small airways occurring in children < 3 years of age. RSV is the 1° agent, although PIV (especially type 3), adenovirus, influenza, and rhinovirus have also been implicated. Most cases occur in late fall to early spring. Risk factors for severe disease include prematurity (< 35 weeks' gestation), low birth weight, age < 12 weeks, chronic pulmonary disease, CHD, and immunodeficiency states.

All that wheezes is not asthma.

SIGNS AND SYMPTOMS

- Presents with rhinorrhea, sneezing, cough, and low-grade fever followed a few days later by tachypnea and wheezing.
- Signs of respiratory distress, including nasal flaring, retractions, and intermittent cyanosis, may be present.
- Apnea may be the presenting sign in premature or young infants.

DIFFERENTIAL

Asthma, pneumonia, heart failure, laryngomalacia, foreign body aspiration, GERD, CF.

WORKUP

- The diagnosis is based primarily on clinical signs and symptoms. Thus, in routine cases, it is not recommended that labs or radiologic studies be ordered for diagnostic purposes.
- CXR can demonstrate hyperinflation (flat diaphragm, ↑ AP diameter) but should be obtained only for ill or hypoxic patients or for those with recurrent episodes of wheezing.
- RSV can be identified in nasopharyngeal washes by direct fluorescent antibody (DFA) testing or culture. Although commonly tested for, it rarely changes the nature of management, as treatment consists primarily of supportive care. However, such testing can be useful for purposes of disease surveillance and for the grouping of RSV-⊕ patients in hospital wards to ↓ disease transmission.

*What is the best way to prevent the spread of RSV in the hospital? Wash your hands before and after **every** patient encounter!*

TREATMENT

- Primarily supportive (oral hydration, antipyretics).
- Hospitalize those with a resting respiratory rate of > 50–60/min, hypoxemia, apnea, inability to tolerate oral feeding, chronic cardiopulmonary disease, or an unreliable home environment.
- Supplemental O$_2$ and contact isolation are appropriate for hospitalized patients.

Breast-feeding has been shown to ↓ an infant's chance of developing bronchiolitis.

- Bronchodilators (nebulized albuterol or racemic epinephrine) may transiently improve respiratory symptoms but are no longer recommended. Some pediatricians offer a trial dose to determine if they are of any benefit (particularly in the presence of a family history of asthma, as it may be difficult to distinguish bronchiolitis from an initial asthma exacerbation).
- Inhaled steroids are not recommended, as no benefit has been shown to be derived from their use. The use of ribavirin aerosol should be reserved for severely affected or high-risk children.
- During RSV season, high-risk infants < 2 years of age can be treated prophylactically with RSV IVIG or palivizumab (the latter is preferred, as it is a monoclonal antibody and not a blood product).

REFERENCES

- Ngai P, Bye MR. Bronchiolitis. *Pediatr Ann* 31:90–97, 2002. A good review of a common pediatric airway problem.
- Subcommittee on Diagnosis and Management of Bronchiolitis. American Academy of Pediatrics clinical practice guideline: Diagnosis and management of bronchiolitis. *Pediatrics* 118:1774–1793, 2006. An excellent review of current literature accompanied by clear-cut clinical guidelines for the management of bronchiolitis.

Listen for a seal-like bark

in croup.

Croup

Viral croup (laryngotracheobronchitis) is an acute inflammatory disease of the larynx, trachea, and bronchioles that especially affects the subglottic space (see Figure 7-4). Parainfluenza types 1 and 3 are the most common cause; other organisms include RSV, influenza virus, rubeola virus, adenovirus, and *M. pneumoniae*.

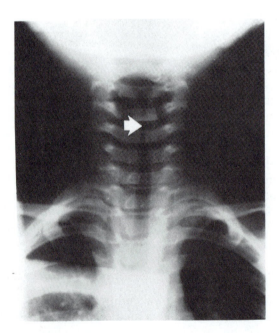

FIGURE 7-4. Croup.

(Reproduced, with permission, from Saunders C. *Current Emergency Diagnosis & Treatment*, 4th ed. Stamford, CT: Appleton & Lange, 1992: 448.)

HIGH-YIELD FACTS

PEDIATRICS

SIGNS AND SYMPTOMS

- Presents with inspiratory stridor that worsens with agitation.
- Also characterized by a hoarse voice and a seal-like, barking cough.
- May be preceded by a prodrome of mild fever and coryza.
- Diminished breath sounds, restlessness, altered mental status, or cyanosis may be seen if the child becomes hypoxic.

DIFFERENTIAL

- **Infectious:** Epiglottitis, bacterial tracheitis, retropharyngeal abscess, foreign body aspiration (see Table 7-22). Consider tracheitis if the patient does not respond to aerosolized racemic epinephrine.
- **Other:** Foreign body aspiration, angioneurotic edema.

WORKUP

- CXR and neck x-ray if the diagnosis is in doubt.
- A PA radiograph of the neck shows subglottic narrowing known as the "steeple sign" (see Figure 7-4).

Although now rare owing to routine administration of the Hib vaccine, epiglottitis remains a life-threatening emergency that must be ruled out in the differential of stridor. Patients are typically toxic appearing, with difficulty swallowing, drooling, and severe progressive respiratory distress. **Urgent intubation** *for airway protection is indicated.*

TABLE 7-22. Characteristics of Croup, Epiglottitis, and Tracheitis

	CROUP	EPIGLOTTITIS	TRACHEITIS
Age affected	Three months to five years.	Two to seven years.	Older children.
Etiologic agent	Viral, commonly parainfluenza.	Group A strep, *S. aureus*, viral.	Often *S. aureus*.
Onset	Develops over 2–3 days.	Rapid onset over several hours.	Acute decompensation after two- to three-day gradual onset.
Fever	Low grade.	High grade.	High grade.
Respiratory distress	Usually mild to moderate.	Commonly severe.	Commonly severe.
Position preference	Prefers sitting up, leaning against the parent's chest.	"Tripod" position with neck extended.	May have position preference.
Response to aerosolized racemic epinephrine	Stridor improves.	No response.	No response.
Imaging	"Steeple sign" on PA neck films.	"Thumb sign" on lateral neck films.	Subglottic narrowing.

TREATMENT

- **Mild cases** (no stridor at rest): Supportive measures, oral fluids, cool-mist therapy, humidity (using a humidifier or exposure to steam from a hot bath).
- **Moderate cases** (with stridor at rest): Corticosteroids.
- **Severe cases** (respiratory distress, hypoxia): IV hydration, systemic steroids, nebulized racemic epinephrine, supplemental O_2 and intubation if necessary (rare; only for < 1% of hospitalized patients).

REFERENCE

Stroud RH, Friedman NR. An update on inflammatory disorders of the pediatric airway: Epiglottitis, croup, and tracheitis. *Am J Otolaryngol* 22:268–275, 2001. A review paper that compares and contrasts three major pediatric airway disorders.

Cystic Fibrosis (CF)

A multisystem autosomal-recessive disorder characterized by dysfunctional exocrine gland function that results from a mutation in the CFTR gene, which is located on chromosome 7 and is involved in chloride conductance. CF is the most common lethal genetic disease affecting Caucasians (1 in 3000 live births). Roughly 93% of patients are diagnosed in childhood.

SIGNS AND SYMPTOMS

Patients present with respiratory, GI, reproductive, endocrine, and orthopedic signs and symptoms, which are outlined in Table 7-23. The most common presentations include meconium ileus at birth (~15% of all CF patients), recurrent respiratory infections, FTT, or positive newborn screen.

WORKUP

- A sweat test shows a chloride concentration > 70 mEq/L.
- PFTs reveal obstructive and restrictive disease.
- Sputum/throat cultures.
- CXR may show blebs.
- Some states have newborn screening programs (screening for ↓ amounts of trypsin) that identify roughly 10% of cases.
- Genetic testing for some of the most common mutations in the CFTR gene can also facilitate diagnosis (e.g., > 70% of all CF cases result from the ΔF508 mutation).

TREATMENT

- Aerosolized deoxyribonuclease (DNase) to ↑ mucus clearance.
- Chest physiotherapy with postural drainage.
- Bronchodilators and antibiotics if acute declines in lung function or pneumonia is suspected.
- Intermittent aerosolized tobramycin (BID × 4 weeks) for *Pseudomonas*.
- Pulmonary exacerbations require hospital for IV antibiotics.
- H_2 blockers, antacids.
- Pancreatic enzyme supplements; vitamin A, D, E, and K supplements.
- A high-calorie, high-protein diet with supplemental NG or gastrostomy tube feedings if oral intake is inadequate.
- Most patients will ultimately require double-lung transplantation between the second and third decade of life.

TABLE 7-23. Signs and Symptoms of CF

SYSTEM	PRESENTATION
Respiratory	Asthma with clubbing of the digits.
	Nasal polyps.
	Chronic pansinusitis.
	Recurrent pneumonia (especially staphylococcal).
	Chronic atelectasis, chronic pulmonary disease, pneumothorax, bronchiectasis, hemoptysis, or chronic cough.
	Colonization with mucoid *Pseudomonas aeruginosa*.
	X-rays showing persistent hyperaeration or atelectasis.
GI	Meconium ileus (pathognomonic).
	Intestinal obstruction (meconium plug or recurrent intussusception).
	FTT (protein-calorie malnutrition).
	Steatorrhea or chronic diarrhea.
	Rectal prolapse.
	Prolonged jaundice.
	Hepatic cirrhosis and portal hypertension.
	Recurrent pancreatitis.
Musculoskeletal	Bone pain and joint effusion due to hypertrophic osteoarthropathy.
Reproductive	Infertility in men (due to obliteration of the vas deferens); infertility in women (due to thick, spermicidal cervical mucus).
Miscellaneous	Hypoproteinemia and edema.
	Fat-soluble vitamin deficiencies (vitamins A, D, E, and K).
	Hypoprothrombinemia.
	"Salty" taste or salt crystals on skin.
	Unexplained hyponatremic hypochloremic metabolic alkalosis.
	Impaired glucose tolerance or type 1 DM.

HIGH-YIELD FACTS

PEDIATRICS

REFERENCE

Davis PB. Cystic fibrosis. *Pediatr Rev* 22:257–264, 2001. A user-friendly and thorough review of the basic science and clinical aspects of CF.

TOXICOLOGY

Lead Poisoning

Most lead exposure comes from lead-containing paint remaining in buildings constructed before the 1970s. Other sources of exposure include industrial plants, lead solder in pipes, lead-containing pottery, paint on some imported toys and household items, and some traditional herbal remedies. Lead poisoning requiring medical evaluation refers to levels > 20 μg/dL, but levels of 10–19 μg/dL can also be toxic, and recent data have shown some neurocognitive effects at levels < 10 μg/dL. Lead levels > 70 μg/dL are considered severe.

SIGNS AND SYMPTOMS

- Irritability, hyperactivity, listlessness, a decline in school performance, behavioral difficulties, attention disorders, and even developmental delay may be seen.
- Anorexia, abdominal discomfort, vomiting, and constipation are also common.
- Lead encephalopathy is associated with ↑ ICP, headache, vomiting, ataxia, seizures, coma, or even death in severe cases.
- Other clinical findings include the following:
  - Peripheral neuropathy (wrist and foot drops).
  - Burton's lines (blue lines on the gums).
  - Red-brown discoloration of the urine.
  - Proximal tubule dysfunction (aminoaciduria, glycosuria, and hyperphosphaturia).
  - Pica.

WORKUP

- Obtain lead levels for all children at 12 months and two years of age, and in others based on risk factors.
- A peripheral smear shows basophilic stippling and hypochromic microcytic anemia (often with concomitant iron deficiency).
- X-rays reveal lead lines.

Check lead levels at 12 and 24 months in all children.

TREATMENT

- Chelation therapy with succimer/DMSA or calcium disodium EDTA for lead levels > 45 µg/dL.
- Chelation therapy with EDTA and dimercaprol/BAL for lead levels > 70 µg/dL or signs and symptoms of acute encephalopathy.
- Correct iron deficiency if present.

REFERENCE

Committee on Environmental Health. American Academy of Pediatrics policy statement: Lead exposure in children—prevention, detection, and management. *Pediatrics* 116(4):1036–1046, 2005.

TRAUMA

Child Abuse and Neglect

Most clinicians will encounter at least one case of child abuse at some point in their careers. Almost half of reported cases occur in children < 1 year of age. Children at ↑ risk for abuse include those with special needs or behavioral problems, premature infants, and children of single, teenage, or substance-abusing parents. The presence of spousal abuse ↑ the risk of child abuse in the same household. Even after intervention, the abuse often continues, and the mortality rate for abused children is 5%.

SIGNS AND SYMPTOMS

- Injury is inconsistent with the description of events, or the history elicited changes over time.
- There is unexplained delay in obtaining care.

Suspect child abuse if the story and the injuries don't match.

- Mandibular fractures, rib fractures (often multiple and posterior in location), scapular fractures, and long bone spiral fractures are seen, often in different stages of healing.
- Head injuries can lead to apnea, seizures, subdural hematomas, retinal hemorrhages, or coma.
- Burn marks with straight lines, symmetry, and unusual geometry are seen.
- Sexual abuse may lead to genital trauma, STIs, recurrent UTIs, encopresis, or enuresis. Rectal or genital pain, discharge, or bleeding may also be seen. Sleeping/eating disorders as well as behavioral and school difficulties may be present, as may sexualized behavior with peers or objects.
- Neglect can lead to FTT; ↓ subcutaneous fat in the cheeks, extremities, and buttocks; diaper rash; and impetigo. Look for unwashed skin and clothing.
- Delayed social and speech development may be seen.
- Behavioral changes may include avoidance of eye contact, depressed affect, and absence of a cuddling response.

WORKUP

- Skeletal survey, bone scan, ophthalmologic exam.
- Osteogenesis imperfecta, bleeding disorders, and bullous skin disorders must be ruled out.
- Obtain a UA, a urine culture, and a stool culture if sexual abuse is suspected.
- Laboratory and clinical studies may be conducted without parental permission.
- Photograph and document injuries.

Tests can be ordered without parental permission if abuse is suspected.

TREATMENT

- Immediately report suspected abuse to state protection agencies.
- Stabilize injuries as needed.

REFERENCES

- American Academy of Pediatrics Committee on Child Abuse and Neglect. Shaken baby syndrome: Rotational cranial injuries—technical report. *Pediatrics* 108:206–210, 2001. Discusses current knowledge about "shaken baby syndrome."
- Kini N, Lazoritz S. Evaluation for possible physical or sexual abuse. *Pediatr Clin North Am* 45:205–219, 1998. A review article with definitions, common injuries, and tips for the history and physical exam.

COMMON CLERKSHIP TOPICS

The following is a list of core topics that you are likely to encounter in the course of your pediatrics rotation and on a shelf examination.

- **Well-child care:**
    - Anticipatory guidance and safety
    - Developmental milestones
    - Failure to thrive
    - Growth parameters
    - Immunizations
    - Infant nutrition
    - Tanner staging

- **Cardiology:**
    - Arrhythmias (supraventricular tachycardia, long QT syndrome, Wolff-Parkinson-White syndrome) (see Internal Medicine)
    - Congenital heart disease
    - Congestive heart failure
    - Pericardial disease
- **Dermatology:**
    - Atopic dermatitis
    - Diaper rash
    - Impetigo
    - Neonatal rashes (acne neonatorum, erythema toxicum, milia)
    - Psoriasis
    - Scabies and lice
    - Seborrheic dermatitis
    - Viral exanthems
- **Endocrinology:**
    - Adrenal dysfunction (congenital adrenal hyperplasia)
    - Diabetes
    - Thyroid dysfunction
- **Gastroenterology:**
    - Appendicitis (see Surgery)
    - Constipation
    - Gastroesophageal reflux
    - Hirschsprung's disease
    - Intussusception
    - Malrotation and volvulus
    - Meckel's diverticulum
    - Pyloric stenosis
- **Genetic disorders:**
    - Autosomal trisomies (21, 18, 13)
    - Common associations (CHARGE, VATER)
    - Common syndromes (DiGeorge, Marfan's, Noonan's, Prader-Willi, Williams)
    - Sex chromosome disorders (Turner's, Klinefelter's, fragile X)
- **Hematology and oncology:**
    - Anemia
    - Sickle cell disease
    - Thalassemia
    - Childhood cancers (acute lymphocytic leukemia, Wilms' tumor, neuroblastoma)
- **Immunology:**
    - Autoimmune disorders (Henoch-Schönlein purpura, idiopathic thrombocytopenic purpura, juvenile idiopathic arthritis, Kawasaki disease)
    - Immunodeficiencies (T cell, B cell, combined, complement, phagocytic, HIV)
- **Infectious disease:**
    - Acute otitis media
    - Cellulitis
    - Fever management
    - Gastroenteritis
    - Meningitis
    - Orbital and periorbital cellulitis
    - Osteomyelitis
    - Pneumonia
    - Sexually transmitted infections (see Obstetrics and Gynecology)

- Sinusitis
- Streptococcal pharyngitis
- Urinary tract infection
- **Neonatology:**
  - Apgar score
  - Congenital infections
  - Neonatal hyperbilirubinemia
  - Prematurity
  - Respiratory distress syndrome
- **Nephrology/urology:**
  - Cryptorchidism
  - Fluid and electrolyte management (see Practical Information for All Clerkships)
  - Hematuria and proteinuria
  - Hemolytic-uremic syndrome
- **Neurology:**
  - Cerebral palsy
  - Febrile seizures
  - Hydrocephalus
  - Neural tube defects
  - Seizure disorders
- **Orthopedics:**
  - Developmental hip dysplasia
  - Limp
  - Nursemaid's elbow (subluxation of the radial head)
  - Pediatric fractures
- **Psychiatry:**
  - Attention-deficit hyperactivity disorder (see Psychiatry)
  - Learning disorders (see Psychiatry)
  - Mental retardation (see Psychiatry)
- **Pulmonology:**
  - Apnea/apparent life-threatening event/sudden infant death syndrome
  - Asthma (reactive airway disease)
  - Bronchiolitis
  - Croup
  - Cystic fibrosis
  - Epiglottitis
- **Toxicology:**
  - Acetaminophen and salicylate toxicity
  - Ingestions
  - Lead poisoning
- **Trauma:**
  - Child abuse
  - Head injury

HIGH-YIELD FACTS

PEDIATRICS

Psychiatry is the study and management of behavioral disorders. Given ongoing advances in the neurobiological understanding of major psychiatric disorders, together with continuing additions to the psychiatrist's pharmacologic arsenal, many find psychiatry to be an increasingly exciting field in which to practice and conduct research. Even if you do not intend to enter psychiatry, the rotation will offer you valuable exposure to common psychiatric disorders (e.g., depression, schizophrenia, bipolar disorder, anxiety disorders, dementia, delirium) that you will see for the rest of your career, regardless of the specialty you choose.

What Is the Rotation Like?

In general, the psychiatry core rotation is more relaxed than other clerkships. Thus, if you have the option of choosing the order in which to take your third-year core rotations, psychiatry would be a good rotation to take after surgery or OB/GYN as a means of helping you "catch your breath."

Psychiatry is a more relaxed rotation but can be emotionally intense.

On the other hand, the expectations and mechanics of this rotation are much different from those of the more conventional clerkships. For example, medical students' exposure to the outpatient setting is often limited owing to the private nature of the activity. Consultation and liaison, as well as emergency crisis services, also play an important role in most psychiatric departments. Medical schools that are associated with a VA or children's hospital will allow students to focus on a unique psychiatric population, and students may rotate through any one or combination of these services.

Outpatient psychiatry encompasses a spectrum of activities ranging from one-time consultations and brief crisis intervention to medication management and long-term psychotherapy. Patients who require psychiatric hospitalization are admitted to an inpatient psychiatric service. Patients on other hospital services as well as those in the ER may develop or have a psychiatric illness, and these services may consult psychiatry for advice.

How Do I Excel in Psychiatry?

Emphasizing the biopsychosocial model, modern psychiatry incorporates biological, experiential, and sociocultural factors into a single paradigm. Doing well in psychiatry therefore requires the development of interviewing skills, the study of psychopathology, and the acquisition of knowledge about psychopharmacology. Generally, psychiatry emphasizes the doctor-patient relationship in the healing process. Thus, the development of empathic skills and an ability to listen are critical to excelling in this rotation. The use of open-ended questions to acquire information about a patient's psychopathology is also a must.

Good listening and observational skills are a must on the psych rotation.

In addition to developing interviewing skills, it is important that you acquire a solid fund of psychiatric knowledge. You will also need to hone your observational skills in order to monitor abnormalities in a patient's appearance, behavior, and affect. Specifically, this rotation will provide you with an opportunity to learn about disorders of feeling, thinking, and behavior that interfere with the way a person functions and relates to others. At the same time, you must also learn how to present a psychiatric history. As a medical student, you will often have more recent experience on medicine wards than any other member of the team. You can therefore prove to be a real asset in helping the team manage medical problems in psychiatric patients.

Many students find themselves initially disoriented by the unique organization and expectations of the psychiatry clerkship. Here are some tips from students and residents:

- Keep an open and inquiring mind. Psychiatric training benefits doctors in all fields.
- Be organized. For each patient, keep a card that includes a short history, a thorough medication list, and a checklist of things to do.
- Make a card with the generic and trade names, common dosages, and side effects of the most frequently used psychiatric drugs, as well as a card with an outline of the mental status exam (MSE).
- When interviewing a patient, obtain a thorough medication history, including dates of use, effectiveness, and side effects.
- Be friendly with the support staff, especially the nurses!
- Remember—safety first. If you feel threatened, leave the room immediately and get help. While on this rotation, you may witness a "takedown" in which the staff physically pins down a violent, labile patient. This may look frightening and unpleasant at first, but it is often the safest and kindest option available.
- When interviewing a patient, try to convene in a location that respects the patient's confidentiality while also allowing for an unobstructed departure from the room should this become necessary. If the patient is potentially dangerous, leave the door to the interview room open. In such instances, a third person might be asked to stand inside or outside the room to be available if trouble arises.
- Take the initiative. When discussing your patient, think ahead and consider issues such as housing, finances, social support, time of discharge, cultural issues, and community services.
- Try to pick up on how your patient makes you feel (e.g., depressed, anxious). You'll find that your patient often has similar feelings.
- You may not need your white lab coat or any kind of uniform on this rotation. Some institutions even ban ties and necklaces, as patients can use them to strangle the caretaker. However, bring your white coat on the first day of your rotation, and wear it until you are told that you can leave it at home.
- Don't joke with your patients.
- Don't touch your patients. Touch is a powerful and volatile tool that should be used only after you have gained more experience. With appropriate discussion and information, however, consent can be acquired from patients in situations where contact may be clinically indicated (e.g., in patients suffering from emotional trauma or paranoia).
- Don't share details of your life with your patients.
- Before you interview a patient, discuss the goals of your encounter with your resident or attending. Is the goal to gather information or to treat? Are there any sensitive topics from which you should steer clear?

You will often experience a mix of feelings when dealing with psychiatric patients. Be open to exploring these feelings with your team. Having such feelings will not be seen as a sign of weakness, but failing to deal with them can be detrimental.

Never let a labile patient get between you and the door.

What Is the DSM-IV?

The DSM-IV, or the *Diagnostic and Statistical Manual of Mental Disorders*, 4th edition, is published by the American Psychiatric Association. The DSM is the standard diagnostic classification system used by all U.S. mental health workers (both clinicians and researchers) as well as by insurance companies and the federal government. The DSM, which is revised roughly once a decade to incorporate new research findings, consists of long lists of criteria that are required to assign specific psychiatric diagnoses to patients. At first glance, the DSM-IV may appear lengthy, complex, and confusing. However, you do not need to know the details of all the criteria it describes. The more important criteria will be found here under the appropriate headings.

It is important to note that despite its precise and detailed diagnostic criteria, the DSM-IV is not meant to be used by nonpsychiatrists in a "check the appropriate boxes" or "cookbook" fashion. To the contrary, the DSM-IV merely offers guidelines for trained psychiatrists to apply with a view toward ensuring better diagnostic agreement among clinicians and researchers. Practically speaking, the DSM-IV also provides useful criteria for billing for psychiatric care, and in some institutions this is its primary use. Regardless of the attention paid to the DSM-IV criteria, including an assessment of the five axes will impress your attendings and residents on rounds.

Key Notes

The psychiatric admit note is similar to its medicine counterpart except for the emphasis it places on past psychiatric history and the patient's personal history. Large portions of a psychiatric history often need to be obtained from other sources. At a minimum, you must talk to a family member and to the patient's regular doctor and review any old charts that may exist. Other pertinent information is outlined below.

DSM-IV CLASSIFICATION

The DSM-IV uses a "multiaxial classification," which is just an elaborate way of saying that information is broken down into five categories (which should be used for presenting patients in rounds, write-ups, and the like):

1. **Axis I:** Psychiatric disorders.

2. **Axis II:** Personality disorders and mental retardation.

3. **Axis III:** Physical and medical problems.

4. **Axis IV:** Social and environmental problems/stressors.

5. **Axis V:** The Global Assessment of Functioning (GAF), which rates a patient's overall level of social, occupational, and psychological functioning (current and best in the past year) on a scale of 1 (completely nonfunctional) to 100 (extremely high level of functioning in a wide number of areas).

Key:

A&O × 4 = alert and oriented to person, place, time, and situation

AH = auditory hallucinations

BAD = bipolar affective disorder

BID = twice daily

CAD = coronary artery disease

CC = chief complaint

C/C/E = clubbing/ cyanosis/edema

CM = Caucasian male

CN = cranial nerve

CTAB = clear to auscultation bilaterally

CV = cardiovascular

d/o = disorder

DTRs = deep tendon reflexes

EOMI = extraocular movements intact

EtOH = alcohol

FH = family history

FT = fine touch

FTN = finger to nose

HEENT = head, eyes, ears, nose, and throat

HI = homicidal ideation

h/o = history of

HPI = history of present illness

HSM = hepatosplenomegaly

HTN = hypertension

HTS = heel to shin

IVDU = intravenous drug use

SAMPLE PSYCHIATRY ADMIT NOTE

ID/CC: TM is a 20-year-old CM college student brought into the ER by his parents because he has been bedridden and increasingly isolative for 2 weeks.

Source of information: Parents, who are reliable.

HPI: This is the patient's 1st inpatient admission for symptoms. Patient was in his USOH until 3 years ago, when he became depressed after failing a college class. Also at that time, he thought he was being "followed" and that "whispers were talking behind his back." A first diagnosis of schizophrenia of the paranoid type was made at that time by Dr. Jones, who started patient on Zyprexa (titrated up to 20 mg/day), which was effective. He has since seen 4 additional psychiatrists and has tried Prozac for depressive symptoms with no success. Patient has been able to continue school part time and to function fairly well. However, for the last 2 weeks, his parents report that he has isolated himself in his room and does not leave except to use the restroom. He continually lies in bed with the sheets over his head and the blinds drawn. According to his parents, the patient was "mute and tearful, answering questions with single words and acting differently from his usual social self." At time of admission, patient endorses a running debate in his head from a single, unrecognized voice. The conversation revolves around daily activities and decisions such as choosing a seat. Patient denies VH/HI/SI. No prior h/o suicide attempts.

Patient reports that he currently has no appetite (eats only a small sandwich a day), sleeps 4 hours per night, and is not participating in any of his usual activities. He has been noncompliant with his Zyprexa for the past 3–4 months. He endorses a history of alcohol and cocaine use, but denies using for the last 3 months.

Past psychiatric history: See HPI.

Substance use: Tobacco: 1/2 ppd × 4 years; EtOH: drinks approx. 12 beers/week × 6 years; cocaine: intranasal cocaine 2 times/week × 5 years; denies h/o IVDU.

PMH:

Childhood illnesses: None.

Medical illnesses: None.

Surgeries: None.

Hospitalizations: None.

Trauma: Head injury due to bicycle accident with brief LOC in 1995. No retrograde or anterograde amnesia. No hospitalization or treatment at that time.

Allergies: None.

Medications: Zyprexa 20 mg QD.

No herbs, supplements, or vitamins.

FH: H/o depression in all paternal male relatives, including father. One paternal uncle committed suicide at age 40. Mother with heavy EtOH use. No h/o schizophrenia or other psychiatric illnesses. No h/o CAD, HTN, MI, or cancer.

SH: Patient was raised by his mother and father. Parents state that childhood development was normal, and he was a good student with A's and B's until his diagnosis 3 years ago. He currently lives at home with his parents in Los Angeles and attends a local junior college. He has been unemployed × 1 month and worked most recently at a grocery store. He has held multiple odd jobs over the past 3 years; his longest job was 6 months. No h/o arrests or legal problems. No current girlfriend, and patient is not sexually active. He has enjoyed playing the guitar since age 13.

ROS: Poor sleep, appetite, and energy. No recent weight change. Otherwise unremarkable except as above.

PE:

> Gen: Disheveled 20-year-old male sitting in a chair in NAD.
>
> VS: T 36.8, RR 18, orthostatic BP: sitting 150/82 P 104; standing 156/87 P 107.
>
> Skin: Tattoo on left shoulder; no rashes, scars, or lesions noted.
>
> HEENT: NC/AT, PERRL, EOMI, no nystagmus, conjunctiva clear, O/P clear with good dentition.
>
> Neck: Supple, no LAD.
>
> Lungs: CTAB, no W/R/R.
>
> CV: Tachycardic, regular rhythm, no M/R/G, normal S1/S2.
>
> Abd: Soft, NT/ND, NABS, no masses or HSM.
>
> Ext: Warm and well perfused with cap refill < 2 sec. No C/C/E. Distal pulses 2+ bilaterally.
>
> Neuro: MS: A&O × 4; CN: II–XII intact; motor: normal tone, bulk, and power throughout; sensory: FT/PP/temp intact and symmetric; cerebellar: FTN and HTS intact, Romberg ⊖; DTRs 2+ and symmetric; gait: normal, able to tandem gait.

MSE:

- Appearance: Clean shaven, but hair and clothing are disheveled.
- Behavior: Marked psychomotor retardation with poor eye contact.
- Attitude: Cooperative with interview and questions, but somewhat withdrawn and guarded.
- Speech: Slowed and hypophonic with prolonged speech latency. Coherent but with paucity of content.
- Mood: "Anxious."
- Affect: Blunted—patient tells stories with limited emotional expression.
- Thought process: Linear and goal directed, without circumstantiality or tangentiality.
- Thought content: No SI/HI.
- Perception: Endorses AH; has "voices inside that are debating about where to sit," making it difficult to make decisions. Denies VH/TH.

Key:

LAD = lymphadenopathy

LOC = loss of consciousness

MDD = major depressive disorder

MMSE = Mini-Mental Status Exam

M/R/G = murmurs/rubs/ gallops

MS = mental status

NABS = normoactive bowel sounds

NAD = no acute distress

NC/AT = normocephalic/ atraumatic

NR = normal range

NT/ND = nontender, nondistended

O/P = oropharynx

P = pulse rate

PE = physical examination

PERRL = pupils equal, round, and reactive to light

PMH = past medical history

PO = by mouth

PP = pin prick

ppd = pack per day

PRN = as needed

QAM = every morning

QD = every day

QHS = every night

r/o = rule out

ROS = review of systems

RPR = rapid plasma reagin

Key:

RR = respiratory rate

RUA = routine urinalysis

SAD = schizoaffective
  disorder

SH = social history

SI = suicidal ideation

TH = tactile hallucinations

TSH = thyroid-stimulating
  hormone

USOH = usual state of
  health

VH = visual hallucinations

VS = vital signs

W/R/R = wheezes/
  rhonchi/rales

■ Cognition: MMSE 28/30. Missed 2 points on serial sevens. (Note: If the patient has greater than a high school education, he/she should be asked to do "serial sevens"—ask the patient to start at 100 and repeatedly subtract seven, e.g., 100, 93, 86, 79, 72.)

■ Judgment: Poor—patient wants to leave the hospital without treatment.

■ Insight: Poor—patient does not feel that he is ill or that taking medication will help him.

Labs:

HIV ⊖

RPR NR

TSH 1.6

RUA ⊖

$$\begin{array}{c|c|c} 138 & 98 & 10 \\ \hline 3.8 & 24 & 0.9 \end{array}\!\!\diagup 106$$

$$\diagdown\!\!\begin{array}{c} 16.2 \\ 9.5 \diagonal 247 \\ 41.7 \end{array}$$

Assessment: TM is a 20-year-old male with a 3-year h/o depressive and paranoid symptoms, noncompliant with Zyprexa, now with 2 weeks of increasing isolation and auditory hallucinations.

Axis I: Schizophrenia of paranoid type with depressive features—patient is exhibiting key features of schizophrenia of the paranoid type, including history of hallucinations and delusions for approximately 3 years. Patient is also showing concurrent features of a depressive episode, including lack of interest in normal activities, ↓ appetite, and ↓ sleep. At this time, it is unclear if there is concurrent schizophrenia and MDD; further information on concentration, level of energy, and overall mood (patient now denies being depressed) must be explored.

■ R/o MDD with psychotic features.

■ R/o BAD vs. SAD.

■ R/o substance-related/induced mood d/o.

Polysubstance abuse.

Axis II: Deferred.

Axis III: None.

Axis IV: Poor social support, substance dependence, lives at home, has difficulty
  holding jobs.

Axis V: GAF 35–40.

Plan:

■ Risperidone 2 mg PO QAM and QHS.

■ Cogentin 1 mg PO BID.

■ Wellbutrin SR 100 mg PO QAM.

■ Ativan 1 mg PO q 4 h PRN anxiety.

■ Tylenol 650 mg PO q 6 h PRN headache, fever, or pain.

■ Colace 100 mg PO BID, PRN constipation.

- Monitor sleep, food intake, and activity level.

- Around-the-clock sitter for 24 hours; then reassess the need for constant observation. Elopement risk currently moderate.

- Continue to explore and understand the patient's internal debate.

- Encourage milieu participation and attendance at all groups.

- Involve social work in planning outpatient rehab and a family meeting.

- **Chief complaint (CC)/reason for admission:** Some psychiatric patients may not have a primary complaint, while others may voice a complaint that is incoherent, obscene, or irrelevant—so it is often necessary to briefly state how and why the patient ended up in the hospital or ER in addition to the patient's perception of what happened.

- **History of present illness (HPI):** This includes symptoms, precipitants, time course, any medication changes or medication noncompliance, effects on function at home and work, and current treatment.

- **Past psychiatric history:** This includes age at onset of symptoms, first psychiatric contact, first psychiatric hospitalization, number of hospitalizations, the date and duration of the most recent hospitalization, suicide attempts (when, how, seriousness), substance abuse (what, how much, how often, how long, any withdrawal, shared needles), and medications (what, how much, how long, what helped, side effects, why did the patient stop taking them).

- **Past medical history (PMH):** The PMH should be obtained with the same thoroughness as in other specialties. However, a history of seizures, CNS infections, endocrine difficulties (e.g., thyroid dysfunction), head trauma, or allergies, as well as the presence of acute or chronic pain, are particularly important to obtain.

- **Social history (SH):** In psychiatry, heavy emphasis is placed on the social/personal history, as a patient's health, lifestyle, and social interactions may heavily influence his or her current psychiatric illness. It is therefore important to flesh out the details of a patient's birth, childhood, school performance, marriage, education, religious and cultural beliefs, occupational history, family and social relations, sexual history, hobbies and special interests, community supports, and current living arrangements. The patient's legal history, any history of violence, and a history of physical or sexual abuse should be documented as well. Attention should also be paid to family structure and significant interpersonal dynamics (e.g., whether the patient is divorced or adopted).

- **Family history (FH):** Ask about any psychiatric illnesses that run in the family. Get details on diagnoses, severity, outcomes, and what medications helped. Also ask about nonpsychiatric illnesses that run in the family.

Key Procedures

The MSE is the single most important procedure medical students must learn. Like the physical exam, the MSE provides a way to objectively document mental function and behavior. Although most often used in psychiatry, some form of MSE should be a part of all medical exams. It is therefore helpful to create an MSE template that can be filled in during the interview. Al-

Memorize the MSE as soon as possible in your rotation.

ways rule out organic causes of mental illness when evaluating psychiatric disorders.

What Do I Carry in My Pockets?

You will want to carry a psychiatry handbook (see Top-Rated Review Resources) as well as your drug guide. You will rarely need your stethoscope.

Read about these topics before you start the rotation. Most are discussed in this chapter. A full list of common clerkship topics can be found at the end of this chapter.

❑ **Mental status exam, Mini-Mental Status Exam,** five axes.
❑ **Mood disorders:** Major depressive disorder, bipolar disorder.
❑ **Psychotic disorders:** Schizophrenia.
❑ **Anxiety disorders:** Generalized anxiety disorder, panic disorder, social phobia, obsessive-compulsive disorder.
❑ **Substance abuse, dependence, withdrawal, alcoholism.**
❑ **Adjustment disorder.**
❑ **Eating disorders:** Anorexia nervosa, bulimia nervosa.
❑ **Suicidality.**

MENTAL STATUS EXAM AND MINI-MENTAL STATUS EXAM

Table 8-1 offers a brief outline of the key components of a complete MSE. You may want to use this table as a guide in creating a template. You should, however, refer to a text or manual for a complete treatment of this subject. You should also gain a familiarity with the Mini-Mental Status Examination (MMSE), which is rapidly administered, reliable, and both sensitive and specific for diagnosing dementia and delirium in hospitalized patients.

MOOD DISORDERS

Mood disorders are composed of episodes, each with a certain set of symptoms representing the patient's dominant mood state. These episodes—major depressive episode (MDE), mania, hypomania, and mixed—are not themselves diagnostic. However, they are used by psychiatrists to help make the diagnosis of a mood disorder.

Major Depressive Disorder (MDD)

MDD is the most prevalent psychiatric disorder, with a lifetime risk of 15–20%. The female-to-male ratio is 2:1, with an average age of onset in the mid-20s. Chronic illness and stress ↑ the risk of MDD, and concurrently, MDD can complicate the treatment of chronic disease. Left untreated, MDEs typically last > 4 months, and the recurrence rate is > 50% after one episode.

Although it has recently fallen into disfavor, perhaps the most widely known theory regarding the etiology of MDD is the biogenic amine theory, which holds that depression is due to low levels of amine neurotransmitters (e.g., norepinephrine and serotonin [5-HT]) in the synaptic cleft. This theory has

TABLE 8-1. Mental Status Exam

COMPONENT	COMMENTS
Appearance/ behavior	Grooming, appropriateness of dress, eye contact.
Attitude	The manner in which the patient interacts with the interviewer (e.g., cooperative, hostile).
Motor	Psychomotor agitation, psychomotor depression, tremor, posturing, mannerisms.
Speech	Rate, rhythm, tone, fluency, enunciation, volume, clarity, amount, abnormalities (e.g., aphasia).
Emotions	Mood (e.g., dysthymic, euphoric, irritable, euthymic, anxious) and affect (e.g., flat, blunted or restricted, labile, full, expansive).
Form of thought	The form of expression of a patient's thought, including quality, quantity, associations, and fluency of speech. Abnormalities include circumstantiality, tangentiality, flight of ideas, thought blocking, echolalia, neologisms, clanging, loosening of associations, and perseveration.
Thought content	The content of a patient's thoughts, including suicidal ideation, homicidal ideation, delusions, major themes, preoccupations, obsessions, ideas of reference, and poverty of thought.
Perception	Hallucinations or illusions.
Cognition	Evaluation of various brain functions and level of consciousness (e.g., alert, drowsy, stuporous, and comatose). Includes the MMSE.
Abstraction	Can the patient think abstractly? Ask the patient to explain the meaning of a proverb.
Judgment	Does the patient understand the consequences of his or her actions?
Insight	How aware is the patient of his or her illness, its etiology, and treatment options?

been supported by evidence that antidepressants ↑ the functional quantity of amine neurotransmitters that can bind postsynaptic receptors in the CNS.

SIGNS AND SYMPTOMS

The signs and symptoms of MDD are outlined in the mnemonic **SIG E CAPS.**

Symptoms of depression—

SIG E CAPS

Sleep—↑ or ↓
Interest—anhedonia (loss of interest or pleasure)
Guilt or worthlessness
Energy—↓
Concentration—difficult or disturbed
Appetite—↑ or ↓
Psychomotor changes
Suicidal ideation

MINI-MENTAL STATUS EXAM

Orientation:

1. What is the year, month, date, day of the week, season? (5 points)

2. Where are we? Country, state, city, hospital, floor? (5 points)

Registration:

1. Name three objects and ask the patient to repeat the three objects. Repeat until the patient learns all three, and record the number of trials. (1 point each)

Attention and calculation:

1. Serial sevens: Start with 100 and subtract seven; stop after five answers. (1 point each)

2. Spell *world* backward (an alternative that should be used only if the patient has a low educational level; not a substitute if the patient is uncooperative).

Recall:

1. Recall the three objects that the patient repeated earlier. (1 point each)

Language:

1. Name two objects the interviewer points out. (naming, 2 points)

2. Repeat the phrase "No ifs, ands, or buts." (repetition, 1 point)

3. Follow a three-step command: "Take a paper in your right hand, fold it in half, and put it on the floor." (3 points)

4. Read and obey the command "Close your eyes." (1 point)

5. Write a sentence. (1 point)

Visual/spatial:

1. Copy a design (e.g., interlocking pentagons). (1 point)

Total score:

24–30 = normal

18–23 = mild/moderate cognitive impairment

0–17 = severe cognitive impairment

Note: Validity is questionable if the patient has less than an eighth-grade education, is hearing impaired, or is not a fluent English speaker.

In diagnosing major depressive disorder, it is important to rule out hypothyroidism, as this condition is both common and treatable. Always check a TSH level.

DIFFERENTIAL

- **Psychiatric:** Mood disorder due to a general medical condition, substance-induced mood disorder, cocaine withdrawal, bereavement, schizoaffective disorder, dysthymia, dementia, bipolar disorder (depressed or mixed episode), adjustment disorder with depressed mood.
- **Organic:** Hypothyroidism, AIDS, MS, Parkinson's disease, Addison's disease, Cushing's disease, anemia (especially pernicious anemia), infectious

MAJOR DEPRESSIVE DISORDER VS. GRIEF

- Normal bereavement begins immediately or a few months after the loss of a loved one.
- The symptoms of bereavement are similar to those of MDD, but the latter is not diagnosed unless symptoms persist beyond two months or if excessive depressive symptoms (e.g., suicidal ideation, excessive guilt, or preoccupation with worthlessness) are present.
- Bereavement may vary by culture.

mononucleosis, neuroborreliosis, influenza, malnutrition, malignancies (e.g., pancreatic cancer).
- **Pharmacologic:** OCPs, cimetidine, steroids, some β-blockers.

WORKUP

- DSM-IV criteria for the diagnosis of MDD are as follows:
    - At least five symptoms of depression, at least one of which must be depressed mood or anhedonia.
    - Symptoms must persist for at least two weeks; must lead to significant social or occupational dysfunction; and must not be caused by drugs, medications, medical conditions, or bereavement.
- Distinguishing bereavement from MDD may be difficult in patients with a normal response lasting > 2 months.
- If a patient has one or more episodes of major depression during a two-year period, a diagnosis of "double depression" is made.

TREATMENT

- A combination of pharmacotherapy and psychotherapy is the most effective approach. Antidepressants often take a minimum of 2–3 weeks to take effect, so do not discontinue or assume inefficacy until at least eight weeks of treatment have elapsed (for most antidepressants).
- SSRIs and atypical antidepressants (bupropion, venlafaxine, mirtazapine, trazodone) are well tolerated and are considered first-line therapy for depression.
- Alternative medical agents include TCAs and MAOIs. Electroconvulsive therapy (ECT) is generally reserved for refractory or catatonic depression.
- Psychoanalytically oriented (psychodynamic) therapy is perhaps the most commonly used psychological therapy, but cognitive-behavioral therapy (CBT) and interpersonal therapy are also effective.

COMPLICATIONS

- MDD is associated with high recurrence rates—50% after one episode, 70% after two episodes, and 90% after three episodes.
- Side effects of antidepressants are as follows:
    - **SSRIs:** **Sexual side effects,** insomnia, headache, tremor.
    - **Atypical antidepressants:** Lack sexual side effects, but can cause sedation, weight changes, a ↓ **seizure threshold** (bupropion), and **priapism** (trazodone).

An ↑ risk of suicide has been reported, especially among young adults, immediately following the initiation of pharmacotherapy for MDD. This population should therefore be closely monitored after antidepressant treatment is started.

Discontinue all SSRIs at least five weeks before starting an MAOI and vice versa in light of the risk of serotonin syndrome, which presents with fever, myoclonus, mental status change, and cardiovascular collapse.

KEY ANTIDEPRESSANT MEDICATIONS

Selective serotonin reuptake inhibitors (SSRIs):

- **Drugs:** Fluoxetine (Prozac), sertraline (Zoloft), paroxetine (Paxil), fluvoxamine (Luvox), citalopram (Celexa), escitalopram (Lexapro).

- **Mechanism:** 5-HT-specific reuptake inhibitors.

- **Clinical use:** Endogenous depression in adults. SSRIs have been associated with an ↑ suicide risk in children and adolescents in the early stages of treatment. Currently, only fluoxetine is approved for use in children (must be ≥ 8 years of age).

- **Side effects:** Agitation, neuromuscular restlessness (akathisia), insomnia, sexual dysfunction, GI distress, anorexia, and multiple drug interactions, including serotonin syndrome (restlessness, confusion, hyperthermia, muscle rigidity, cardiovascular collapse, death) when used with other serotonergic medications (e.g., MAOIs). Avoid in pregnancy.

- **Pros:** Relatively well tolerated, so you can usually start at the therapeutic dose. Safe in overdose, with fewer side effects than TCAs. Citalopram is commonly used in patients who have multiple comorbid conditions, as it has very few drug interactions.

- **Cons:** Sexual dysfunction is very common and is often the cause of noncompliance. Like all antidepressants, they take 2–3 weeks to have an effect.

Tricyclic antidepressants (TCAs):

- **Drugs:** Amitriptyline (Elavil), imipramine (Tofranil), desipramine (Norpramin), clomipramine (Anafranil), nortriptyline (Pamelor), doxepin (Sinequan).

- **Mechanism:** Block reuptake of norepinephrine and 5-HT.

- **Clinical use:** Endogenous depression, bed-wetting (imipramine), OCD (clomipramine), and chronic pain.

- **Side effects:** Anticholinergic effects (dry mouth, blurred vision, constipation, urinary retention, delirium, worsening glaucoma), sedation, α-blocking effects (orthostatic hypotension), cardiac arrhythmias (widened QRS, prolonged PR and QTc, potential for SVT/VT/VF), seizures, respiratory depression, confusion, and hallucinations in the elderly. 3° TCAs (imipramine, amitriptyline) have more anticholinergic side effects and sedation than do 2° TCAs (nortriptyline). Desipramine is the least sedating.

- **Pros:** Inexpensive, well studied, and effective in severe depression.

- **Cons:** Poor compliance owing to side effects. Lethal in overdose, so must titrate slowly. The **"3 C's"** of TCA toxicity are **C**onvulsions, **C**oma, and **C**ardiac arrhythmias.

- **Labs:** Check an ECG before starting, after a few days, and at the therapeutic dose. Check blood levels if no response is obtained, excessive side effects occur, or there is suspected noncompliance.

Monoamine oxidase inhibitors (MAOIs):

- **Drugs:** Phenelzine (Nardil), tranylcypromine (Parnate), isocarboxazid.

- **Mechanism:** Nonselective MAO inhibition.

- **Clinical use:** Atypical depression, anxiety, and hypochondriasis.

- **Side effects:** Hypertensive crisis ("tyramine reaction" or "cheese and wine reaction"; avoid aged cheeses, red wine, cured foods, yeast extracts, meperidine, and common sympathomimetic "cold and pain" drugs); headache, dizziness, insomnia, orthostatic hypotension, and weight gain.

- **Pros:** Inexpensive; efficacious; highly effective for atypical depression.

- **Cons:** Dietary restrictions and poor tolerability of side effects. Contraindicated for use with β-agonists, SSRIs, or meperidine.

Atypical/heterocyclic antidepressants:

Second- and third-generation antidepressants have varied mechanisms of action. They are costly and rarely first-line therapy and should be avoided in pregnancy.

- **Bupropion (Wellbutrin):** Also used in smoking cessation (as Zyban). Rarely lethal in overdose and has few sexual side effects. Other side effects include tachycardia, agitation, dry mouth, aggravation of psychosis, and a tendency to lead to seizures.

- **Venlafaxine (Effexor):** Inhibits norepinephrine and 5-HT reuptake. Can also be used in generalized anxiety disorder (GAD). Side effects include stimulant effects (insomnia, anxiety, agitation, headache, and nausea) and ↑ DBP. BP must be monitored.

- **Mirtazapine (Remeron):** An α_2-antagonist (↑ norepinephrine and 5-HT neurotransmission) and a potent 5-HT$_2$ receptor antagonist. Has fewer sexual side effects, although it leads to marked sedation, ↑ appetite, and weight gain (which could be of use in underweight patients with depression).

- **Nefazodone (Serzone)/trazodone (Desyrel):** Primarily inhibit serotonin reuptake by a mechanism different from that of the SSRIs. Both have short half-lives. Side effects are sedation (especially trazodone), postural hypotension, and priapism (trazodone only). Because of the side effect of sedation, trazodone in combination with another antidepressant may be effective in depressed patients with insomnia.

- **Duloxetine (Cymbalta):** The newest approved antidepressant; acts as a multiple reuptake inhibitor with strong norepinephrine action. Also useful in diabetics with peripheral neuropathic pain. In particular, it may improve symptoms of apathy and fatigue. Associated with a risk of interaction with thioridazine; requires slow taper to prevent withdrawal syndrome. Avoid in renal failure.

ELECTROCONVULSIVE THERAPY (ECT)

Despite its infamous reputation, ECT is safe and effective for use in MDD. Patients usually require 6–12 treatments. ECT can be done on an outpatient basis and can be lifesaving for refractory or catatonic depression. It can also be used in bipolar disorder (for mania and depression) and acute psychosis.

- **Pre-ECT evaluation:** Conduct a history and physical (H&P); obtain an ECG, electrolytes, CBC, LFTs, UA, TFTs, CXR, a spinal x-ray series, and a head CT. Alert anesthesiology in advance. Informed consent is required.

- **Procedure:** The patient is kept NPO for at least eight hours. A short-acting barbiturate (methohexital) is given for anesthesia. Prior to the induction of muscle paralysis with succinylcholine, a tourniquet is placed around an extremity to prevent paralysis in that area in order to monitor the seizure.

- **Contraindications:** Recent MI, recent stroke, or intracranial mass. ECT is also a relative contraindication in patients who are a high anesthesia risk.

- **Side effects:** Postictal confusion, arrhythmias, headaches (resolve in hours), retrograde amnesia (usually no longer than six months), and sore muscles.

Treat TCA overdose with sodium bicarbonate.

- **TCAs:** Can be lethal in overdose and can lead to prolonged QRS intervals on ECG.
- **MAOIs:** Less frequently used because they can lead to hypertensive crisis if taken with high-tyramine foods (e.g., aged cheese, wine).

REFERENCES

- Moore JD, Bona JR. Depression and dysthymia. *Med Clin North Am* 85: 631–644, 2001. A review of the diagnosis, pathophysiology, and treatment of depressive disorders. Also discusses management issues for special groups, including children, pregnant women, and the elderly.
- Whooley MA, Simon GE. Managing depression in medical outpatients. *NEJM* 343:1942–1950, 2000. An excellent, easy-to-read summary about the diagnosis (including suicide assessment) and treatment of depression. Includes excellent tables and flow charts.

Dysthymic Disorder

Has a 6% lifetime prevalence and a twofold greater incidence among females than males. Patients have chronic depression of > 2 years' duration that is not severe enough to meet the criteria for MDD. Lacks psychotic features, does not lead to social or occupational dysfunction, and does not require hospitalization.

Dysthymia is the presence of at least two years of chronic depression that is not severe enough to meet the criteria for major depression.

DIFFERENTIAL

Similar to that of MDD.

To meet DSM-IV criteria for dysthymic disorder, in addition to depressed mood more days than not, a patient must exhibit **two or more** of the following six symptoms **for more days than not over a period of at least two years:**

- ↑ or ↓ appetite
- ↑ or ↓ sleep
- ↓ energy or fatigue
- ↓ self-esteem
- Difficulty concentrating or disturbed concentration
- Hopelessness

TREATMENT

Antidepressants that are effective in treating MDD may also be effective in dysthymic disorder. Supportive psychotherapy and psychoeducation (teaching patients and their families about this illness) are helpful as well.

Bipolar Disorder

BIPOLAR I DISORDER

Bipolar I disorder, or manic-depression, is an affective disorder with a 0.5–1.5% lifetime prevalence. Men and women are affected equally, and the average age of onset is 21 years. As in MDD, there is a strong genetic component, with a 70% concordance in monozygotic twins. The recurrence rate after one manic episode is 90%, and 10–15% of patients will commit suicide.

SIGNS AND SYMPTOMS

- DSM-IV criteria for the diagnosis of a manic episode include the presence of an elevated, expansive, or irritable mood with at least three (or four, if the mood is irritable) signs and symptoms from the **DIG FAAST** mnemonic.
- Symptoms of a **manic** or **mixed** episode (i.e., one that meets the criteria for both an MDE and a manic episode) must be present for at least one week (or less if hospitalization was required).
- Only a single manic episode is required for diagnosis.
- Patients may initially present with depression.
- More commonly associated with substance abuse than other psychiatric disorders.

DIFFERENTIAL

- **Psychiatric:** Schizophrenia, schizoaffective disorder, cyclothymia, borderline personality disorder, ADHD.
- **Organic:** Brain tumors, CNS syphilis, encephalitis, metabolic disorders, hyperthyroidism, MS.
- **Pharmacologic:** Cocaine, amphetamines, corticosteroids, anabolic steroids, phenylpropanolamine, INH, captopril, antidepressants.

TREATMENT

- Assess patients for suicidal and homicidal ideation and the need for hospitalization. Treat with a combination of pharmacotherapy and psychotherapy.

Bipolar I subtypes:

- Some 20% of bipolar I patients suffer from **rapid cycling,** in which at least four mood episodes (MDE, mania, hypomania, or mixed) occur in 12 months. This subtype carries a poorer prognosis.
- **Bipolar I with psychotic features** can feature mood-congruent or mood-incongruent delusions or hallucinations.

Signs and symptoms of mania—

DIG FAAST

Distractibility
Insomnia—↓ need for sleep
Grandiosity—inflated self-esteem
Flight of ideas
↑ in goal-directed **A**ctivity; psychomotor **A**gitation
Pressured **S**peech
Thoughtlessness—seeks pleasure without regard for consequence (e.g., substance abuse, hypersexual behavior, shopping sprees)

HIGH-YIELD FACTS

PSYCHIATRY

What is unique about the presentation of early-onset bipolar disorder? Unlike adults, who show well-defined, distinct episodes of depression and mania, children may present with both classes of symptoms within the same day.

- **Acute mania:** Give mood stabilizers (e.g., lithium, valproic acid, carbamazepine). Low-dose antipsychotics may be required. Benzodiazepines or other anxiolytics may be useful in refractory agitation.
- **Bipolar depression:** Use mood stabilizers +/– an antidepressant. Start mood stabilizers first to avoid inducing mania with an antidepressant. Antidepressants alone can also precipitate rapid cycling.

■ **Prophylaxis and maintenance:**
  - Lifelong prophylaxis with a mood stabilizer is warranted after the second episode, after a first episode that is severe or life-threatening, or in the presence of a strong family history.
  - Lithium and valproic acid are considered first-line therapy; carbamazepine and lamotrigine are second-line agents if first-line treatments fail.
  - ECT is effective but is reserved for patients who are refractory to pharmacotherapy or when a more immediate treatment response is required.
  - Psychotherapy focuses on helping patients understand and accept their illness, cope with its consequences, and maintain medication compliance.

*A 28-year-old woman being treated for bipolar disorder presents with ataxia, coarse tremor, and nystagmus. She appears dehydrated on PE. Why? Think **lithium toxicity** leading to nephrotoxicity (e.g., nephrogenic diabetes insipidus).*

BIPOLAR II DISORDER

Patients must have at least one MDE and one hypomanic episode to be diagnosed with bipolar II disorder; mixed and manic episodes are absent. Has a lifetime prevalence of 0.5%, with an incidence that is slightly greater for women.

SIGNS AND SYMPTOMS

- DSM-IV criteria require at least four days of abnormally elevated, expansive, or irritable mood **and** at least three signs and symptoms (or four, if the mood is irritable) from the **DIG FAAST** mnemonic.
- Changes are not severe enough to require hospitalization, cause psychotic features, or lead to social or occupational dysfunction.
- Can also show rapid cycling.

TREATMENT

Similar to that of bipolar I disorder.

REFERENCES

Bipolar II disorder requires the presence of at least one MDE and one hypomanic episode.

- Keck PE et al. Bipolar disorder. *Med Clin North Am* 85:645–661, 2001. An excellent review article that discusses subtypes within the bipolar spectrum, criteria for diagnosis, and currently available treatment options.
- Levin FR, Hennessy G. Bipolar disorder and substance abuse. *Biol Psychiatry* 15;56(10):738–748, 2004. A review of treatment strategies for patients with bipolar disorder and comorbid substance abuse.
- Maj M. Diagnosis and treatment of rapidly cycling bipolar disorder. *Eur Arch Psychiatry Clin Neurosci* 251(Suppl. 2):II/62–II/65, 2001. A review showing recent evidence that lithium is an effective treatment for rapid-cycling bipolar disorder.

KEY MOOD STABILIZERS

Lithium:

- **Clinical use:** The mainstay of treatment for bipolar disorder and mania (acute episodes and prophylaxis). Also has mild antidepressant effects.

- **Side effects:** Fine tremor, nausea, acne, weight gain, benign leukocytosis, arrhythmias, other ECG cardiac changes (flattened T waves or T-wave inversion), hypothyroidism, nephrogenic DI (lithium is an ADH antagonist), CKD, and teratogenesis.

- **Pros:** Inexpensive and well studied for long-term use.

- **Cons:** Regular lab studies are required because long-term renal damage is possible. Dosage must be titrated owing to the narrow therapeutic index; aim for a level of 0.8–1.2 mEq/L in acute mania and 0.6–1.0 mEq/L for maintenance. NSAIDs, ACEIs, and diuretics (when first started) ↑ plasma lithium level.

- **Signs of toxicity:** Coarse tremor, arrhythmias, dysarthria, ataxia, nausea, diarrhea, nystagmus (level of 1.5 mEq/L); seizures and coma (2.5 mEq/L); and death (≥ 3 mEq/L). Patients may require dialysis.

Valproate (Depakote):

- **Clinical use:** As effective as lithium in bipolar disorder and better in mixed mania, substance abuse, and rapid cycling. Can be used for acute episodes and prophylaxis.

- **Side effects:** GI distress, sedation, hepatotoxicity (e.g., rare hepatitis, ↑ LFTs, ↑ ammonia), pancreatitis (rare), and thrombocytopenia (rare).

- **Pros:** Well tolerated, broad therapeutic index, and relatively benign in overdose. Patients can start at the therapeutic dose, and fewer blood tests are required once the dosage is established.

- **Cons:** LFTs, platelets, and valproic acid levels should be checked at regular intervals.

Carbamazepine (Tegretol):

- **Clinical use:** Second-line agent used in patients who do not respond to lithium.

- **Side effects:** Rare but serious side effects include Stevens-Johnson syndrome, agranulocytosis, aplastic anemia, and hepatitis.

- **Cons:** A CBC is needed before starting and should be obtained on a monthly basis for the first 3–6 months and then once every 3–6 months.

- **Signs of toxicity:** Ataxia, confusion, and tremors.

Cyclothymia

A mild form of bipolar disorder consisting of recurrent mood disturbances alternating between hypomania and dysthymia. Some 30% of patients have a family history of bipolar disorder.

SIGNS AND SYMPTONS

- DSM-IV criteria require at least two years of cycling hypomanic and dysthymic episodes without major depressive, manic, or mixed episodes. The patient must not be symptom free for > 2 months at a time.
- Symptoms are less severe than those of bipolar I and II but may cycle more rapidly.
- Patients may also have borderline personality disorder; one-third to one-half will develop a mood disorder (usually bipolar II).

TREATMENT

The treatment of choice is a mood stabilizer. Antidepressants alone may ↑ the rate of cycling and precipitate manic episodes.

PSYCHOTIC DISORDERS

Psychotic disorders are defined by the presence of psychosis, which is a "gross impairment in reality testing."

Schizophrenia

A psychotic disorder that is characterized by a disruption in thought, affect, volition, social behavior, and motor activity in which the patient becomes increasingly preoccupied with his or her internal environment. Its prevalence is approximately 1%, and the male-to-female ratio is 1:1. Peak onset in men is earlier (15–25 years as opposed to 25–35 years in women) and is of greater severity. In general, patients exhibit a chronic and progressive course. Risk factors and etiologies are as follows:

Approximately 10–15% of patients with schizophrenia die by suicide, while 40–50% of patients make a suicide attempt.

- An ↑ prevalence of the disease has been observed among lower socioeconomic classes in the United States, likely due to a "downward drift" of these patients into the lower classes as a result of impairment from their disease.
- Dizygotic twins and children of a single schizophrenic parent have a 12% prevalence of schizophrenia, and the prevalence ↑ to 40% and 47% with two parents with schizophrenia or a monozygotic twin, respectively.
- Various neurotransmitter abnormalities have also been identified in association with schizophrenia.
    - An imbalance of dopamine (the "dopamine hypothesis"), the most widely favored theory, posits that ↑ dopamine activity and receptors in the limbic system correlate with the symptoms of disease.
    - This is supported by the observation that dopamine receptor antagonists (antipsychotic medications) alleviate psychotic symptoms, while dopamine agonists (e.g., cocaine and amphetamines) may induce such symptoms.

KEY TERMS

- **Affect:** The outward expression, including facial expression, of the patient's internal emotional state.

- **Circumstantiality:** Indirect speech that is delayed in reaching the point but does eventually reach the desired goal (i.e., ability to "get from point A to point B" after some period of time).

- **Clanging:** Association of words with similar sounds but not similar meaning.

- **Compulsions:** Conscious, stereotyped behaviors or thoughts that the patient manifests to prevent the distress or anxiety induced by an obsession.

- **Delusions:** Fixed false beliefs that are not consistent with the patient's cultural background and cannot be altered by reasoning.

- **Depersonalization:** A state in which the self is felt to be unreal or detached from reality.

- **Derealization:** Perception of the world around a person as unreal.

- **Echolalia:** Persistent repetition of the words or phrases of another person.

- **Flight of ideas:** Rapid, continuous use of words with constant shifting between connected ideas.

- **Hallucinations:** False sensory perceptions.

- **Ideas of reference:** A patient's belief that an object (e.g., a radio or television) is speaking to or about him or her.

- **Illusions:** Misinterpretations of actual stimuli.

- **Loosening of associations:** Flow of thought with random shifting of ideas from one subject to another.

- **Mood:** The patient's subjective, internal emotional state.

- **Neologisms:** New words, often created by combining syllables of other words.

- **Obsessions:** Recurrent, intrusive thoughts, impulses, or images that lead to anxiety and that the patient attempts to suppress or neutralize in order to ↓ anxiety.

- **Perseveration:** Persistent response to a previous stimulus when a new stimulus is presented.

- **Poverty of thought:** Having only a few thoughts, which lack variety and richness.

- **Pressured speech:** Rapid speech that is ↑ in amount and difficult to understand or interrupt.

- **Tangentiality:** Inability to have goal-directed thought (i.e., inability to "get from point A to point B" at all).

- **Thought blocking:** Abrupt interruption in a train of thought before the thought or idea is completed.

- **Thought broadcasting:** Belief that one's thoughts are being transmitted to others.

SIGNS AND SYMPTOMS

- According to the DSM-IV, patients must present with at least two of the following signs and symptoms for at least six months:
  - ⊕ **symptoms:** The presence of unusual thought, behaviors, or perceptions, including hallucinations (usually auditory or visual), delusions, bizarre behavior (e.g., echolalia, echopraxia, odd dress), and disordered thought (e.g., ideas of reference, tangentiality, loose associations).
  - ⊖ **symptoms:** Lack of normal social and/or mental function, including flat affect, poverty of thought and/or speech, apathy, anhedonia, and lack of purposeful actions.
- These symptoms must lead to social and/or occupational dysfunction. Depression, if present, is brief in comparison to the duration of the illness.

DIFFERENTIAL

- **Psychiatric:** Other psychotic disorders (e.g., schizoaffective, schizophreniform), mood disorders (e.g., bipolar disorder, severe melancholia, mood disorder with psychotic features), delusional disorder, delirium, dementia, Cluster A personality type, developmental disorders (e.g., Asperger's syndrome, autism).
- **Organic:** Early Huntington's disease, early Wilson's disease, complex partial seizures (e.g., temporal lobe epilepsy), frontal or temporal lobe tumors, early MS, early SLE, acute intermittent porphyria, electrolyte imbalances, hepatic encephalopathy, HIV encephalopathy, viral encephalitis, neurosyphilis, endocrine abnormalities (e.g., Cushing's disease, calcium imbalance, thyroid dysfunction, hypoglycemia).
- **Pharmacologic:** Substance abuse (e.g., amphetamines, cocaine, or PCP), medications (e.g., digoxin, ACTH, INH, L-dopa).

WORKUP

- According to the DSM-IV, the criteria for diagnosis of schizophrenia include the presence of two or more of the above signs and symptoms for a period of at least one month, with continuous evidence of social and/or occupational dysfunction 2° to psychiatric disturbance for at least six months.
- These symptoms cannot be due to a preexisting medical condition, a substance-related condition, or another psychiatric condition. Subtypes of schizophrenia are outlined in Table 8-2.
- Imaging studies are not necessary, although schizophrenic brains may show abnormal findings such as enlarged ventricles and cortical atrophy.

TREATMENT

- Treatment consists primarily of antipsychotic (neuroleptic) medications. The side effects of typical antipsychotics include extrapyramidal symptoms (EPS), hyperprolactinemia, and anticholinergic effects.
- Psychosocial intervention includes supportive treatment such as vocational rehabilitation and arranged social support in the community.
- Hospitalization may be required, especially during psychotic episodes.

If medication is discontinued, the two-year relapse rate for schizophrenia approaches 75–80%.

REFERENCE

Goff CC et al. Schizophrenia. *Med Clin North Am* 85:663–689, 2001. A review of the pathophysiology, diagnosis, and treatment of schizophrenia. Provides insight into the difficulty of treating the schizophrenic patient with comorbidities.

TABLE 8-2. Schizophrenia Subtypes

SUBTYPE	COMMENTS
Paranoid	Delusions or hallucinations (frequently auditory). Lacks disorganized speech, disorganized or catatonic behavior, and ⊖ symptoms. Relatively good self-care. Has the best prognosis—relatively good preservation of thought, personality, and function over time.
Disorganized	Prominent disorganized speech, disorganized behavior (poor personal appearance), and flat/inappropriate affect (e.g., disinhibited). Does not involve catatonic behavior. Associated with the worst prognosis.
Catatonic	Diagnosis requires at least two the following: ■ Motor immobility (rigidity) ■ Excessive motor activity ■ Extreme negativism or mutism ■ Peculiar voluntary movement and bizarre posturing (waxy flexibility) ■ Echolalia or echopraxia
Undifferentiated	Has characteristics of > 1 subtype.
Residual	The patient meets the criteria for schizophrenia in the past but now lacks delusions and hallucinations. The patient has residual ⊖ symptoms or attenuated hallucinations, delusions, and other thought disorders.

Schizophreniform Disorder

The prevalence of schizophreniform disorder is slightly less than that of schizophrenia (0.2%). Many patients will eventually develop schizophrenia, while others will develop a mood disorder.

SIGNS AND SYMPTOMS

■ Patients with schizophreniform disorder meet the criteria for schizophrenia, except that the **duration of illness is > 1 month but < 6 months** (instead of > 6 months as in schizophrenia).
■ Social and/or occupational function may or may not be impaired
■ Males and females are equally affected.

TREATMENT

Methods of psychotherapy, family and social-vocational therapies, and pharmacotherapy used in schizophrenia may all be considered in schizophreniform disorder.

■ *Schizophrenia: At least six months of psychotic features.*
■ *Schizophreniform disorder: Requires 1–6 months of psychotic features.*
■ *Brief psychotic disorder: One day to one month of psychotic features.*
■ *Schizoaffective disorder: Combines symptoms of schizophrenia with a major affective disorder (MDD or bipolar disorder).*

HIGH-YIELD FACTS

PSYCHIATRY

KEY ANTIPSYCHOTIC MEDICATIONS

Antipsychotic medications are usually divided into "typical" and "atypical" medications. Atypicals produce fewer EPS, have a better side effect profile, and do not ↑ prolactin levels but are very expensive.

Typical antipsychotics:

- **Drugs:** Can be divided into high, medium, and low potency.
    - **High:** Haloperidol (Haldol), fluphenazine (Prolixin), thiothixene (Navane), droperidol.
    - **Medium:** Trifluoperazine (Stelazine) and perphenazine (Trilafon).
    - **Low:** Thioridazine (Mellaril) and chlorpromazine (Thorazine).
- **Mechanism:** Block dopamine receptors (mostly D_2 and D_4 subtypes).
- **Clinical use:** Most effective in treating ⊕ symptoms.
- **Side effects:** Similar for all typical agents. Higher-potency drugs have more EPS, while lower-potency drugs have more anticholinergic, sedative, and orthostatic hypotensive effects.
    - **EPS:**
        - **Acute dystonia:** Early, sudden-onset twisting of the neck or rolling of the eyes (torticollis and oculogyric crisis, respectively), occurring mainly in young men after 10–14 days of treatment. Treat with IM anticholinergics such as benztropine (Cogentin), trihexyphenidyl (Artane), or diphenhydramine (Benadryl).
        - **Akathisia:** A subjective sense of inner restlessness in the legs that may or may not lead to objective manifestations of restlessness (e.g., walking around or difficulty remaining still). Treat with β-blockers (e.g., propranolol) or benzodiazepines (e.g., clonazepam, diazepam).
        - **Parkinsonism:** Resting tremor, cogwheel rigidity, bradykinesia, shuffling gait, and masklike facies. Treat with oral anticholinergics and possibly amantadine (a dopamine-releasing agent).
        - **Tardive dyskinesia:** Involuntary, abnormal lip smacking, tongue protrusion, and writhing movements of the limbs or trunk. Occurs in 10–30% of long-term neuroleptic users (especially elderly patients, women, and patients with mood disorders). Treatment involves withdrawing neuroleptics or changing to clozapine. Often irreversible.
    - **Neuroleptic malignant syndrome:** Fever, rigidity, autonomic instability, and clouding of consciousness. Can give rise to rhabdomyolysis, myoglobinuria, and renal failure; in this case, CPK is usually markedly ↑. The condition is uncommon but life-threatening (20% mortality). Treat by withdrawing neuroleptics, by initiating supportive measures, and sometimes by administering dantrolene, bromocriptine, or amantadine.

HIGH-YIELD FACTS

PSYCHIATRY

- **Hyperprolactinemia:** Causes amenorrhea, galactorrhea, and gynecomastia. A pituitary tumor must be ruled out.
- **Anticholinergic effects:** Include dry mouth, urinary retention, constipation, and orthostatic hypotension.
- **Other:** Orthostatic hypotension, weight gain, sedation, seizures, and ECG changes or arrhythmias (e.g., conduction delays).

Atypical antipsychotics:

- **Drugs:**
  - **Clozapine (Clozaril):** Thought to be more effective for treatment-resistant schizophrenia and ⊖ symptoms. A dangerous side effect is **agranulocytosis,** which occurs in 0.5–1.0% of patients, thus mandating a weekly CBC for the first six months of treatment and every other week thereafter. Other side effects include severe sedation, anticholinergic effects, orthostatic hypotension, vertigo, weight gain, seizures, arrhythmias, and eosinophilia.
  - **Risperidone (Risperdal):** Does not lead to agranulocytosis. Side effects include a low incidence of EPS, hyperprolactinemia, fatigue, tachycardia, sedation, orthostatic hypotension, and weight gain.
  - **Olanzapine (Zyprexa):** Particularly effective in treating ⊖ symptoms and in treating more agitated patients. Has a low incidence of EPS; the most common side effects are drowsiness, akathisia, weight gain, insomnia, and dry mouth. No hepatotoxicity.
  - **Quetiapine (Seroquel):** This medication has a very low incidence of EPS. Side effects include somnolence and orthostasis. Usually dosed more than once daily.
  - **Ziprasidone (Geodon):** Side effects include QT prolongation, insomnia, and restlessness.
  - **Aripiprazole (Abilify):** A D_2 and 5-HT$_{1A}$ partial agonist and an HT$_{2A}$ antagonist with rapid onset of action and a lower rate of weight gain than other medications, together with a very low rate of hyperprolactinemia or cardiotoxicity.
- **Mechanism:** All medications of this class have some degree of 5-HT$_2$ receptor antagonism, but each has a different combination of receptor blockade.
- **Clinical use:** Atypical antipsychotics have fewer anticholinergic symptoms and EPS. Because of this, they are currently used as first-line drugs in newly diagnosed schizophrenia. These agents can be effective in treating patients with ⊕ and ⊖ symptoms as well as those who are refractory to typical antipsychotics.
- **Side effects:** These drugs do not lead to agranulocytosis but may be less effective than clozapine in treatment-resistant patients. Key side effects of the atypicals as a class include weight gain, type 2 DM, and QT prolongation on ECG.

Brief Psychotic Disorder

This diagnosis carries a better prognosis than schizophrenia.

SIGNS AND SYMPTOMS

Patients exhibit one or more of the following symptoms for one day to one month: delusions, hallucinations, disorganized speech, grossly disorganized behavior, and catatonic behavior.

DIFFERENTIAL

Since the differential diagnosis of an acute psychotic episode is broad and this disorder is rare, it is key to rule out other causes. It should be noted that this disorder can occur with or without the presence of stressors, including parturition (episode within four weeks of giving birth).

TREATMENT

- Brief hospitalization if necessary.
- A short course of neuroleptics or benzodiazepines.

Schizoaffective Disorder

Unlike schizophrenia and schizophreniform disorder, schizoaffective disorder is said to be present when a patient concurrently meets the criteria for schizophrenia and for MDE, manic episode, or mixed episode. The lifetime prevalence is 0.5–0.8%, with a peak age of onset in the late teens and early 20s.

WORKUP

Mood symptoms must be present for a significant portion of the disease, but acute psychotic symptoms (e.g., delusions, hallucinations) must be present for at least two weeks in the absence of mood symptoms. This disorder also has bipolar and depressive subtypes.

TREATMENT

- Give a combination of an antipsychotic and a mood stabilizer.
- Antidepressants and possibly ECT may be indicated for acute depressive types.

Delusional Disorder

Like schizophrenia, delusional disorder is chronic. Unlike schizophrenia, however, its hallmark feature is nonbizarre (or plausible) delusions. The prevalence is 0.03%, with males and females equally affected. The age of onset is variable but generally peaks in the 40s.

What is the prognosis for delusional disorder? Some 10–15% of cases resolve over time, whereas 40–55% worsen and 30–50% do not change.

WORKUP

- To fulfill DSM-IV criteria, delusions must be present for at least one month in the absence of hallucinations, disorganized speech, disorganized behavior, or ⊖ symptoms.
- The subtypes of delusional disorder are defined by the predominant delusional content and are as follows:
  - **Persecutory:** Delusions that the individual is being harassed or malevolently treated.

- **Grandiose:** Delusions that the individual possesses exaggerated power, money, or knowledge.
- **Erotomanic:** Delusions that another person, usually of higher status, is in love with the individual.
- **Somatic:** Delusions that the individual has a physical defect or a medical condition.
- **Jealous:** Delusions that the individual's partner is unfaithful.
- **Mixed:** Delusions that are of > 1 type.
- **Unspecified.**

TREATMENT

Effective treatment is difficult, as most patients are refractory to neuroleptics. Psychotherapy may provide some benefit.

Anxiety disorders are a group of disorders in which anxiety—the presence of a sense of impending doom or threat—is the prominent feature. The patient's anxiety is poorly based in reality, is out of proportion to the actual threat, and is vague or poorly defined. The anxiety disorders are the most prevalent of all psychiatric disorders.

Generalized Anxiety Disorder (GAD)

Has a prevalence of nearly 5%, with a female-to-male ratio of 2:1. GAD commonly coexists with other psychiatric disorders. Patients may report excessive worry as adolescents, but the disorder generally becomes prominent when patients reach their 20s.

SIGNS AND SYMPTOMS

- The defining symptom is **chronic, excessive anxiety or worry** about a number of actual life events
- Somatic manifestations are common and include palpitations, lightheadedness, dizziness, clammy hands, dry mouth, dysphagia, ↑ urinary frequency, difficulty breathing, abdominal pain, and diarrhea.

DIFFERENTIAL

- **Psychiatric:** Other anxiety disorders (e.g., panic disorder, OCD, social phobia, hypochondriasis), mood disorders (e.g., depression, dysthymia), psychotic disorders.
- **Organic:** Hyperthyroidism; pheochromocytoma; abnormalities of calcium, glucose, or phosphate.
- **Pharmacologic:** Substance-induced anxiety disorder (e.g., intoxication with caffeine, cocaine, or amphetamines); substance withdrawal (e.g., benzodiazepines, alcohol).

WORKUP

According to DSM-IV criteria, the patient must have excessive anxiety on more days than not for six or more months, along with at least three of the six following symptoms:

- Restlessness or a feeling of being "on edge"
- Easy fatigability

KEY ANTIANXIETY MEDICATIONS

Benzodiazepines:

- **Drugs (by half-life):**

    - **Long (> 100 hours):** Clonazepam (Klonopin), clorazepate (Tranxene), chlordiazepoxide (Librium), diazepam (Valium), flurazepam (Dalmane).

    - **Intermediate (10–20 hours):** Alprazolam (Xanax), lorazepam (Ativan), temazepam (Restoril).

    - **Short (3–8 hours):** Oxazepam (Serax), triazolam (Halcion).

- **Mechanism:** Bind to $GABA_A$ receptors ($\uparrow$ GABA-binding affinity and $\uparrow$ frequency of chloride channel opening).

- **Clinical use:** Used for a broad spectrum of anxiety disorders (e.g., GAD, social phobia, panic disorder) and sleep disorders (e.g., insomnia) as well as for alcohol detoxification, seizures, catatonia, and mood/adjustment/psychotic disorders with anxiety components. Also used as muscle relaxants.

- **Side effects:** Sedation, slurred speech, ataxia, dizziness, tolerance, cross-tolerance, dependence, anterograde amnesia, and respiratory depression (especially with other sedatives or in COPD patients).

- **Pros:** Lorazepam, oxazepam, and temazepam are not metabolized by the liver and are safe in patients with hepatic dysfunction.

- **Cons:**

    - The potentiation of alcohol and other CNS depressants $\uparrow$ the risk of sedation and respiratory depression. **There is a high risk of dependence and abuse even in patients without a history of substance abuse.** Generally not indicated for long-term treatment of anxiety disorders because of the increasing tolerance and dependence with which they are associated. SSRIs and other psychotropics are better suited for long-term management of anxiety.

    - P-450 inhibitors (e.g., cimetidine, fluoxetine, INH, estrogen) $\uparrow$ levels, while drugs such as carbamazepine and rifampin $\downarrow$ levels.

    - Lorazepam, alprazolam, and diazepam are most frequently abused in patients with a history of alcohol and drug abuse.

    - Withdrawal symptoms are more severe and abrupt with shorter-acting agents.

Buspirone (BuSpar):

- **Mechanism:** Partial agonist for $5\text{-}HT_{1A}$ receptors.

- **Clinical use:** GAD. Not useful in panic disorder. Can augment antidepressant treatment in MDD or OCD.

- **Side effects:** Infrequent sedation, dizziness, headache, and GI upset.

- **Pros:** Safe and without the tolerance, dependence, withdrawal, and respiratory depression of benzodiazepines. Favored in patients with a history of substance abuse.

- **Cons:** Slow onset of action. Thus, **not** useful in panic disorder. Less reliable than benzodiazepines in the treatment of anxiety disorders.

ACUTE PHARMACOTHERAPY FOR GENERALIZED ANXIETY DISORDER

- Like most psychiatric medications, SSRIs and the "atypical" agents require several weeks to show a significant clinical effect. In the interim, patients may be given a benzodiazepine-buspirone combination.

- Benzodiazepines with longer half-lives are used, including clonazepam and diazepam. These medications take effect immediately but lead to dependence and withdrawal with > 2–3 weeks of use.

- Difficulty concentrating or "mind going blank"
- Irritability
- Muscle tension
- Sleep disturbance (insomnia)

TREATMENT

- Combination pharmacotherapy and psychotherapy.
- External stressors (e.g., caffeine, nicotine, sleep disturbances) should be eliminated. First-line pharmacotherapy includes SSRIs, venlafaxine, and buspirone. Avoid benzodiazepines in patients dealing with substance abuse.
- SSRIs and TCAs may be used for the treatment of GAD with depressive symptoms. CBT, with a focus on relaxation techniques, is a useful adjunct.

REFERENCE

Gliatto MF. Generalized anxiety disorder. *Am Fam Physician* 62:1591–1600, 2000. A brief review of GAD.

Panic Disorder

Characterized by unexpected, discrete periods of terror (panic attacks) as well as by anticipatory anxiety about future attacks. The lifetime prevalence is 1.5–3.5%, and women have a threefold ↑ in risk compared to males. The peak age of onset is in the mid-20s, and the disorder rarely presents after the age of 45.

SIGNS AND SYMPTOMS

- The DSM-IV has two criteria for the diagnosis of panic disorder: recurrent, unexpected panic attacks that begin suddenly, peak in intensity within 10 minutes, and include a sensation of intense fear along with at least four of the following symptoms:
    - Palpitations or ↑ heart rate, sweating, trembling, shaking, shortness of breath, or a feeling of choking.
    - Chest pain or discomfort; nausea or abdominal distress; dizziness or lightheadedness.
    - Derealization or depersonalization.
    - Fear of losing control or "going crazy"; fear of dying.
    - Paresthesias, chills, hot flashes.

For which two major comorbid conditions should panic disorder patients be screened? MDD (50%) and agoraphobia (50%).

HIGH-YIELD FACTS

PSYCHIATRY

- At least one attack must be followed for one month or more by one of the following:
  - Persistent worry about additional attacks (anticipatory anxiety).
  - Worry about the implications of the attack.
  - A change in baseline function 2° to the attack.
- Agoraphobia (i.e., fear and avoidance of places or situations where escape might be embarrassing or difficult) is present in 30–50% of cases.

DIFFERENTIAL

- **Psychiatric:** GAD, social phobia, OCD, PTSD.
- **Pharmacologic:** Substance-induced anxiety disorder (e.g., caffeine, cocaine, amphetamines).
- **Organic:** Pheochromocytoma, arrhythmia, pulmonary embolism, hypoxia, angina, hyperthyroidism.

TREATMENT

- Treat with combination pharmacotherapy and psychotherapy.
- The most effective psychotherapy is CBT with a focus on relaxation techniques and reversal of symptom misinterpretation.
- SSRIs are first-line treatment; TCAs and MAOIs are second-line choices. MAOIs are more effective than TCAs, although they are limited in use owing to their side effects.
- Benzodiazepines (often alprazolam and clonazepam) may be used for immediate relief, but long-term use should be avoided in light of their addiction potential. In addition, most panic attacks last less than the time it takes for benzodiazepines to become active, and thus benzodiazepines are seldom useful in acute management.
- Buspirone is **not** effective in panic disorder.

Social Phobia

Defined as at least six months of persistent, intermittent fear of a social or public situation in which the patient is exposed to unfamiliar persons or to situations in which his or her performance will be scrutinized.

- Affects 3–13% of the population, with a female-to-male ratio of 1:1.
- Onset is usually in adolescence and is preceded by childhood shyness.

SIGNS AND SYMPTOMS

- Can be **situational** (most commonly public speaking or meeting new people) or **generalized** (fear of nearly all social situations). Phobic situations usually provoke a panic attack and impair social or occupational functioning.
- Patients recognize that their fear is excessive and irrational.

TREATMENT

- CBT with relaxation techniques.
- Pharmacotherapy consists of MAOIs, SSRIs, and occasionally β-blockers (e.g., for stage fright). Benzodiazepines are indicated if SSRIs are not effective.

Specific Phobia

The most common psychiatric disorder among females and the second most common in males (after substance abuse disorder). The lifetime prevalence is 10–25%, with a female-to-male ratio of 2:1. Most cases begin in childhood. Significant impairment and distress are rare, but comorbid anxiety disorders are common.

SIGNS AND SYMPTOMS

- Common specific phobias encountered in the medical setting involve fear of blood or injections (often with vasovagal syncope). Others include situations such as airplane trips or heights.
- Patients recognize that they have an excessive, irrational fear.

DIFFERENTIAL

- **Psychiatric:** OCD, GAD, panic disorder, social phobia, avoidant personality disorder.
- **Other:** Normal shyness or fear appropriate to the situation.

TREATMENT

- Most childhood specific phobias resolve without treatment.
- Treat persistent phobias by initiating behavioral therapy with flooding (sudden exposure to the feared object or situation) or gradual desensitization through incremental exposures.
- Relaxation and breathing techniques, hypnosis, insight-oriented psychotherapy, or CBT can also be used.

Obsessive-Compulsive Disorder (OCD)

OCD has a lifetime prevalence of 2–3%. Although men and women are equally affected, men tend to develop OCD at an earlier age. The disorder usually begins during adolescence or early adulthood and shows a gradual progression. Issues complicating treatment and diagnosis are concomitant depression, reluctance to discuss symptoms, and substance abuse.

SIGNS AND SYMPTOMS

- The DSM-IV requires that the patient have either obsessions or compulsions and that **the patient recognize them as excessive and irrational.**
  - **Obsessions:** Persistent, unwanted, and **intrusive ideas, thoughts, impulses, or images** that lead to significant anxiety or distress. Common obsessions include cleanliness, contamination, or a fear of harm to self or loved ones.
  - **Compulsions: Repeated mental acts or behaviors** that neutralize anxiety from obsessions—e.g., excessive cleaning (hands may be chafed $2°$ to frequent washing), elaborate rituals for conducting ordinary tasks (e.g., walking through the doorway), or excessive checking (e.g., multiple trips back home to check that the door is locked).
- Obsessions and compulsions must be time-consuming (take up > 1 hour per day), be associated with marked distress, and interrupt normal social or occupational function.

- OCD is **ego dystonic**—
  patients know their
  behavior is problematic.
- OCPD is **ego syntonic**—
  symptoms are part of a
  person's personality, and
  patients are usually
  unaware of their
  problematic perfectionist
  behavior.

DIFFERENTIAL

- **Psychiatric:** GAD, specific phobia, trichotillomania, body dysmorphic disorder, obsessive-compulsive personality disorder (OCPD) (which, in comparison, is ego syntonic and lacks separate obsessions and compulsions), Tourette's syndrome, schizophrenia (which can include obsessions and compulsions, but with hallucinations and delusions), MDD (usually with obsessive rumination).
- **Organic:** Brain tumor or temporal lobe epilepsy.
- **Drugs:** Substance-induced anxiety disorder (e.g., cocaine, amphetamines, caffeine).

TREATMENT

- SSRIs are effective first-line treatment, usually at higher doses than those used for MDD. Clomipramine is also used.
- Behavioral therapy involves exposure-response prevention, thought stopping, and flooding.

Post-Traumatic Stress Disorder (PTSD)

PTSD can occur after an individual is exposed to a traumatic event that is associated with intense fear or horror and that involves actual or threatened harm. Its lifetime prevalence is roughly 8% and is highest among young adults. In populations exposed to combat or assault, however, its prevalence approaches 60%.

SIGNS AND SYMPTOMS

- **Reexperiencing of traumatic events** through intrusive thoughts, flashbacks, and nightmares.
- Persistent **avoidance** of stimuli associated with the trauma.
- A **numbing of responsiveness** indicated by at least three of the following symptoms: anhedonia, amnesia, restricted affect, or detachment.
- ↑ **arousal** as indicated by two of the following: hypervigilance, insomnia, ↑ startle response, poor concentration, and irritability.
- Associated symptoms include survivor guilt, personality change, dissociation, aggression, depression, substance abuse, and suicidality.
- Symptoms must be present for > 1 month and are classified according to their duration:
  - **Acute:** Symptoms present for < 3 months.
  - **Chronic:** Symptoms present for > 3 months.
  - **Delayed onset:** Symptoms start > 6 months after the traumatic event.

DIFFERENTIAL

Acute stress disorder, MDD, OCD, anxiety disorder, adjustment disorder, malingering, borderline personality disorder.

TREATMENT

- SSRIs and mood stabilizers are first-line therapy (higher-than-normal doses of antidepressants are required). Buspirone is occasionally helpful.
- Anxiolytics such as β-blockers, benzodiazepines, and α$_2$-agonists may be used if first-line treatment fails. Benzodiazepines are generally less effec-

*What is acute stress disorder?
It is similar to PTSD, but
symptoms occur within one
month of the traumatic event
and last two days to one
month.*

tive but may be helpful in the early stages; their use must be balanced with the high risk of addiction and abuse potential.
■ CBT and support groups are also effective.

REFERENCE

Yehuda R. Post-traumatic stress disorder. *NEJM* 346:1081–1114, 2002. A brief but excellent review of the epidemiology, pathophysiology, diagnosis, and treatment of PTSD in light of the September 11 tragedy.

PERSONALITY DISORDERS

Personality disorders (see Table 8-3) are maladaptive patterns of perceiving, relating to, and thinking about oneself, other people, and the environment. They typically begin in childhood, crystallize by late adolescence, and affect all facets of the personality, including cognition, mood, behavior, and interpersonal style. However, they are not diagnosed in individuals < 18 years of age. Personality disorders are coded on Axis II and often coexist with, and affect the treatment of, acute psychiatric illnesses (Axis I).

SIGNS AND SYMPTOMS

■ A stable, enduring pattern of experiences and behaviors that deviates markedly from cultural expectations
■ Behaviors are persistent, inflexible, and maladaptive, leading to significant impairment in social or occupational function. Hallmark features are summarized in the mnemonic **MEDIC**.

DIFFERENTIAL

■ Normal variants of an individual's personality or environmental stressors.
■ Substance abuse.
■ Axis I psychiatric disorders (e.g., schizophrenia, MDD, bipolar disorder, delusional disorder, anxiety disorders).

TREATMENT

Long-term psychotherapy is usually the treatment of choice. Pharmacotherapy with anxiolytics and/or low-dose antipsychotics may be necessary for anxiety or agitation.

SUBSTANCE ABUSE AND DEPENDENCE

Substance abuse and dependence have a 13% lifetime prevalence in the United States, and alcohol is the most commonly abused substance (excluding tobacco and caffeine). Alcohol abuse and dependence have a lifetime prevalence of 6% in the general U.S. population. Males are affected nearly four times more frequently than females, but the incidence of alcoholism in women is increasing.

SIGNS AND SYMPTOMS

■ **Substance dependence:** Defined as at least three of the following for at least one year:
  ■ **Tolerance:** Using progressively larger amounts to obtain the same effect.

Personality disorders are pervasive, persistent, maladaptive patterns of behavior.

Features of personality disorders—

MEDIC

Maladaptive
Enduring
Deviates from norm
Inflexible
Causes impaired social functioning

Personality disorders are typically ego syntonic, and patients therefore have little insight into their disorders.

The highest prevalence of alcoholism occurs in males 21–34 years of age.

TABLE 8-3. Classes of Personality Disorders

CLUSTER	EXAMPLE	CHARACTERISTICS	CLINICAL DILEMMA	COPING STRATEGY
Cluster A: "weird"	Paranoid	Persistent distrust and suspicion that others are harming or deceiving the patient. Patients are reluctant to confide in others and perceive attacks on character that are not apparent to others.	Patients are suspicious of physicians and do not trust them. Patients rarely visit the physician.	Use a clear, honest attitude and a noncontrolling, nondefensive approach. Avoid humor and maintain distance. Patients' defense mechanisms are projection and fantasy.
	Schizoid	Social isolation and restricted emotional range (cold and detached). Patients lack close friends, lack interest in sexual experiences, and are indifferent to praise.		
	Schizotypal	Odd beliefs, speech, behavior, or appearance; magical thinking, ideas of references, and unusual "out-of-body" perceptual experiences.		
Cluster B: "wild"	Borderline	Marked impulsivity; unstable sense of self and interpersonal relationships; recurrent suicidal ideation. Inability to control mood lability and chronic feelings of emptiness.	Patients will change the rules on the physician. They are clingy, demand attention, and feel that they are special. Patients will manipulate the physician and staff ("splitting").	**Be firm:** Stick to the treatment plan. **Be fair:** Do not be punitive or derogatory. **Be consistent:** Do not change the rules. Patients' defense mechanisms are dissociation, denial, splitting, and acting out.
	Histrionic	Excess emotionality and attention seeking with a constant need to be the "center of attention." Inappropriate sexual or provocative behavior, self-dramatization, and suggestibility.		

TABLE 8-3. **Classes of Personality Disorders** *(continued)*

CLUSTER	EXAMPLE	CHARACTERISTICS	CLINICAL DILEMMA	COPING STRATEGY
	Narcissistic	Persistent grandiosity about self and accomplishments; need for excessive admiration; sense of entitlement, envy of others, and lack of empathy.		
	Antisocial	Blatant disregard for the rights of others with failure to conform to social norms and lawful behavior. Impulsivity, deceitfulness, and lack of remorse. Disregard for the safety of self and others, aggression, and irresponsibility.		
Cluster C: "worried and wimpy"	Obsessive-compulsive	Preoccupation with details, cleanliness, order, and control over all aspects of life. Perfectionism is evident in excessive devotion to work over leisure. Patients have inflexibility in morals and values, inability to discard objects, miserliness, and rigidity.	Patients may subtly sabotage their own treatment. They are very controlling, with words not necessarily consistent with actions.	Avoid power struggles. Passive wins over active. Give clear treatment recommendations, but do not push patients into a decision. Patients' defense mechanisms are hypochondriasis, passive aggression, and isolation.
	Avoidant	Social inhibition; feelings of inadequacy; excessive shyness and hypersensitivity to rejection. Avoidance of activities and relationships for fear of being disliked or ridiculed.		
	Dependent	Submissive and clinging behavior; a need to be "taken care of"; and difficulty making decisions, expressing disagreement, and initiating projects. Uncomfortable with being alone.		

- **Withdrawal:** Symptoms occur when not taking the substance.
- Persistent desire or attempts to cut down.
- Considerable time and energy spent trying to obtain the substance, use the substance, or recover from its effects.
- Important social, occupational, or recreational activities given up or reduced because of substance use.
- Continued use despite awareness of the problems that it causes.
- **Substance abuse:** Defined as > 1 of the following for at least one year (see also Table 8-4):
  - Failure to fulfill major obligations at work, school, or home.
  - Recurrent substance use in physically hazardous situations.
  - Recurrent substance-related legal problems.
  - Continued use despite problems caused by use.

TABLE 8-4. Signs and Symptoms of Substance Abuse

DRUG	RECEPTOR/MECHANISM	INTOXICATION	WITHDRAWAL
Alcohol	GABA$_A$ and glutamate	Disinhibition, emotional lability, incoordination, slurred speech, ataxia, coma, blackouts (retrograde amnesia).	Tremor, tachycardia, hypertension, malaise, nausea, seizures, DTs, tremulousness, agitation, hallucinations.
Opioids	Opioid receptor (μ, δ, κ) agonism	CNS depression, nausea and vomiting, constipation, pupillary constriction, seizures, respiratory depression (overdose is life-threatening).	Anxiety, insomnia, anorexia, sweating, fever, rhinorrhea, piloerection, nausea, stomach cramps, diarrhea.
Amphetamines (dextroamphetamine, methamphetamine)	Norepinephrine, dopamine, and 5-HT release and reuptake inhibition	Psychomotor agitation, impaired judgment, pupillary dilation, hypertension, tachycardia, euphoria, prolonged wakefulness and attention, cardiac arrhythmias, delusions, hallucinations, fever.	Postuse "crash," including anxiety, lethargy, headache, stomach cramps, hunger, severe depression, dysphoria, fatigue, and insomnia/hypersomnia.
MDMA ("Ecstasy")	5-HT release and reuptake inhibition, dopamine reuptake inhibition	Euphoria; excessive empathy, trust, sociability; anorexia, hyperthermia.	"Serotonin dip" (dysphoria, fatigue, memory problems, ↓ libido).
Cocaine	Norepinephrine, acetylcholine, 5-HT, and dopamine reuptake inhibition	Euphoria, psychomotor agitation, impaired judgment, tachycardia, pupillary dilation, hypertension, hallucinations (including tactile), paranoid ideations, angina, hyperthermia, arrhythmias, respiratory depression, convulsions, death.	Hypersomnolence, fatigue, depression, malaise, suicidality.

TABLE 8-4. **Signs and Symptoms of Substance Abuse** *(continued)*

DRUG	RECEPTOR/MECHANISM	INTOXICATION	WITHDRAWAL
Phencyclidine piperidine (PCP)	NMDA and acetylcholine antagonism	Altered ability to differentiate between self and nonself; belligerence, impulsiveness, fever, psychomotor agitation, vertical and horizontal nystagmus, tachycardia, ataxia, homicidality, psychosis, delirium.	Recurrence of symptoms due to reabsorption from lipid stores; sudden onset of severe violence.
Lysergic acid diethylamide (LSD)	5-HT$_2$ agonism	Marked anxiety or depression, delusions, visual hallucinations, flashbacks.	
Marijuana	Opioid, acetylcholine, norepinephrine, and dopamine release	Euphoria, anxiety, paranoid delusions, slowed sense of time, impaired judgment, social withdrawal, ↑ appetite, dry mouth, conjunctival injection, persecutory delusions, hallucinations, amotivation.	
Barbiturates	GABA$_A$ agonism	Respiratory depression (major).	Anxiety, seizures, delirium, life-threatening cardiovascular collapse.
Benzodiazepines	GABA$_A$ agonism	Alcohol interactions, amnesia, ataxia, sleep, respiratory depression.	Rebound anxiety, seizures, tremor, insomnia, hypertension, tachycardia.
Caffeine	Adenosine antagonism, norepinephrine release	Restlessness, insomnia, diuresis, muscle twitching, arrhythmias.	Headache, lethargy, depression, weight gain.
Nicotine/tobacco	β-subunit acetylcholine agonism, dopamine release	Restlessness, insomnia, anxiety, arrhythmias.	Irritability, headache, anxiety, weight gain, tachycardia.

Adapted, with permission, from Le T et al. *First Aid for the USMLE Step 2 CK,* 5th ed. New York: McGraw-Hill, 2006: 336.

DIFFERENTIAL

Delirium, Axis I disorders (schizophrenia, MDD, bipolar disorder, anxiety disorders).

WORKUP

■ A complete history is key. It is often necessary to consult collateral sources (e.g., family, friends), since substance use is often denied or underreported.

↑ *GGT and* ↑ *MCV suggest what type of substance abuse?*

Chronic alcohol abuse (GGT from liver damage; MCV from folate or B$_{12}$ deficiency, leading to macrocytic anemia).

- Use the **CAGE** questionnaire (see mnemonic) to screen for alcoholism.
- Toxicology screen, CBC, electrolytes, LFTs, and a Breathalyzer or serum ethanol level.
- Always offer HIV testing to substance abusers (especially IV drug abusers), as they often engage in high-risk behaviors.

TREATMENT

- Treatment depends on the substance abused and the context in which it is used (see Table 8-5). The first goal is usually abstinence/detoxification; the rehabilitation process then targets the patient's physical, psychological, and social well-being.
- The treatment of alcohol withdrawal includes the following:
  - Rule out any medical complications (e.g., hepatic dysfunction, Wernicke's encephalopathy) by physical exam and laboratory tests.
  - Start a benzodiazepine taper for withdrawal symptoms (e.g., chlordiazepoxide). Lorazepam, temazepam, or oxazepam should be used if the patient has liver dysfunction.
  - Give multivitamins with thiamine (before glucose) and folate. Correct any electrolyte abnormalities.
  - Check vital signs and give fluid replacement if necessary.
  - For patients with an alcohol seizure history, give anticonvulsants. Avoid neuroleptics, which ↓ seizure threshold.
  - Alcohol dependence can be treated with group therapy (Alcoholics Anonymous), disulfiram, and naltrexone.

COMPLICATIONS

- ↑ risk of accidental and traumatic injuries, especially motor vehicle accidents.
- IV drug abusers are at ↑ risk of acquiring HIV, HBV, HCV, endocarditis, cellulitis (especially among "skin poppers"), and STDs.

ALCOHOL WITHDRAWAL SYNDROMES

- **Uncomplicated withdrawal:** Occurs within several hours (usually 6–8 hours) after cessation of drinking; characterized by tremulousness, tachycardia, hypertension, diaphoresis, anxiety, nausea, insomnia, hypervigilance, hyperreflexia, weakness, tinnitus, blurred vision, paresthesias, and numbness.

- **Alcohol hallucinosis:** Occurs within two days after cessation of or ↓ in drinking and is characterized by auditory hallucinations that persist after the withdrawal symptoms have disappeared. The sensorium is clear (no delirium). Delusions or paranoid ideation may be present.

- **Delirium tremens (DTs):** Occur approximately 1–8 days after cessation of drinking (most often within 24–72 hours after cessation) and can be life-threatening (has an untreated mortality of 15–20%). DTs are characterized by disorientation, fever, agitation, tremor, delusions, seizures, memory deficits, insomnia, visual and tactile hallucinations, and autonomic instability.

TABLE 8-5. Management of Intoxication

DRUG	MANAGEMENT
Hallucinogens (e.g., LSD)	If severe, benzodiazepines or traditional antipsychotics; otherwise, provide reassurance.
Cocaine	Severe agitation is treated with haloperidol, benzodiazepines, antiemetics, antidiarrheals, and NSAIDs (for muscle cramps).
PCP	If severe, benzodiazepines; otherwise, provide reassurance.
Amphetamines	Same as that for cocaine.
Opioids	Naloxone/naltrexone block opioid receptors, reversing their effects. Beware of the antagonist being cleared before the opioid, particularly with longer-acting opioids such as methadone.

■ Substance abusers are often exceptionally destructive both to themselves and to their families. Always ask about the care of their children (you may need to contact child protection agencies) and how they obtain their drug money (this may give you clues to other potential medical and legal problems).

REFERENCE

McRae AL et al. Alcohol and substance abuse. *Med Clin North Am* 85: 779–801, 2001. An overview of the various drugs of abuse, associated symptoms of intoxication and withdrawal, and treatment options for individual substances.

CHILDHOOD AND ADOLESCENT DISORDERS

Many of these disorders are more common in boys and often coexist with other conditions. In addition, childhood disorders can persist into adulthood or parallel similar disorders in adults. In many cases, the combination of gender, maladaptive interactions between the child and the environment, and unconscious or conscious prompting by parents can play a role in these disorders. Interviewing a child poses a unique dilemma; pictures, role playing, and storytelling are techniques that can be used to facilitate the interview.

Attention-Deficit Hyperactivity Disorder (ADHD)

A disorder of attention that occurs almost nine times more often in boys than in girls, with 7% of school-age children and an estimated 4% of adults in the United States affected. ADHD generally presents in children between 3 and 13 years of age and typically manifests as poor performance in school. There is a genetic predisposition to this condition.

What proportion of children with ADHD show symptom resolution by adulthood? Nearly 40%.

SIGNS AND SYMPTOMS

- Inattention in work/school/play, hyperactivity, distractibility, and/or impulsivity that lead to significant impairment in academic and social function.
- Many children also have associated learning disabilities.

DIFFERENTIAL

- **Psychiatric:** Learning disability, major depression, bipolar disorder, cyclothymic disorder, anxiety disorders, intermittent explosive disorder, oppositional defiant disorder.
- **Organic:** Head trauma.
- **Pharmacologic:** Bronchodilators and sedatives (sleeping pills may exhibit paradoxic stimulant effect in children).
- **Other:** Normal active child.

WORKUP

The diagnosis and treatment of ADHD is controversial, particularly in adults. This may stem from the use of behavior to diagnose a presumably cognitive problem that may not always significantly impair functioning.

- Diagnosis requires six or more symptoms of inattention or six or more symptoms of hyperactivity and impulsivity (listed below) in at least two settings that lead to clinically significant impairment in social and academic functioning.
- Symptoms cannot be accounted for by another Axis I disorder and must present before age seven.
- ADHD is classified as predominantly inattentive type, predominantly hyperactive/impulsive type (more common in boys), or combined.
  - **Inattentive:**
    - Makes careless mistakes owing to inability to pay attention to detail.
    - Has difficulty maintaining attention in schoolwork or at play.
    - Has difficulty listening even when spoken to directly.
    - Fails to follow instructions or complete tasks or schoolwork.
    - Has difficulty organizing tasks and activities.
    - Avoids or dislikes tasks requiring concentration or sustained mental effort.
    - Loses items necessary for completion of school tasks (e.g., pencils, paper, books).
    - Is easily distracted by external stimuli.
    - Is forgetful in daily activities.
  - **Hyperactive/impulsive:**
    - Fidgety (e.g., squirms in seat).
    - Unexpectedly leaves desk in classroom.
    - Runs about excessively in inappropriate situations.
    - Has difficulty playing quietly.
    - Is often "on the go" or acts as if "driven by a motor."
    - Talks excessively.
    - Blurts out answers before questions have been completed.
    - Has difficulty waiting his or her turn.
    - Often interrupts or intrudes on others.

TREATMENT

- First-line treatment for ADHD is conservative. Address associated learning disabilities and maladaptive family behavior patterns. Behavioral modification techniques are often useful.
- Pharmacologic treatment is used for cases in which impairment is significant and is not improved by conservative measures:

KEY ADHD MEDICATIONS

Psychostimulants:

- **Drugs:** Methylphenidate (Ritalin, Concerta), dextroamphetamine (Dexedrine), pemoline (Cylert), and dextroamphetamine + racemic amphetamine (Adderall).

- **Clinical use:** Treatment of ADHD in children and adolescents.

- **Side effects:** Insomnia, ↓ appetite, irritability, tachycardia, hypertension, exacerbation of tics, ↓ growth velocity.

- **Pros:** Long history of clinical use.

- **Cons:** Methylphenidate is a schedule II controlled substance.

Nonstimulants—atomoxetine (Strattera):

- **Mechanism:** Selective norepinephrine reuptake inhibitor.

- **Clinical use:** Treatment of ADHD in children, adolescents, and adults.

- **Side effects:** GI distress, nausea, dry mouth, and severe liver injury (rare). Avoid MAOIs.

- **Pros:** Minimal anorexia; QD or BID dosing; no abuse potential.

Antidepressants:

- **Drugs:** Nortriptyline, imipramine, and bupropion.

α_2-agonists:

- **Drugs:** Clonidine and guanfacine (better for hyperactivity and impulsivity than for inattention).

- **Psychostimulants:** Methylphenidate (has abuse potential); dextroamphetamine. Side effects include insomnia, ↓ appetite, tic exacerbation, and ↓ growth velocity. These drugs have high abuse potential and high street value. Amphetamines may also have long-term effects on neural development.
- **Other:** Antidepressants and α_2-agonists can also be used.

REFERENCES

- Herrerias CT et al. The child with ADHD: Using the AAP Clinical Practice Guideline. *Am Fam Physician* 63:1803–1810, 2001. A review article on the criteria for diagnosis of ADHD. Includes excellent flow charts.
- Smucker WD, Hedayat M. Evaluation and treatment of ADHD. *Am Fam Physician* 64:817–830, 2001. A brief, easy-to-read review of the diagnosis and treatment of ADHD.

Pervasive Developmental Disorders

Pervasive developmental disorders are severe, persistent impairments in developmental areas (e.g., communication, social interaction) or stereotypical, repetitive behaviors or interests. They encompass a number of disorders, including autism, Asperger's syndrome, Rett syndrome, and childhood disintegrative disorder.

*Contrary to some popular media reports, extensive research has concluded that childhood vaccination does **not** lead to autism.*

Nearly 75% of autistic children have comorbid mental retardation, and approximately 25% have seizures.

Other pervasive developmental disorders:

- **Asperger's syndrome:** *An autism-like disorder without marked language or cognitive delays.*
- **Rett syndrome:** *A genetic neurodegenerative disorder of females with progressive impairment (language, coordination) after several months of normal development.*
- **Childhood disintegrative disorder:** *Severe developmental regression after < 2 years of normal development.*
- **PDD NOS (not otherwise specified):** *Diagnosis for people who are well described by the "PDD" label but cannot be categorized by any other disorder.*

Autism, like schizophrenia, involves a preoccupation with the internal world. Autism has an incidence of 2–6 in 10,000 live births, frequently presents before the age of four, and is 3–4 times more common in males. It is organic in nature, **not** a reaction to a cold and distant mother, and is associated with familial transmission, tuberous sclerosis, and fragile X syndrome.

SIGNS AND SYMPTOMS

Autism generally presents with three hallmark features: deficiencies in social interaction, communication, and behavior. Impairing symptoms and restricted activities/interests should be evident before age three.

- **Impaired social interaction:** Failure to develop nonverbal communication skills such as a social smile; impaired ability or desire to create relationships (with parents or peers) or show enjoyment.
- **Communication deficiencies:** Impaired language development, inability to start or sustain a conversation, and use of repetitive or idiosyncratic language (e.g., echolalia, pronoun reversals, abnormalities in speech quality).
- **Behavioral deficiencies:** Represent patients' fixation on the internal world. Patients may show ritualized behaviors (e.g., staring at the flushing toilet), stereotyped motor movements (e.g., body rocking), and preoccupation with a restricted area of knowledge (e.g., sports trivia). They may also show self-injurious behavior (e.g., biting oneself) and compulsive behavior (e.g., arranging objects in a certain way).

The American Academy of Pediatrics recommends that all children be screened for autism at well-child checks at 18 and 24 months. Key points to note include no babbling by 12 months, no gesturing by 12 months, no single words by 16 months, no two-word spontaneous phrases by 24 months, and any loss of language/social skills at any age.

DIFFERENTIAL

- **Psychiatric:** Mental retardation, childhood psychosis, language disorders, OCD, Tourette's syndrome, other pervasive developmental disorders.
- **Organic:** Congenital deafness or blindness, congenital CMV, hepatic encephalopathy, fragile X syndrome.

WORKUP

- Obtain a complete history and an MSE.
- Monitor developmental milestones and delays.
- Evaluate vision and hearing.

TREATMENT

- Provide a highly structured educational setting to help patients learn communication and living skills.
- Behavioral management to help reduce stereotyped behaviors.
- Psychotherapy may be of benefit both to the parents and to the patient.
- Unless a comorbid disorder is present, medications are rarely useful. Neuroleptics may be given for aggressive and self-injurious behaviors, and anticonvulsants may be used for concurrent seizure disorder.

Conduct Disorder

Defined as a repetitive and persistent pattern of inappropriate conduct for six months or more in which patients < 18 years of age ignore or violate the rights of others. Patients frequently have comorbid ADHD or learning disorders.

SIGNS AND SYMPTOMS

- Behavior can be aggressive (e.g., violence, destruction, theft) or nonaggressive (e.g., violation of rules, lying).
- Patients may or may not form social bonds, but if they do, bonding with a loyal group often manifests in gang formation.
- If behavior continues as an adult, it is defined as antisocial personality disorder.

TREATMENT

Individual and family therapy is necessary to address emotional conflicts and sociocultural factors.

Mental Retardation

Defined as intellectual functioning significantly below that expected for a child's developmental stage, with cognitive performance below the third percentile of the general population. Mental retardation has a prevalence of 1–2% and is two times more common in males than in females. Causes include genetic disorders, congenital infections, teratogens, and disease acquired after birth. Down syndrome and fragile X syndrome are common causes.

SIGNS AND SYMPTOMS

- IQ (defined as mental age divided by chronological age) ≤ 70 (see Table 8-6).
- Concurrent deficiencies in multiple areas of adaptive functioning (e.g., social skills, self-hygiene, communication).
- Onset of symptoms before the age of 18.

DIFFERENTIAL

Learning disorders, depression, seizure disorders, ADHD, schizophrenia.

TABLE 8-6. Levels of Mental Retardation

LEVEL	IQ SCORE	EDUCATIONAL POTENTIAL
Mild	50–69	Educable
Moderate	35–49	Trainable
Severe	20–34	Limited
Profound	< 20	Very limited

Patients with oppositional defiant disorder do not show blatant disregard for the rights of others. Instead, such patients demonstrate disruptive, annoying behavior inappropriate for their mental age.

Fragile X syndrome is the most common heritable form of mental retardation. Fetal alcohol syndrome is the most common potentially preventable cause of mental retardation.

■ Physical exam (including neurologic exam).
■ IQ testing. Levels of severity are borderline (IQ 70–79), mild (IQ 50–69, 85% of cases), moderate (IQ 35–49), severe (IQ 20–34), and profound (IQ < 20).
■ Brain imaging and EEG (if seizure disorder is suspected).

TREATMENT

Management depends on severity. Family counseling and support, speech and language therapy, occupational/physical therapy, behavioral therapy, and educational assistance may all be useful.

■ **Mild:** Patients may be able to function in society and maintain employment.
■ **Moderate:** Patients should be able to perform activities of daily living and live in a group home.
■ **Severe:** Patients are unable to care for themselves and usually suffer a premature death.

Learning Disorders

Learning disorders are relatively common, affecting roughly 5% of school-aged children. Males are at a two- to fourfold greater risk than females. Such disorders are also more common in those of low SES. Diagnosis is usually made around the fourth or fifth grade.

SIGNS AND SYMPTOMS

■ There are three categories of learning disorders: reading, mathematics, and written expression.
■ In comparison to mental retardation, learning disorders are deficiencies in a particular area that place the child below the expected performance for his or her chronological age, intelligence, and education (often measured by standardized test achievement).

DIFFERENTIAL

Mental retardation, communication disorders, ADHD, depression, anxiety disorders (e.g., school phobia), physical disorders (e.g., abnormal hearing or sight), cultural factors (e.g., language barriers), poor education.

WORKUP

Involves intelligence and subject-specific achievement testing.

TREATMENT

Management involves learning strategies to overcome deficits, academic remediation, and, if possible, teaching in environments that support patients.

Tourette's Syndrome

More common in males, and has a genetic predisposition. Associated with ADHD, learning disorders, and OCD, both clinically and in functional MRI studies of patients with these disorders.

- Onset is before age 18.
- Presents with multiple motor tics (e.g., blinking, grimacing) and vocal tics (e.g., grunting, coprolalia) occurring many times throughout the day, recurrently, for > 1 year.

TREATMENT

- Haloperidol, pimozide, or clonidine. Counseling can aid in social adjustment and coping.
- Psychostimulants (treatment for ADHD) can worsen tics, but with severe ADHD, treatment with stimulants should nonetheless be considered.

MISCELLANEOUS DISORDERS

Adjustment Disorder

- A state in which emotional ideas and actions are the result of a particular stressor.
- The disorder must arise within three months of experiencing the stressor and, unless the stressor is chronic, must resolve within six months.
- To qualify as an adjustment disorder, Axis I or bereavement criteria must not be met.

Anorexia Nervosa

An eating disorder affecting 0.5–1.0% of females with a female-to-male ratio of nearly 20:1. The peak ages of onset are 14 and 18, although the disorder has been diagnosed in much younger girls. Nearly two-thirds of patients have a history of a depressive episode.

SIGNS AND SYMPTOMS

- A body weight < 85% of ideal body weight (for age and height).
- Patients have a distorted body image (patients perceive themselves, incorrectly, as fat) and an intense fear of gaining weight.
- Patterns of dieting include **restricting** (e.g., fasting, dieting, or exercising excessively) or engaging in **binge-eating/purging** behavior.
- Amenorrhea (absence of three consecutive cycles) and ↓ sexual activity/interest are common.
- Patients may exhibit lanugo, dry skin, bradycardia, lethargy, hypotension, electrolyte disturbances (e.g., metabolic acidosis due to vomiting and/or metabolic alkalosis due to laxatives), cold intolerance, anemia and leukopenia, osteoporosis, nephrolithiasis, and low thyroid function.
- A rigid personality, obsessive-compulsive features (e.g., counting calories), and a need to control the social environment are also seen.

DIFFERENTIAL

- **Psychiatric:** MDD, social phobia, OCD, bulimia nervosa, body dysmorphic disorder.
- **Organic:** AIDS, malignancies, superior mesenteric ischemia (all of which lead to vomiting or weight loss without a distorted body image), Addison's disease, DM, hyperthyroidism, drug abuse.

Mortality rates approach 10–15% for patients who have been hospitalized for anorexia nervosa.

Rapid refeeding following anorexic starvation can precipitate a syndrome of hypermetabolic hypophosphatemia, so feeding should be done in a slow, controlled manner, and labs should be checked regularly.

Unlike patients with anorexia nervosa, bulimic patients usually maintain a normal or only slightly decreased body weight.

What musculoskeletal complaint may frequently be reported by patients with bulimia? Muscle spasms due to low serum potassium and sodium.

WORKUP

- Conduct a complete H&P and psychiatric evaluation with attention to any comorbid disorders.
- Obtain height and weight measurements.
- Labs/studies include CBC, serum albumin ($\downarrow$), electrolytes (hypocalcemia, hypokalemia, hyponatremia), endocrine tests, and an ECG.

TREATMENT

- Early treatment involves monitoring caloric intake to stabilize weight and achieve weight gain.
- In severe cases, hospitalization may be required to restore nutritional status and/or to correct electrolyte imbalances.
- Later treatment includes individual, family, and/or group psychotherapy.
- SSRIs may help treat comorbid depression.

REFERENCE

Golden NH. Eating disorders in adolescence and their sequelae. *Best Pract Res Clin Obstet Gynaecol* 17(1):57–73, 2003. An excellent assessment of anorexic complications, focusing on management of amenorrhea and osteomalacia.

Bulimia Nervosa

Bulimia nervosa has a prevalence of 1–3% in young females and 0.1–0.3% in males. It is characterized by recurrent episodes of bingeing (eating excessive amounts of food in a two-hour period) during which the patient feels a lack of self-control. Most patients have a history of dieting, and many have coexisting personality or impulse-control disorders.

SIGNS AND SYMPTOMS

- Presents with dental enamel erosion (from vomiting), enlarged parotid glands, and scars on the dorsal surfaces of the hands (from inducing vomiting).
- Menstrual irregularities are also seen.
- Emetic abuse can lead to cardiomyopathy, and laxatives can damage GI mucosa.

WORKUP

- To fulfill DSM-IV criteria for bulimia, bingeing and compensatory behavior must occur at least twice a week for three months.
- Binge eating takes place rapidly and secretly. Bulimic patients tend to be more disturbed by and ashamed of their behavior than anorexic patients.
- Patients try to compensate for binge behaviors through vomiting, excessive exercise, or laxatives in order to prevent weight gain.
- Electrolyte abnormalities (hypochloremic hypokalemic metabolic alkalosis 2° to vomiting) may be seen.

TREATMENT

- Bulimic patients are more easily engaged in therapy than anorexic patients.
- Psychotherapy and CBT are the most effective treatments and focus on behavior and body self-image modification.
- Antidepressants such as fluoxetine, imipramine, and desipramine are effective in both depressed and nondepressed patients.

Somatoform and Related Disorders

The principal characteristics of somatoform and related disorders are outlined in Tables 8-7 and 8-8.

TABLE 8-7. Somatoform Disorders

DISORDER	COMMENTS
Somatization disorder (Briquet's syndrome)	A history of many physical complaints beginning before age 30 and occurring over a period of several years. Affects up to 1% of the population, with a 5:1 female-to-male predominance. Individual symptoms must include four pain symptoms, two GI symptoms, one sexual symptom, and one pseudoneurologic symptom. Symptoms cannot be explained by organic causes and are in excess of exam findings. Patients may have had multiple procedures or surgeries and often "doctor shop." Psychotherapy and regular, planned, brief 1° care visits may be beneficial.
Conversion disorder	One or more **neurologic** complaints (e.g., paralysis, paresthesia, blindness, pseudoseizures) that cannot be explained by a medical disorder. Psychological factors must be associated with symptom onset in order for the diagnosis to be made. Patients often show a characteristic lack of concern (*"la belle indifférence"*). Conversion is most common in women, usually affecting adolescents and young adults. Men have been noted to experience this disorder after battlefield trauma. May spontaneously remit, but anxiolytics may help. Symptoms are not intentionally produced or feigned.
Hypochondriasis	Preoccupation with and fear of having a serious disease leading to significant psychological distress and/or impaired social or occupational functioning for > 6 months. Based on misinterpretation of bodily symptoms. Men and women are equally affected; onset is most common between 20 and 30 years of age. Group therapy and frequent reassurance from the physician are necessary for treatment.
Body dysmorphic disorder	Preoccupation with an imagined physical defect or abnormality (e.g., facial features, hair, body build) or, if a defect is present, excessive concern about that defect. The preoccupation must lead to significant distress or impaired social and occupational functioning. Patients often present to dermatologists or plastic surgeons. Women are affected slightly more often than men, with an average onset at 15–20 years of age. May be associated with depression. Antidepressants such as SSRIs and clomipramine may be effective.

TABLE 8-8. Nonsomatoform Disorders

DISORDER	COMMENTS
Malingering	Occurs when a patient intentionally feigns illness for 2° gain (e.g., financial compensation, avoiding work, obtaining food or shelter). It differs from factitious disorder (defined below) in that what is sought is concrete and is usually related to material gain.
Factitious disorder (Munchausen syndrome)	Conscious simulation or creation of psychiatric or physical symptoms or illness for 1° gain in order to play the sick role and receive attention from medical personnel. It is most common in men and among health care personnel. **Munchausen by proxy** involves simulation of illness in another person, usually in a child by a parent.

Suicidality

Suicide is the eighth leading cause of death in the United States and is the second leading cause of death (after accidents) in people between the ages of 15 and 24. In general, women are more likely to attempt suicide than men, but men are more likely to complete suicide. Men are also more likely to commit suicide by violent means such as firearm use; women are more likely to commit suicide by drug ingestion. Risk factors include the following:

Suicide risk factors—

SAD PERSONS

Sex (male)
Age
Depression
Previous attempt
Ethanol
Rational thought
Sickness
Organized plan
No spouse
Social support lacking

- A previous suicide attempt.
- Male gender.
- Increasing age.
- Depression (depressed patients are 30 times more likely to commit suicide than the general population) or other psychiatric illness; recent recovery from suicidal depression (since patients have regained the energy to kill themselves) or recovery from a first episode of schizophrenia (since patients have developed insight).
- Alcohol or substance abuse.
- The presence of rational thought or an organized plan.
- A family history of suicide.
- A recent severe stressor (e.g., bereavement, job loss, examinations).
- Chronic medical conditions or illnesses (e.g., terminal cancer, HIV).
- Divorced parents, unmarried status, poor social support.
- **Other demographics:** Caucasians commit suicide more frequently than do African-Americans; Protestants have a higher suicide rate than do Catholics. Police officers and physicians have a higher suicide rate than that of any other occupation.

*Asking the patient about suicide will **not** "plant" the idea in the patient's thoughts.*

WORKUP

- Ask the patient about a ⊕ family history, a previous attempt, ambivalence about death, and feelings of hopelessness. Ask specifically about suicidal ideation, intent, and plan.
- Assess if the patient has an available means of committing suicide.
- Perform a complete MSE.

TREATMENT

■ Patients who express the desire to kill themselves, or who you believe may do so, require emergent inpatient hospitalization even if it is against their wishes. The actively suicidal patient needs intensive monitoring, close contact, and ongoing assessment.

■ When the patient is stable, identification of the underlying stressor/disorder is necessary. Patients frequently require intensive psychotherapy and hospitalization as well as antidepressant and antipsychotic medication.

■ ECT may be used as a second-line treatment for actively suicidal patients who are refractory to medications and psychotherapy. Severely depressed patients are often at greatest risk for suicide in the first few weeks after starting an antidepressant, as their energy may return before the depressed mood lifts.

Sexual and Physical Abuse

Most frequently affect women < 35 years of age. Many women affected have a partner who is a substance abuser and/or abuse substances themselves, or have a restraining order against a current or previous spouse or significant other. Women who are abused are also often experiencing marital discord, are of low SES, or are pregnant. Victims of childhood abuse are more likely to be abused as adults and are at risk of becoming abusers.

SIGNS AND SYMPTOMS

■ Frequent ER visits with multiple somatic complaints, bruising, unexplained injuries, and delayed medical treatment.

■ Look for unequal power in interactions between victim and partner.

■ Patients may act afraid or hostile, deny abuse, and avoid eye contact.

■ Children may present with premature sexual behavior, genital or anal trauma, STDs, UTIs, and psychiatric trauma.

TREATMENT

■ Emotional support and counseling.

■ Medical care.

■ Provide information to the patient about available support services, and encourage them to contact such services. Document the encounter.

COMMON CLERKSHIP TOPICS

The following is a list of core topics that you are likely to encounter in the course of your psychiatry rotation and on a shelf examination:

■ **Mental status exam, Mini-Mental Status Exam, five axes**
■ **Mood disorders:**
   ■ Major depressive disorder
   ■ Dysthymic disorder
   ■ Bipolar disorder
   ■ Cyclothymia
■ **Psychotic disorders:**
   ■ Schizophrenia
   ■ Schizophreniform disorder
   ■ Brief psychotic disorder
   ■ Schizoaffective disorder
   ■ Delusional disorder

- **Anxiety disorders:**
  - Generalized anxiety disorder
  - Panic disorder
  - Social phobia
  - Specific phobia
  - Obsessive-compulsive disorder
  - Post-traumatic stress disorder
- **Personality disorders**
- **Substance abuse, dependence, withdrawal**
- **Childhood and adolescent disorders:**
  - Attention-deficit hyperactivity disorder
  - Pervasive developmental disorders—autism
  - Conduct disorder
  - Mental retardation
  - Learning disorders
  - Tourette's syndrome
- **Miscellaneous disorders:**
  - Adjustment disorder
  - Anorexia nervosa
  - Bulimia nervosa
  - Somatoform and factitious disorders
  - Suicidality
  - Sexual and physical abuse
  - Dementia
  - Delirium
  - Pathologic grief
  - Sleep disturbances
  - Issues regarding the dying patient

Surgery

The general surgery rotation is among the most challenging experiences of medical school, largely because of the vast amount of clinical information that must be assimilated along with the significant demands made on students' time and energy. Many students thus look toward their surgery rotations with unbridled enthusiasm, extreme trepidation, or, more commonly, a combination of both. Your success on this rotation will hinge on your accumulation of knowledge, your performance of appropriate scut work, and your interactions with the clinical team, nursing staff, and ancillary personnel. At the same time, the culture of surgery will likely color your experience and perceptions of the field as a whole and, in so doing, may help you make the big career decision of "medicine or surgery." In either case, most students finish their surgery rotation with a vastly increased fund of knowledge, more confidence in their clinical skills, and, inevitably, a newfound appreciation for food and sleep.

What Is the Rotation Like?

The surgery clerkship is designed to expose students to the principles of basic surgical management, including the evaluation of patients to determine the need for surgery; pre- and postoperative care; and hands-on experience in basic bedside procedures, sterile technique, and operating room (OR) tasks (although such tasks are often limited to cutting sutures, retracting tissue, and suctioning). The structure of the rotation will vary from service to service and even, at times, within the same facility, depending on the patient population served, the nature of the surgical illnesses managed, and the specific emphases of the attendings on a given service. As with your other rotations, your experience in surgery will be heavily influenced by the team of residents and attendings with whom you work. The following outline summarizes the nature and responsibilities of the clerkship:

- **Clinical experience:**
  - Inpatient and ambulatory experience in general surgery.
  - Trauma/emergency service.
  - Surgical subspecialties, often including otolaryngology, cardiothoracic surgery, urology, orthopedics, neurosurgery, and plastic surgery.
- **Didactic instruction:**
  - Conferences and lectures on basic principles of patient management and surgical disease.
  - Departmental grand rounds, weekly multidisciplinary conferences (e.g., gastroenterology, oncology), and lectures organized by the faculty for the students.
  - Weekly service conferences in which the house staff present details of the patient census, operative and perioperative complications, and patient cases that illustrate interesting clinical issues.
  - Informal teaching sessions from the house staff as time permits.
  - In what little time you have left over, you will be expected to read and assimilate as much material as possible throughout the course of your rotation.
- **Responsibilities:**
  - Prerounding on all patients.
  - Presenting patients on ward rounds.

- Writing the admission history and physical (H&P) for new patients.
- Writing notes (preoperative, operative, postoperative) on the patients whose surgeries you are involved with.
- **You should:**
  - Try to follow patients from the beginning of their admission through their surgery and postsurgical care. Such longitudinal care will allow you to cultivate a better relationship with your patients while simultaneously enabling you to see the complete picture. The residents will love you for doing this!
  - Always keep in mind that competence is only half the story; knowing your patients will impress not only the patients themselves but your residents and attendings as well.
  - **Try to plan out** which surgery you want to participate in the next day; then read up on the procedure and relevant anatomy, and **learn something about the patient's history and presentation.**
  - Practice some basic suturing and knot-tying skills in the event that you are presented with the opportunity to help close an incision.
  - Learn some of the medical jargon common to surgeries, and be willing to **ask questions** pertaining to the technique involved or to the prognosis of the surgery being performed.
  - Be ready to **answer questions** about the basic anatomy, surgical procedure, and prognosis of the surgery being performed.
  - Strive to create a balanced experience—one in which you spend enough time in the OR to understand sterile technique and get a basic handle on the issues of intraoperative care while devoting most of your time to helping residents take care of patients and reading relevant material.

Who Are the Players?

Attendings. Every service is staffed by several attendings, each of whom has senior responsibility for patient management. Patients on the surgical service are either private patients followed by the attending in his or her private clinic or patients who were admitted to the service by the ward team (e.g., from the ER or other services from which patients are referred for surgical management). In the latter case, the attending who is "on call" for new admissions (i.e., patients who are not admitted electively by their own attending physicians) will be responsible for patient management.

The attending physicians bear ultimate responsibility for the perioperative management of their patients as well as for what takes place during the surgery itself. At most teaching institutions, much of the operating is done by the chief and senior residents under the guidance of the attending. The extent to which this is the case, however, depends on the nature of the service (i.e., whether it is an elective general surgery service at a private hospital, a trauma service at a county hospital, or a vascular service at a VA) as well as on the nature of the surgical disease and the complexity of the surgery. Simple procedures such as hernia repairs and appendectomies, for example, are frequently performed by interns and junior residents, whereas complicated operations such as the Whipple procedure (pancreaticoduodenectomy for pancreatic cancer) are usually performed by the chief resident and attending. As a general rule, an attending is present for every surgery performed, although some procedures are done entirely by the residents under the attending's umbrella of guidance and responsibility.

Chief resident. If the attending is the "chairman of the board" of the service, the chief resident functions as the chief executive officer, assuming responsibility for the management of the entire service as well as for the day-to-day running of the ward team. All patients on the service are managed by the chief resident, regardless of their individual attendings; therefore, the chief resident must be aware of every important issue affecting each patient on the service, including lab and x-ray results, plans for wound/dressing/line care, plans for advancing patients' diets, and dispositions. Since each attending on a service may have specific preferences for certain management issues (e.g., staples out on day five, advance from NPO to clear liquids vs. a soft diet), the chief must be well informed about these issues, as he or she must answer to the attendings if things go wrong.

Because culpability tends to roll downhill, it is in the best interests of all the residents and students to ensure that things function as smoothly as possible and that the chief is kept abreast of any problems that may arise. Chiefs spend most of their time in the OR, although they often have significant administrative and didactic responsibilities as well. They are generally in charge of arranging patient presentations for conferences and may schedule teaching sessions for the students on their service. They also arrange admissions and oversee consultations to other services. As a student, you may find that the chief resident bears significant responsibility for your evaluation. The onus is therefore on you to **ensure that your efforts do not go unnoticed by your chief.**

Surgery fosters a more formal pecking order.

Senior resident(s). On a given surgery service, there may be one or two senior residents (residents in their third or fourth clinical year) who assist the chief resident in the management of the service. Typically, the senior resident is responsible for running rounds in the morning and updating the service for the chief, since the chief may or may not walk on rounds with the team each morning. Also, when issues come up during the day that cannot easily be managed by the interns and junior residents, the senior resident may be called on to assume responsibility, as the chief may be busy operating. Of course, senior residents do their fair share of operating as well, handling less complex cases such as bowel resections for cancer and mastectomies. You may find yourself working more closely with your senior resident than with your chief on a daily basis. If this is the case, your senior(s) will play a critical role in your ultimate evaluation.

Help your interns!

Interns and junior residents. These are the "scut monkeys" of the surgery service (as is the case on other services, but with surgery there is usually much more scut work to be done). Interns and second-year residents are responsible for the minutiae of patient care—e.g., writing notes, checking labs, writing and dictating discharge summaries, checking wounds, and changing dressings. They also respond to pages from the nursing staff when patients are crashing. They are thus harried, get little sleep, and often have no lives, so part of your job is to make their days easier.

Subinterns ("sub-I's"). Sub-I's include acting interns and fourth-year medical students. As a general rule, if there are sub-I's on your team, their goal will be to go into surgery. This means that sub-I's will be working hard to function at an intern level as well as to shine in the eyes of their chiefs and attendings. As a third-year student, you may be intimidated by the idea of working on a service with sub-I's and being compared to them. Bear in mind, however, that the expectations of a third-year student's performance differ from those of a sub-I. Also keep in mind that you are more than likely capable of performing most of the tasks that the sub-I's do; you're just on a steeper portion of the learning curve. A typical sub-I will be expected to take call on a schedule comparable to that of an intern (again, services vary in their expectations), will assume some responsibility for evaluating patients on consults or in the ER, will take on a fair amount of daily scut work, and will try to squeeze into the OR whenever they can. As acting interns, however, sub-I's should also assume some responsibility for the education of the service, particularly the third-year students. So use your sub-I's as a resource, as they may have valuable advice to give you about performing well on the rotation—not to mention more knowledge about surgical diseases.

How Is the Day Set Up?

On OR days, the chief/senior residents and attendings will spend most of the day in surgery. Although some of the surgical cases may be simple outpatient procedures such as breast biopsies and hernia repairs, most will be procedures in which patients are admitted for postoperative care that lasts one to several days. On clinic days, new patients are seen for their referred problems, established patients are worked up for their preoperative evaluations, and postoperative patients are seen for follow-up. On both operative and clinic days, the entire inpatient service will need to be rounded on, and most teams will try to write all the progress notes on morning rounds before heading off to the OR or to clinic. This, of course, means that the workday starts especially early on a surgery service—usually anywhere from 5:00 to 6:00 A.M. Here is the overall structure of a typical OR day on a general surgery service:

5:00–6:00 A.M.	Prerounds
6:00–7:30 A.M.	Morning rounds
7:30–8:00 A.M.	OR preoperative preparation of patients
8:00 A.M.–12:00 noon	Surgery or work time
Noon–1:00 P.M.	Noon conference
1:00–6:00 P.M.	Surgery or work time
6:00–7:30 P.M.	"Afternoon" rounds
7:30 P.M.–?	Postrounds scut work

On clinic days, the morning schedule is usually similar, as rounds must be completed before the start of clinic. The evening schedule may be lighter depending on whether clinic is scheduled in the afternoon and on how many patients need to be worked up or admitted for surgery the next day. On days in which there is not a great deal of scut work, the intern/residents on call may offer to complete the work so that the rest of the team can leave for the day.

On operative days, the senior and chief residents will usually be tied up in the OR, so the responsibility for scut work, consults, and procedures will fall to the junior resident(s), intern(s), and students. You may therefore find yourself shuttling from the OR to the ward between cases to help the interns write orders, check labs, change dressings, see consults, get films read, and so on. Because your role in the OR is usually minimal, you may be expected to spend the bulk of your time doing scut work, especially if you are on a scut-heavy service with a high census (e.g., vascular surgery). In the OR, you may be able

Balance your time between the OR and the wards.

to participate in a case or you may find yourself relegated to observing from outside the surgical field, depending on the attendings' and residents' preferences, your own interest in getting hands-on surgical experience, and the need for your help in taking care of patient issues on the floor.

What Do I Do During Prerounds?

The daily tasks on a surgery service begin with prerounding. The team will expect you to preround on your patients, which on average will involve following 2–3 patients. Keep in mind that interns will also follow these patients in order to check your work, but you will have the responsibility to present them during rounds. On other services, the team may simply round as a group on everyone and write patient notes while in transit from room to room. As a rule, each patient should be seen in the morning and the following information updated:

- **Basic information:** This includes diagnosis, surgical procedure, hospital day number, postoperative day number, antibiotic day number(s), and so on.
- **Events overnight:** Have there been any episodes of respiratory distress? Fever? Problems with pain management? Nausea or vomiting? Wound-site bleeding?
- **Subjective data:** How is the patient's pain control (on a scale of 1 to 10)? Has he/she passed gas or had a bowel movement? (This is relevant for postoperative feeding.) Is the patient tolerating PO?
- **Vitals:** This includes maximum and current temperature, BP, heart rate, respiratory rate, O_2 saturation, and weight. Some chiefs may want the 24-hour ranges as well (use your discretion).
- **I/Os:** Record the total intake and output, and divide the input into PO intake (is the patient NPO, on clear liquids, or on solid food?) and IV fluids (type and rate of fluid repletion, boluses given). Divide output into urine output (including Foley status), stool output, emesis and NG output, and output of indwelling drains.
- **Other data:** What kind and amount of pain medication is the patient getting? Is he/she on a patient-controlled analgesia (PCA) device or receiving boluses of pain meds from the nurses? Which antibiotics is the patient taking, and how many days remain in the regimen? Are any other significant medications being given (e.g., steroid taper, antiemetics, promotility agents)? Is the patient diabetic, and if so, how high has his or her blood glucose been running, and how much insulin does he or she require?
- **Physical exam:** You should perform a focused, directed exam based on the patient's overall well-being and presenting problem. In general, all patients should receive a brief respiratory, cardiac, and abdominal exam in addition to a global assessment of mental status every morning. In addition, postoperative patients will require an assessment of urinary status (look at the Foley bag), drain output, and wound healing. Look at the dressing/wound and ask yourself the following questions: Is there wound drainage? Purulent exudate? Excessive peri-incisional tenderness or erythema? Do the sutures or staples need to come out? Is there any sign of wound dehiscence?
- **Assessment and plan (A&P):** You should construct an A&P for rounds even if it is incorrect. It shows that you have been thinking. Things to consider include diet, antibiotics, wound healing, and ultimate disposition.

On services where the medical student is not assigned specific patients to see before rounds, you will often be expected to engage in a modified preround activity on the entire service. In this situation, you will examine each patient's chart and begin writing a patient note before rounds begin. Specifically, you should begin writing the note by recording the patient's vitals, I/Os, and lab data over the past 24 hours. There is no need to see the patient beforehand if he or she will be seen during rounds with the team. If this is your role during prerounding, then your role during formal rounds will often consist of reading the information you wrote to the team before the team goes to see the patient.

How Do I Excel in Surgery?

Your role on the surgery service will be a hodgepodge of scut work, reading, and simply being with the team. The following are some guidelines for excelling on this service:

- **Always show up on time.**
- **Communicate frequently.**
- **Be visible.** Expect to stay late for evening rounds (unless you are excused by your chief). Your residents may expect you to follow 2–3 patients closely and take primary responsibility for their management with direct supervision from the intern(s). Alternatively, a "team approach" may be taken wherein the entire team shares responsibility for each patient—in which case you obviously won't be expected to know as much detail about every patient, but you may have more information to keep track of.
- **Become a "Highly Absorbent Information Sponge."** Reading about perioperative care, the pathophysiology of surgical illnesses, the basics of trauma evaluation, and the like will occupy a significant portion of your time, but necessarily so.
- **Know the expectations.** It is wise to ask your attending or chief resident to sit down with you early in the clerkship to discuss his or her expectations with regard to third-year students on the service. You may be expected to participate in many intern-level tasks, which may include performing preoperative H&Ps in clinic, checking labs and x-rays, following patients' I/Os, taking out sutures and staples postoperatively, writing discharge paperwork, evaluating patients in the ER, placing and changing arterial and venous lines, assisting in the OR, writing medication orders, and giving presentations on rounds and in conferences. The balance of these activities will depend on your own initiative and on the demands of your service.
- **Work quickly, independently, and efficiently.** Order lab tests, make necessary phone calls, and write notes on patients. In addition, remain focused, organized, and brief when presenting each patient.
- **Be assertive.** Ask good questions (you should know something about the subject matter before asking the questions), know other patients on the service (for your own learning and in case you are asked to fill in), take the initiative to ask for demonstrations of procedures, volunteer for drawing blood (you need to practice anyway), and **ask for feedback** from your residents and chiefs both at the midpoint of the rotation and at the end.
- **Be a team player.** Be helpful to your interns and residents. This may require that you do a little extra scut work on other patients for some "quid pro quo" teaching from the interns, but it will be well worth your while. In general, you will have a successful surgery experience if you **show interest,** accept responsibility eagerly and fulfill it competently, make your interns' lives easier, **laugh and smile** a lot, follow your patients closely, give crisp and succinct oral presentations, and **make an extra effort** to read and present interesting issues to the rest of the team. Do anything less and you will almost certainly pass the rotation but may get overshadowed by overly enthusiastic classmates or by solicitous sub-I's. Protect yourself by working hard. **Unless policies are being broken, never complain about the workload.** Hard work, after all, is what surgery is all about.

Efficiency, efficiency, efficiency!

TIPS FOR SUCCESS

The blueprint for survival and success on surgery focuses on several key factors:

- Enthusiasm
- Assertiveness
- Voracious reading
- Efficiency, efficiency, efficiency
- Respect for authority
- Appropriate humility

Key Notes

After prerounds, you will need to complete a brief **S**ubjective data/**O**bjective data/**A**ssessment and **P**lan (**SOAP**) progress note on each patient. These SOAP notes will follow the typical format but will usually be significantly shorter on a surgery service, as seen below. Other types of chart notes you may encounter on the surgery rotation include the admission H&P, the operative note, the procedure note, and the postoperative check.

Admission H&P. If this is a preoperative H&P for an elective surgery, you should include a succinct history of present illness (HPI), a brief past medical history (PMH) with particular attention paid to illnesses that have significance for perioperative management (e.g., a history of atrial fibrillation, COPD, or diabetes), and information on medications and allergies. Your exam should be comprehensive but should focus on the particular organ system involved (e.g., a thorough abdominal exam for GI cases and a detailed peripheral vascular exam for vascular cases) and should always include a rectal exam as well as a breast exam for women. In addition, the admission H&P should document that the attending/chief resident has discussed with each patient the risks, benefits, alternatives, and expectations of the surgical procedure, and that the patient understands these issues and grants consent.

SOAP note. This will serve as the daily progress note for each patient on the service. SOAP notes should follow the format given in the boxed item on page 391.

Operative note. This is a note that is entered into the chart at the completion of a surgical procedure documenting the findings and events of the case. It is usually a brief summary and should include pertinent data regarding the participants, the pre- and postoperative diagnoses (which are usually the same but are sometimes different, particularly in exploratory cases), total fluid exchange, disposition, and any complications. A sample operative note is shown on page 392.

Postoperative orders. Interns and sub-I's are normally responsible for writing postoperative orders. If you are comfortable writing postop orders, **this is an area in which you can shine.** A sample set of postoperative orders is shown on page 393.

What is the most common cause of fever on postoperative day 1? Atelectasis.

SAMPLE SOAP NOTE

55 yo WM admitted for perforated peptic ulcer, HD#3, POD#2 s/p Graham patch, NPO, abx = Ancef D#1/5, Flagyl D#1/5, central line D#1.

S: Pt ambulating, pain well controlled on PCA. c/o peri-incisional pain (3:10 this A.M.), no drainage. No flatus or bowel movements. Good use of incentive spirometer ($\uparrow$ 1500 cc). No other overnight issues.

O: VS T_m 38^3 / T_c 38^1 BP 110/63 P 86 RR 16 O_2 sat 99% 2 L NC.

24 hr I/O 2100/2000 (3000/2800—yesterday's I/O); UO 1500 (24 hr total) = 2.3 cc/kg/hr.

D5 1/2 NS @ 80 cc/hr, JP output → 15 cc—12 hr total. (If the patient is in the ICU, also document pulmonary artery catheter readings.)

PE: Gen: WD/WN male in NAD, A&O × 3.

CV: RRR, nl S1/S2, no M/R/G.

Chest: CTAB, no W/R/R, right chest tube suction intact with no air bubbles and moderate serosanguineous drainage.

Abd: Soft, NT/ND, hypoactive bowel sounds, no HSM, dressing C/D/I, staples intact, no induration/erythema.

Foley catheter in place; 300 cc of yellow fluid present in Foley bag.

Labs:

Hb/Hct 9.2/29 (10.1/30—i.e., yesterday's Hb/Hct).

Wound Cx pending.

CT scan, x-rays, etc.

A/P: 55 yo WM POD#2 s/p Graham patch for perforated peptic ulcer, doing well. Low-grade temperature most likely 2° to atelectasis.

1. Continue antibiotic regimen.

2. Encourage OOB, ambulation, and incentive spirometry.

3. Consider D/C PCA; switch to oral analgesics.

4. Keep NPO for now; will advance to clear fluids when flatus passed.

5. D/C JP drain, D/C Foley.

Key:

A&O × 3 = alert and oriented to person, place, and time

A/P = assessment and plan

abx = antibiotics

C/D/I = clean, dry, and intact

c/o = complains of

CTAB = clear to auscultation bilaterally

Cx = culture

D/C = discontinuing

Hb = hemoglobin

Hct = hematocrit

HD = hospital day

HSM = hepatosplenomegaly

JP = Jackson-Pratt drain

M/R/G = murmur/rubs/gallops

NAD = no acute distress

NC = nasal cannula

nl = normal

NPO = nothing by mouth

NS = normal saline

NT/ND = nontender and nondistended

O = objective data

OOB = out of bed

P = pulse rate

PE = physical exam

POD = postoperative day

RR = respiratory rate

RRR = regular rate and rhythm

S = subjective data

s/p = status post

T_c = current temperature

T_m = maximum temperature

UO = urine output

VS = vital signs

WD/WN = well developed and well nourished

WM = white male

W/R/R = wheezes/rhonchi/rales

Postoperative check. Generally, patients will need to be seen 2–4 hours after surgery to be evaluated for immediate complications (e.g., hypotension, hemorrhage, dyspnea), adequacy of urine output, level of comfort, and the like. A brief postoperative note—presented again in the standard SOAP format—should then be written. The subjective section of the note should primarily address the patient's postoperative pain control; the objective portion should include vital signs, intraoperative and postoperative blood loss and fluid intake, urinary output, wound drainage, appearance of the incision and dress-

Key:

CBD = common bile duct

dx = diagnosis

EBL = estimated blood loss

GB = gallbladder

GETA = general
endotracheal anesthesia

IOC = intraoperative
cholangiogram

LR = lactated Ringer's
solution

BRIEF OPERATIVE NOTE: BLUE SURGERY TEAM

Preop dx: Biliary colic.

Postop dx: Cholelithiasis.

Procedure: Laparoscopic cholecystectomy + intraoperative cholangiography.

Surgeons: Attending, resident (PGY-5), intern (PGY-1), med student (MS-3).

Anesthesia: GETA.

Fluids: 1400 cc LR.

Blood transfusions: None (no cell saver).

EBL: 200 cc.

Findings: Distended gallbladder with slightly thickened wall, multiple stones within GB, no CBD stones by IOC.

Specimens: GB to path (no cultures taken).

Drains: None.

Complications: None apparent.

Disposition: To recovery room in stable condition, awake and extubated.

---

*Don't forget to get and
document informed consent.*

ings, postoperative lab results from the recovery room, and any significant abnormalities on physical exam. Always communicate abnormal findings and/or laboratory values to your team.

Procedure note. Frequently, surgical patients will undergo other procedures, such as central line insertion, chest tube placement/removal, extubation, incision and drainage of abscesses, thoracentesis, paracentesis, lumbar puncture, and suturing of lacerations. When these are done as bedside procedures, they should be documented in the medical chart with an appropriate procedure note. This procedure note should follow the standard format. Remember to get informed consent and document having done so in the chart.

Key Procedures

Because surgery is principally an intervention-oriented specialty, you should gain hands-on experience with procedures that may be relevant to you in other specialties. These include suturing lacerations (including learning techniques of local anesthesia), knot tying and suture cutting, gowning and gloving in sterile fashion, arterial line placement, starting IVs, ABGs, paracentesis, thoracentesis, chest tube placement, incision and drainage of abscesses, staple and suture removal, dressing changes, Foley catheterization, NG tube insertion, central venous cannulation, and drain pulling (see the boxed item on page 394). You should also become familiar with the process of patient preparation and transfer to and from the operating suite. Surgical knots are best learned from a resident and then practiced at home. Of course, you'll get plenty of practice at retraction in the OR. Do not kill yourself trying to do all of these procedures, but make use of the opportunities that present them-

POSTOPERATIVE ORDERS

Admit to: 3-West, General Surgery; attending: Dr. Jones; interns Lee (×46789) and Smith (×97850); MS-3 Stone (×57689).

Diagnosis: Perforated peptic ulcer.

Condition: Stable.

Vitals: Per routine.

Allergies: NKDA.

Activity: As tolerated, OOB TID.

Nursing orders:

Strict I/Os.

DVT prophylaxis: Heparin 1000 units SQ, SCDs.

Foley catheter to gravity.

Incentive spirometer 10 times/hr while awake.

Diet: NPO.

IV fluids: D5 1/2 NS + 20 KCl to run at 100 cc/hr.

Medications:

Abx: Cefotaxime 1 g IV q 8 h.

Analgesics: PCA.

(Do not forget to list all the patient's preoperative and PRN medications.)

Studies: CXR in A.M.

Labs: CBC, chem 7, UA in A.M.

Call house officer if: HR > 100 or < 60; BP > 180/100 or < 90/60; RR > 25 or < 12; or temp > 39.5.

When considering the causes of fever in a postoperative patient, use the **"5 W's"** mnemonic.

Key:

CBC = complete blood count

CXR = chest x-ray

DVT = deep venous thrombosis

NKDA = no known drug allergies

PRN = as required

SCD = sequential compression device

SQ = subcutaneously

TID = three times daily

UA = urinalysis

---

selves. Remember, if you fall in love with surgical procedures, you can always do a subinternship in your fourth year and go into surgery.

Operating Room Etiquette

Interestingly enough, one of the most challenging (and often frustrating) concepts that a student must learn during his or her surgical ward rotation is the maintenance of a sterile field in the OR. This includes making sure you are not contaminating the operating field (or yourself) and staying out of the way of other team members in the OR (e.g., residents, scrub nurse, circulating nurse, x-ray technicians). Since you will probably be the least experienced member of the group, it is important to know some of the points of etiquette associated with working in the OR. These include the following:

Postoperative fever etiologies—

The 5 W's

Wind: atelectasis, pneumonia
Water: UTI
Wound: infection
Walking: pulmonary embolus arising from a DVT
Wonder drug: drug fever

TUBES AND DRAINS

Jackson-Pratt (JP) drain: Used to drain surgical wounds and keep bacteria and blood from building up; drains are usually attached to bulb suction. You will see the resident "strip" or milk these tubes, which means pulling along the length of the clear tube filled with blood to prevent clotting.

Penrose drain: A yellow-colored tube used to drain large abscesses for cases in which a JP drain is ineffective. No suction.

NG tube: A tube leading from the nasopharynx to the stomach; used to drain the stomach of fluids (gastric decompression). It can also be used for feeding when the patient's GI tract starts working after surgery.

G-tube or gastrostomy tube: Goes from the stomach to the outside; resembles a permanent NG tube used for feeding patients with an obstruction above the stomach, or for decompression in patients with pyloric outlet obstruction.

J-tube or jejunostomy tube: Primarily used for feeding.

GJ-tube/Moss tube: Has two ports—one to the stomach and the other to the jejunum. Acts like one G-tube and one J-tube. J- and GJ-tubes are often used in patients at high risk for aspiration.

T-tube: A biliary tube shaped like a "T."

- **Introduce yourself** both to the OR circulating nurse and to the scrub nurse when you first enter the OR and before you scrub in, and tell them that you will be scrubbing in on the case. Tell the circulating nurse what size gown you will need. Pull your gloves and give them to the scrub nurse yourself—ask for help the first time! If you don't know your glove size, follow this general guideline: size 6 = small; size 7 = medium; size 8 = large.
- Remember to **double-glove** to protect yourself against needle sticks. In double-gloving, many people prefer that the outer set of gloves be a half size larger than the inner set so that they aren't too tight.
- Ask the circulating nurse or resident if he or she needs any help in moving or positioning the patient on the operating table or "prepping" the patient for surgery. In some hospitals, the nurses will prep the patient; in other facilities it may be up to you (ask your resident or sub-I prior to your first OR case).
- Before scrubbing, place your beeper on one of the nonsterile side tables with a piece of paper attached to it giving your name. This will not only allow the circulating nurse to return your pages but also help you find the beeper if you accidentally leave it in the OR after the case is over.
- Remember to **take off any jewelry you might have** (e.g., rings, bracelets, watches, earrings) and put on your mask, cap, and safety eyewear before you start scrubbing.
- Although there is no specific rule on how long to scrub, a good rule of thumb is to scrub for five minutes prior to the first case of the day. For subsequent cases, be sure to scrub **1–2 minutes longer than your attending** so that he or she won't be able to criticize you for not scrubbing thoroughly enough.
- Offer to help with the draping of the patient after you are gowned. If no help is needed, quietly stand out of the way of others who are doing so.

- Try to **keep your hands above your waist and below your shoulders.** Place your hands on the draping during the surgery to ensure that your gloves remain sterile.
- Do not reach over or pass any instrument unless you are specifically instructed to do so.
- When the surgeon is using the bovie (electrocautery device) to incise fat, muscle tissue, and fascia, use the suction device to suck up the smoke and noxious odor associated with it.
- When you return needles or blades back to the scrub nurse, always announce out loud the presence of any sharps on the field that are being returned to the instrument tray (e.g., "needle down," "knife back"). It is also helpful to announce to the anesthesiologist when the initial incision has been made so that he or she knows when the surgery has started and can document the time of incision. At the end of the case, ask the anesthesiologist for the estimated blood loss and how much fluid the patient received intraoperatively (this information is then recorded on the operative note).
- Try to **make yourself helpful** by paying attention to minor details such as providing adequate retraction, adjusting the overhead lights, and suctioning excess blood from the area of dissection. These measures will allow the surgeon to have good visualization of the operative field.
- Those of you who wear eyeglasses should be aware that the easiest way to contaminate yourself is to accidentally adjust your glasses with your sterile glove. Work to avoid that habit in the OR.
- If you do end up contaminating your gown, glove, or sleeve, step out of the operating field and let the scrub nurse know so that he or she can replace the contaminated parts and help ensure that you do not end up contaminating anything else.
- If you follow these basic principles of OR etiquette, you are likely to find that your OR experience is more enjoyable and far less stressful. One last thing: Don't forget to carry a pen in the pocket of your scrubs so that you can write the operative note and postoperative orders when the case is complete.

How to Suture Like a Pro

One way to get more out of your OR experience is to become highly proficient at suturing and surgical knot tying. Unfortunately, the only way to do so is to practice, practice, practice! The best way to sharpen your suturing technique is to go to the ER/OR supply room and obtain the following:

- **Sutures of different types and sizes:** The most common sutures with which to practice surgical knot tying are 3–0 silk suture ties. Ideally, however, you should try to become proficient in suturing with many different types of sutures, such as 5–0 nylon (most commonly used when suturing up the skin), 1–0 Vicryl (most commonly used when suturing up deep fascia and muscle layers), and 4–0 Vicryl (most commonly used when closing up the subcutaneous layer). It is also helpful to remember which sutures are absorbable (e.g., Vicryl, polydioxanone [PDS], Dexon, chromic, catgut) as opposed to nonabsorbable (e.g., nylon and silk); which are natural (e.g., silk, catgut) as opposed to synthetic (e.g., nylon, PDS); and which are monofilament (e.g., nylon) as opposed to braided (e.g., silk, Dexon, Vicryl).
- **A "laceration tray" from the ER:** Specific instruments you will need include a needle holder, a pair of pickups, and a pair of suture scissors. Laceration trays usually have many of these instruments in varying sizes.

- **A box of gloves:** Remember that when you are suturing on a patient, you should be double-gloved to protect against needle sticks. It would thus make sense to practice suturing and surgical knot tying with two sets of gloves on so that the process won't prove to be too awkward when you work on an actual patient.
- **A suture removal kit:** This should include a pair of forceps as well as a fine-pointed pair of scissors for taking out sutures.

The next step is to find a fourth-year medical student (e.g., a sub-I) or an intern (ideally one who is not very busy) who would be willing to show you how to suture and tie surgical knots. The types of suture methods that you should learn include the following:

- Simple interrupted sutures (most commonly used to close up skin lacerations)
- Vertical mattress sutures (used to close skin that is under tension)
- Horizontal mattress sutures (also used to close skin that is under tension)
- "Buried" (subcutaneous) sutures
- Figure-of-eight sutures (used to tie off a bleeding vessel)
- Running sutures (used to quickly close deep fascial layers)

As for surgical knot tying, focus on learning how to tie surgical knots by the "instrument tie" and the two-handed tie before progressing to the more advanced one-handed surgical knot tie. Good materials to practice suturing on include pigs' feet (for the classic diehard surgeon-to-be), chicken breast, orange peels, banana peels, and two-sided sponges.

What Do I Carry in My Pockets?

As with any rotation, surgery has its necessary gear. Unlike most residents, however, surgery residents try to carry as little extraneous material as possible with them, as they tend to shift rapidly from OR to clinic to ward to cafeteria and must therefore remain as unencumbered as possible. As a student, you should adopt this minimalist stance as well. This means not carrying around too many handbooks and not wearing a fanny pack laden with tuning forks, otoscopes, and the like. The main requirements for the surgery rotation include the following:

- **White coat:** Always wear one on the first day. Find out if you're expected to wear it daily or just in clinic.
- **Stethoscope:** Essential on any rotation. However, be aware of the fact that many surgeons frown on wearing the stethoscope as a necklace ("dog collar"), as this is a sign of an internal medicine resident. To be safe, carry your stethoscope in the pocket of your white coat.
- **Penlight:** Critical for its common uses (checking pupils) and for examining wounds and the like.
- **Trauma scissors:** Trauma scissors, or surgical shears, are a pair of heavy-duty scissors that are used primarily to cut through a patient's clothing during an acute trauma situation or to cut through bulky dressings on rounds. These handy, all-purpose scissors will prove useful during both your general surgery and your inpatient OB/GYN rotations. To score points with your chief/senior resident, cut your patients' dressings open when you preround so that they can be easily and quickly removed on rounds.
- **Index cards/clipboard/patient data sheets:** You will need something portable to manage information (e.g., lab data) on each patient. Figure out which method works most effectively and efficiently for you, and then stick

with it and abandon extraneous gear. Keep in mind that clipboards can and often do get lost.

- **Wound care accessories:** Sometimes it is helpful to carry spare gauze (Kerlix rolls and 4 × 4 cotton gauze pads), surgical tape, and other wound care accessories for rapid dispensing at the request of your chief resident on rounds. Many students use a bucket or tray stocked full of the items the team may conceivably need for wound checks and dressing changes on morning rounds.
- **Drug guide:** A must-have throughout your medical training (until you get to the level where you don't have to look up drug doses—which won't come for several years).
- **Antimicrobial guide:** *Sanford's Guide to Antimicrobial Therapy* is an excellent pocket resource for bacterial susceptibilities and drug dosing for common infections.
- **Surgery handbook:** There are a number of useful, concise pocket guidebooks for surgery students and residents. It is advisable that you spend some time evaluating these books before purchasing one, as they differ markedly in style and organization (but are generally consistent in content). Some of the more popular handbooks are reviewed in the Top-Rated Review Resources section.
- You should probably purchase the above items if you don't already own them. Most will come in handy for other rotations, and a good pocket handbook is great to have as a quick reference before conferences or teaching (pimping) rounds.

HIGH-YIELD CLINICAL TOPIC CHECKLIST

Read about these topics before you start the rotation. Most are discussed in this chapter. A full list of common clerkship topics can be found at the end of this chapter.

- ❑ Acute abdomen
- ❑ Small bowel obstruction
- ❑ Colorectal cancer
- ❑ GI bleeding
- ❑ Gallbladder disease
- ❑ Pancreatic cancer
- ❑ Hernias (direct, indirect, hiatal)
- ❑ Breast cancer
- ❑ Lung cancer
- ❑ Abdominal aortic aneurysm

GASTROINTESTINAL DISEASE

Acute Abdomen

The workup of a patient with an acute abdomen is a diagnostic challenge as well as a key component of the surgical rotation. Early diagnosis is critical, as early intervention is required to prevent significant morbidity and mortality.

SIGNS AND SYMPTOMS

A thorough H&P is indispensable in making the diagnosis of acute abdomen and should thus include the following information:

What is Kehr's sign? Pain referred to the left shoulder due to irritation of the left hemidiaphragm, often associated with splenic rupture.

All female patients with an acute abdomen need a pelvic exam and a pregnancy test to rule out PID, ectopic pregnancy, ovarian torsion, and the like.

What is Fitz-Hugh–Curtis syndrome? Perihepatitis associated with chlamydial infection of the cervix.

- **HPI:**
  - The onset, duration, and progression of the pain (e.g., maximal at onset, intermittent, constant, worsening).
  - The location of the pain both at onset and at presentation.
  - The quality (burning, cramping, sharp, aching) and severity of the pain.
  - Aggravating and alleviating factors.
  - GI complaints (nausea, vomiting, anorexia, hematemesis, hematochezia, melena, or change in bowel function).
  - Gynecologic complaints and last menstrual period.
  - Any similar episodes in the past.
- **PMH:**
  - Metabolic or endocrine disease (e.g., diabetes, Addison's disease, porphyria).
  - CAD, heart failure, abdominal surgery, hernias, gallstones, EtOH abuse, PUD.
  - Prior surgical history (e.g., cholecystectomy, appendectomy, hysterectomy).
- **Medications.**
- **PE:** Begin with general observation. How ill is the patient? Is he/she writhing in pain or lying motionless?
- **Abdominal exam:**
  - **Inspect:** Look for distention, symmetry, scars, trauma, and obesity. Ask the patient to point to the location of maximal pain.
  - **Auscultate:** Absent or hypoactive bowel sounds may mean ileus. Listen for high-pitched sounds or tinkles (obstruction) and bruits (aneurysm).
  - **Palpate:** Start at the quadrant farthest from maximal pain. First touch lightly, and then gradually ↑ to deep palpation. Assess for tenderness to palpation, rebound tenderness, referred pain, guarding (voluntary or involuntary), masses, and hernias (inguinal, femoral, incisional). Assess the patient for flank tenderness (indicative of renal inflammation or a retrocecal appendix).
  - **Percuss:** Shifting dullness or a fluid wave indicates ascites. Percuss the liver and spleen to assess for hepatosplenomegaly.
- **Rectal exam:** Look for occult blood, mass lesions, tenderness, sphincter tone, and the presence or absence of stool in the rectal vault.
- **Pelvic exam:** Check for adnexal tenderness, masses, cervical discharge, cervical motion tenderness, and uterine size and consistency.

DIFFERENTIAL

See Table 9-1 and Figure 9-1 for the differential diagnosis of acute abdomen according to abdominal quadrants. Additional disorders to consider in the differential diagnosis of acute abdomen include the following:

- **GI:** Small bowel obstruction (SBO), large bowel obstruction (LBO), paralytic ileus, ischemic bowel disease.
- **Endocrine:** DKA, addisonian crisis, uremic crisis.
- **Hematologic:** Acute intermittent porphyria, sickle cell crisis.
- **Cardiac:** Pericarditis, angina/MI.
- **GU:** Obstructive uropathy.
- **Toxins:** Lead, venom.

TABLE 9-1. **Differential of Acute Abdomen by Location**

RUQ	LUQ	Epigastrium	RLQ	LLQ
Acute cholecystitis/ biliary colic	Acute pancreatitis	GERD	Acute appendicitis	Diverticulitis
PUD	Perforated viscus	Pancreatitis (acute/ chronic)	IBD	Sigmoid volvulus
Gastritis	MI	PUD	Meckel's diverticulum	Colorectal cancer
Cholangitis	Splenic rupture/ infarction	Angina, MI	Acute cholecystitis	Mesenteric ischemia
Hepatitis	GERD/gastritis	Gastroenteritis	Pyelonephritis, nephrolithiasis	Colitis
Pneumonia	PUD	Perforated viscus	Diverticulitis	Pyelonephritis, nephrolithiasis
Pleurisy		Esophagitis/gastritis	Ovarian torsion, cyst	Ovarian torsion, cyst
		Abdominal aortic aneurysm (AAA)	Ruptured ectopic pregnancy, PID	Ruptured ectopic pregnancy/PID
		Early appendicitis	Intussusception	
		Acute bowel obstruction	Colon cancer	

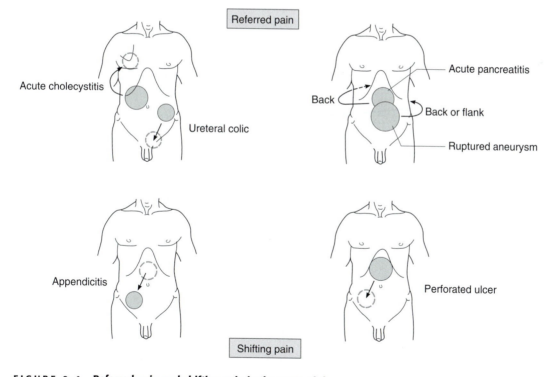

FIGURE 9-1. **Referred pain and shifting pain in the acute abdomen.**

Solid circles indicate the site of maximal pain; broken lines indicate sites of lesser pain. (Reproduced, with permission, from Way LW, Doherty GM. *Current Surgical Diagnosis & Treatment,* 11th ed. New York: McGraw-Hill, 2003: 505.)

WORKUP

- **Labs:**
    - CBC, electrolytes, LFTs, amylase and lipase, UA, urine microscopic exam, and urine culture.
    - Urine pregnancy test in women.
- **Imaging:**
    - CXR and AXR to look for free air.
    - Kidneys, ureters, and bladder (KUB).
    - Abdominal CT scan and/or RUQ ultrasound.

TREATMENT

- First determine whether the condition represents a surgical abdomen (i.e., an abdomen in need of emergent surgical treatment) or whether it can be treated with expectant management.
- **Expectant management:**
    - NPO.
    - NG suction in cases of nausea and vomiting, hematemesis, or suspected GI tract obstruction.
    - Aggressive IV fluid hydration and correction of electrolyte abnormalities.
    - Monitoring of vital signs and serial abdominal exams.
    - Foley catheterization to evaluate fluid status and response to rehydration therapy.
    - Serial laboratory exams, including CBC and electrolytes.
- **Surgery: Exploratory laparotomy** is appropriate for unstable patients in whom a surgically correctable or identifiable cause is suspected.

REFERENCE

Makary MA. *General Surgery Review*, 2nd ed. Arlington, VA: Ladner-Drysdale, 2008, www.shelfexam.com. A good overview of clinical presentations that appear on the shelf exam.

GI Bleeding

UPPER GI BLEEDING (UGIB)

Defined as bleeding proximal to the ligament of Treitz, which includes the esophagus, stomach, and duodenum. Risk factors include alcohol and smoking; a PMH of PUD or bleeding disorders; use of medications such as aspirin/ NSAIDs, anticoagulants, and steroids; burn injuries; and trauma. Etiologies are as follows:

- Peptic ulcer (45%)
- Gastric erosions (23%)
- Varices (10%)
- Mallory-Weiss tear (7%)
- Esophagitis/duodenitis (6%)

SIGNS AND SYMPTOMS

- **Hematemesis:** Vomiting bright red blood or coffee-ground emesis (blood exposed to gastric acid).
- **Melena:** Black, tarry stools due to an upper GI bleeding source.

- **Hematochezia:** Bright red blood per rectum (BRBPR) may be seen in cases of vigorous upper GI bleeding.
- **Other:** Dehydration (pallor, tachycardia, orthostasis, syncope), shock, epigastric discomfort, and guaiac-$\oplus$ stools are commonly seen.

DIFFERENTIAL

In addition to the disease entities listed above, consider gastric cancer, splenic vein thrombosis, epistaxis, and hemoptysis.

WORKUP

- **Labs:**
  - CBC, electrolytes, LFTs, PT/PTT.
  - Type and cross-match for 4–6 units of packed RBCs.
  - NG lavage, stool guaiac.
- **Imaging:** KUB, upper endoscopy (EGD).

TREATMENT

- **Resuscitate:**
  - Using two large-bore IVs (16–18 gauge), resuscitate with LR (2 L) followed by packed RBCs until the patient is hemodynamically stable.
  - Use a Foley catheter to assess fluid status.
  - Assess the magnitude of the hemorrhage using vital signs, serial hematocrits, O_2 saturation, and evidence of active bleeding.
  - Correct any underlying coagulopathy with FFP/vitamin K. Give platelets for severe thrombocytopenia.
- **Identify the bleeding source:**
  - **NG lavage:** If aspiration yields bright red blood or coffee grounds, perform saline lavage of the GI tract to remove blood clots until clear fluid returns. A nonbloody bilious aspirate suggests a source distal to the ligament of Treitz or lower GI bleeding.
  - **Endoscopy (EGD):** Identify the site of bleeding and coagulate the bleeding vessels.
  - **Angiography:** If GI bleeding is to be identified with angiography, the rate of bleeding must be > 0.5 cc/min. If a source is identified, perform selective sclerotherapy or embolization.
- **Control bleeding:**
  - Sclerotherapy or embolization should be used during the localization procedure.
  - Vasopressin is often used to improve hemodynamic stability. It is specifically used in the presence of varices to ↓ mesenteric circulation and ultimately to ↓ flow to the varices. Bear in mind that vasopressin leads to vasoconstriction of the enteric circulation but also causes coronary vasoconstriction. Therefore, it is commonly given with nitroglycerin to ↓ the risk of MI. Somatostatin is also being used.
  - Balloon tamponade (with a Levine tube) can be used as a temporary measure (< 48 hours) in cases of refractory variceal hemorrhage.

REFERENCE

Pianka JD, Affronti J. Management principles of gastrointestinal bleeding. *Prim Care* 28:557–575, 2001. A good review of the management of UGIB along with a list of answers to commonly encountered clinical questions.

INDICATIONS FOR SURGICAL TREATMENT OF UPPER GI BLEEDING

In 80–85% of cases, bleeding will stop spontaneously; approximately 20% will require surgery.

- **PUD:** In general, surgery is indicated if patients require six or more units of blood in the first 24 hours or if they rebleed while receiving maximal medical therapy.

- **Esophageal varices:** If bleeding continues despite medical measures, consider performing a transjugular intrahepatic portosystemic shunt (TIPS) procedure. In this case, interventional radiology staff pass a stent via the jugular vein and the IVC to bridge the liver into the portal venous system and decompress the portal hypertension.

What is the most common cause of LGIB in adults and in children? Diverticulosis in adults and angiodysplasia in children.

LOWER GI BLEEDING (LGIB)

Defined as bleeding distal to the ligament of Treitz, including the jejunum, ileum, colon, and rectum. Most cases occur in the colon. Etiologies include the following:

- **Acute:** Diverticulosis, angiodysplasia (AVM, telangiectasia), IBD and ischemic colitis, intussusception/volvulus, UGIB.
- **Chronic:** Colorectal cancer, hemorrhoids/fissures.

SIGNS AND SYMPTOMS

- Anorexia, fatigue, abdominal pain, and a change in bowel habits.
- Hematochezia (BRBPR) or melena.

WORKUP

- CBC, electrolytes, PT/PTT, type and cross 4–6 units of packed RBCs.
- Stool guaiac.

TREATMENT

- **Resuscitate:** Guidelines are the same as those for UGIB. In 90% of cases, bleeding will stop spontaneously following two units of transfusion.
- **Identify the bleeding source:**
    - NG lavage yields bilious GI contents in the case of LGIB.
    - DRE, anoscopy, and/or sigmoidoscopy to rule out hemorrhoids or polyps.
- **Colonoscopy:** A technetium-labeled RBC scan is sensitive for slow bleeds but is less specific than angiography.
- **Angiography:** As with UGIB, brisk bleeding (> 0.5 cc/min) is required to make the diagnosis.
- **Control the bleeding source:**
    - Vasopressin injection is often performed during angiography.
    - Laser coagulation or electrocoagulation can be used.
- **Surgical indications** are as follows:
    - Persistent bleeding despite angiographic or endoscopic therapy.
    - Segmental colectomy if the bleeding site is well localized.
    - If it is not possible to localize the bleeding site, consider total colectomy with ileorectal anastomosis or a temporary ileostomy and a Hartmann pouch (in which the distal rectal stump is sutured closed).

Small Bowel Disease

SMALL BOWEL OBSTRUCTION (SBO)

Defined as blocked passage of bowel contents through the duodenum, jejunum, or ileum. Fluid and gas build up proximal to the obstruction, leading to fluid and electrolyte imbalances and significant abdominal discomfort. The obstruction can be complete or partial and may be dangerous if strangulation of the bowel occurs. Etiologies are as follows:

- Adhesions from a prior abdominal surgery (60% of cases)
- Hernias (10–20% of cases)
- Neoplasm (10–20% of cases)
- Intussusception
- Gallstone ileus
- Stricture from IBD

What is the leading cause of SBO in adults and in children? Adhesions and hernias, respectively.

SIGNS AND SYMPTOMS

- **History:**
  - **Cramping abdominal pain:** Pain follows a recurrent crescendo-decrescendo pattern at intervals of 5–10 minutes (see Figure 9-2).

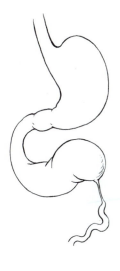 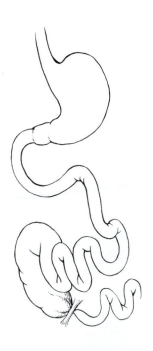 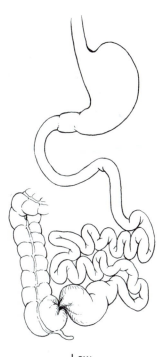

High	Middle	Low
Frequent vomiting. No distention. Intermittent pain but not classic crescendo type.	Moderate vomiting. Moderate distention. Intermittent pain (crescendo, colicky) with free intervals.	Vomiting late, feculent. Marked distention. Variable pain; may not be classic crescendo type.

FIGURE 9-2. Small bowel obstruction.

Signs and symptoms vary with the level of blockage. (Reproduced, with permission, from Way LW, Doherty GM. *Current Surgical Diagnosis & Treatment,* 11th ed. New York: McGraw-Hill, 2003: 685.)

- **Vomiting:** Nonfeculent in the setting of proximal obstruction; feculent in the presence of distal obstruction. Keep in mind that feculence is 2° to bacterial overgrowth, not actual emesis of feces.
- **Obstruction:** Suspect complete obstruction if no flatus or stool is passed; suspect partial obstruction with continued passage of flatus but no stool.
- **PE:** High-pitched bowel sounds and peristaltic rushes. Bowel sounds become hypoactive and eventually absent as the obstruction progresses.
- **Abdominal exam: Distention,** abdomen tympanic to percussion, tenderness, prior surgical scars, or hernias.
- **General:** Fever, hypotension, and tachycardia (due to dehydration) are not uncommon.

DIFFERENTIAL

- **Acute appendicitis:** Should **always** be near the top of the differential for an acute abdomen.
- **Adynamic ileus:** Postoperative ileus after abdominal surgery, hypokalemia, or medications.
- **Other:** LBO; IBD; mesenteric ischemia; renal colic/pyelonephritis.

WORKUP

- **Labs:**
  - **CBC:** Leukocytosis = strangulation.
  - **Electrolytes:** Potassium and sodium abnormalities due to dehydration; metabolic alkalosis 2° to vomiting.
- **Imaging:** Abdominal films show a **stepladder** pattern of **dilated small bowel loops** and **air-fluid levels** (see Figure 9-3). It is possible to see an **absent colon gas pattern.**

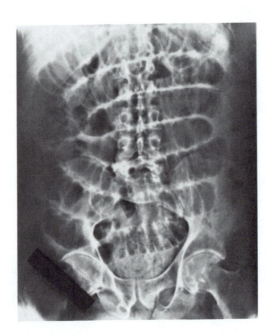

FIGURE 9-3. Small bowel obstruction on supine AXR.

Note the dilated loops of the small bowel in a ladderlike pattern. Air-fluid levels may be seen if an upright x-ray is done. (Reproduced, with permission, from Way LW, Doherty GM. *Current Surgical Diagnosis & Treatment,* 11th ed. New York: McGraw-Hill, 2003: 686.)

STRANGULATED VS. NONSTRANGULATED SMALL BOWEL OBSTRUCTION

■ Nonstrangulated SBO carries a total mortality of approximately 2%, while the risk of death from strangulated SBO ↑ in proportion to time from diagnosis to operative therapy, with a peak of roughly 25%.

■ A second-look laparotomy or laparoscopy may be performed 18–36 hours after initial surgical treatment to reevaluate bowel viability.

TREATMENT

■ **Medical management:**
  ■ Appropriate for partial SBO in stable patients.
  ■ NPO, NG tube decompression, IV hydration, correction of electrolyte abnormalities, pain management.
■ **Surgical management:**
  ■ Appropriate for complete SBO, vascular compromise, hemodynamic instability, or SBO of > 3 days' duration without resolution.
  ■ Exploratory laparotomy may be performed with lysis of adhesions and resection of necrotic bowel as well as running the bowel (inspection of the entire length of bowel) with evaluation for stricture, tumor, IBD, and hernias.

Large Bowel Disease

DIVERTICULAR DISEASE

Prevalent in 35–50% of the general population; more common in the elderly and in industrialized nations. Risk factors include a low-fiber diet, chronic constipation, and a ⊕ family history. Distinguished as follows (see also Table 9-2):

■ **Diverticulosis:** Herniation of the mucosa and submucosa through the muscular layer, forming **false, or pulsion, diverticula.** Caused by weakness in the bowel wall related to areas where blood vessels enter and leave the colon as well as by ↑ intraluminal pressure. Most commonly found in the **sigmoid portion** (95%) with sparing of the rectum.
■ **Diverticulitis:** Inflammation of a diverticulum that may lead to perforation and typically results in peritonitis.

What is the most common cause of LGIB in patients > 40 years of age? Diverticulosis.

REFERENCE

Farrell RJ et al. Diverticular disease in the elderly. *Gastroenterol Clin North Am* 30:475–496, 2001. A review of the epidemiology, pathogenesis, diagnosis, and management of diverticulosis and diverticulitis, including a thorough discussion of the complications of diverticular disease.

Massive LGIB is common with diverticulosis but rare with diverticulitis. Colonoscopy and barium enema are contraindicated in diverticulitis in light of the risk of perforation.

COLORECTAL CANCER

The **third leading cause of cancer mortality** in the United States after breast, prostate, and lung cancer. Affects approximately 150,000 new patients per

TABLE 9-2. Diverticulosis vs. Diverticulitis

	DIVERTICULOSIS	**DIVERTICULITIS**
Symptoms	Often **painless** (80%); presents with rectal bleeding.	**LLQ pain;** constipation or diarrhea; fever, chills, anorexia, nausea/vomiting.
Workup	H&P. ↓ hematocrit due to bleeding. Barium enema and/or colonoscopy.	H&P. ↑ WBC count. AXR reveals ileus, air-fluid levels, or free air if perforated. CT is the study of choice. Barium enema/colonoscopy are contraindicated.
Treatment	High-fiber diet; stool softeners; resuscitation in the presence of massive bleeding.	**Mild:** IV fluids; broad-spectrum antibiotics. **Severe:** If emergent, resection of bowel and creation of colostomy and a Hartmann pouch. If elective, resection of bowel and a 1° anastomosis.

What are the three most common causes of cancer mortality in the United States? Breast cancer (women) and prostate cancer (men); lung cancer; and colorectal cancer.

year and accounts for 50,000–60,000 deaths annually. Incidence ↑ with age, with a peak incidence at 70–80 years.

SIGNS AND SYMPTOMS

- In the absence of screening, colorectal cancer typically presents symptomatically only after a prolonged period of silent growth (see Figure 9-4).
- **Abdominal pain** is the most common presenting complaint (see Table 9-3 and Figure 9-5).

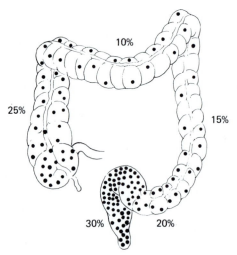

FIGURE 9-4. Distribution of cancer of the colon and rectum.

(Reproduced, with permission, from Way LW, Doherty GM. *Current Surgical Diagnosis & Treatment*, 11th ed. New York: McGraw-Hill, 2003: 716.)

TABLE 9-3. Presenting Symptoms of Colorectal Cancer by Location

	MASS CHARACTERISTICS	COMMON PRESENTING SYMPTOMS
Right-sided lesions	Bulky, fungating, ulcerating masses.	Anemia from chronic occult blood loss. Weight loss, anorexia, weakness. Obstruction is rare.
Left-sided lesions	"Apple-core" obstructing mass (see Figure 9-5).	Obstruction, since feces in the left colon are more solid and the wall is less distensible. Change in bowel habits.
Rectal lesions	Can coexist with hemorrhoids.	BRBPR. Rectal pain, tenesmus.

WORKUP

- Labs:
  - CBC often shows microcytic anemia.
  - Stool is ⊕ for occult blood.
  - CEA is nonspecific but useful for follow-up after treatment to screen for recurrence.

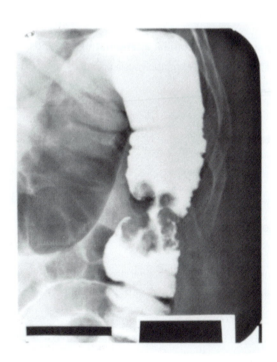

FIGURE 9-5. Barium enema x-ray showing the classic "apple-core" lesion of an encircling carcinoma in the descending colon.

Note the loss of mucosal pattern and the "hooks" at the margins of the lesion due to undermining. (Reproduced, with permission, from Way LW, Doherty GM. *Current Surgical Diagnosis & Treatment*, 11th ed. New York: McGraw-Hill, 2003: 720.)

- **Imaging:**
  - **Sigmoidoscopy** should be performed and all suspicious lesions biopsied.
  - **Colonoscopy** with barium enema.
  - Transrectal ultrasound to determine depth of invasion for rectal cancer.
  - Abdominal CT/MRI to stage colon cancer.
- **Metastatic workup:**
  - LFTs, CXR, abdominal CT.
  - Metastases may arise from the following:
    - **Hematogenous spread:** Blood-borne metastases commonly go to the liver (40–50% of cases), lungs, bone, and brain.
    - **Lymphatic spread:** Pelvic lymph nodes are often affected.
    - **Direct extension:** Local viscera.
    - **Peritoneal spread.**

TREATMENT

- **Colonic lesions:**
  - Surgical resection of the lesion with bowel margins of 3–5 cm.
  - Resection of the lymphatic drainage and mesentery at the origin of the arterial supply.
  - 1° anastomosis of bowel can usually be performed.

What are the common metastatic locations for colorectal cancer? Liver, lungs, and bone.

KEY POINT

RISK FACTORS AND SCREENING FOR COLORECTAL CANCER

- **Risk factors:**

  - Age.

  - **Hereditary syndromes: Familial adenomatous polyposis** (100% risk), Gardner's disease, hereditary nonpolyposis colorectal cancer (HNPCC).

  - Family history.

  - **IBD:** Ulcerative colitis >> Crohn's disease.

  - **Adenomatous polyps:** Villous polyps progress more often than tubular polyps and sessile more often than pedunculated. Lesions > 2 cm carry an ↑ risk.

  - A past history of colorectal cancer.

  - A high-fat, low-fiber diet.

- **Screening:**

  - A DRE should be performed yearly after age 55. Up to 10% of lesions are palpable with a finger.

  - Stool guaiac for occult blood should be performed every year for patients > 55 years of age. Up to 50% of ⊕ guaiac tests are due to colorectal cancer.

  - It is possible to visualize and biopsy 50–75% of lesions with sigmoidoscopy, which should be carried out every 3–5 years for those > 55 years of age.

  - Colonoscopy is indicated every 10 years beginning at age 40 in patients with a family history of colon cancer or polyps.

- Rectal lesions:
    - **Abdominoperineal resection:** For **low-lying lesions** near the anal verge, remove the rectum and anus and provide a permanent colostomy.
    - **Low anterior resection:** For **proximal lesions,** perform a 1° anastomosis of the colon to the rectum.
    - **Wide local excision:** For small, low-stage, well-differentiated tumors in the lower one-third of the rectum.
    - Ileoanal anastomosis spares the patient an abdominal ileostomy; pouch procedures ("continent ileostomy") provide a reservoir to maintain fecal continence.
- **Adjuvant therapy:**
    - Chemotherapy in cases of colon cancer with $\oplus$ lymph nodes.
    - In contrast to its role in rectal cancer, radiation has proven ineffective for colon cancer.
- **Follow-up:**
    - LFTs; serial CEA levels.
    - Colonoscopy.
    - CXR; abdominal CT or liver ultrasound (for metastases).

REFERENCES

- Blumberg D, Ramanathan RK. Treatment of colon and rectal cancer. *Clin Gastroenterol* 34:15–26, 2002. A comprehensive review of existing surgical, radiologic, and chemotherapeutic treatment options for colon and rectal cancer.
- Ponz de Leon M. Pathogenesis of colorectal cancer. *Dig Liver Dis* 32: 807–821, 2000. A useful review of the genetics and pathophysiology of colorectal cancer.

Inflammatory Bowel Disease (IBD)

A chronic, often progressive inflammatory disease of the small bowel, colon, and rectum. The two principal disorders, Crohn's disease and ulcerative colitis, differ in their histologic and clinical manifestations, their natural course, and their modes of therapy (see Table 9-4 and Figures 9-6 and 9-7).

DUKES' STAGING (ASTLER-COLLER MODIFICATION)

Dukes' staging has been supplanted by TNM staging but is still a favorite pimp topic.

Stage	Description	Five-Year Survival
A	Tumor limited to submucosa	> 90%
B1	Tumor invades into muscularis propria	70–80%
B2	Tumor invades through muscularis propria	50–65%
C1	B1 plus nodes	40–55%
C2	B2 plus nodes	20–30%
D	Distant metastasis/unresectable local spread	< 5%

TABLE 9-4. Crohn's Disease vs. Ulcerative Colitis

VARIABLE	ULCERATIVE COLITIS	CROHN'S DISEASE
Site of involvement	The **rectum** is always involved. May extend proximally in a **continuous fashion.** Inflammation and ulceration are **limited to the mucosa and submucosa.**	May involve **any portion** of the GI tract, particularly the **ileocecal region,** in a **discontinuous pattern** ("skip lesions"). The rectum is often spared. **Transmural** inflammation.
Symptoms and signs	**Bloody diarrhea,** lower abdominal cramps, tenesmus, urgency. Exam may reveal orthostatic hypotension, tachycardia, abdominal tenderness, frank blood on rectal exam, and extraintestinal manifestations.	Abdominal pain, abdominal mass, low-grade fever, weight loss, watery diarrhea. Exam may reveal fever, abdominal tenderness or mass, **perianal fissures, fistulas,** and extraintestinal manifestations.
Extraintestinal manifestations	Aphthous stomatitis, episcleritis/uveitis, arthritis, **1° sclerosing cholangitis, toxic megacolon,** erythema nodosum, and pyoderma gangrenosum.	Same as ulcerative colitis, as well as nephrolithiasis and fistulas to the skin, biliary tract, or urinary tract or between bowel loops.
Workup	CBC, AXR, stool cultures, O&P, stool assay for *C. difficile.* Colonoscopy can show diffuse and continuous rectal involvement, friability, edema, and **pseudopolyps.** Definitive diagnosis can be made with biopsy.	Same laboratory workup as ulcerative colitis. Colonoscopy may show aphthoid, linear, or stellate ulcers, strictures, **"cobblestoning,"** and **"skip lesions."** "Creeping fat" may also be present. Definitive diagnosis can be made with biopsy.
Treatment	**Sulfasalazine** or **5-ASA** (mesalamine); corticosteroids and immunosuppressants for refractory disease. **Total colectomy is curative** for long-standing or fulminant colitis or toxic megacolon.	**Sulfasalazine;** corticosteroids and immunosuppression are indicated if no improvement is seen. Surgical resection may be necessary for suspected perforation; **may recur** anywhere in the GI tract.
Incidence of cancer	**Markedly ↑ risk of colorectal cancer** in long-standing cases (monitor with frequent fecal occult blood screening and colonoscopy after eight years of disease).	Incidence of 2° malignancy is much lower than in ulcerative colitis.

HIGH-YIELD FACTS

SURGERY

REFERENCES

■ Chutkan RK. Inflammatory bowel disease. *Prim Care* 28:539–556, 2001. A comprehensive comparative review of the clinical presentation of IBD, its pathology (including images), and medical and surgical therapy.
■ Stotland BR et al. Advances in inflammatory bowel disease. *Med Clin North Am* 84:1107–1124, 2000. A thorough review of recent advances in diagnostics and therapies for IBD, along with an extensive bibliography.

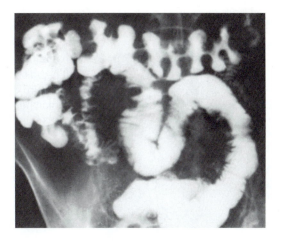

FIGURE 9-6. Crohn's disease on barium x-ray, showing spicules, edema, and ulcers.

(Reproduced, with permission, from Way LW, Doherty GM. *Current Surgical Diagnosis & Treatment*, 11th ed. New York: McGraw-Hill, 2003: 691.)

HEPATOBILIARY DISEASE

The four major disease processes to be aware of in the biliary system are cholelithiasis, acute cholecystitis, choledocholithiasis, and acute cholangitis. Figure 9-8 illustrates the basic anatomy of the gallbladder.

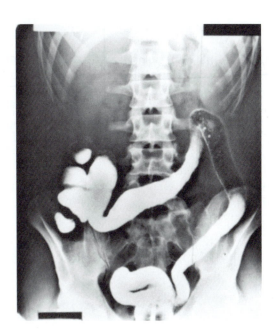

FIGURE 9-7. Ulcerative colitis on barium enema x-ray of the colon.

Note the short-ended colon, the "lead pipe" appearance due to loss of haustral markings, and the fine serrations at the edge of the bowel wall, which represent multiple small ulcers. (Reproduced, with permission, from Way LW, Doherty GM. *Current Surgical Diagnosis & Treatment*, 11th ed. New York: McGraw-Hill, 2003: 742.)

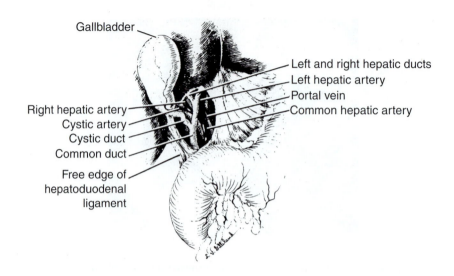

FIGURE 9-8. Anatomy of the gallbladder.

(Reproduced, with permission, from Way LW, Doherty GM. *Current Surgical Diagnosis & Treatment*, 11th ed. New York: McGraw-Hill, 2003: 597.)

Cholelithiasis and Biliary Colic

Transient obstruction of the cystic duct **without acute inflammation or infection** leading to recurrent bouts of postprandial abdominal pain.

SIGNS AND SYMPTOMS

- History:
    - Postprandial abdominal pain (usually in the RUQ) radiating to the right subscapular area or epigastrium. Pain is typically abrupt in onset with gradual relief and is self-limited but recurrent.
    - Nausea and vomiting.
    - Fatty food intolerance, dyspepsia, bloating, and flatulence are also common.
- PE:
    - Possible mild abdominal tenderness.
    - Patients generally do not present with fever or peritoneal signs.
    - Gallstones may be **asymptomatic in up to 80%** of patients.

DIFFERENTIAL

- GI: Acute cholecystitis, PUD, pancreatitis, GERD, appendicitis, hepatitis.
- Cardiac: MI.

WORKUP

- Labs:
    - CBC, electrolytes, amylase, lipase.
    - LFTs, bilirubin.
- Imaging:
    - RUQ ultrasound may show gallstones (90% sensitive), a dilated bile duct, and thickness of the gallbladder wall.
    - Plain x-rays are rarely diagnostic (only 10–15% of stones are radiopaque).

> **The 5 F's (risk factors) of cholelithiasis:**
>
> **F**emale
> **F**at
> **F**ertile
> **F**orty
> **F**latulent

KEY POINT ESSENTIALS OF GALLSTONES

- Stone formation requires (1) imbalance of the ratio of cholesterol/lecithin/bile salts, (2) a nucleating nidus, and (3) stasis.
- Subtypes are as follows:
  - **Cholesterol stones (80%):** Radiolucent and arise when bile becomes supersaturated with cholesterol, leading to cholesterol precipitation.
  - **Pigmented stones (20%):** Radiopaque.
    - **Black stones:** Contain calcium bilirubinate and are caused by hyperbilirubinemia due to chronic hemolysis or cirrhosis.
    - **Brown stones:** Associated with biliary tract infection and may have gram-⊖ bacteria in their core.

- CXR and ECG to rule out cardiopulmonary processes.
- HIDA scan to assess the patency of the cystic duct and, after cholecystokinin (CCK) administration, gallbladder ejection fraction (normal > 35%). A ⊕ HIDA usually indicates cholecystitis.

Only 10–15% of gallstones are radiopaque.

TREATMENT

- Dietary modification (avoid triggering substances such as fatty foods).
- Ursodiol (Actigall) desaturates the bile, impairing cholesterol nidus formation. This is effective in only 50% of patients, and recurrence is frequent.
- Lithotripsy uses extracorporeal shock waves to break up stones and is followed by dissolution therapy of the small fragments.
- **Cholecystectomy** (usually laparoscopic) represents definitive and curative therapy.

REFERENCE

Kalloo AN, Kantsevoy SV. Gallstones and biliary disease. *Prim Care* 28: 591–606, 2001. A thorough review of the definition, epidemiology, and pathophysiology of gallstones, acute cholecystitis, choledocholithiasis, and gallstone pancreatitis.

Acute Cholecystitis

Acute inflammation of the gallbladder caused by stone impaction in the cystic duct. May be accompanied by sepsis, gallbladder necrosis, or abscess formation. Obstruction of the cystic duct leads to gallbladder distention, inflammation, and infection.

SIGNS AND SYMPTOMS

- History:
  - Symptoms are similar to those of biliary colic but are more severe and of longer duration.
  - Include nausea, vomiting, and RUQ pain with or without fever/chills and jaundice.

What is Murphy's sign? Arrest of inspiration while palpating or placing an ultrasound probe on the RUQ.

- **PE:**
  - Presents with fever and abdominal guarding and/or rebound tenderness.
  - ⊕ **Murphy's sign:** Inspiratory arrest with subcostal palpation (30–98% sensitive).
  - ⊕ **Boas' sign:** Pain referred from the gallbladder to the right scapular region (< 7% sensitive).
  - Palpable gallbladder.

DIFFERENTIAL

- **GI:** Biliary colic, cholangitis, pancreatitis, PUD, GERD, hepatitis, appendicitis.
- **Cardiac:** MI.
- **Pulmonary:** Pneumonia.
- **GU:** Renal colic.

WORKUP

Ultrasound is the gold standard for the diagnosis of gallstones. Ultrasound and physical examination are the gold standards for cholecystitis. HIDA is used when ultrasound is equivocal.

- **Labs:**
  - CBC (leukocytosis), electrolytes, amylase, lipase.
  - **LFTs and bilirubin** often reveal mild hyperbilirubinemia (1–2 mg/dL).
- **Imaging:**
  - **Ultrasound** often shows stones, biliary sludge, pericholecystic fluid, a thickened gallbladder wall, and Murphy's sign.
  - HIDA scan shows nonfilling of the gallbladder, indicating cystic duct obstruction.

TREATMENT

- NPO, IV fluids.
- IV antibiotics (often cefazolin).
- **Cholecystectomy** (commonly laparoscopic) should be done as early as possible into the course of the infection, but not after three days of symptoms.

COMPLICATIONS

Abscess formation (15–20%), sepsis/perforation, gallbladder gangrene, gallstone ileus.

Choledocholithiasis

The presence of gallstones in the **common bile duct** can lead to cholangitis, pancreatitis, biliary colic, and/or jaundice.

SIGNS AND SYMPTOMS

RUQ pain, abdominal tenderness, biliary colic, jaundice.

WORKUP

- **Labs:**
  - CBC, electrolytes, amylase, lipase.

- ↑ **alkaline phosphatase** on LFTs may be the only abnormal laboratory value in patients without jaundice.
- Bilirubin levels.
- **Imaging:**
  - Ultrasound often shows bile duct dilatation but is only 15–30% sensitive for demonstrating common bile duct stones.
  - MRCP.

TREATMENT

- **ERCP** with sphincterotomy and stone removal.
- Mechanical lithotripsy.
- Extracorporeal shock wave lithotripsy.

Acute Cholangitis

A potentially **life-threatening** infection caused by gallstone or biliary sludge blockage of the common bile duct; can lead to severe septic shock without early intervention. Etiologies are as follows:

- **Obstruction:**
  - Common bile duct stones are the most common cause.
  - Stricture, neoplasm.
- **Infection:** Gram-⊖ bacteria (*E. coli, Klebsiella, Pseudomonas, Enterobacter, Proteus, Serratia*).

SIGNS AND SYMPTOMS

- **Charcot's triad:** RUQ pain, fever, and jaundice (the complete triad is present in only 20% of patients).
- **Reynolds' pentad:** Charcot's triad plus shock and altered mental status.

DIFFERENTIAL

- **GI:** Cholecystitis, pancreatitis, hepatitis.
- **Infection:** Sepsis.

WORKUP

- **Labs:**
  - CBC (leukocytosis), electrolytes, amylase, lipase.
  - LFTs (↑ alkaline phosphatase), ↑ bilirubin (direct more than indirect).
  - Blood cultures are ⊕ in roughly 50% of cases.
- **Imaging:** Ultrasound reveals ductal dilatation and gallstones (95% sensitivity).

TREATMENT

- IV hydration, electrolyte repletion, antibiotics.
- Bile duct decompression via endoscopic sphincterotomy, percutaneous transhepatic drainage, or operative decompression.

What is Charcot's triad? RUQ pain, fever, and jaundice—a triad that is pathognomonic for acute cholangitis.

Gas in the biliary tree supports the diagnosis of cholangitis.

HIGH-YIELD FACTS

SURGERY

Causes of acute pancreatitis—

BAD HITS

Biliary (gallstones obstructing the pancreatic ductal system—40%)
Alcohol (30%)
Drugs (steroids, estrogens, thiazide diuretics)
Hypercalcemia, **H**yperlipidemia, **H**yperparathyroidism
Idiopathic, **I**atrogenic (ERCP)
Trauma
Scorpion stings

What are the two most common causes of acute pancreatitis? Gallstones and alcohol.

Acute Pancreatitis

Acute inflammation of the pancreas. Etiologies are described in the mnemonic **BAD HITS**.

SIGNS AND SYMPTOMS

- History:
  - **Epigastric abdominal pain** often **radiating to the back** (present in 90% of cases).
  - Nausea/vomiting.
  - Fever.
- PE:
  - Dehydration, hypovolemia, tachycardia, tachypnea, hypotension, and shock.
  - An abdominal mass may be suggestive of a pseudocyst, abscess, or phlegmon.
  - Dullness over the left lower lung suggests a pleural effusion or pseudocyst.
  - **Grey Turner's sign:** Ecchymotic discoloration of the flank from pancreatic hemorrhage; seen in 1–2% of cases.
  - **Cullen's sign:** Ecchymosis of the periumbilical area from pancreatic hemorrhage; seen in 1–2% of cases.

DIFFERENTIAL

- **GI:** Perforated peptic ulcer, cholecystitis, appendicitis, mesenteric ischemia, SBO, hepatitis.
- **Cardiac:** MI; ruptured AAA.
- **GU:** Nephrolithiasis, pyelonephritis.

WORKUP

- Labs:
  - CBC (moderate leukocytosis), electrolytes, LFTs, PT/PTT.
  - **Amylase:** ↑ in > 90% of cases.
  - **Lipase: More specific** for pancreatitis than amylase.
- Imaging:
  - **CT:** The preferred diagnostic test. Can demonstrate pancreatic edema, necrosis, phlegmon, calcifications, and pseudocysts.
  - **CXR:** Shows basilar atelectasis indicative of a pleural effusion.
  - **AXR:** Shows sentinel loop or colon cutoff signs (a distended colon to the midtransverse colon with no air distally).
  - **Ultrasound:** Good for identifying pseudocyst, abscess, gallstones, and bile duct dilatation.

TREATMENT

Can be operative or nonoperative depending on the severity of the disease and on the presence of operable complications such as hemorrhage, pancreatic necrosis, or pseudocyst formation.

- Medical management:
  - NPO. Consider NG intubation in cases with abdominal distention and/or emesis.
  - Fluid and electrolyte repletion.

- **Pain control:** Meperidine (Demerol) may cause less spasm of the sphincter of Oddi than morphine (controversial) but is not typically used.
- **Nutrition:** Patients may require TPN if they are to be NPO for more than several days.
- Initiate **alcohol withdrawal prophylaxis** (benzodiazepines).
- There is no benefit to using antibiotics except in cases of pancreatic necrosis/abscess or sepsis.
- **Surgical management:**
  - **Pancreatic necrosis:** Surgical debridement.
  - **Noninfected pseudocysts:** Operative drainage via cystogastrostomy, cystojejunostomy, or cystoduodenostomy (usually not performed in the acute setting).
  - **Infected pseudocysts:** Must drain externally.
  - **Pancreatic hemorrhage:** Operative hemostasis.
  - **Gallstone pancreatitis:** ERCP and sphincterotomy with stone extraction followed by interval cholecystectomy (done after pancreatitis has resolved).
  - **If diagnosis is uncertain:** Diagnostic laparotomy.

COMPLICATIONS

- The mortality rate for acute pancreatitis is 10–20%. The prognosis worsens with a higher **Ranson's score** (see the boxed item below) or coexistent hemorrhage, respiratory failure, or severe persistent hypocalcemia.
- Complications include pseudocyst (10%); DIC/hemorrhage; sepsis, ARDS, and renal failure; and pleural effusion.

Chronic Pancreatitis

Chronic inflammation of the pancreas with damage to the parenchyma and resulting **endocrine and exocrine dysfunction.** Etiologies are outlined in the discussion of acute pancreatitis.

RANSON'S CRITERIA

The risk of mortality is 20% with 3–4 signs, 40% with 5–6 signs, and 100% with ≥ 7 signs.

On Admission	At 48 Hours after Admission
Age > 55 years	Hematocrit fall > 10%
WBC > 16,000/mL	BUN rise > 5 mg/dL
SGOT (AST) > 250 IU/dL	Serum Ca^{2+} < 8 mg/dL
Serum LDH > 350 IU/L	Arterial P_{O_2} < 60 mmHg
Blood glucose > 200 mg/dL	Estimated fluid sequestration > 6 L
	Base excess > 4 mEq/L

What is the most common cause of chronic pancreatitis in the United States? Alcohol abuse (70–80%).

HIGH-YIELD FACTS

SURGERY

SIGNS AND SYMPTOMS

- Recurrent epigastric pain that often radiates to the back.
- Weight loss.
- **Steatorrhea** due to lipase insufficiency from destruction of the exocrine pancreas.
- **Diabetes** due to insulin insufficiency from destruction of the endocrine pancreas.

WORKUP

- Labs:
  - CBC, electrolytes, LFTs, PT/PTT.
  - **Amylase, lipase.**
- Imaging:
  - CT is the preferred diagnostic test.
  - KUB may reveal calcifications.
  - ERCP/MRCP may show ductal dilatation and strictures ("chain of lakes" pattern).

TREATMENT

- **Medical management:** Similar to that of acute pancreatitis, plus insulin and pancreatic enzyme replacement in light of endocrine and exocrine dysfunction.
- **Surgical management:** Indicated after failure of medical therapy as well as failed ERCP with pancreatic sphincterotomy and endostent placement.
  - Pancreatectomy.
  - Pancreaticojejunostomy leading to decompression of the pancreatic ducts.

REFERENCES

- Cooperman AM. Surgery and chronic pancreatitis. *Surg Clin North Am* 81:431–455, 2001. A comprehensive discussion of the evaluation and surgical management of chronic pancreatitis.
- Vlodov J, Tenner SM. Acute and chronic pancreatitis. *Prim Care* 28: 607–628, 2001. Comprehensive yet manageable reviews of both of these topics.

Pancreatic Cancer

Most often characterized by adenocarcinoma arising from the **duct cells.** Tumors are most often found in the **head of the pancreas.** The prognosis is very poor for these patients, with only a 15–25% five-year survival rate. More common in men and in those > 65 years of age; additional risk factors include smoking, diabetes, alcohol abuse, high-fat and high-protein diets, African-American ethnicity, and industrial exposure.

SIGNS AND SYMPTOMS

- Jaundice, pruritus, dark urine, light stools.
- Anorexia and weight loss.
- Midepigastric abdominal pain and back pain.
- **Courvoisier's sign:** A nontender, distended gallbladder (50% of pancreatic cancer patients).

WORKUP

- **Labs:**
  - CBC, electrolytes, LFTs, PT/PTT.
  - Amylase and lipase are often not ↑.
  - CEA and CA 19-9.
- **Imaging:** CT, ERCP or MRCP, endoscopic ultrasound, staging laparoscopy or laparotomy.

TREATMENT

- **Whipple procedure** (pancreaticoduodenectomy): For tumors in the head of the pancreas.
- **Distal pancreatectomy with or without splenectomy:** For tumors of the body and tail of the pancreas.
- **Unresectable disease:** Palliation of biliary obstruction with endoprosthesis, percutaneous catheter, or biliary bypass (hepaticojejunostomy or choledochojejunostomy).

HERNIAS

Defined as abnormal protrusions of structures through the tissues that normally contain them. Hernias are the most common surgical disease in men and are 8–9 times more common in males than in females.

Inguinal Hernia

Protrusion of abdominal contents (usually the small intestine) into the inguinal region through a weakness or defect in the abdominal wall. Defined as direct or indirect according to their relationship to the inguinal canal (see Table 9-5).

COMPLICATIONS

- The recurrence rate after repair is 1–3%.
- Risk factors for recurrence include excessive suture line tension, use of an absorbable suture, failure to properly identify the hernia sac, postoperative wound infection, and chronic conditions that ↑ intra-abdominal pressure (e.g., constipation, morbid obesity, prostatism, chronic cough).

Femoral Hernia

An abnormal protrusion of abdominal contents **through the femoral canal** medial to the femoral vein. More common in women (85%); carries the **highest risk of incarceration and strangulation** owing to the narrow and unforgiving femoral canal, which is bordered superiorly by the inguinal ligament.

Hiatal Hernia

Present in 80% of patients with **GERD.** Subtypes are as follows:

- **Type I: Sliding hiatal hernias** (> 90%):
  - The gastroesophageal junction and the fundus of the stomach are displaced into the mediastinum.
  - **Signs/Sx:** Common symptoms include reflux, dysphagia, and esophagitis, but patients can be asymptomatic.

Inguinal hernias occur much more often in men than in women.

What is the most common hernia in both men and women? Indirect inguinal hernia.

Femoral hernias occur more often in women than in men.

419

TABLE 9-5. Direct vs. Indirect Inguinal Hernia

	DIRECT INGUINAL HERNIA	INDIRECT INGUINAL HERNIA
Definition	Herniation of abdominal contents through the **floor of Hesselbach's triangle** (see Figure 9-9).	Herniation of abdominal contents through the **internal inguinal ring** of the inguinal canal.
Defect	Acquired defect in the **transversalis fascia** from mechanical breakdown.	Congenital **patent processus vaginalis.**
Risk factors	Age.	The **most common hernia** in both men and women.
Characteristics	Does not traverse the internal inguinal ring. Herniates directly through the abdominal wall; contained within the aponeurosis of the external oblique muscle.	Traverses the external inguinal ring and ends up in the scrotum.
Treatment (surgical unless medically contraindicated)	High ligation of the hernia sac with correction of the defect in the transversalis fascia with Bassini repair, McVay repair, or mesh repair.	Isolation and ligation of the hernia sac with repair or enlarged internal ring.

- Tx: Antacids, small meals, head elevation.
- Type II: Paraesophageal hernias (< 5%):
  - The fundus herniates alongside the esophagus while the gastroesophageal junction remains in a normal position.
  - Tx/Cx: Incarceration and strangulation are common complications, and surgical repair is therefore indicated.

Other Hernias

- **Sliding hernia:** One wall of the inguinal hernia sac is formed by a viscus (cecum or sigmoid colon).
- **Pantaloon hernia:** A combination of a direct and an indirect inguinal hernia.
- **Richter's hernia:** Only one wall of the viscus lies within the hernia sac.
- **Spigelian hernia:** A ventral hernia occurring at the junction of the semilunar line and the lateral edge of the rectus muscle.

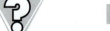

What is the most common cancer in women? Breast cancer.

Breast Cancer

The most common cancer and the second most common cause of cancer death in women (next to lung cancer). Approximately 10% of women in the United States will be diagnosed with breast cancer during their lifetimes. Al-

INGUINAL HERNIA ANATOMY AND KEY TERMS

■ **Anatomy:**

■ **Layers of the abdominal wall:** Skin, subcutaneous fat, Scarpa's fascia, external oblique muscle, internal oblique muscle, transversus abdominis muscle, transversalis fascia, and peritoneum.

■ **Inguinal (Poupart's) ligament:** The thickened lower border of the aponeurosis of the external oblique muscle, which runs from the anterior superior iliac spine to the pubic tubercle on each side.

■ **Inferior epigastric artery:** The branch of the external iliac artery that supplies the lower portion of the abdominal wall.

■ **Hesselbach's triangle:** An area formed by the inguinal ligament inferiorly, the lateral border of the rectus abdominis muscle medially, and the inferior epigastric vessels laterally (see Figure 9-9).

■ **Superficial (external) inguinal ring:** A defect in the external oblique aponeurosis through which the spermatic cord or round ligament passes en route to the scrotum/labia majora.

■ **Deep (internal) inguinal ring:** A defect in the transversalis fascia lateral to Hesselbach's triangle through which the spermatic cord emerges from the peritoneal cavity.

■ **Key terms:**

■ **Reducible hernia:** The contents of the hernia sac return to the abdomen with manual pressure.

■ **Incarceration:** The hernia cannot be reduced by external manipulation.

■ **Strangulation:** The blood supply to the contents of an incarcerated hernia is compromised, leading to ischemia.

though women are most commonly affected, a small number of men get breast cancer as well. Risk factors include the following:

■ Female gender, increasing age, postmenopausal obesity.
■ Early menarche (before age 12), late menopause (after age 50), nulliparity, first pregnancy after age 30.
■ A previous history of breast cancer.
■ A ⊕ family history of breast cancer.
■ A history of ductal carcinoma in situ (DCIS) and/or lobular carcinoma in situ (LCIS).
■ A history of ovarian/endometrial cancer.
■ BRCA1/2 genes.

SIGNS AND SYMPTOMS

■ A breast mass that does not change in size with menstrual cycle.
■ Breast mass tenderness.

What is the most common cause of cancer death in women? Lung cancer. Breast cancer is the second leading cause of cancer death in women.

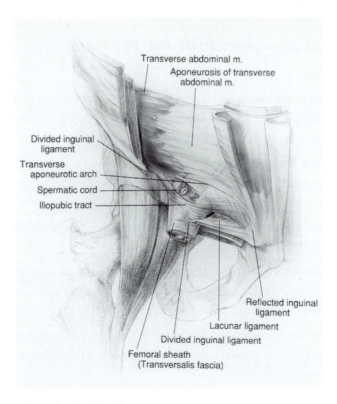

FIGURE 9-9. Hesselbach's triangle.

(Reproduced, with permission, from Schwartz SI et al (eds). *Principles of Surgery*, 7th ed. New York: McGraw-Hill, 1999: 1588.)

↑ *exposure to estrogen* ↑ *the risk of breast cancer.*

- Nipple discharge or retraction.
- A change in breast appearance, contour, or symmetry.

DIFFERENTIAL

- **Benign masses:** Well circumscribed, mobile, and tender; change in size with the menstrual cycle.
    - **Fibrocystic change (the most frequent breast lesion):** Painful (↑ before menses); fluctuate in size; often multiple/bilateral. Associated with an ↑ breast cancer risk only in the presence of ductal/atypical hyperplasia.
    - **Fibroadenomas:** Firm, round, mobile, and **nontender (the most common breast mass in women < 30 years of age).**
    - **Intraductal papilloma:** The most common cause of bloody nipple discharge.
    - **Other:** Lipoma, breast abscess, fat necrosis, mastitis.
- **Malignant masses:** Hard, irregular, and fixed; associated with nipple retraction, dimpling of the skin, edema, and lymphadenopathy (see Figure 9-10).
    - **Ductal carcinoma:** The most common breast malignancy (75% of breast cancer cases).
    - **Lobular carcinoma:** Approximately 8–10% of cases.
    - **Paget's carcinoma:** Infiltrating ductal carcinoma in the nipple. Symptoms include itching/burning of the nipple with superficial ulceration or erosion.

422

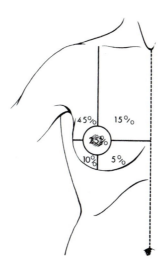

FIGURE 9-10. Frequency of breast cancer at various anatomic sites.

(Reprinted, with permission, from Way LW, Doherty GM. *Current Surgical Diagnosis & Treatment*, 11th ed. New York: McGraw-Hill, 2003: 323.)

- **Inflammatory carcinoma:** The most aggressive lesion; poorly differentiated and rapidly lethal. Symptoms include diffuse induration, warmth, erythema, edema, and axillary lymphadenopathy.

WORKUP

- Clinical breast examination.
- Mammography.
- Ultrasound for palpable masses or equivocal mammographic findings (e.g., microcalcifications).
- Needle aspiration of a palpable cystic lesion (with or without ultrasound guidance).
- If no fluid is aspirated, perform fine-needle aspiration (FNA) of a palpable lump.
- If FNA is nondiagnostic, perform core needle biopsy.
- Open excisional biopsy (with or without needle wire localization) is definitive but most invasive.
- Ductography and cytology are often performed for nipple discharge.

TREATMENT

- **Wide local excision (lumpectomy) plus radiation of remaining breast tissue:** Complete excision of the tumor with margins and axillary node dissection, followed by radiotherapy. Contraindicated in any of the following conditions:
  - A large cancer or a small breast.
  - Inability to obtain a clean margin.
  - Diffuse microcalcifications.
  - Previous radiation to the breast.
- **Simple mastectomy:** Removal of the breast and nipple only. Can be used as prophylaxis, but does not represent adequate treatment of breast cancer.
- **Modified radical mastectomy:** Removal of the breast and nipple with axillary node dissection (spares the chest wall muscles).

- **Radical mastectomy:** Removal of the breast, nipple, axillary nodes, and chest wall muscles. No longer commonly used to treat breast cancer.
- **Adjuvant therapy:** Carried out to eliminate micrometastases responsible for late recurrence. Determined by the following:
  - **Estrogen receptor status:** Use **tamoxifen for estrogen-sensitive tumors** and combination chemotherapy for non-estrogen-receptive tumors.
  - **Nodal involvement:** If there is evidence of ⊕ nodes, use combination chemotherapy.

REFERENCES

- Apantaku LM. Breast cancer diagnosis and screening. *Am Fam Physician* 62:596–602, 605–606, 2000. A complete review of the epidemiology, symptomatology, and diagnosis of breast cancer.
- Jatoi I. The natural history of breast cancer. *Surg Clin North Am* 79: 949–960, 1999. An article addressing the history of breast cancer screening, diagnosis, and management.

VASCULAR SURGERY

Abdominal Aortic Aneurysm (AAA)

Abnormal dilation of the abdominal aorta that develops from weakness or a defect in the wall of the vessel. Most AAAs are infrarenal. Risk factors include atherosclerosis, hypertension, smoking, age > 60, and male gender.

SIGNS AND SYMPTOMS

- Often asymptomatic.
- May present with **abdominal pain radiating to the back** and with a **pulsatile abdominal mass** in the midepigastrium or LUQ.
- Hypotension is also seen with rupture.

DIFFERENTIAL

- **Cardiac:** Aortic dissection, MI.
- **GI:** Pancreatitis, diverticulosis.
- **GU:** Renal colic.

WORKUP

- AXR may demonstrate a calcified outline of the AAA.
- Ultrasound is the best test for screening and follow-up of known small AAAs.
- CT is appropriate only for hemodynamically stable patients. Contrast allows full evaluation of aneurysmal size and possible dissection.
- ECG; tests of renal and pulmonary function to evaluate the risk of surgical repair.

TREATMENT

- **Ruptured AAAs are surgical emergencies.**
- **Medical management:** Control BP; provide IV access (two large-bore IVs); administer O_2.
- **Surgical management:**
  - Elective surgical repair to prevent rupture is indicated if the AAA is > **5 cm.**

What is the most common cause of AAA? Atherosclerosis.

Risk of rupture with AAA:

- **5 cm:** *5% per year*
- **6 cm:** *7% per year*
- **7 cm:** *15–20% per year*

- The operative mortality rate for nonruptured AAAs is < 5%, whereas that for ruptured AAAs is > 50%.
- Prosthetic graft placement.

Peripheral Vascular Disease

Caused by occlusive atherosclerotic plaques in the lower extremities. The most commonly involved artery is the **superficial femoral artery** in the adductor (Hunter's) canal. Risk factors include atherosclerosis, hyperlipidemia, diabetes, smoking, and hypertension.

SIGNS AND SYMPTOMS

- **Claudication:** Reproducible leg pain produced by walking a certain distance, with relief of the pain on resting. Rest pain represents a more severe progression of peripheral vascular disease.
- **Other:** Absent pulses, impaired sensation, bruits, muscular atrophy, ↓ hair growth, impotence, tissue infection.

WORKUP

- The **ankle-brachial index (ABI)** measures the ratio of systolic BP at the ankle to that of the arm.
  - **ABI 1.0–1.2:** Normal.
  - **ABI 0.4–0.9:** Moderate arterial obstruction, often associated with claudication.
  - **ABI < 0.4:** Advanced ischemia.
  - **Note:** ABI is falsely elevated in DM owing due to arterial calcification.
- Doppler ultrasound.

Rest pain typically occurs with an ABI < 0.4.

TREATMENT

- Exercise, diet.
- Smoking cessation is critical to the long-term success of any vascular reconstruction.
- Treatment of hypertension.
- Pentoxifylline.
- Bypass graft (autologous vein or prosthetic).

REFERENCE

Newman AB. Peripheral arterial disease: Insights from population studies of older adults. *J Am Geriatr Soc* 48:1157–1162, 2000. A review of the epidemiology, symptomatology, natural history, and management of peripheral vascular disease.

Acute Arterial Occlusion

Insufficient arterial blood flow to meet the metabolic demands of tissue can lead to limb-threatening ischemia. The most common site of occlusion is the common femoral artery. Etiologies include embolism, vascular trauma, and thrombosis of an atherosclerotic lesion.

SIGNS AND SYMPTOMS

Presents with the "6 P's" (see mnemonic) plus ischemic ulcers and limb gangrene.

> **The 6 P's of acute arterial occlusion:**
>
> **P**ain
> **P**aralysis
> **P**allor
> **P**aresthesia
> **P**oikilothermia
> **P**ulselessness

ABI, Doppler ultrasound, angiography, MRI.

TREATMENT

- Anticoagulation (i.e., IV heparin).
- Surgical thrombectomy/embolectomy or arterial bypass. Compartment syndrome is a possible sequela to revascularization; check compartment pressures and perform fasciotomy if > 30 mmHg.
- Amputation.

UROLOGIC DISEASE

Prostate Cancer

The most common visceral malignant neoplasm affecting U.S. males, with the risk of disease approximating 1 in 5 in that population. The mortality rate is decreasing, with a current annual risk of approximately 3%. Roughly 95% of masses are adenocarcinomas. Risk factors include the following:

- Increasing age (rarely diagnosed before age 50; 85% of diagnoses are made in patients > 65 years of age).
- African-American ethnicity (African-Americans also have a higher mortality rate even after adjusting for age and SES).
- A family history of prostate cancer.
- Prostate cancer susceptibility genes.
- Dietary fat, especially polyunsaturated fats.

DIAGNOSIS

- Localized prostate cancer rarely causes symptoms at earlier stages, since the disease usually occurs at the periphery of the gland away from the urethra. Therefore, screening is vital to increasing detection and decreasing mortality. Screening involves annual DRE and PSA tests starting at age 50.
- Abnormalities on DRE (nodularity, induration) or an elevated PSA (usually > 4 ng/mL) can prompt the use of prostate biopsy for histologic diagnosis.
- Grading and staging:
  - **Tumor grade:** Elucidated from prostate biopsy. The Gleason grading system classifies cancers by describing the low-magnification architecture of the biopsy specimen. The Gleason score is considered predictive of prognosis and disease extent.
  - **Tumor stage:** Most often classified by means of the TNM staging system; can be either clinical (using pretreatment parameters) or pathologic (determined following prostate removal and careful histologic analysis).

TREATMENT

- Radical prostatectomy:
  - The gold standard for clinically localized (< T2N0M0) disease. Usually performed by the retropubic approach.
  - Involves complete removal of the prostate gland and seminal vesicles along with modified pelvic lymph node dissection. Anatomic nerve-sparing dissection is performed if the surgeon is comfortable with the technique and disease is limited.

TNM STAGING FOR PROSTATE CANCER

- **T (tumor):**

    - **T1:** A nonpalpable tumor; not evidenced by imaging, and found incidentally during tissue removal.

        - **T1a:** < 5% of transurethrally resected (TUR) tissue is cancerous and Gleason grade < 7.

        - **T1b:** > 5% of TUR tissue is cancerous or Gleason grade > 7.

        - **T1c:** The tumor is found after a biopsy prompted by an elevated PSA.

    - **T2:** A palpable tumor on DRE; limited to the prostate.

        - **T2a:** The tumor involves only one lobe.

        - **T2b:** The tumor involves more than one lobe.

    - **T3:** A palpable tumor that goes beyond the prostate.

        - **T3a:** Extends past the prostate capsule on one side.

        - **T3b:** Extends past the prostate capsule on both sides.

        - **T3c:** Involves the seminal vesicles.

    - **T4:** The tumor is fixed or involves adjacent structures (other than the seminal vesicles).

        - **T4a:** The tumor involves the bladder neck, the external sphincter, and/or the rectum.

        - **T4b:** The tumor involves the levator muscle and/or the pelvic wall.

- **N (node):**

    - **N0:** No regional lymph node metastasis.

    - **N1:** Single regional node involvement < 2 cm.

    - **N2:** Single regional node involvement 2–5 cm or multiple regional nodes < 5 cm.

    - **N3:** Single or multiple regional node involvement > 5 cm.

- **M (metastasis):**

    - **M0:** No distant metastasis.

    - **M1:** Distant metastasis.

        - **M1a:** Metastasis to nonregional lymph nodes.

        - **M1b:** Metastasis to bones.

        - **M1c:** Metastasis to other distant sites.

- Complications include bleeding, impotence, incontinence, and rectal injury.
- **Radiation therapy:** Can be delivered by an external beam or through implantation of radioactive seeds (brachytherapy). Complications include functional urinary complaints, impotence, hematuria, strictures, and rectal complaints.
- **Androgen ablation:** Usually reserved for extraprostatic disease, in cases of refractory disease, or for patients who do not seek other modalities of treatment. Often used as neoadjuvant therapy in conjunction with surgery or radiation for T2 disease or as nonadjuvant 1° therapy for more progressive disease.

REFERENCE

Wein AJ et al. *Campbell-Walsh Urology*, 9th ed. Atlanta: Elsevier, 2007. Regarded as the "Bible of urology."

COMMON CLERKSHIP TOPICS

The third-year surgery clerkship often involves time not only in general surgery but also in some of the surgical specialties. The following three questions can help you focus on the specific topics at hand:

- What is the natural history and appropriate evaluation of the current surgical problem?
- How do surgeons make the decision to intervene and prioritize the various therapeutic options?
- How do surgeons evaluate the risks and benefits of those therapeutic options in the context of a patient's problems, overall status, and life expectancy?

Given these considerations, the following list outlines common diseases and key topics that you are likely to encounter in the course of your surgery rotation.

- **Gastrointestinal disease:**
  - Acute abdomen
  - Esophageal disorders (achalasia, esophageal varices, esophageal rupture, esophageal cancer)
  - Stomach disorders (gastritis, gastroenteritis, gastric cancer, GERD [see Internal Medicine], peptic ulcer disease [see Internal Medicine])
  - GI bleeding
    - Upper GI bleeding
    - Lower GI bleeding
  - Small bowel disease
    - Small bowel obstruction
    - Neoplasms
      - Benign (adenomas, hemangiomas, leiomyomas, lipomas)
      - Malignant (adenocarcinoma, carcinoid, lymphoma, metastatic)
  - Large bowel disease
    - Colitis
    - Diverticular disease
    - Fistulas

- Hemorrhoids
- Intussusception (see Pediatrics)
- Colorectal cancer
- Inflammatory bowel disease (Crohn's vs. ulcerative colitis)
- Appendicitis (see Emergency Medicine)
- **Hepatobiliary disease:**
  - Cholelithiasis and biliary colic
  - Acute cholecystitis
  - Choledocholithiasis
  - Acute cholangitis
  - Hepatocellular carcinoma
- **Pancreatic disease:**
  - Acute pancreatitis
  - Chronic pancreatitis
  - Pancreatic pseudocysts
  - Pancreatic cancer
  - Splenic rupture
- **Hernias:**
  - Inguinal hernia
  - Femoral hernia
  - Hiatal hernia
  - Other hernias
- **Breast disease (also see OB/GYN):**
  - Breast cancer
  - Fibrocystic disease
  - Fibroadenoma
- **Cardiothoracic surgery:**
  - Coronary artery disease (see Internal Medicine)
  - Congenital and valvular heart disease (see Internal Medicine)
  - Lung cancer (see Internal Medicine)
  - Pulmonary emboli (see Internal Medicine)
  - Potentially life-threatening injuries and their treatment (pneumothorax, tamponade [see Emergency Medicine])
- **Otolaryngology:**
  - Head and neck tumors
  - Hyperthyroidism
  - Hyperparathyroidism
- **Urology:**
  - Benign prostatic hypertrophy
  - Incontinence
  - Prostate cancer
  - Renal and ureteral stones
- **Vascular surgery:**
  - Abdominal aortic aneurysm
  - Carotid vascular disease, carotid endarterectomy (see Neurology)
  - Peripheral vascular disease, diabetic vascular disease, acute arterial occlusion, deep venous thrombosis, varicose veins, lymphedema
- **Other:**
  - Anesthesiology (intubation)
  - Burns (see Emergency Medicine)
  - Fluids and acid-base balance (see Practical Information for All Clerkships)
  - Wound healing/surgical infection
  - Trauma and shock (see Emergency Medicine)

SECTION 3

Top-Rated Review Resources

This section is a database of recommended books and study guides for use during wards rotations. For each book, we list the **Title** of the book, the **First Author** (or editor), the **Current Publisher**, the **Copyright Year**, the **Edition**, the **Number of Pages**, the **ISBN Code**, and the **Approximate List Price** of the book. Entries also include Summary Comments that describe the various books' style and utility for study and review. Finally, each book receives a **Rating.** The books are sorted into a general section as well as into sections corresponding to the seven clinical rotations (emergency medicine, internal medicine, neurology, OB/GYN, pediatrics, psychiatry, and surgery). Also included are review sections devoted to pocket drug references; pocket cards; ECG books; resources on fluids, electrolytes, and acid-base physiology; radiology books; and PDA resources. Within each section, books are arranged first by Rating, then by Author, and finally by Title.

For this fourth edition of *First Aid for the Wards*, the database of review books has been completely revised, with in-depth summary comments. A letter rating scale with six different grades reflects detailed student evaluations. Each book receives a rating as follows:

A+	Excellent for the wards.
A	
A–	Very good for the wards; choose among the group.
B+	
B	Good, but use only after exhausting better sources.
B–	

The **Rating** is meant to reflect the overall usefulness of the book. This is based on a number of factors, including the following:

- The cost of the book
- The readability of the text
- The appropriateness and accuracy of the book
- The quality and appropriateness of the illustrations (e.g., graphs, diagrams, photographs)
- The length of the text (longer is not necessarily better)
- The quality and number of other books available in the same discipline

Many books with low ratings are well written and informative but are not ideally suited to the wards experience. We have also avoided listing or commenting on the wide variety of general textbooks available in the clinical sciences.

Evaluations are based on the cumulative results of formal and informal surveys of hundreds of medical students from medical schools across the country. The summary comments and overall ratings represent a consensus opinion, but there may have been a large range of opinions or limited student feedback on any particular book.

Please note that the data listed are subject to change because:

- Publishers' prices change frequently.
- Individual bookstores often charge an additional markup.

- New editions come out frequently, and the quality of updating varies.
- The same book may be reissued through another publisher.

We actively encourage medical students and faculty to submit their opinions and ratings of these books so that we may update our database (see "How to Contribute," p. xiii). In addition, we ask that publishers and authors submit review copies of clinical science resources, including new editions and books not included in our database, for evaluation. We also solicit reviews of new books or suggestions for alternate modes of study that may be useful for the wards, such as flash cards, computer-based tutorials, and Internet Web sites.

DISCLAIMER/CONFLICT-OF-INTEREST STATEMENT

No material in this book, including the ratings, reflects the opinion or influence of the publisher. All errors and omissions will gladly be corrected if brought to the attention of the authors through the publisher.

A

Bates' Pocket Guide to Physical Examination   **$39.95**
and History Taking
BICKLEY
Lippincott Williams & Wilkins, 2007, 5th ed., 455 pages,
ISBN 9780781793483
A concise yet thorough overview of the physical exam, written in full
color with numerous illustrations and organized into two columns
for rapid reference. A compact version of *Bates' Guide*, the book is
probably all one needs to master the physical exam from children to
pregnant women. Also contains a free PDA download.

A

DeGowin's Diagnostic Examination   **$49.95**
DEGOWIN
McGraw-Hill, 2004, 8th ed., 1077 pages, ISBN 9780071409230
A classic handbook divided into physical exam, lab tests, and common disease patterns. Gives clear explanations of pathophysiology
and provides differentials for nearly every physical finding imagin-
able. Includes brief discussions of the pathophysiology of abnormal
lab values. The section on diagnostic clues highlights signs and
symptoms along with abnormal labs found in specific diseases. Much
too big to carry in the pocket; ideally used as a supplement to *Bates'
Guide* or another more basic exam book.

A⁻

Boards and Wards: A Review for the   **$36.95**
USMLE Steps 2 & 3
AYALA
Lippincott Williams & Wilkins, 2003, 2nd ed., 416 pages,
ISBN 9781405103411
A good overview of every major rotation. Excellent for reading both
before and at the end of each rotation. Written in outline format
with great tables, charts, and algorithms. Appendices include reviews
of zebras and syndromes, toxicology, and vitamins and nutrition. Fits
in the pocket. Not a complete resource for any specific rotation, as it
lacks necessary details, but useful for a quick and comprehensive review of high-yield information for end-of-rotation written exams.
May be helpful for USMLE preparation as well. The clinical vignettes and practice questions included at the end of each chapter
could be expanded.

A– ***History and Physical Examination***   ***$14.95***

CHAN

Current Clinical Strategies, 2002, 10th ed., 99 pages,
ISBN 9781929622283

A concise outline pocketbook that contains advice on pertinent things to include in an H&P for a particular chief complaint. Can be helpful in the formulation of differentials as well as for questioning on rounds. Good for writing admit notes. Offers limited coverage of disease, but a useful resource for its price.

A– ***Fundamentals of Clinical Medicine***   ***$34.95***

CHAUDHRY

Lippincott Williams & Wilkins, 2004, 4th ed., 443 pages,
ISBN 9780781751926

A good introductory book for the transition from classroom to wards. Contains helpful yet concise information on history taking, progress notes, diagnostic tests, and the basic pathophysiology of numerous diseases, organized by system. Small enough to fit in a pocket, and provides a great overview of the wards for beginning third-year medical students.

A– ***Clinician's Pocket Reference***   ***$39.95***

GOMELLA

McGraw-Hill, 2007, 11th ed., 722 pages, ISBN 9780071454285

A good overall wards orientation that makes excellent use of tables, graphs, and diagrams to explain concepts. Provides an effective reference for procedures, and includes useful algorithms, protocols for medical emergencies, interpretations of abnormal lab values, and a chapter on commonly used drugs with dosages and contraindications. Practical sections on basic ECG reading and critical care medicine are also provided. Does not emphasize pathophysiology or differential diagnoses. General and light on coverage of diseases; fits tightly in most coat pockets. Most beneficial for students entering the wards.

REVIEW RESOURCES

GENERAL

436

A⁻

Maxwell's Quick Medical Reference

$7.95

MAXWELL

Maxwell Publishing, 2006, 5th ed., 32 pages,
ISBN 9780964519138

Popular, compact, spiral-bound fact cards detailing ACLS algorithms, various in-house notes, normal lab values, basic formulas, the H&P, and the psychiatric and neurologic exams. Especially important at the beginning of the clinical years, but not as critical toward the end, when students have become better acquainted with the wards. The most frequently used features are the common lab values, formulas, and sample notes. Great for quick reference, and small enough to fit in any pocket.

A⁻

Pocket Guide to Diagnostic Tests

$39.95

NICOLL

McGraw-Hill, 2007, 5th ed., 512 pages, ISBN 9780071489683

A concise and useful reference for common diagnostic tests in quick-flip tabular format. Discusses physiologic bases for and interpretation of lab results. Includes useful sections focusing on microbiology, drug monitoring, ECG interpretation, and diagnostic radiology. A good size for the pocket, but relatively heavy, so students may want to carry it in a backpack for quick reference whenever needed.

A⁻

Interpretation of Diagnostic Tests

$69.95

WALLACH

Lippincott Williams & Wilkins, 2007, 8th ed., 1200 pages,
ISBN 9780781730556

A text that is organized by organ system with summaries of available tests for most diseases. Discusses the interpretation of abnormal labs and differentials, and includes tables comparing test results from similar diseases. Similar to *Pocket Guide to Diagnostic Tests* but larger and more comprehensive, with excellent, encyclopedic coverage. Will not fit in the pocket; better for use as a reference.

B⁺

On Call Procedures

$36.95

ADAMS

Elsevier, 2006, 2nd ed., 300 pages, ISBN 9781416024446

A quick, concise resource on basic and advanced procedures, including endotracheal intubation, central line placement, and fluid taps. Includes indications, contraindications, precautions, step-by-step techniques, complications, and guidelines for removal. Good diagrams are provided for anatomy and approach. Although there is no substitute for actual hands-on experience, the book provides a clear picture of the invasive medical and surgical procedures one is likely to encounter on the wards.

REVIEW RESOURCES

GENERAL

Differential Diagnosis of Common Complaints
$38.95

SELLER

Elsevier, 2007, 5th ed., 468 pages, ISBN 9781416029069

A detailed discussion of 36 common complaints or problems and their associated diagnoses, including ways to differentiate between them. Best used for patients with common complaints but complicated clinical pictures or for reviewing the general management of common complaints.

Blackwell's Survival Guide for Interns
$9.95

HAMMAD

Lippincott Williams & Wilkins, 2002, 1st ed., 130 pages, ISBN 9780632045891

A pocketbook written for residents and interns on the wards. Not particularly useful for junior medical students, but may serve as a good introduction to subinternships.

Blueprints Clinical Procedures
$42.95

MARBAS

Lippincott Williams & Wilkins, 2004, 1st ed., 227 pages, ISBN 9781405103886

An easy-to-read instruction book for common procedures pertinent to inpatient care. Contains advice on reading charts, entering orders, writing various in-house notes, performing basic procedures, and organizing data and presentations. Some information given is common sense. Not as useful once students have become more advanced in their clinical education.

On Call Principles and Protocols
$40.95

MARSHALL

Elsevier, 2005, 4th ed., 528 pages, ISBN 9780721639024

A practical guidebook designed for the intern or resident on call. Not as useful for the junior medical student, but may come in handy for the subintern. Attempts to cover a broad range of problems, which makes it superficial in its scope. Most useful for internal medicine and surgery. Divided into phone-call management, elevator thoughts, threats to life, and bedside care.

**Saint-Frances Guide to Clinical Clerkships: The Answer
Book**
WIESE
Lippincott Williams & Wilkins, 2006, 1st ed., 529 pages,
ISBN 9780781737548
An all-purpose approach toward success in the clinical clerkships.
One-third of the text offers general tips for medical clerkships, from
charting to navigating the hospital environment to communicating
and gathering information. A third is devoted to a detailed review of
the physical exam. The final third of the text describes specific tips
and characteristics of the individual clerkships. Designed to help students succeed on the wards, the book is of limited utility for more
advanced students but is ideal for those about to enter their first
clerkship.

$32.95

Ferri's Differential Diagnosis
FERRI
Elsevier, 2006, 1st ed., 378 pages, ISBN 9780323040938
An extensive list of the differential diagnoses of common disorders
and syndromes, organized by symptom. Particularly helpful for diagnosing unusual symptoms or combinations of findings, but not as
useful for studying common disorders or for boards review. Conve-
nient size and format for carrying in a coat pocket.

$23.95

Rapid Review Laboratory Testing in Clinical Medicine
GOLJAN
Elsevier, 2008, 1st ed., 456 pages, ISBN 9780323036467
A text that focuses on the pathophysiology underlying abnormal laboratory values and common clinical tests, including pulmonary function tests and peripheral blood smears. Presented in outline format.
Includes 212 USMLE-style questions along with free access to the
online question bank. Useful as a review text, but too large and detailed to be used as an everyday reference guide.

$39.95

The Right Test
SPEICHER
Elsevier, 1998, 3rd ed., 350 pages, ISBN 9780721651231
A handbook that is organized into five broad sections with discussions of frequently encountered disorders. Each section consists of
chapters that include a textual description of the diagnostic approach
and clinical thinking, followed in most cases by a review and a clinical vignette. Includes a limited number of figures and tables. Educational but oversimplified, the text may be too superficial to be of
value by the time one reaches clinical rotations.

$41.95

The Sanford Guide to Antimicrobial Therapy

$12.95

GILBERT

Antimicrobial Therapy, 2007, 37th ed., 202 pages,
ISBN 9781930808386

The gold-standard pocket antimicrobial reference guide, updated yearly. Includes dosage, coverage, sensitivities, length of therapy, renal dosing, and drugs of choice for common and uncommon infections. Presented in tabular format. The small print is sometimes difficult to read. Remember to see if your own institution has its own guidelines or formulary. Otherwise, a pocket-worthy guide for any rotation.

Tarascon Pocket Pharmacopoeia: Classic Shirt-Pocket Edition

$11.95

GREEN

Tarascon Publishing, 2008, 22nd ed., 160 pages,
ISBN 9781882742554

An excellent pocket reference book of drugs indexed by generic and trade names. Includes drug class, typical dosing, metabolism, safety in pregnancy and lactation, relative cost, tables, and conversion factors. Also included is a short summary of ACLS protocols, emergency drug infusions, and pediatric dosing. A must-have for the wards, especially for subinterns. Compact and inexpensive.

Clinician's Pocket Drug Reference

$11.95

GOMELLA

McGraw-Hill, 2007, 1st ed., 286 pages, ISBN 9780071477680

Related to *Clinician's Pocket Reference*, this pocketbook is slightly larger than the shirt-pocket edition of *Tarascon Pharmacopoeia* but smaller than the deluxe version. Organized in alphabetical order, it contains information on 900 commonly used medications. Also included are descriptions of common uses, mechanisms of action, precautions and contraindications, and common side effects. Useful tables near the end of the book compare similar drugs.

REVIEW RESOURCES

POCKET DRUG REFERENCES

Nelson's Pocket Book of Pediatric Antimicrobial Therapy

$19.95

NELSON

AWWE, 2007, 16th ed., 152 pages, ISBN 9789507623035

A specialized pediatric version of *Sanford* with a quick-reference guide to the selection and use of antimicrobials in children. Given that much of pediatrics is infectious disease, this text can serve as a good reference for students, especially subinterns. The format makes it easy to find pathogens, diseases, and recommended drugs of choice.

Handbook of Clinical Drug Data

$49.95

ANDERSON

McGraw-Hill, 2002, 10th ed., 1148 pages, ISBN 9780071363624

A comprehensive drug guide written from primary literature. Includes mechanisms of action, patient instructions, pharmacokinetics, interactions, adverse effects, drug monitoring, and abundant tables that compare each drug within a therapeutic class. A good but costly resource for those interested in a detailed pharmacology reference. Too bulky to be used as a pocket drug manual.

Medi-Data

$9.95

RODRIGUEZ

Rodram, 2002, 6th ed., 58 pages, ISBN 9789686277920

A small, concise pocketbook with extensive listings of normal lab values and diagnostic tests.

REVIEW RESOURCES

POCKET DRUG REFERENCES

Adult History and PE-Pro $8.75

Medical Information Systems, 2001, 1st ed., 2 cards,
ISBN 1981953419

A thorough two-card reference set summarizing the essentials of the H&P in an expanded outline format that includes a detailed review of systems and a comprehensive physical examination section. Although most applicable to a medicine or surgery rotation, this card set also contains an extensive amount of neurology, including the Mini-Mental Status Examination, a Glasgow Coma Scale discussion, and a summary of the neurologic exam. Most helpful for students beginning their clinical rotations and for those who seek a quick review of the H&P before their patient encounters.

ECG Pocketcard $3.95

Börm Bruckmeier Publishing, 2005, 2nd ed., 1 card,
ISBN 9781591030287

A pocket card similar to *EKG Interactive* in both scope and content. The small type is somewhat difficult to read.

EKG Interactive $5.95

RODRIGUEZ

Rodram, 2003, 3rd ed., 1 card, ISBN 9780972305877

A detailed pocket card containing normal ECG values, criteria for diagnosing specific ECG abnormalities, and a ruler for measuring intervals. Too advanced for the junior medical student beginning clinical rotations, as students need prior knowledge of ECG interpretation if they are to make best use of the card. Would be helpful as a quick reference for the cardiology subintern. Includes a bonus CD containing a clinical calculator.

H&P Interactive $5.95

RODRIGUEZ

Rodram, 2003, 3rd ed., 1 card, ISBN 9780972305884

A well-organized pocket card for the H&P that includes a bonus CD containing a clinical calculator. More compact than *Adult History and PE-Pro* but not as detailed, particularly in the physical exam section.

REVIEW RESOURCES

POCKET CARDS

History & Physical Exam Pocketcard

$3.95

Börm Bruckmeier Publishing, 2005, 2nd ed., 1 card,
ISBN 9781591030225

Offers a nice table layout with a breakdown of each section of the H&P in its own separate box. Not as comprehensive as other available cards.

History and Physical Exam Guide

$4.50

Medical Information Systems, 2001, 1st ed., 1 card,
ISBN 8804956658

A condensed version of *Adult History and PE-Pro,* written in an expanded outline format. Includes only a minimal description of the key features of the HPI. Disproportionate attention is focused on the cardiac exam, including the differential of heart murmurs, as compared to the other components of the physical exam.

Normal Values Guide

$4.50

Medical Information Systems, 1999, 1st ed., 1 card,
ISBN 8804950552

Contains normal lab values for electrolytes, hematology, urine, CSF, toxicology, ABGs, and protein electrophoresis. Also includes a small table of fluid composition and conversion factors. A pupil-size gauge is included in the back along with a ruler. Omits normal cardiac enzyme levels. Maxwell's pocket reference is more comprehensive and useful.

Normal Values-Pro

$8.75

Medical Information Systems, 2002, 1st ed., 2 cards,
ISBN 8819980096

An expanded version of the *Normal Values Guide* that includes a diagram for acid-base disturbances along with additional normal lab values. Not as useful as it could potentially be with the addition of an extra card. Too many lab values are listed where the normal is "negative," such as those for RPR or HCV serologies.

ECG Ruler Pocketcard

$3.95

Börm Bruckmeier Publishing, 2002, 1st ed., 1 card,
ISBN 9781591030027

A pocket card with one side dedicated to the proper placement of leads and the other side containing a systematic check-off list of steps toward ECG interpretation. Contains no normal values or criteria for diagnosing ECG abnormalities.

B– ***Pocket PE: Physical Examination Study Cards***   *$22.95*
MATTHEWS
Lippincott Williams & Wilkins, 2000, 1st ed., 33 cards,
ISBN 9780781723695
A collection of cards with detailed information on physical signs, ex-
amination, and charts/tables. Individual cards may be bulky to carry
and are often unsuitable for quick review.

The Only EKG Book You'll Ever Need
THALER

$59.95

Lippincott Williams & Wilkins, 2007, 5th ed., 342 pages,
ISBN 9780781773157

A text that stresses basic electrophysiology and simple ECG interpretation, organized according to problem. Includes useful chapter summaries and a comprehensive review of important principles. Also offers case presentations, tables, graphs, and sample 12-lead ECGs. Concise and highly readable, but would benefit from more practice ECGs. Good for beginners looking for simple explanations and descriptions, but may be too superficial for those who seek to seriously master ECG interpretation.

Marriott's Practical Electrocardiography
WAGNER

$69.95

Lippincott Williams & Wilkins, 2008, 11th ed., 488 pages,
ISBN 9780781797382

A thorough ECG reference that includes normal and abnormal ECG findings. May be too detailed for junior medical students. Includes illustrations, literature references, ECG tracings, and a glossary. Excellent for cardiology subinterns and for those interested in going to the next level of ECG interpretation. Somewhat costly, but includes a DVD reference.

Rapid Interpretation of EKGs
DUBIN

$38.00

Cover Publishing, 2000, 6th ed., 368 pages,
ISBN 9780912912066

Presented as a "workbook," this classic reference facilitates the rapid acquisition of ECG fundamentals, emphasizing active learning with fill-in-the-blank exercises and visual aids on each page. Includes excellent quick-reference pages at the end that can be copied and placed in one's coat pocket. Can easily be read in a weekend. Although its content has not changed significantly in several years, this book is still considered a basic stepping stone for the junior student. However, it falls somewhat short on practice ECGs, and another book will likely be needed for more advanced ECG interpretation.

150 Practice ECGs: Interpretation and Review $39.95
TAYLOR

Wiley, 2006, 3rd ed., 272 pages, ISBN 9781405104838

A spiral-bound workbook with sections dedicated to basic electrophysiology and practice. Excellent for medical students wishing to practice, but can be difficult to use, as reviews for the ECGs are randomly organized and some are highly advanced. Lacks thorough explanations of ECG pathology and physiology, but frequently focuses on clinical management.

Basic Electrocardiography in 10 Days $39.95
FERRY

McGraw-Hill, 2007, 2nd ed., 266 pages, ISBN 9780071465625

A good discussion of how to interpret ECGs. Organized by pathology, with illustrations of the heart showing where the corresponding lesions should be located along with a vector cardiographic loop approach. Designed at an appropriate level for junior and senior medical students. Each section is followed by several ECGs for the student to diagnose. Overall, a weighty book that contains numerous ECG samples to practice but lacks more detailed explanations in some parts.

Rapid ECG Interpretation $45.95
KHAN

Elsevier, 2003, 2nd ed., 255 pages, ISBN 9780721603285

Presents ECGs organized by abnormality with explanations of the pathophysiology and differentials of aberrant waveforms. Well organized, with consistent presentation of an 11-step method for rapid ECG diagnosis. Readable and helpful but not outstanding.

Quick and Accurate 12-Lead ECG Interpretation $44.95
DAVIS

Lippincott Williams & Wilkins, 2005, 4th ed., 464 pages, ISBN 9781582553795

A good introductory text for ECG interpretation. Covers basic electrophysiology and the pathophysiology of ECG findings. Not as high yield as some other resources, and not designed for more advanced reading of complex ECGs.

B

ECG Made Easy $31.95
HAMPTON
Elsevier, 2003, 6th ed., 160 pages, ISBN 9780443072529
An extremely quick review of major ECG findings. Includes tables
and a few rhythm strips, but does not offer practice problems or case
discussions. Examples might be more informative if they showed an
entire 12-lead ECG rather than just one lead and if arrows were used
to point to the exact abnormalities. Can fit in a coat pocket.

B

ECG Workout: Exercises in Arrhythmia Interpretation $41.95
HUFF
Lippincott Williams & Wilkins, 2006, 5th ed., 384 pages,
ISBN 9780781782302
A practical workbook with more than 500 actual ECGs. Includes updated ACLS guidelines. Emphasizes arrhythmias with no discussion
of MI, ischemia, or hypertrophy. Includes good tables, illustrations,
and self-assessment problems. Best used in conjunction with a primary ECG reference. Too advanced for the junior medical student
seeking to learn the basics of ECG interpretation.

B⁻

Pocket Guide to ECG Diagnosis $56.95
CHUNG
Wiley, 2001, 2nd ed., 528 pages, ISBN 9780865425897
A highly technical, comprehensive pocketbook with a good introductory overview of the principles of electrophysiology. Coverage of
some disorders is far too advanced for the junior medical student and
probably for the subintern as well. A potential pocket reference for
residents who wish to become cardiologists.

B+

Understanding Acid-Base $29.95
ABELOW
Lippincott Williams & Wilkins, 1998, 1st ed., 333 pages,
ISBN 9780683182729
A text that places heavy emphasis on physiology and little on clinical relevance, although treatment plans for different acid-base disorders are discussed. Includes a self-assessment quiz at the end of each section. Best for highly dedicated students.

B+

Acid-Base, Fluids, and Electrolytes Made Ridiculously Simple $18.95
PRESTON
MedMaster, Inc., 1998, 1st ed., 160 pages, ISBN 9780940780316
A concise, practical approach toward solving problems of acid-base, fluid, and electrolyte abnormalities. Easy to read and well organized with good use of tables, but more diagrams and figures would be of benefit, and some mnemonics are a stretch. Several questions with detailed explanations at the end of each section reinforce key principles. Reasonably priced in view of the amount and complexity of material covered.

B

Fluid, Electrolyte, and Acid-Base Physiology $85.00
HALPERIN
Elsevier, 1999, 3rd ed., 532 pages, ISBN 9780721670720
A well-written clinical approach toward recognizing, diagnosing, and treating common metabolic abnormalities. Presented in case-based fashion with numerous clinical vignettes and clinically oriented questions. Good illustrations integrate basic science principles into the discussion of metabolic disorders. However, may be too advanced and expensive for students looking for basic information in a limited amount of time.

Radiology 101

$69.95

ERKONEN

Lippincott Williams & Wilkins, 2005, 2nd ed., 402 pages, ISBN 9780781751988

A good overview of radiology with special emphasis on the normal anatomy of different organ systems. Contains numerous radiographic illustrations and easy-to-understand explanations for the clinical aspects of various imaging modalities. As its name suggests, the book is geared toward students who want to understand the fundamentals of reading films, but it is also useful in anatomy. Expensive, so consider checking out a copy at the library.

Clinical Radiology: The Essentials

$59.95

DAFFNER

Lippincott Williams & Wilkins, 2007, 3rd ed., 544 pages, ISBN 9780781799683

Specifically designed for third- and fourth-year medical students, this book outlines basic information on different imaging modalities, organized by organ system. It discusses more pathology than *Radiology 101* but is heavier reading and includes fewer illustrations.

Clinical Radiology Made Ridiculously Simple

$30.95

OUELLETTE

MedMaster, Inc., 2006, 2nd ed., 109 pages, ISBN 9780940780750

A good, concise introduction to the basics of radiology in easy-to-understand terms. Covers the essentials of the CXR, AXR, bone films, and head CT. However, it omits many other important components of clinical radiology, including ultrasound, body CTs, MRIs, and angiograms, and it offers fewer illustrations and figures than most radiology texts. An easy-to-read text that covers the basics, but not comprehensive.

Lecture Notes on Radiology

$35.95

PATEL

Wiley, 2005, 2nd ed., 320 pages, ISBN 9781405120678

A good general overview of diagnostic radiology, presented in a disease-specific manner. A double-page-spread format with radiographs of a specific disorder on one page and a succinct explanatory text on the other allows for immediate cross-reference. Covers the basic physics of the different radiographic forums as well as treatment options for radiographically detected diseases.

REVIEW RESOURCES

RADIOLOGY

Radiology Secrets

$41.95

KATZ

Elsevier, 2006, 2nd ed., 656 pages, ISBN 9780323034050

A comprehensive overview of radiology presented in a question-and-answer format typical of the *Secrets* series. Discussions are broken down by organ system and include well-explained correlations between radiographic findings and medical disorders. Covers all imaging modalities, with a large number of radiographs interspersed within the text. Too lengthy to be used as a basic introduction; more appropriate for quick reference and review by students who are interested in radiology.

Blueprints in Radiology

$36.95

UZELAC

Lippincott Williams & Wilkins, 2006, 2nd ed., 170 pages, ISBN 9781405104609

A text review of radiologic findings for common diseases, organized by organ system (e.g., thorax, abdomen) and by common disease processes associated with each. Includes a number of plain radiographs as well as ultrasound and CT images along with 25 questions at the end. A fairly superficial review of basic radiology topics; more useful as an overview than for test preparation.

Epocrates Rx

www.epocrates.com

A quick, accurate, and comprehensive drug resource that is updated continually. Provides accurate and up-to-date information on clinical indications, adult and pediatric dosing, contraindications, adverse reactions, mechanisms of action, forms of administration, potential interactions, and prices for virtually any pharmaceutical product. At no cost, a must for all medical students and residents.

Free — Palm and Pocket PC

Griffith's 5-Minute Clinical Consult 2006

www.handheldmed.com

An excellent PDA program for the wards that provides a quick summary of both common and obscure medical conditions. Great for last-minute presentations and preparation before rounds. Well organized, making use of lists and summaries with an easy-to-use interface and search function. Discussions are divided into disease basics, differential, treatment, medications, follow-up, and miscellaneous. Not a substitute for a textbook, but surprisingly comprehensive. May be combined with other programs from Handheldmed for a discount.

$64.95 — Palm and Pocket PC

MedCalc

www.med-ia.ch/medcalc

A great program with more than 80 formulas that will calculate whatever you need to know, including the A-a gradient, creatinine clearance, corrected electrolytes, Fe_{Na}, water deficit, BMI, and epidemiologic data (e.g., sensitivity, specificity, number needed to treat). Also includes a pregnancy wheel that will be helpful on the obstetrics and gynecology rotation.

Free — Palm

MedMath, Version 2.01

Available from many Web sites, including http://handheld.softpedia.com/

Similar in scope to *MedCalc*. Users need only correctly plug in relevant lab and clinical values into the appropriate sections to get the calculation immediately. Brief explanations of formulas are provided along with normal ranges of lab values. Like *MedCalc*, it contains some rarely used formulas.

Free — Palm

REVIEW RESOURCES

PDA RESOURCES

Schwartz's Principles of Surgery, PDA Edition

www.usbmis.com/surg

$49.95   Palm and Pocket PC

A PDA version of the reference textbook for the serious surgery student. Well organized and comprehensive, with a good discussion of surgical disease processes and explanations of the diagnosis and treatment of surgical problems. Features a user-friendly interface that allows users to bookmark certain sections and take notes. Also has great figures depicting important anatomic relationships and surgical procedures. A good investment for those considering a surgical career, and a valuable quick reference with which to prepare for the inevitable intraoperative pimping sessions. A free 14-day demo is available.

The Sanford Guide to Antimicrobial Therapy 2007 PDA Edition

www.sanfordguide.com

$29.95   Palm and Pocket PC

A brand-new PDA version of the popular handbook for treatment of infectious diseases. Users can find the diagnosis and appropriate therapy by scrolling through a hierarchical menu (e.g., to find the treatment of diverticulitis, tap on "gastrointestinal" and then "diverticulitis"). Also includes the all-important table comparing the spectra of each antibiotic against a variety of pathogens. One can simplify the table by tapping on the drugs and bugs of interest. Not as detailed as and much more expensive than the pocket-sized print edition ($10).

Tarascon Pocket Pharmacopoeia

www.tarascon.com

$29.95 for 1 year

A PDA version of the ubiquitous shirt-pocket edition of the *Pharmacopoeia*. Similar to *Epocrates Rx* and equally comprehensive. Includes pediatric and adult dosing information for each drug, dose forms, adverse reactions, and cost information. Drugs are also grouped by class (e.g., cardiovascular drugs, GI drugs) for easy navigation. Also includes additional tools, including a medical calculator (less comprehensive than *MedCalc* and *MedMath*) and summaries of a few high-yield topics (e.g., a review of anticoagulation and a summary of the antimicrobial spectra of various antibiotics).

Johns Hopkins Antibiotic Guide

www.hopkins-abxguide.org

Free   Palm

Put together by infectious disease experts and the makers of the *Physician's Desk Reference*, this guide focuses on the up-to-date management of community- and hospital-acquired infections. Information is accessible via three menus: diagnosis, pathogen, or antibiotic. A great resource, especially considering that it is free. Similar to the *Sanford Guide*. A major weakness, however, is the lack of a table comparing the spectra of various antibiotics.

Washington Manual of Medical Therapeutics, PDA edition

www.skyscape.com

An excellent resource outlining the pathophysiology and diagnosis of common diseases. Includes 26 chapters and 8 appendices that are similar to those in the print edition. Like the print version, it is aimed toward medical residents but is also highly useful for medical students, especially subinterns. Relatively easy to access, and can be cross-indexed with any other Skyscape product.

$59.95 Palm and Pocket PC

Epocrates Essentials

www.epocrates.com

A package that combines Epocrates products for drug reference, laboratory testing, and diagnosis. Includes a database of more than 1000 diseases and conditions, including the signs and symptoms, causes, diagnosis, treatment, and prognosis of each. Information is adapted from *Griffith's 5-Minute Clinical Consult*. Uses the same format as other Epocrates programs, with easy-to-navigate tabs and menus. Also offers a database of lab tests, normal reference values, and collection information (e.g., what color tube to use for blood collection for a specific test). Very helpful for interpreting general data; however, users should be mindful that reference values often vary by institution. The collection information can be useful, especially in the event that you have to draw blood on a patient when the phlebotomist or nurse is unsuccessful. Much less comprehensive diagnostically than *Griffith's 5-Minute Clinical Consult*.

$149 for 1 year, $249 for 2 years Palm and Pocket PC

Pocket Companion to Cecil Textbook of Medicine

www.skyscape.com

A guide that allows users to find a topic of interest by scrolling through the alphabetical index or the table of contents (which lists topics by system). Descriptions are concise but surprisingly complete. Great for a quick review of a topic, providing adequate preparation for potential pimp questions during rounds. Good for reference of known diagnoses.

$59.95 Palm and Pocket PC

Pocket Emergency Medicine

www.skyscape.com

A resource that present 57 chief complaints in an easy-to-read bulleted format, presented in a layout similar to that of the *Pocket Companion to Cecil Textbook of Medicine*. Includes historical clues and physical and lab findings that are typical of each disease process. Also included with each topic are clinical pearls that students are certain to be pimped on; this is perhaps the greatest strength of the program. Notes can be added within topics to customize the information for the user.

$39.95 Palm and Pocket PC

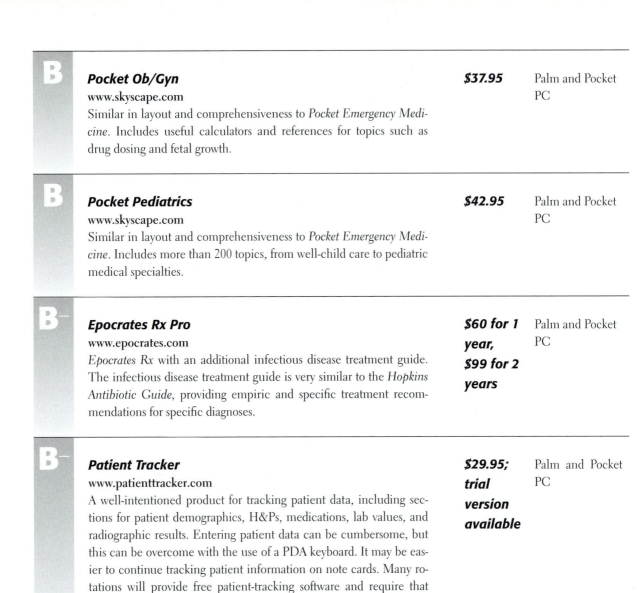

B

Pocket Ob/Gyn
www.skyscape.com
Similar in layout and comprehensiveness to *Pocket Emergency Medicine*. Includes useful calculators and references for topics such as drug dosing and fetal growth.

$37.95   Palm and Pocket PC

B

Pocket Pediatrics
www.skyscape.com
Similar in layout and comprehensiveness to *Pocket Emergency Medicine*. Includes more than 200 topics, from well-child care to pediatric medical specialties.

$42.95   Palm and Pocket PC

B−

Epocrates Rx Pro
www.epocrates.com
Epocrates Rx with an additional infectious disease treatment guide. The infectious disease treatment guide is very similar to the *Hopkins Antibiotic Guide*, providing empiric and specific treatment recommendations for specific diagnoses.

$60 for 1 year, $99 for 2 years   Palm and Pocket PC

B−

Patient Tracker
www.patienttracker.com
A well-intentioned product for tracking patient data, including sections for patient demographics, H&Ps, medications, lab values, and radiographic results. Entering patient data can be cumbersome, but this can be overcome with the use of a PDA keyboard. It may be easier to continue tracking patient information on note cards. Many rotations will provide free patient-tracking software and require that you keep a log of your patients, so downloading this program may be unnecessary.

$29.95; trial version available   Palm and Pocket PC

HANDBOOK/POCKETBOOK

NMS Clinical Manual of Emergency Medicine
BIDDINGER

$19.95

Lippincott Williams & Wilkins, 2002, 2nd ed., 283 pages,
ISBN 9780781735513

A text that is thin enough to carry everywhere and contains crucial information commonly encountered during the emergency medicine clerkship. Organized by system, with each chapter subdivided alphabetically. Also offers numerous table and figures for easy reference.

Pocket Emergency Medicine
WALLS

$44.95

Lippincott Williams & Wilkins, 2003, 1st ed., 311 pages,
ISBN 9780781743518

A pocket text that is organized in loose-leaf binders with room for more notes. Contains key clinical information organized by symptom-based presentation. A concise, helpful, and popular resource. Not as well referenced as its sibling, *Pocket Medicine*.

Current Essentials of Emergency Medicine
STONE

$36.95

McGraw-Hill, 2005, 1st ed., 520 pages, ISBN 9780071440585

Organized by organ system, this book contains a succinct summary of each disease, focusing on practical clinical information. One disease and pearl is offered on each page. Good for quick reference and review. Easy to read, although it would benefit from a more extensive discussion of pathophysiology.

SOAP for Emergency Medicine
BOND

$24.95

Lippincott Williams & Wilkins, 2005, 1st ed., 232 pages,
ISBN 9781405104425

A thin pocketbook that presents information in a SOAP-note format. Organized by organ system, the book focuses heavily on clinical problems, not on diagnosis. The "S" (subject) section contains a helpful list of questions to ask when interviewing patients and writing notes. The book would be most helpful in guiding day-to-day management and in formulating an assessment and plan for patients with a known diagnosis. Would benefit from some figures or diagrams.

A

Emergency Management of the Trauma Patient: Cases, Algorithms, Evidence

$31.95

BISANZO

Lippincott Williams & Wilkins, 2006, 1st ed., 180 pages, ISBN 9781405104876

Although not intended for boards review or fundamental wards preparation, this text would be of benefit for students who are interested in learning more about trauma management. Presents scenarios and then emphasizes the role of clinical judgment and the ACLS protocol in making appropriate management decisions.

A

Emergency Management of the Coding Patient: Cases, Algorithms, Evidence

$31.95

SENECAL

Lippincott Williams & Wilkins, 2005, 2nd ed., 170 pages, ISBN 9781405104555

Although not intended for boards review or fundamental wards preparation, this text would be of benefit for students who are interested in learning more about the management of a coding patient. Presents scenarios and then emphasizes the role of clinical judgment and the ACLS protocol in making appropriate management decisions.

A⁻

First Aid for the Emergency Medicine Clerkship

$41.95

STEAD

McGraw-Hill, 2006, 2nd ed., 416 pages, ISBN 9780071448734

A comprehensive overview of pertinent topics in emergency medicine, written in outline format and intended for NBME shelf and USMLE Step 2 exam study. Covers essential high-yield information and common procedures in a succinct, systematic manner. Includes well-organized tables as well as helpful figures. High-yield mnemonics and clinical scenarios are provided in the margins. Overall, an excellent review of the broad field of emergency medicine. This publication is not affiliated with the authors of *First Aid for the Wards*.

In A Page Emergency Medicine

$32.95

CATERINO

Lippincott Williams & Wilkins, 2003, 1st ed., 272 pages,
ISBN 9781405103572

A concise review of more than 250 diseases, organized by organ system. Each disease pathology is explained in one page, from etiology to prognosis. Provides a big picture and high-yield information; best suited for quick review before seeing a patient or preparing for a pimp session. The book is thin enough to carry around everywhere but lacks figures and tables, so students will need to refer to other textbooks for more detailed information.

Underground Clinical Vignettes: Emergency Medicine

$22.95

KIM

Lippincott Williams & Wilkins, 2007, 4th ed., 200 pages,
ISBN 9780781768344

A well-organized review of clinical vignettes commonly encountered on NBME shelf and USMLE Step 2 exams. Includes a focused, high-yield discussion of pathogenesis, epidemiology, management, and complications. Black-and-white images are included where relevant. Also offers several "minicases" in which only key facts related to each disease are presented. An entertaining, easy-to-use supplement for studying during the clinical rotation. May benefit from increased coverage of surgical subspecialties, including ophthalmology, anesthesiology, and pediatric surgery.

Emergency Medicine Secrets

$41.95

MARKOVCHICK

Elsevier, 2006, 4th ed., 748 pages, ISBN 9780323035873

A great, easy-to-use text that covers the most important topics of all aspects of emergency medicine, presented in a question-and-answer format similar to that of others in the *Secrets* series. Best used as a supplement to a more comprehensive text. Rather large for a pocket.

Blueprints in Emergency Medicine

$36.95

MICK

Lippincott Williams & Wilkins, 2005, 2nd ed., 300 pages,
ISBN 9781405104616

A text that covers the essentials of the field but does not go into extensive detail. Features 75 boards-format questions and answers with explanations. Great for a general introduction to the field, but best used in conjunction with a more comprehensive text. Intended for clerkship preparation as well as for boards review.

BRS Emergency Medicine

$36.95

STEAD

Lippincott Williams & Wilkins, 2000, 1st ed., 673 pages,
ISBN 9780683306170

This book is organized in the same manner as its counterpart USMLE prep series (*BRS*). Although it contains substantial information on different disorders with accompanying questions at the end of each section, it is a bit dry and features few figures or tables. Not designed for quick reference.

First Exposure to Emergency Medicine Clerkship

$33.95

HOFFMAN

McGraw-Hill, 2004, 1st ed., 467 pages, ISBN 9780071417167

Organized by symptom as well as by organ system, this book offers a thorough discussion of each emergency medicine topic at a level of detail that is probably appropriate for a month-long clerkship. Because of its prose-style writing, it is not the best book for a quick reference. Common procedures in the ER are included at the end. Although a comprehensive source of information, the text would benefit from more tables and bulleted lists for easier reading.

Emergency Medicine Recall

$34.95

WOODS

Lippincott Williams & Wilkins, 2000, 1st ed., 529 pages,
ISBN 9780683306101

Written in a quick question-and-answer format typical of the *Recall* series, this book reviews many high-yield facts that are covered on the shelf and USMLE Step 2 exams. It lacks clinical vignettes, and some of the topics covered can be obscure while others are not given enough attention. Useful as a quick-review supplement for another, more detailed text.

A–

Blueprints Clinical Cases in Emergency Medicine   *$29.95*
FILBIN

Lippincott Williams & Wilkins, 2006, 2nd ed., 160 pages,
ISBN 9781405104975

Organized by common presenting signs and symptoms, this book contains 60 symptom-based clinical cases followed by thought questions and a discussion. Also provides 100 USMLE-style questions. A popular question book that is very high yield for both wards and shelf preparation.

REVIEW RESOURCES

EMERGENCY MEDICINE

TEXTBOOK/REFERENCE

A

Current Emergency Diagnosis & Treatment

$69.95

STONE

McGraw-Hill, 2008, 6th ed., 1030 pages, ISBN 9780071443197

A text that discusses common emergency problems while also providing trauma-based and medical cases. Focuses on practical clinical information and includes several problem-oriented cases. The new edition contains more illustrations than the previous version.

A⁻

Introduction to Emergency Medicine

$46.95

MITCHELL

Lippincott Williams & Wilkins, 2005, 1st ed., 708 pages,
ISBN 9780781732000

A resource that falls between a review book and a text in terms of its
length and content. A few figures and tables interspersed throughout
make it easier to understand. Organized by system and common presenting symptom; contains a series of questions at the end of some
chapters with which students can prepare for the shelf and USMLE
exams. Geared toward medical students.

A⁻

Emergency Medicine: A Comprehensive Study Guide

$195.00

TINTINALLI

McGraw-Hill, 2004, 6th ed., 2042 pages, ISBN 9780071388757

A classic, highly comprehensive textbook covering almost all aspects
of medicine. Organized by organ system, the book is heavy on text
with only a few tables, figures, and algorithms.

HANDBOOK/POCKETBOOK

A   *The Washington Manual of Medical Therapeutics*   **$47.95**
COOPER

Lippincott Williams & Wilkins, 2007, 32nd ed., 862 pages,
ISBN 9780781765176

An excellent handbook outlining the pathophysiology and diagnosis of common diseases. Contains highly detailed descriptions of various therapeutic options. Aimed toward medical residents, but highly useful for medical students as well, especially subinterns. Fits tightly in most coat pockets. Contains references for the retrieval of primary sources.

A   *Practical Guide to the Care of the Medical Patient*   **$42.95**
FERRI

Elsevier, 2007, 7th ed., 1120 pages, ISBN 9780323048361

A well-organized but fat pocketbook covering common diseases, written at an appropriate level for medical students. Includes a discussion of etiology, differentials, diagnostic approach, laboratory interpretation, and management. Excellent tables and algorithms are available for the wards. The outline format focuses on enhancing readers' understanding of disease processes and their evaluation. Some treatment sections are better covered in more specialized handbooks.

A   *Pocket Medicine*   **$44.95**
SABATINE

Lippincott Williams & Wilkins, 2008, 3rd ed., 288 pages,
ISBN 9780781771443

A small pocketbook with great overviews of most diseases encountered in inpatient settings along with the latest management approaches. Offers up-to-date references to primary literature after each subject. Also includes handy tables, charts, and algorithms, although the small print may be a drawback. Note cards can easily be added to the ring-bound pocketbook, but pages can rip out of the binder. Limited in detail owing to its size and scope, but easy to carry everywhere. Great for a quick reference before and after seeing patients. Compare with *Practical Guide to the Care of the Medical Patient* and *Washington Manual of Medical Therapeutics*.

Saint-Frances Guide to Inpatient Medicine

SAINT

$36.95

Lippincott Williams & Wilkins, 2003, 2nd ed., 533 pages,
ISBN 9780781737289

An excellent, cheap, and concise pocketbook emphasizing the development of a basic, organized approach toward many common diseases. Makes good use of tables and charts, and devotes a substantial portion of its text to medical mnemonics. However, it cannot be used as a primary resource because it lacks extensive discussion of pathophysiology, diagnostic evaluation, management, and treatment. Best used as prerotation reading, as it offers a good overview of differential diagnosis and simplifies complex medical issues. Its small size makes it easy to carry around.

Saint-Frances Guide to Outpatient Medicine

SAINT

$36.95

Lippincott Williams & Wilkins, 2008, 2nd ed., 752 pages,
ISBN 9780781765022

Like its inpatient counterpart, this pocketbook contains numerous medical mnemonics and useful algorithms applicable to an office-care environment. The last part of each section provides useful recommendations on follow-up, which is significant for outpatient medicine. Its portability makes this text an excellent supplement to a more thorough and detailed textbook.

The Internal Medicine Peripheral Brain

TALREJA

$36.95

Lippincott Williams & Wilkins, 2005, 1st ed., 928 pages,
ISBN 9780781728065

A pocketbook similar in content to *Harrison's Manual* that deals with all aspects of medicine. Each chapter is consistently organized, highlighting etiology, epidemiology, pathophysiology, treatment, and prognosis. The outline format makes it easy to read, but its style is somewhat monotonous and features few figures and tables.

Harrison's Manual of Medicine

$52.95

BRAUNWALD

McGraw-Hill, 2005, 16th ed., 1087 pages, ISBN 9780071444415

A "baby" pocket version of the parent book, this manual focuses on commonly encountered diseases, providing a wealth of information on pathophysiology, clinical manifestations, and therapeutics. Useful for quick reading on established diagnoses, although its dense copy and large blocks of text make it difficult to skim. Not as practical for day-to-day wards problems, as it lacks thorough explanations of the approach toward diagnosis and management. Great as a pocket reference book for reviewing diseases that students have encountered on the wards or are considering on their differential.

Internal Medicine on Call

$39.95

HAIST

McGraw-Hill, 2005, 4th ed., 656 pages, ISBN 9780071439022

A quick-reference guidebook giving a step-by-step approach toward most commonly encountered medical "on-call" problems. Organized by common presenting symptoms, this book is most useful for formulating differential diagnoses and appropriate management plans when new patients are encountered on call. Includes sections on laboratory interpretation, procedures, fluids and electrolytes, ventilator management, and commonly used drugs. Would benefit from more diagrams and tables.

Tarascon Internal Medicine & Critical Care Pocketbook

$14.95

LEDERMAN

Tarascon Publishing, 2007, 4th ed., 226 pages,
ISBN 9781882742509

A small, cheap, pocket-sized book containing a great deal of information. Excellent tables, graphs, and algorithms present the diagnostic workup and treatment of common emergency problems encountered in internal medicine. A section at the end is dedicated to a description of commonly used drugs in the critical care setting. Occasionally too complex, as information is presented in a highly technical manner with little discussion; geared more toward those with a prior knowledge of the highlighted diseases. Useful for subinterns during their ICU rotations.

Current Essentials of Medicine

$36.95

TIERNEY

McGraw-Hill, 2005, 3rd ed., 688 pages, ISBN 9780071438322

An abridged version of *Current Medical Diagnosis & Treatment* that provides a quick reference for wards and outpatient medicine, organized into bulleted lists containing the essentials of diagnosis, differentials, and treatment. Each medical disorder has its own dedicated page, enlightening clinical pearl, and general primary reference with the goal of highlighting crucial points of each disease. Detailed discussions of pathophysiology, diagnosis, and management are beyond the scope of this book, limiting its usefulness on the wards. Consider as a quick-review supplement to its parent book or another textbook.

SOAP for Internal Medicine

$25.00

UZELAC

Lippincott Williams & Wilkins, 2005, 1st ed., 280 pages, ISBN 9781405104364

A thin pocketbook that presents information in a SOAP note format. Organized by organ system, the book focuses heavily on clinical problems, not diagnoses. The "S" (subject) section contains a list of helpful questions to ask when interviewing patients and writing notes. The book would be most helpful in guiding day-to-day management and in formulating an assessment and plan for patients with a known diagnosis. Similar to *Internal Medicine on Call* in concept, but the focus here is more on treatment plans than on differentials. Would benefit from more figures and diagrams. Contains some errors.

A

Step-Up to Medicine $39.95
AGABEGI
Lippincott Williams & Wilkins, 2005, 1st ed., 564 pages,
ISBN 9780781747875
A text that is similar in format to *First Aid for the Medicine Clerkship*
but makes for slightly heavier reading. Offers marginal notes for quick
reference and clinical vignettes with which to reinforce learned
knowledge. Also includes a section on ambulatory medicine. Great
for both the clerkship and preparation for the USMLE Step 2, but requires significant time commitment.

A

First Aid for the Medicine Clerkship $41.95
STEAD
McGraw-Hill, 2006, 2nd ed., 416 pages, ISBN 9780071448758
A good overview of pertinent topics in internal medicine, written in
outline format and intended for NBME shelf and USMLE Step 2
exam study. Covers essential high-yield information in a succinct,
well-written manner. Few figures and photographs are provided. May
contain slightly less pathophysiology than the *Blueprints* series, but
easier to read and more clinically relevant. Overall, an excellent review of the broad field of internal medicine. This publication is not
affiliated with the authors of *First Aid for the Wards*.

A‑

Parkland Manual of In-Patient Medicine: An Evidence- $42.95
Based Approach
KATZ
F. A. Davis, 2006, 1st ed., 649 pages, ISBN 9780803613973
Organized by subspecialty, this book comprehensively reviews disorders related to inpatient medicine and their treatment, with extensive
citations from the literature. Written in a bulleted format with many
figures and tables; good for the review of subspecialty topics and patient management supported by the literature. Covers only inpatient
management and critical care. Can be carried in a coat pocket.

A‑

Case Files Family Medicine $29.95
TOY
McGraw-Hill, 2007, 2nd ed., 507 pages, ISBN 9780071471886
A comprehensive look at the diagnosis and treatment of virtually all
important conditions in obstetrics and gynecology. Makes good use of
figures and tables, with illustrations of surgical fields and exam maneuvers. Also includes algorithms for medical management with coverage of relevant topics in women's health. Covers the epidemiology,
etiology, prevention, presentation, diagnosis, treatment, and prognosis of common disorders.

REVIEW RESOURCES

INTERNAL MEDICINE

A−

Case Files Internal Medicine
$29.95

TOY

McGraw-Hill, 2007, 2nd ed., 528 pages, ISBN 9780071463034

A compilation of more than 60 case series accompanied by extended discussions of each case, definitions of key terms, clinical pearls, a primer on how to approach problems, and a short section consisting of USMLE-style questions. Although the format is similar to that of the *Underground Clinical Vignettes* series, this book is much more comprehensive, placing greater emphasis on pathophysiology and management plans. Originally designed for USMLE Step 2 preparation, the text could also serve as a useful companion for the clerkship as well as a source of practice cases for the shelf exam. Drawbacks include busy organization and a lack of figures and tables.

B+

Cecil Essentials of Medicine
$67.95

ANDREOLI

Elsevier, 2007, 7th ed., 1296 pages, ISBN 9781416029335

A great condensed version of the parent book. Offers clear, detailed explanations of pathophysiology, but not as useful as a treatment reference or for differential diagnosis. More useful for reference than for practical wards work. Contains many effective tables and charts. Not portable.

B+

Hospital Medicine Secrets
$42.95

GLASHEEN

Elsevier, 2007, 1st ed., 464 pages, ISBN 9780323040877

A review of many critical topics in hospital medicine accompanied by discussions of important issues such as patient safety, the subtleties of patient management, and evidence-based medicine. Highly useful for those interested in careers in medicine. Includes many helpful tips and equations for the effective use and interpretation of diagnostic tests. Also provides pertinent questions along with concise answers.

B+

Common Medical Diagnosis: An Algorithmic Approach
$44.95

HEALEY

Elsevier, 2006, 4th ed., 256 pages, ISBN 9781416025429

An interesting book dedicated solely to algorithms, organized by body system and presenting sign. The text guides readers from the background through the differential to the appropriate clinical workup, helping students organize their strategies for addressing medical problems. Only "bread-and-butter" medical problems are covered, requiring that other books be used for uncommon conditions, but overall a good resource for the seasoned medical student.

Kelley's Essentials of Internal Medicine

HUMES

$59.95

Lippincott Williams & Wilkins, 2001, 2nd ed., 920 pages, ISBN 9780781719377

A condensed version of *Kelley's Textbook*, written at the medical student level with the basics needed for patient workup and diagnosis. Offers good tables and algorithms for a problem- or symptom-based approach to evaluation and differential diagnosis. Slightly less detailed than *Cecil Essentials*.

High-Yield Internal Medicine

NIRULA

$26.95

Lippincott Williams & Wilkins, 2007, 3rd ed., 128 pages, ISBN 9780781781695

Part of a popular USMLE Step 1 prep series that offers a review book for each clerkship. Typical of its format, the book contains high-yield information in a clear and concise outline form organized by organ system. Could benefit from more tables and figures.

Internal Medicine Clerkship Guide

PAAUW

$39.95

Elsevier, 2008, 3rd ed., 302 pages, ISBN 9780323045582

Designed specifically for medical students beginning their internal medicine clerkships, this text is divided into sections addressing the basic skills needed for the clerkship, common symptoms or signs, and common diseases. Provides practical core knowledge of common medical conditions, with basic questions and answers helping guide students in their transition to clinical thinking. Not useful for looking up detailed information, but an effective introduction to clinical problem solving and diagnosis.

Crash Course: Cardiovascular System

RUSS

$29.95

Elsevier, 2006, 1st ed., 192 pages, ISBN 9780323043458

A helpful review book divided into two sections, the first reviewing basic cardiovascular physiology from the first two years of medical school, and the second emphasizing the clinical assessment of cardiovascular diseases. Not comprehensive, but useful for USMLE exam review.

B+

Crash Course: Gastroenterology

$29.95

THULUVATH

Elsevier, 2006, 1st ed., 248 pages, ISBN 9781416029922

A review book divided into three sections: a symptoms-based approach toward gastroenterology; a review of common gastroenterologic diseases; and a review of the basic H&P and diagnostic tests. Includes more information than needed for the basic medicine clerkship, but would undoubtedly be of benefit when read in conjunction with a GI elective.

B+

Blueprints in Medicine

$36.95

YOUNG

Lippincott Williams & Wilkins, 2007, 4th ed., 352 pages, ISBN 9781405105002

A good basic review that students can read early in the rotation to learn the fundamentals of internal medicine. Easy to read, with good tables and charts to illustrate key points. Although some students feel it is too simplistic and not comprehensive enough for the NBME shelf exam, it may be adequate for the USMLE Step 2. Compare with NMS Medicine. Consider using as a supplement to textbooks or for more advanced review.

B

Medicine

$42.95

FISHMAN

Lippincott Williams & Wilkins, 2003, 5th ed., 654 pages, ISBN 9780781725439

A highly readable and approachable text organized by body system. Sometimes simplistic and lacking in detail. Makes good use of tables, but offers few illustrations. Not a replacement for a medicine reference book, but adequately presents the basics.

B

Internal Medicine Pearls

$45.95

HEFFNER

Elsevier, 2000, 2nd ed., 275 pages, ISBN 9781560534044

Contains detailed clinical vignettes with laboratory and radiographic findings, followed by a discussion of clinically important pearls. Questions focus on clinical decision making and management. Only selected topics are covered, so the text is not comprehensive, and discussions may be too detailed for review purposes. A good, clinically focused supplement.

In A Page Signs & Symptoms

$32.95

KAHAN

**Lippincott Williams & Wilkins, 2004, 1st ed., 224 pages,
ISBN 9781405103688**

Organized by common presenting signs and symptoms, this book focuses on differential diagnosis and workups. Like its counterpart (*In A Page Medicine*), the book explains each symptom with lists in one page. Excellent for quick review, and a great companion to use while on call, providing guidelines on how to work up "fresh" patients.

NMS Medicine

$39.95

MYERS

**Lippincott Williams & Wilkins, 2004, 5th ed., 776 pages,
ISBN 9780781754682**

A text that is organized by system with easy-to-read chapters in outline form. Includes questions at the end of each chapter to solidify concepts just learned as well as a comprehensive exam at the end. Geared toward NBME shelf exam and USMLE Step 2 study, but can be used to review topics on the wards. Offers few diagrams, tables, and illustrations; not always up to date. Thorough and highly detailed, although its inclusion of some esoteric information may make it difficult for readers to find the essentials. For highly motivated students.

In A Page Inpatient Medicine

$32.95

PERKINS

**Lippincott Williams & Wilkins, 2008, 2nd ed., 239 pages,
ISBN 9780781764995**

A review of 200 diseases, organized by organ system. Each disease pathology is explained in one page, from etiology to prognosis, in list format. Provides a big picture and high-yield information; best suited for quick review before seeing a patient or preparing for a pimp session. The book is thin enough to carry around everywhere but lacks figures and tables, so students will need to refer to other textbooks for more detailed information.

B

Underground Clinical Vignettes: Internal Medicine, Vol. 1

SWANSON

Lippincott Williams & Wilkins, 2007, 4th ed., 256 pages,
ISBN 9780781768351

$19.95

A well-organized review of clinical vignettes commonly encountered on the NBME shelf and USMLE Step 2 exams. Includes a focused, high-yield discussion of pathogenesis, epidemiology, management, and complications. Black-and-white images are included where relevant. Also contains several "minicases" in which only key facts related to each disease are presented. An entertaining and easy-to-use supplement for studying during the clinical rotation. Covers cardiology, endocrinology, gastroenterology, hematology, and oncology.

B

Underground Clinical Vignettes: Internal Medicine, Vol. 2

SWANSON

Lippincott Williams & Wilkins, 2007, 4th ed., 256 pages,
ISBN 9780781768368

$19.95

See the above review of *Underground Clinical Vignettes: Internal Medicine, Vol. 1*. This volume covers dermatology, infectious disease, nephrology, urology, pulmonary disease, and rheumatology.

B⁻

Medicine Recall

BERGIN

Lippincott Williams & Wilkins, 2008, 3rd ed., 832 pages,
ISBN 9780781794145

$38.95

A good but not-so-portable book for rapid review and answering pimp questions. Follows the standard *Recall*-series question-and-answer format of high-yield information, organized by medical specialty. Requires significant time commitment to complete. No images are provided, and some information is incorrect or out of date. Not as useful on the wards as its counterpart, *Surgical Recall*. Useful as a supplement to other resources.

B⁻

Color Atlas and Text of Clinical Medicine

FORBES

Elsevier, 2003, 3rd ed., 536 pages, ISBN 9780723431947

$57.95

A sizable softcover text that gives a broad overview of medicine in an excellent and readable format. Although it offers great figures and tables, the text's strength lies in its more than 1500 color photos. Excellent illustrations include physical signs of disease, radiographic images, and pathology slides. Not meant for in-depth review, but highly effective both as an introductory clinical text and as a visual encyclopedia. An excellent investment and supplement to more traditional reference textbooks.

Most Commons in Medicine

$34.95

GOLJAN

Elsevier, 2000, 1st ed., 857 pages, ISBN 9780721687599

A resource that breaks information down into several tables of the most common causes, clinical findings, complications, and treatment options of a wide range of medical disorders. Not designed for primary learning so much as for quick review on the wards when one has spare time. Explanations given for answers are short and limited if presented at all. Offers decent preparation for wards pimp questions.

Pathophysiology of Disease: An Introduction

$59.95

MCPHEE

McGraw-Hill, 2006, 5th ed., 784 pages, ISBN 9780071441599

A concise, interdisciplinary reference text of the pathophysiology of common diseases, organized by system. Offers excellent explanations of disease processes. Not designed for the wards or for dealing with treatment and management issues, but useful as an adjunct to a more traditional textbook. Some students may find it more appropriate for pathophysiology classes during preclinical years.

Medical Secrets

$39.95

ZOLLO

Elsevier, 2005, 4th ed., 608 pages, ISBN 9781560533870

An interesting but dense compilation of useful and clinically relevant information presented in a question-and-answer format. Designed for surviving wards pimping sessions, although inevitably one is seldom asked the majority of these questions. Excellent tables are good for quick review. May not be a prudent buy if the student does not like the format.

PreTest Internal Medicine

$26.95

BERK

McGraw-Hill, 2006, 11th ed., 356 pages, ISBN 9780071455534

A collection of 500 multiple-choice questions covering a wide range of topics in internal medicine. Includes clinical vignette–style questions, and provides detailed paragraph-format explanations for each answer. Probably the most widely used preparation for shelf exams. Good for last-minute review before the exam.

Blueprints Clinical Cases in Medicine

$29.95

LI

Lippincott Williams & Wilkins, 2007, 2nd ed., 425 pages, ISBN 9781405104913

Organized by common presenting signs and symptoms, this book contains symptom-based clinical cases accompanied by 200 USMLE-style questions. The format is similar to that of the *Case Files* series but places less emphasis on discussions and greater focus on questions. May contain some errors.

Blueprints Q&A Step 2 Medicine

$19.95

SHINAR

Lippincott Williams & Wilkins, 2005, 2nd ed., 176 pages, ISBN 9781405103893

The new edition of this book contains more than 200 USMLE-style questions (increased from 100 from the previous edition) with explanations for both correct and incorrect answers, although explanations are not as detailed and well referenced as the ones in the *PreTest* series. The book was originally designed for Step 2 preparation, but since the format of the shelf exam is similar, this would be a useful companion for clerkship preparation as well. The book is thin enough to carry around in the pocket and could easily be read in a few days.

A+

Harrison's Principles of Internal Medicine
$199.00

BRAUNWALD

McGraw-Hill, 2008, 17th ed., 2650 pages, ISBN 9780071466332

An excellent, comprehensive reference considered by many to be the "gold standard" of internal medicine textbooks. Makes excellent use of tables, graphs, illustrations, and radiographs. Not for quick reference, but rather for in-depth home reading on specific topics. Requires serious concentration and reading time, but provides some of the most thorough reviews of disease processes that one can find. A great reference for those considering internal medicine as a career. Available as a single- or double-volume text. The new edition is in full color and provides free Web site access to cases, a test bank, and an image library.

A+

Cecil Textbook of Medicine
$149.00

GOLDMAN

Elsevier, 2008, 23rd ed., 3120 pages, ISBN 9781416028055

One of the classic textbooks of medicine. As comprehensive and detailed as *Harrison's* but easier to read, making good use of tables and an ample number of colorful pictures. Available as a single- or double-volume text. Equal in utility to *Harrison's* as an alternative reference for internists.

A

Current Medical Diagnosis & Treatment
$80.00

TIERNEY

McGraw-Hill, 2007, 47th ed., 1672 pages, ISBN 9780071494304

A clinically oriented reference that is concise yet detailed and highly readable for medical students. Well organized with excellent descriptions of pathophysiology, clinical findings, and treatment. The beginning of each section offers the essentials of diagnosis. The text is revised annually and thus offers useful tables and up-to-date references. Includes more thorough coverage of ambulatory care than that found in more conventional textbooks.

A−

The Merck Manual of Diagnosis & Therapy
$65.00

BEERS

Merck, 2006, 18th ed., 3000 pages, ISBN 9780911910186

Offers clear discussions of a wide variety of diseases, but with limited tables, charts, and illustrations. Well organized, comprehensive, and well indexed. May be used as a reference book, but not as extensive as *Harrison's or Cecil*. Useful as an adjunctive, quick home-reference textbook.

REVIEW RESOURCES

INTERNAL MEDICINE

Kelley's Textbook of Internal Medicine $110.00
Humes
Lippincott Williams & Wilkins, 2000, 4th ed., 3254 pages,
ISBN 9780781717878
Offers well-organized, straightforward discussions of pathophysiology, clinical findings, diagnosis, and management. Not yet on the same level as *Harrison's or Cecil,* but subsequent editions have improved. The recent edition places more emphasis on evidence-based medicine, with specialized "clinical decision guides" based on the most recent research.

Textbook of Internal Medicine $150.00
Stein
Elsevier, 1998, 5th ed., 2515 pages, ISBN 9780815186984
A comprehensive reference book that is not at the same level of detail as the previously mentioned textbooks but is more approachable and friendly. Offers effective explanations of pathophysiology with good sections on diagnostic evaluation. A slightly older reference than the other textbooks.

REVIEW RESOURCES

INTERNAL MEDICINE

HANDBOOK/POCKETBOOK

On Call Neurology
MARSHALL

$36.95

Elsevier, 2007, 3rd ed., 505 pages, ISBN 9781416023753

A compact book addressing on-call neurologic issues a physician is likely to encounter. The structure of the book effectively models the process of working up a patient in a hospital setting: phone-call management (pertinent questions and orders), elevator thoughts (differential diagnoses), major threats to life, bedside management (neuro exam, labs), and management. Not high yield for studying for a shelf exam, but well designed (though a little large) as a pocket reference for students on a rotation or a subinternship.

Neurology (House Officer Series)
WEINER

$39.95

Lippincott Williams & Wilkins, 2004, 7th ed., 336 pages, ISBN 9780781747479

A clinically oriented pocketbook organized by signs and symptoms. Concise chapters offer clinically relevant material, although the text is somewhat short on tables and diagrams. Covers most topics thoroughly, but lacks detail. Written for interns and residents, but can also be useful for medical students during their initial patient encounters.

Primer of Clinical Neurology
CAMPBELL

$32.95

Lippincott Williams & Wilkins, 2002, 1st ed., 411 pages, ISBN 9780781724814

Specifically designed for medical students on the clerkship, this book places significant emphasis on the neurologic history, the physical exam, and the reasoning underlying differential diagnoses. Consequently, less space is devoted to a discussion of disorders, which are simply divided into those above and those below the foramen magnum. Great to read before the rotation to get a good handle on the clerkship.

Neurologic Pearls
DEVINSKY

$23.95

F. A. Davis, 2000, 1st ed., 309 pages, ISBN 9780803604339

A concise pocketbook that presents simple, clear explanations of the approach to neurologic disorders. Chapters are organized by clinical presentation with useful clinical pearls interspersed throughout. More illustrations of neuroanatomy and pathways would increase the quality of the discussion.

Manual of Neurologic Therapeutics

$59.95

SAMUELS

Lippincott Williams & Wilkins, 2004, 7th ed., 592 pages,
ISBN 9780781746465

A spiral-bound pocketbook written in expanded outline format and
patterned after the *Washington Manual*. Strikes an excellent balance
between concise, practical information and reference-level detail.
Better for clinical management than for review of pathophysiology.
An appendix lists agencies that provide support and education for patients with specific neurologic problems.

Little Black Book of Neurology

$54.95

LERNER

Elsevier, 2008, 5th ed., 656 pages, ISBN 9780323039505

An alphabetically organized pocketbook with a format similar to that
of a dictionary. Presented in essay format without an index or a table
of contents, detracting from its utility as a quick reference. Written
more for residents than for medical students. Best used for review by
advanced neurology students.

Merritt's Neurology Handbook

$64.95

MAZZONI

Lippincott Williams & Wilkins, 2006, 2nd ed., 707 pages,
ISBN 9780781762700

A volume that follows its parent text, *Merritt's Neurology*, chapter by
chapter with an abbreviated text in a pocket-sized format. Accordingly, a wide range of topics is covered but with little depth. No images of scans are included. Better as a quick reference for a resident
or attending than for a medical student.

A

Clinical Neurology $47.95
AMINOFF

McGraw-Hill, 2005, 6th ed., 401 pages, ISBN 9780071423601

A well-organized, clinically oriented reference that is detailed
enough to serve as a student textbook. Emphasizes essential information with excellent use of tables and diagrams. A great introductory
neurology text for the motivated student. Highly useful appendices
offer guides on how to perform an extensive neurologic exam.

A⁻

Neurological Examination Made Easy $37.95
FULLER

Elsevier, 2004, 3rd ed., 260 pages, ISBN 9780443074202

A review of the neurologic exam for medical students, written from
the author's perspective of what to do, what one finds, and what it
means. Excellent flow diagrams guide the reader through the process
of examining the patient. Good for the non-neurologist who wishes
to learn the neurologic exam extremely well, or for the serious neurology student who wants to start off with an excellent foundation.

A⁻

Neurology and Neurosurgery Illustrated $87.95
LINDSAY

Elsevier, 2004, 4th ed., 608 pages, ISBN 9780443070563

Offers extensive coverage of a wide variety of topics, with great line
drawings illustrating key aspects of pathophysiology, clinical features,
and treatment. Not for reading cover to cover during a short rotation,
but can be used as a reference for the essential features of neurologic
disease. Sections are organized both by presenting complaint and by
specific disorder.

B⁺

Neurology $49.95
COLLINS

Elsevier, 1997, 1st ed., 201 pages, ISBN 9780721659923

A concise, thorough review of neurology that examines the most
common symptoms and diseases of the nervous system. A number of
tables and interesting historical facts are interspersed throughout the
text. The focus on theory may not be practical for wards application
but would be of interest to students considering a career in neurology.

REVIEW RESOURCES

NEUROLOGY

Lecture Notes on Neurology

$44.95

GINSBERG

Wiley, 2005, 8th ed., 199 pages, ISBN 9781405114370

A good, concise review of key points with great tables, figures, and illustrations. May be read from cover to cover during a short rotation. Organized primarily by pathology rather than by presenting complaint.

The Four-Minute Neurologic Exam

$12.95

GOLDBERG

MedMaster, Inc., 1999, 1st ed., 58 pages, ISBN 9780940780057

A brief, practical guide that is best reviewed before the rotation to help students understand the fundamentals of the neurologic screening examination. Can be read in a few hours to provide a good foundation for physical exam skills, but too simplistic to be of long-term value. Discusses only how to conduct a physical exam; provides little explanation of what findings could mean.

Underground Clinical Vignettes: Neurology

$22.95

KIM

Lippincott Williams & Wilkins, 2007, 4th ed., 256 pages, ISBN 9780781768375

A well-organized review of clinical vignettes commonly encountered on the NBME shelf and USMLE Step 2 exams. Includes a focused, high-yield discussion of pathogenesis, epidemiology, management, complications, and associated diseases. Black-and-white images are included where relevant. Also contains several "minicases" in which only key facts related to each disease are presented. An entertaining, easy-to-use supplement for studying during the clinical rotation, although it is neither as comprehensive nor as relevant for day-to-day wards activities.

In A Page Neurology

$32.95

BRILLMAN

Lippincott Williams & Wilkins, 2005, 1st ed., 200 pages, ISBN 9781405104326

A dry review of more than 150 diseases, organized by type of neurologic condition. Each disease pathology is explained in one page, from etiology to prognosis with lists. Provides a big picture and high-yield information; best suited for quick review before seeing a patient or preparing for a pimp session. The book is thin enough to carry around but is not pocket-sized. No figures or tables are included, and readers will need to refer to other textbooks for more detailed information.

High-Yield Neuroanatomy

$26.95

Fix

Lippincott Williams & Wilkins, 2005, 3rd ed., 142 pages,
ISBN 9780781758994

An outline review designed for the USMLE Step 1 exam preparation. Best used for prerotation study for those interested in getting a
head start. Not comprehensive, but some students consider it a good
"minimalist" reference for short neurology rotations. Good for pathways and review of general pathophysiology, but lacks a discussion of
management issues.

Neurology Recall

$34.95

Miller

Lippincott Williams & Wilkins, 2003, 2nd ed., 340 pages,
ISBN 9780781745888

A text written in a question-and-answer format typical of the *Recall*
series. A good reference for students preparing for pimping on wards,
it provides fast, easy-to-read reviews of disorders. Not as detailed as
Neurology Secrets, so future neurologists will need another reference
for in-depth discussion of disease.

Neurology Secrets

$39.95

Rolak

Elsevier, 2005, 4th ed., 480 pages, ISBN 9781560536215

A quick-reference text in a question-and-answer format consistent
with the *Secrets* series. Although not useful as a comprehensive text,
it is of value in helping students prepare for pimping on rounds.
Covers the most commonly encountered neurologic disorders, and
offers good explanations of clinically relevant questions, although
some obscure information is also included.

Neurology: An Illustrated Colour Text

$51.95

Fuller

Elsevier, 2006, 2nd ed., 148 pages, ISBN 9780443100710

An introductory-level text of common neurologic disorders with
good, cartoon-style images illustrating how to evaluate different aspects of the neurologic exam. Includes more color line drawings
than color photographs or radiographs of disease. May lack the level
of detail necessary for use as a reference during the clinical rotation,
particularly with respect to management.

Manter & Gatz's Essentials of Clinical Neuroanatomy and Neurophysiology   ***$33.95***

GILMAN

F. A. Davis, 2003, 10th ed., 281 pages, ISBN 9780803607729

An extensive, in-depth review of neuroanatomy and neurophysiology that is too detailed for most medical students and would be difficult to read during such a short rotation. Offers excellent pathway diagrams. Only for the highly motivated student with a deep interest in the basic sciences.

A⁻

PreTest Neurology
ANSCHEL

McGraw-Hill, 2006, 6th ed., 384 pages, ISBN 9780071455503

$26.95

A collection of 500 multiple-choice questions covering a wide range of topics in neurology. Includes clinical vignette–style questions and provides detailed paragraph-format explanations for each answer. Probably the most widely used preparatory text for shelf exams. Good for last-minute review before the exam.

B⁺

Blueprints Clinical Cases in Neurology
JOSHI

Lippincott Williams & Wilkins, 2003, 1st ed., 152 pages, ISBN 9780632046133

$25.95

Organized by common presenting signs and symptoms, this book contains symptom-based clinical cases accompanied by 200 USMLE-style questions. The format is similar to that of the *Case Files* series but places less emphasis on discussions and greater focus on questions.

A

Adams and Victor's Principles of Neurology
ROPPER

$140.00

McGraw-Hill, 2005, 8th ed., 1382 pages, ISBN 9780071416207

A comprehensive reference text with detailed discussions of disease from a clinical perspective. Uniquely organized, with chapters transitioning from a general patient approach to cardinal manifestations of neurologic disease to specific diseases. Tables and figures are somewhat sparse. Most appropriate for students considering neurology as a specialty.

A⁻

Merritt's Neurology
ROWLAND

$129.00

Lippincott Williams & Wilkins, 2005, 11th ed., 1271 pages, ISBN 9780781753111

A reference textbook that covers the entire spectrum of neurologic disease in depth, although not in as much detail as *Principles of Neurology*. Concise chapters are accompanied by a number of clinical radiographs.

B

Netter's Concise Neurology
MISULIS

$48.95

Elsevier, 2007, 1st ed., 565 pages, ISBN 9781929007899

A full-color illustrated atlas that uses excellent, familiar Netter-style illustrations. A brief overview of each disease is supplemented by classic drawings. May be more suitable for premedical students than for medical students on rotation, but several useful tables and flowcharts are included.

REVIEW RESOURCES

NEUROLOGY

HANDBOOK/POCKETBOOK

Benson & Pernoll's Handbook of Obstetrics and Gynecology

$46.95

BENSON

McGraw-Hill, 2001, 10th ed., 908 pages, ISBN 9780071356084

A handbook comprehensive enough to serve as a mini-reference. Excellent tables and graphics offer thorough discussions of etiology, pathophysiology, clinical findings, and management. Too bulky to fit in the pocket, and the small print makes for labored reading. Good to have for relatively detailed explanations when carrying a big textbook is impractical. Includes a section on breast disease.

Current Clinical Strategies: Gynecology and Obstetrics

$16.95

CHAN

Current Clinical Strategies, 2006, 3rd ed., 167 pages, ISBN 9781929622634

A quick, readable pocketbook containing essential high-yield information. Its outline format includes signs and symptoms, differential, treatment, and complications. Inexpensive and remarkably compact; great for both management and quick review on the wards. Includes an excellent, concise oncology section with classifications.

Pocket Ob/Gyn

$29.95

NAYLOR

Lippincott Williams & Wilkins, 2000, 1st ed., 72 pages, ISBN 9780781717700

Organized in loose-leaf pocket binders with room for more notes. Contains key clinical information that is easy to carry and suitable for quick reference.

Obstetrical Pearls

$27.95

BENSON

F. A. Davis, 1999, 3rd ed., 225 pages, ISBN 9780803604322

A practical, easy-to-read, clinically oriented pocketbook that can be used as prerotation orientation material on the wards. Gives basic wards survival information, but does not cover the full spectrum of information that is necessary for in-depth study or exams. Clinical pearls and current controversies in management are highlighted in the text. Contains excellent tidbits that can be read in a few dedicated hours.

REVIEW RESOURCES

OBSTETRICS AND GYNECOLOGY

B⁺

Manual of Obstetrics $44.95
EVANS

Lippincott Williams & Wilkins, 2000, 7th ed., 720 pages,
ISBN 9780781796965

A good pocketbook in the same format as the *Washington Manual*.
Offers a light discussion of pathophysiology, symptoms, and signs but
more detailed coverage of diagnostic approach and therapeutics.
Covers a broad range of topics on obstetrics; useful for quick review.
More appropriate for subinterns than for junior medical students.

B

Gynecologic Pearls $23.95
BENSON

F. A. Davis, 2000, 2nd ed., 243 pages, ISBN 9780803605022

Good prerotation introductory material, but not sufficient for exams
or for the wards. Useful as easy, quick, supplementary reading. Requires separate purchase of its sister book for obstetrics, which makes
the combination expensive. Clinical pearls and current controversies
in management are highlighted in the text.

B

On Call Obstetrics and Gynecology $36.95
CHIN

Elsevier, 2006, 3rd ed., 433 pages, ISBN 9781416023944

A compact guide presented in a format similar to the rest of the *On
Call* series, addressing common problems the on-call physician will
encounter on obstetrics and gynecology. Although not comprehensive enough for study, the pocketbook guides students' clinical thinking and approach toward emergent issues. More for residents on call
than for medical students.

B

Obstetrics & Gynecology (House Officer Series) $29.95
RAYBURN

Lippincott Williams & Wilkins, 2002, 4th ed., 429 pages,
ISBN 9780781728553

A good pocketbook for quick reference as patients are seen in the
hospital. Written in essay form, it is sometimes difficult to sift
through for the main points. Offers basic, broad coverage of most
conditions encountered on the wards and in outpatient clinics.

SOAP for Obstetrics and Gynecology $25.00

UZELAC

Lippincott Williams & Wilkins, 2005, 1st ed., 168 pages,
ISBN 9781405104357

A thin pocketbook that presents information in a SOAP note format.
Focuses heavily on clinical problems, not on the diagnosis. The "S"
(subject) section contains a list of helpful questions to ask when interviewing patients and writing notes. The book would be most helpful in guiding day-to-day management and in formulating an assessment and plan for patients with a known diagnosis. Would benefit
from some figures or diagrams.

Blueprints in Obstetrics & Gynecology $35.95
CALLAHAN
Lippincott Williams & Wilkins, 2004, 3rd ed., 356 pages,
ISBN 9781405104890
A good, concise introductory review for the obstetrics and gynecology rotation. Offers an excellent and easy-to-read synopsis of major topics as well as good figures and tables. Some students feel that this is the best of the *Blueprints* series. Also includes an excellent review test for shelf and USMLE Step 2 exams, but students considering a career in obstetrics and gynecology will need to find a more detailed textbook as well. Contains a section on breast disease.

First Aid for the Obstetrics & Gynecology Clerkships $41.95
STEAD
McGraw-Hill, 2007, 2nd ed., 304 pages, ISBN 9780071448741
A comprehensive overview of pertinent topics in obstetrics and gynecology, written in a concise outline format that covers essential high-yield information often found on shelf and USMLE Step 2 exams. "Exam tips" and "ward tips" are included in the margins of the text. Pathophysiology is not explained fully, and few figures and photographs are provided. Overall, an excellent review for a busy clerkship. This publication is not affiliated with the authors of *First Aid for the Wards*.

Gynaecology Illustrated $67.95
HART
Elsevier, 2000, 5th ed., 443 pages, ISBN 9780443061981
An excellent mini-reference for gynecology, written at an appropriate level for medical students. Provides high-yield information along with good schematic drawings of anatomy, pathology, and procedures. A bit brief with respect to treatment. The fact that one must find another resource for obstetrics detracts from its overall utility. Excellent for reviewing the basics, particularly for those interested in obstetrics and gynecology.

Case Files Obstetrics & Gynecology

$29.95

TOY

McGraw-Hill, 2007, 2nd ed., 456 pages, ISBN 9780071463010

A compilation of more than 60 case series accompanied by extended discussions of each case, definitions of key terms, clinical pearls, a primer on how to approach problems, and a short section consisting of USMLE-style questions. The format is similar to that of the *Underground Clinical Vignettes* series, but this book is much more comprehensive, placing greater emphasis on pathophysiology and management plans. Originally designed for USMLE Step 2 preparation, the text could also serve as a useful companion for the clerkship as well as a source of practice cases for the shelf exam. Drawbacks include busy organization and a lack of figures and tables.

Obstetrics and Gynecology

$49.95

BECKMANN

Lippincott Williams & Wilkins, 2006, 5th ed., 850 pages, ISBN 9780781758062

A concise textbook intended for medical students on their core obstetrics and gynecology rotation, based on the Association of Professors of Gynecology and Obstetrics Instructional Objectives. Features a case-based approach with brief coverage of topics and many questions. Chapters are short enough to finish in one sitting and include some helpful tables, figures, and diagrams. Offers enough information to get by, but lacks the depth of other texts. Some students state that it is too simplistic and somewhat disorganized.

Essentials of Obstetrics and Gynecology

$56.95

HACKER

Elsevier, 2004, 4th ed., 554 pages, ISBN 9780721601793

A well-organized text written at an appropriate level for medical students. Serves as a good introductory resource for those intending to enter the field, although it may prove difficult to finish on a busy service. Contains excellent discussions on patient workups and good background material. Overall very readable, but lacks the depth of a true reference book. Compare with Beckmann's *Obstetrics and Gynecology*.

High-Yield Obstetrics & Gynecology

$26.95

SAKALA

Lippincott Williams & Wilkins, 2006, 2nd ed., 194 pages, ISBN 9780781796309

Part of a popular USMLE Step 1 prep series that offers a review book for each clerkship. Typical of its format, the book contains high-yield information in a clear and concise outline form organized by organ system. It also contains ample figures and tables for easier reading.

In A Page OB/GYN & Women's Health

$32.95

CARR

Lippincott Williams & Wilkins, 2003, 1st ed., 176 pages,
ISBN 9781405103800

A dry review of more than 120 diseases, organized by a woman's life span (from adolescence to postmenopause). Each disease pathology is explained in one page, from etiology to prognosis, with lists. Provides a big picture and high-yield information; best suited for quick review before seeing a patient or preparing for a pimp session. The book is thin but not pocket-sized and also lacks figures and tables, so readers will need to refer to other textbooks for more detailed information.

Underground Clinical Vignettes: OB/GYN

$19.95

KIM

Lippincott Williams & Wilkins, 2007, 4th ed., 256 pages,
ISBN 9780781768405

A well-organized review of clinical vignettes commonly encountered on NBME shelf and USMLE Step 2 exams. Includes a focused, high-yield discussion of pathogenesis, epidemiology, management, complications, and associated diseases. Black-and-white images are included where relevant. Also contains several "minicases" in which only key facts related to each disease are presented. An excellent, entertaining, and easy-to-use supplement for studying during the clinical rotation.

NMS Obstetrics & Gynecology

$39.95

PFEIFER

Lippincott Williams & Wilkins, 2007, 6th ed., 496 pages,
ISBN 9780781770712

A comprehensive review presented in an outline format that may be too dense for regular use. Well organized, but discussions can be lengthy and boring. An excellent comprehensive exam at the end poses questions similar to those found on the shelf and USMLE Step 2 exams. Offers few tables and diagrams.

Obstetrics and Gynecology Secrets

$36.95

BADER

Elsevier, 2003, 3rd ed., 378 pages, ISBN 9781560534754

A text presented in the question-and-answer format typical of the *Secrets* series, with good coverage of many high-yield, clinically relevant topics. Detailed, but contains no vignettes or images. Some explanations appear inadequate. Provides a good clinical context for quick self-testing, but does not serve as a formal topic review.

B–

Obstetrics and Gynecology Recall

$36.95

BOURGEOIS

Lippincott Williams & Wilkins, 2008, 3rd ed., 608 pages,
ISBN 9780781770699

A question-and-answer format in *Recall*-series style set in two columns, making it easy to use for self-quizzing. Reviews many high-yield concepts and facts. Questions emphasize individual facts but do not integrate concepts, and no vignettes or images are included. In addition, some topics are covered only sparingly. Useful as a review of selected material, but not a comprehensive source for wards or end-of-rotation examinations.

B–

Lecture Notes on Obstetrics and Gynaecology

$43.95

CHAMBERLAIN

Wiley, 2004, 2nd ed., 344 pages, ISBN 9781405120661

A mini–review text designed for medical students. Offers excellent coverage of basic science, etiology, and clinical presentation, but its discussion of differentials, diagnostic approach, and therapeutic options is only average, limiting its usefulness on the wards. Portable enough to carry around in the coat pocket if readers wish to use it to study for shelf and USMLE Step 2 exams.

PreTest Obstetrics and Gynecology   *$26.95*
SCHNEIDER
McGraw-Hill, 2006, 11th ed., 368 pages, ISBN 9780071458108
A collection of 500 multiple-choice questions covering a wide range
of topic in obstetrics and gynecology. Includes clinical vignette–style
questions, and provides detailed paragraph-format explanations for
each answer. Probably the most widely used preparatory text for shelf
exams. Good for last-minute review before the exam.

Blueprints Clinical Cases in Obstetrics & Gynecology   *$29.95*
CAUGHEY
Lippincott Williams & Wilkins, 2007, 2nd ed., 418 pages,
ISBN 9781405104906
Organized by common presenting signs and symptoms, this book
contains symptom-based clinical cases accompanied by 200 USMLE-
style questions. The format is similar to that of the *Case Files* series
but places less emphasis on discussions and greater focus on questions.

Blueprints Q&A Step 2 Obstetrics & Gynecology   *$39.95*
TRAN
Lippincott Williams & Wilkins, 2007, 2nd ed., 168 pages,
ISBN 9781405103909
The new edition of this book contains more than 200 USMLE-style
questions (increased from 100 from the previous edition) with explanations for both correct and incorrect answers, although explanations
are not as detailed and well referenced as those in the *PreTest* series.
The book was originally designed for Step 2 preparation, but since
the format of the shelf exam is similar, this would be a useful companion for clerkship preparation as well. The book is thin enough to
carry in the pocket and could easily be read in a few days.

Appleton & Lange Obstetrics & Gynecology   *$39.95*
VONTVER
McGraw-Hill, 2006, 8th ed., 320 pages, ISBN 9780071461399
A question-and-answer book with 1600 multiple-choice questions organized under different topics. Provides detailed, paragraph-length
explanations for each answer. Questions tend to focus on details
rather than following the shelf exam format. A good review of the
topics, but could be overwhelming if used for last-minute preparation.

TEXTBOOK/REFERENCE

A⁻

Williams Obstetrics
CUNNINGHAM

$155.00

McGraw-Hill, 2005, 22nd ed., 1441 pages, ISBN 9780071413152

The definitive book within its field, meant for the serious obstetrics and gynecology student. Organized by organ system; includes good use of graphics to highlight material. Offers more ultrasound pictures than the previous edition contained. Well referenced with updated guidelines and a strong, evidence-based approach. Its usefulness is diminished only by the need to find another reference for gynecology.

A⁻

Danforth's Obstetrics and Gynecology
DANFORTH

$165.00

Lippincott Williams & Wilkins, 2008, 10th ed., 715 pages, ISBN 9780781769372

An excellent core text for residents and students considering careers in obstetrics and gynecology, but too detailed for most others. A well-organized and comprehensive reference for both obstetrics and gynecology, with numerous illustrations. Places increased emphasis on the latest advances, evidence-based medicine, and the most recent clinical guidelines. Also offers good, concise outlines of many diseases, although some key points are not highlighted as well as they should be in view of the book's extensive detail.

B⁺

Current Obstetric & Gynecologic Diagnosis & Treatment
DECHERNEY

$64.95

McGraw-Hill, 2007, 10th ed., 1166 pages, ISBN 9780071439008

A good overall reference book. Makes effective use of graphics and tables, but minimal emphasis is placed on differential diagnosis. A good value, but not very high yield or appropriate for those with less interest in the specialty, especially when compared to other reference textbooks.

HANDBOOK/POCKETBOOK

Saint-Frances Guide to Pediatrics
$32.95

MIGITA

Lippincott Williams & Wilkins, 2003, 1st ed., 736 pages,
ISBN 9780781721462

A concise pocketbook emphasizing the development of a basic, organized approach toward many common diseases. Makes good use of tables and charts, and devotes a substantial portion of its text to medical mnemonics. Good to keep in the pocket during the rotation for a quick reference, as it discusses all major disorders in a concise outline format.

Clinical Handbook of Pediatrics
$39.95

SCHWARTZ

Lippincott Williams & Wilkins, 2003, 3rd ed., 975 pages,
ISBN 9780781736497

A spiral-bound pocket reference focusing on the diagnostic approach toward a broad range of pediatric problems. Contains an extensive differential diagnosis list along with discussions of presenting symptoms and laboratory values. Concepts in treatment are discussed, but specific management details are limited. Easy to read with good algorithms, tables, and figures. Also includes a useful chapter outlining the H&P along with many pearls.

Pediatric Drug Reference
$9.95

GENNRICH

Current Clinical Strategies, 2004, 1st ed., 88 pages,
ISBN 9781929622436

A practical handbook detailing admit orders, specific pharmacologic treatment options, and the management of common pediatric diseases. Includes useful charts on developmental milestones and immunization. An excellent value for its size and price. Useful for subinterns, although its discussion of differential diagnoses is limited.

Manual of Pediatric Therapeutics
$45.95

GRAEF

Lippincott Williams & Wilkins, 2008, 7th ed., 736 pages,
ISBN 9780781771665

A relatively comprehensive spiral-bound manual that adequately covers the general principles, management, and treatment of common pediatric diseases, presented in a concise outline format that makes good use of tables and charts. Includes updated guidelines and a focused drug formulary section. Appropriate for subinterns.

SOAP for Pediatrics

$25.00

POLISKY

Lippincott Williams & Wilkins, 2005, 1st ed., 192 pages, ISBN 9781405104340

A thin pocketbook that presents information in a SOAP note format. Organized according to the visit setting (inpatient vs. outpatient), the book focuses heavily on clinical problems, not on diagnosis. The "S" (subject) section contains a list of helpful questions to ask when interviewing patients and writing notes. The book would be most helpful in guiding day-to-day management and in formulating an assessment and plan for patients with a known diagnosis. Would benefit from some figures or diagrams.

The Harriet Lane Handbook

$54.95

ROBERTSON

Elsevier, 2005, 17th ed., 1168 pages, ISBN 9780323029179

The classic pocketbook designed for residents. Very focused on practical treatment and management, with limited discussion of pathophysiology and differential diagnoses. Includes an extensive drug formulary section with pediatric dosing of common drugs. Numerous well-indexed tables and charts are interspersed throughout the text in an easy-to-read format. Roughly organized by system, including sections on pediatric subspecialties. Too technical for junior students, but good for subinterns and serious pediatric students.

Practical Guide to the Care of the Pediatric Patient

$49.95

ALARIO

Elsevier, 2007, 2nd ed., 976 pages, ISBN 9780323036702

A spiral-bound, student-friendly pocket manual written in outline format with emphasis on high-yield clinical features, diagnostic evaluation, and management of pediatric diseases. Contains sections about the pediatric H&P, development, and routine health maintenance and preventive care. Offers more information on pathophysiology and differentials than does *Harriet Lane*, but not as helpful with pharmacology.

Handbook of Pediatrics

$31.95

MERENSTEIN

McGraw-Hill, 2005, 19th ed., 1029 pages, ISBN 9780838535684

A useful handbook offering good coverage of a variety of diseases. Discusses etiology, pathophysiology, clinical findings, and treatment. Contains a limited drug formulary that is quite cumbersome, but makes excellent use of tables, charts, and algorithms. May be good to read during breaks while on the wards, but a bit bulky to carry around. Has not been updated in several years, so some information is out of date.

On Call Pediatrics

$38.95

NOCTON

Elsevier, 2006, 3rd ed., 480 pages, ISBN 9781416023937

A practical, portable guide to the pediatric problems one is likely to encounter on call. Takes a systematic approach that begins with the phone call and includes preliminary evaluation, differential diagnosis, workup, and initial management. Sections are well organized by common problems, but readers will need to look elsewhere for more detail. Limited in breadth; cannot replace other pocket manuals in pediatrics. Not useful for beginning medical students.

A

Rudolph's Fundamentals of Pediatrics

$72.95

RUDOLPH

McGraw-Hill, 2002, 3rd ed., 848 pages, ISBN 9780838584507

An excellent, well-organized softcover reference book written at an appropriate level for students on their pediatric clerkship. The highly readable text makes good use of algorithms that summarize approaches toward common pediatric diseases. Suffices as a general home reference, but students going into pediatrics should consider a more detailed textbook such as the parent volume. Has not been updated in several years.

A

First Aid for the Pediatrics Clerkship

$39.95

STEAD

McGraw-Hill, 2008, 2nd ed., 464 pages, ISBN 9780071448703

A highly comprehensive overview of pertinent topics in pediatrics, written in outline format and intended for NBME shelf and USMLE Step 2 exam study. Covers essential high-yield information in a manner that is succinct and easy to read. Pearls and high-yield information are highlighted in the margins. Pathophysiology is not explained fully, and few figures and photographs are provided. Overall, an excellent review of the broad field of pediatrics. This publication is not affiliated with the authors of *First Aid for the Wards*.

Oski's Essential Pediatrics

$59.95

CROCETTI

Lippincott Williams & Wilkins, 2004, 2nd ed., 784 pages, ISBN 9780781737708

A good, basic reference text organized by problem. Includes illustrations and tables. Easier to read than *Nelson* and provides a good overview of treatment and management, but lacks detail and depth. Sections vary in their coverage. Useful for the time-limited student. An interesting section at the end describes common syndromes with morphologic abnormalities, including line illustrations of distinctive facial phenotypes.

Blueprints in Pediatrics

$36.95

MARINO

Lippincott Williams & Wilkins, 2007, 4th ed., 303 pages,
ISBN 9781405105019

A handy, concise, easy-to-read resource of high-yield information that is likely to appear on shelf and USMLE Step 2 exams. Presents adequate coverage of the basics, and includes good charts, diagrams, and key points. Not comprehensive enough to be a complete review book; some sections are too detailed and others too simplistic. Offers a good overview of topics students are most likely to encounter while on the rotation.

Nelson Essentials of Pediatrics

$68.95

NELSON

Elsevier, 2006, 5th ed., 1008 pages, ISBN 9781416001591

A condensed softcover version of *Nelson Textbook of Pediatrics* with concise explanations. Still quite lengthy, and better suited as a reference text than as a rapid review resource. Well organized into sections on clinical diagnosis, differential diagnosis, and treatment. Comparable to *Rudolph's Fundamentals of Pediatrics* in terms of quality.

Case Files Pediatrics

$29.95

TOY

McGraw-Hill, 2007, 2nd ed., 576 pages, ISBN 9780071463027

A compilation of more than 60 case series accompanied by extended discussions of each case, definitions of key terms, clinical pearls, a primer on how to approach problems, and a short section consisting of USMLE-style questions. More comprehensive than the *Underground Clinical Vignettes* series, but still fairly basic in terms of case selection. Originally designed for USMLE Step 2 preparation, the text could also serve as a useful companion for the clerkship as well as a source of practice cases for the shelf exam. Page layout is overly busy, and figures and tables are lacking.

Illustrated Textbook of Paediatrics

$69.95

LISSAUER

Elsevier, 2007, 3rd ed., 528 pages, ISBN 9780723433972

A solid, easy-to-understand textbook written at a good introductory level for medical students. Makes excellent use of numerous color photos, diagrams, case histories, and clinical tips. A good basic reference for learning and reviewing the fundamentals of pediatrics.

B+

Underground Clinical Vignettes: Pediatrics $19.95

SWANSON

Lippincott Williams & Wilkins, 2007, 4th ed., 256 pages,
ISBN 9780781768443

A well-organized review of clinical vignettes commonly encountered on NBME shelf and USMLE Step 2 exams. Includes a focused, high-yield discussion of pathogenesis, epidemiology, management, and complications. Black-and-white images are included where relevant. Also offers several "minicases" in which only key facts related to each disease are presented. An excellent, entertaining, and easy-to-use supplement for studying during the clinical rotation, but not meant to be used as a primary text.

B

Pediatrics for Medical Students $42.95

BERNSTEIN

Lippincott Williams & Wilkins, 2003, 2nd ed., 650 pages,
ISBN 9780781729413

An introductory softcover text geared toward junior medical students doing their pediatric clerkship. Divided into common primary care problems and pediatric subspecialty problems. The text is readable but a bit dry and is not as comprehensive as similar books. Some information is out of date, as the book has not been updated for several years. Offers few illustrations and tables.

B

Clinical Paediatrics and Child Health $71.95

CANDY

Elsevier, 2001, 1st ed., 398 pages, ISBN 9780702017261

An introductory textbook designed for medical students on their pediatric clerkship. An excellent and comprehensive section is devoted to normal child development and approaching common illnesses. Also functions as a mini-encyclopedia of disorders, etiologies, clinical findings, and management, although some of the diseases covered are a bit obscure. Overall, a good overview of general disease and pathophysiology, but lacks detail with regard to treatment and management.

B

Mosby's Color Atlas and Text of Pediatrics and Child Health $60.95

CHAUDHRY

Elsevier, 2001, 1st ed., 420 pages, ISBN 9780723424369

A highly visual reference with full-color photographs and radiographs throughout the text. Contains more illustrations than the *Illustrated Textbook of Paediatrics* but is not as detailed in its coverage of pediatric disease manifestations, diagnosis, and treatment, making it less useful as a reference. Has not been updated in several years, but remains a useful basic text.

REVIEW RESOURCES

PEDIATRICS

In A Page Pediatrics

KAHAN

$32.95

Lippincott Williams & Wilkins, 2008, 2nd ed., 384 pages,
ISBN 9780781770453

A dry review of more than 200 diseases, organized by organ system. Each disease pathology is explained in one page, from etiology to prognosis. Provides a big picture and high-yield information; best suited for quick review before seeing a patient or preparing for a pimp session. The book is thin but is not pocket-sized and also lacks figures and tables, so students will need to refer to other textbooks for more detailed information.

Lecture Notes on Paediatrics

NEWELL

$37.95

Wiley, 2008, 8th ed., 304 pages, ISBN 9781405145091

A portable review book on the core knowledge and fundamentals of pediatric diseases. Offers a number of useful tables and figures. Unique sections are dedicated to describing the essentials of the pediatric clinical exam, and self-assessment questions have been added to the new edition. Too superficial for practical wards use given its limited coverage of diagnostic approach and management, but useful as a supplement to other textbooks. Costly for the limited amount of material covered.

Pediatric Secrets

POLIN

$39.95

Elsevier, 2005, 4th ed., 729 pages, ISBN 9781560536277

A text presented in the question-and-answer format typical of the *Secrets* series. Organized by organ system and includes good use of tables, charts, and mnemonics. Designed to prepare students for pimping sessions, although these sessions are infrequent in pediatrics. Best used for quick self-testing during downtime. Some questions are too specific and detailed. Too big to fit in the coat pocket or carry around comfortably.

In A Page Pediatric Signs & Symptoms

TEITELBAUM

$32.95

Lippincott Williams & Wilkins, 2004, 1st ed., 255 pages,
ISBN 9781405104272

Organized by common presenting signs and symptoms, this book focuses on differential diagnosis and workup. As with its counterpart (*In A Page Pediatrics*), each symptom is explained in one page with lists. Best used as a quick review, and a great companion to use while on call, providing guidelines on how to work up "fresh" patients.

Berkowitz's Pediatrics: A Primary Care Approach

$64.95

BERKOWITZ

American Academy of Pediatrics, 2008, 3rd ed., 600 pages,
ISBN 9781581102833

A comprehensive review text with sections focusing on a key symptom or general disease category followed by step-by-step guidelines on diagnostic approach and treatment strategies. Case vignettes and self-assessment questions are included, but the book makes inadequate use of tables and illustrations. The format is somewhat difficult to follow and is not useful for test preparation. Sufficiently broad to help students understand general pediatric issues, but specific treatment regimens must be found in another reference.

BRS Pediatrics

$36.95

BROWN

Lippincott Williams & Wilkins, 2005, 1st ed., 649 pages,
ISBN 9780781721295

This book is organized in the same manner as its counterpart USMLE prep series. Contains substantial information on pediatric disorders with accompanying questions at the end of each section, but the text is a bit too dry for review during the rotation and is not designed for use as a quick reference.

NMS Pediatrics

$39.95

DWORKIN

Lippincott Williams & Wilkins, 2001, 4th ed., 739 pages,
ISBN 9780683306378

A lengthy, detailed review book that covers most important pediatric disorders found on the shelf and USMLE Step 2 exams. Although more comprehensive than the *Blueprints* series, it is occasionally too wordy, and its outline format often lacks organization. Few tables and figures are included to complement the text. Not particularly useful for management issues on the wards. Review questions are available at the end of each chapter, and a comprehensive test is included at the end of the book.

Pediatrics Recall

$36.95

MCGAHREN

Lippincott Williams & Wilkins, 2008, 3rd ed., 508 pages,
ISBN 9780781771184

Like the *Secrets* series, this book is meant for quick self-testing during free time, covering essential bare-bones issues of pediatric health and disease in a question-and-answer format. A bit smaller than previous versions, but still too bulky to carry around in the coat pocket.

PreTest Pediatrics

$26.95

YETMAN

McGraw-Hill, 2006, 11th ed., 464 pages, ISBN 9780071455527

A collection of 500 multiple-choice questions covering a wide range of topics in pediatrics. Includes clinical vignette–style questions and provides detailed paragraph-format explanations for each answer. Probably the most widely used preparatory text for shelf exams. Good for last-minute review before the exam, but not as useful for general clerkship knowledge.

Blueprints Q&A Step 2 Pediatrics

$19.95

FOTI

Lippincott Williams & Wilkins, 2005, 2nd ed., 176 pages, ISBN 9781405103916

The new edition of this book contains more than 200 USMLE-style questions (increased from 100 from the previous edition) with explanations for both correct and incorrect answers, although explanations are not as detailed and well referenced as those in the *PreTest* series. The book was originally designed for Step 2 preparation, but since the format of the shelf exam is similar, this would be a useful companion for clerkship preparation as well. The book is thin enough to carry in the pocket and could easily be read in a few days.

Blueprints Clinical Cases in Pediatrics

$29.95

LONDHE

Lippincott Williams & Wilkins, 2007, 2nd ed., 426 pages, ISBN 9781405104920

Organized by common presenting signs and symptoms, this book contains 50 symptom-based clinical cases accompanied by 200 USMLE-style questions. The format is similar to that of the *Case Files* series but places less emphasis on discussions and greater focus on questions.

REVIEW RESOURCES

PEDIATRICS

Nelson Textbook of Pediatrics $149.00

BEHRMAN

Elsevier, 2007, 18th ed., 3200 pages, ISBN 9781416024507

An authoritative reference book that many consider the "gold standard" of pediatric textbooks. Well organized with clear explanations and comprehensive discussions on the diagnosis and treatment of pediatric disorders. Worth the investment for those pursuing pediatrics as a career; otherwise, best borrowed from the library. Great for preparing complete, detailed presentations.

Oski's Pediatrics: Principles and Practice $149.00

MCMILLAN

Lippincott Williams & Wilkins, 2006, 4th ed., 2600 pages, ISBN 9780781738941

Another authoritative and comprehensive textbook that has been around for many years. Although the book is presented in black-and-white format with few figures or tables, it is still a great resource for motivated students.

Rudolph's Pediatrics $150.00

RUDOLPH

McGraw-Hill, 2003, 21st ed., 2688 pages, ISBN 9780838582855

A comprehensive hardcover reference book for very serious pediatric students. The text is similar in price and scope to *Nelson Textbook of Pediatrics* but may be a bit easier to read. An alternative worth considering. The new, updated version includes more treatment algorithms as well as a greater number of specialty-oriented topics.

Current Diagnosis and Treatment in Pediatrics $64.95

HAY

McGraw-Hill, 2007, 18th ed., 1306 pages, ISBN 9780071463003

An up-to-date, comprehensive reference book with excellent organization of disease entities. Provides clinical information on ambulatory and inpatient medical care from birth to adolescence. Makes excellent use of tables, graphs, and illustrations. High-yield information is presented as essentials of diagnosis at the beginning of each section. Overall, a useful book for home reference. Easier to read than the "classic" texts, but not as detailed.

HANDBOOK/POCKETBOOK

Current Clinical Strategies: Psychiatry

$12.95

HAHN

Current Clinical Strategies, 2008, 3rd ed., 125 pages,
ISBN 9781934323106

A recently updated, concise pocketbook designed for quick reference while on the wards. Contains DSM-IV diagnostic criteria, differential diagnoses, and current treatment guidelines. An excellent psychopharmacology section at the end of the book contains tables comparing drugs and their side effects. Also included is a brief overview of the mental status exam and sample admitting orders for common psychiatric disorders. A good value for its size and price.

Saint-Frances Guide to Psychiatry

$28.95

McCARTHY

Lippincott Williams & Wilkins, 2001, 1st ed., 276 pages,
ISBN 9780683306613

An excellent, cheap, and concise pocketbook emphasizing the development of a basic, organized approach toward many common psychiatric diseases. Makes good use of tables and charts, and devotes a substantial portion of its text to medical mnemonics. However, the text cannot be used as a primary resource because it lacks an extensive discussion of pathophysiology, diagnostic evaluation, management, and treatment. Still a great companion during the rotation, and small enough to carry everywhere.

Kaplan & Sadock's Pocket Handbook of Clinical Psychiatry

$54.95

SADOCK

Lippincott Williams & Wilkins, 2005, 4th ed., 515 pages,
ISBN 9780781762168

This staple quick-reference handbook discusses etiology, epidemiology, clinical features, and therapeutic measures in a well-organized outline format. Contains up-to-date diagnostic criteria and pharmacologic guidelines along with cross-references to its parent book, *Comprehensive Textbook of Psychiatry*. Also includes useful tables, color photographs of commonly used psychiatric drugs, and a general overview of the psychiatric examination. The small print makes it difficult to read.

Practical Guide to the Care of the Psychiatric Patient $46.95

GOLDBERG

Elsevier, 2007, 3rd ed., 608 pages, ISBN 9780323036832

A concise, easy-to-read, spiral-bound handbook patterned after the growing *Practical Care* series. Offers thorough coverage of all major psychiatric areas with DSM-IV criteria and numerous comparative charts and tables. Not comprehensive, but contains the basic information that a medical student needs. Also includes an interesting section on P-450 drug interactions. A drug formulary at the end of the book for commonly prescribed psychiatric medications includes some out-of-place drugs such as allopurinol, INH, and procainamide.

Psychiatry Clerkship Guide $36.95

MANLEY

Elsevier, 2007, 2nd ed., 544 pages, ISBN 9781416031321

A well-designed pocket guide with one section organized by presentation and a second section grouped by known diagnosis, allowing readers to use the reference in either manner. Information within each chapter is organized in a question-and-answer format, with answers given in paragraph style. Covers many questions that come up on rotations, but may not be the quickest on-the-go reference.

Psychiatry (House Officer Series) $39.95

TOMB

Lippincott Williams & Wilkins, 2008, 7th ed., 309 pages,
ISBN 9780781774529

A compact pocketbook of commonly encountered psychiatric disorders, written in essay format with highlighted key words and phrases to facilitate rapid review. Contains good references for further in-depth study, updated management guidelines, a number of useful tables, and a color guide of psychiatric medications. A basic review book that is not comprehensive enough for primary study.

Quick Reference to the Diagnostic Criteria from DSM-IV-TR $35.00

AMERICAN PSYCHIATRIC ASSOCIATION

American Psychiatric Press, 2000, 4th ed., 496 pages,
ISBN 9780890420263

A pocketbook best used for the review of diagnostic criteria rather than for general wards work or application to patient care. Offers comprehensive coverage of all DSM-IV-TR psychiatric diseases, but lacks a discussion of etiologies and therapies, thus negating its clinical usefulness. The same diagnostic criteria for major disorders can be found in other handbooks.

On Call Psychiatry   *$36.95*

BERNSTEIN

Elsevier, 2006, 3rd ed., 308 pages, ISBN 9781416025740

A compact guide with a format similar to that of the rest of the *On Call* series, addressing common problems the on-call physician will encounter in psychiatry. Not comprehensive enough for study, but reviews important basic concepts of clinical thinking. Geared more toward residents on call than toward medical students. Some sections are related less to psychiatry than to general inpatient care.

A

Kaplan & Sadock's Concise Textbook of Clinical Psychiatry

$64.95

SADOCK

Lippincott Williams & Wilkins, 2004, 2nd ed., 669 pages,
ISBN 9780781750332

An excellent, downsized version of Kaplan's *Synopsis* that retains all the clinical psychiatry students need to know minus the behavioral science. Based on DSM-IV and well organized, with practical chapters on psychopharmacology and laboratory tests. A nice addition to the bookshelf of the non-psychiatry-bound student.

A

First Aid for the Psychiatry Clerkship

$41.95

STEAD

McGraw-Hill, 2005, 2nd ed., 179 pages, ISBN 9780071448727

A highly comprehensive overview of pertinent topics in psychiatry, written in outline format and intended for NBME shelf and USMLE Step 2 exam study. Covers essential high-yield information in a succinct, systematic manner. Includes more tables than the previous edition, but few figures and photographs are provided. High-yield mnemonics and clinical scenarios are given in the margins. Overall, an excellent review of the broad field of psychiatry.

Psychiatry

$46.95

CUTLER

Elsevier, 1999, 1st ed., 351 pages, ISBN 9780721667218

An excellent introductory text written at an appropriate level for medical students. Discusses all major psychiatric disorders with numerous clinical vignettes to illustrate how each disorder may present. Contains good quick-reference tables of DSM-IV criteria, but has not been updated in many years. Also includes chapters on the psychiatric interview, psychotherapy, and psychopharmacology.

Blueprints Clinical Cases in Psychiatry

$29.95

HOBLYN

Lippincott Williams & Wilkins, 2008, 2nd ed., 304 pages,
ISBN 9781405104968

Consists of 60 cases divided into adult, geriatric, and child/adolescent categories. Each case is presented in a thorough (but perhaps overly extensive) manner, and the discussion section is in paragraph form but thorough. Each case study is followed by a few brief questions. Questions are not thorough enough to use alone for shelf study, but the cases are for the most part interesting and readable. Includes 100 USMLE-style questions for review.

Blueprints in Psychiatry $36.95

MURPHY

Lippincott Williams & Wilkins, 2007, 4th ed., 144 pages,
ISBN 9781405105026

A brief review text of psychiatry designed for the shelf and USMLE
Step 2 exams. Offers good coverage of high-yield topics with helpful
tables. Short, compact, and easy to read within a few days. Lacks the
detail necessary for rounds and the clinical clerkship, but remains a
great resource for rapid review. The discussion of psychopharmacology is limited.

Case Files Psychiatry $29.95

TOY

McGraw-Hill, 2007, 2nd ed., 408 pages, ISBN 9780071462822

A compilation of more than 60 case series accompanied by extended
discussions of each case, definitions of key terms, clinical pearls, a
primer on how to approach problems, and a short section of
USMLE-style questions. Case presentations are somewhat simplistic, but the format is easy to read and well organized. Contains a basic pharmacology section.

Review of General Psychiatry $49.95

GOLDMAN

McGraw-Hill, 2005, 6th ed., 583 pages, ISBN 9780071410748

A lengthy but engaging introductory text for medical students interested in psychiatry. Includes a discussion of etiology, epidemiology,
DSM-IV classification, differential diagnosis, and treatment modalities. Good clinical vignettes are interspersed throughout the text to
help illustrate key principles. Another reference for specific drug
therapy that includes drug dosing is needed to supplement this book
for practical wards usage.

DSM-IV-TR Casebook $69.00

SPITZER

American Psychiatric Press, 2002, 1st ed., 624 pages,
ISBN 9781585620593

This companion text to DSM-IV-TR consists of short clinical vignettes followed by a discussion of etiology, differentials, and treatment. The text is easy to read but is a long didactic tool for students
interested in psychiatry. Geared more toward exam study than toward practical wards work; useful as a supplement to a more comprehensive review book.

REVIEW RESOURCES

PSYCHIATRY

B+

Clinical Psychiatry for Medical Students

$42.95

STOUDEMIRE

Lippincott Williams & Wilkins, 1998, 3rd ed., 941 pages,
ISBN 9780397584604

A detailed review text for medical students that integrates biological, psychological, and sociological concepts into its discussion of psychiatric disease. Good tables and figures illustrate concepts. Discussions are lengthy but of interest to students who are considering a career in psychiatry. Would benefit from more information on general neurophysiologic processes within the brain, especially when the biological basis of psychiatric disease is discussed. Compare with *Concise Textbook of Clinical Psychiatry*.

B

Underground Clinical Vignettes: Psychiatry

$22.95

KIM

Lippincott Williams & Wilkins, 2007, 4th ed., 187 pages,
ISBN 9780781768467

A well-organized review of clinical vignettes commonly encountered on the shelf and USMLE Step 2 exams. Includes 80 patient cases designed to take students from chief complaint through diagnostic workup and management. Black-and-white images are included where relevant, and the book provides a brief selection of USMLE-style questions. Offers a good discussion of differential diagnoses, but does not contain DSM-IV criteria. Overall, an entertaining, easy-to-use supplement for studying during the clinical rotation.

B

BRS Psychiatry

$36.95

SHANER

Lippincott Williams & Wilkins, 2000, 2nd ed., 419 pages,
ISBN 9780683307665

A concise, easy-to-read, outline-format review book geared toward shelf and USMLE Step 2 exams. Covers a fairly comprehensive number of subjects for a psychiatry review book while highlighting the key points of each disorder, allowing for quick, focused learning. Questions are available after each chapter, and a comprehensive exam is given at the end of the book. More useful and readable than *NMS Psychiatry*.

NMS Psychiatry

$39.95

THORNHILL

Lippincott Williams & Wilkins, 2008, 5th ed., 300 pages,
ISBN 9780781765145

A highly detailed review book geared toward passing the shelf and
USMLE Step 2 exams. Although the book is comprehensive, its
dull, dry outline format makes it difficult to read. Multiple-choice
questions are included after each chapter and at the end of the book,
accompanied by lengthy explanations. Too detailed to be of use as a
quick reference.

Psychiatry Recall

$36.95

FADEM

Lippincott Williams & Wilkins, 2003, 2nd ed., 250 pages,
ISBN 9780781745116

Written in a quick question-and-answer format typical of the *Recall*
series, this book reviews many high-yield facts that are covered on
the shelf and USMLE Step 2 exams. Lacks clinical vignettes, and
some of the topics covered can be obscure while others are not given
enough attention. Useful as a quick-review supplement for another,
more detailed text.

Psychiatric Secrets

$39.95

JACOBSON

Elsevier, 2000, 2nd ed., 500 pages, ISBN 9781560534181

Written in the question-and-answer format typical of the *Secrets* series, this book offers detailed and clear explanations of important
psychiatric concepts. Good for preparation for pimping sessions on
rounds as well as for students interested in psychiatric trivia, but not
a useful resource as a reference text. Can be interesting reading
while waiting on the wards.

Clinical Psychopharmacology Made Ridiculously Simple

$14.95

PRESTON

MedMaster, Inc., 2005, 5th ed., 79 pages, ISBN 9780940780651

A practical review of the pharmacologic treatment of psychiatric disease, written with a patient-oriented perspective. Numerous algorithms are provided on when and how to treat a patient as well as on
common errors to avoid and advice to give to patients. May be best
suited to residents prescribing treatment. Includes a limited discussion of mechanisms of action and adverse effects.

A⁻

PreTest Psychiatry

PAN

$26.95

McGraw-Hill, 2006, 11th ed., 355 pages, ISBN 9780071455541

A collection of 500 multiple-choice questions covering a wide range of topics in psychiatry. Includes clinical vignette–style questions and provides detailed paragraph-format explanations for each answer. Good for last-minute review before the exam, but less useful for general clerkship knowledge.

B⁺

Blueprints Q&A Step 2 Psychiatry

McLOONE

$39.95

Lippincott Williams & Wilkins, 2004, 2nd ed., 96 pages, ISBN 9781405103923

Offers 200 USMLE-style questions with explanations for both correct and incorrect answers, although the explanations are not as detailed and well referenced as those in the *PreTest* series. The book was originally designed for Step 2 preparation, but since the format of the shelf exam is similar, this would be a useful companion for the clerkship preparation as well. The book is thin enough to carry in the pocket and could easily be read in a few days.

B

Lange Q&A: Psychiatry

ORANSKY

$39.95

McGraw-Hill, 2007, 9th ed., 280 pages, ISBN 9780071475679

A question-and-answer book that includes 750 questions along with detailed explanations of each answer. Questions are organized by topic and are accompanied by two comprehensive practice exams at the end of the book. Questions from past editions tended to focus on details, but this new edition successfully replicates the USMLE Step 2 format. Best used as a supplement to the topic review books during the rotation.

A

Kaplan & Sadock's Synopsis of Psychiatry
SADOCK

$99.00

Lippincott Williams & Wilkins, 2007, 10th ed., 1470 pages,
ISBN 9780781773270

A comprehensive reference text pared down from its parent version. Not a good exam review book, as it is too detailed for shelf and USMLE Step 2 study. Offers solid tables, case studies, diagnostic coding tables, and instant online access, but information on some subjects is difficult to find. Provides good integration of information from the basic science and clinical years. A great reference for students going into psychiatry, but students may eventually want to consider the *Comprehensive Textbook* version during residency and practice. Compare with the *Concise Textbook* version for the amount of detail that is needed.

A⁻

Kaplan & Sadock's Comprehensive Textbook of Psychiatry
SADOCK

$299.00

Lippincott Williams & Wilkins, 2005, 8th ed., 3344 pages,
ISBN 9780781734349

The "gold standard" of psychiatric textbooks. Highly comprehensive, with interesting historical perspectives on psychiatric disease and treatment. Because of its size and hefty price, students should buy this text only as a long-term investment if they know they are going to pursue psychiatry. Even then, they may wish to wait and consider the more compact alternatives, as the text may still be too detailed. Available as a two-volume set.

B⁺

Current Diagnosis & Treatment in Psychiatry
EBERT

$59.95

McGraw-Hill, 2008, 2nd ed., 640 pages, ISBN 9780071422925

A well-written text with a format consistent with that of the *Current* series. Offers a concise, easy-to-read reference with each discussion of a disease beginning with the corresponding DSM-IV diagnostic criteria. Separately addresses psychiatry topics for children and adolescents, and includes a discussion of the psychological, biological, and sociological bases for disease. A good contender to *Kaplan & Sadock's Synopsis of Psychiatry*.

B+

Psychiatry: Behavioral Science and Clinical Essentials

$53.95

KAY

Elsevier, 2000, 1st ed., 707 pages, ISBN 9780721658469

A comprehensive review text that discusses the etiology, pathophysiology, clinical features, diagnosis (as per DSM-IV criteria), and treatment of major psychiatric disorders. Includes reviews of the fundamentals of neurobiology, genetics, sleep, and learning and memory. Long clinical vignettes are given at the end of each chapter. Overall, a good, detailed review text that is slightly less comprehensive than *Kaplan & Sadock's Synopsis of Psychiatry*.

B

DSM-IV-TR

$84.00

AMERICAN PSYCHIATRIC ASSOCIATION

American Psychiatric Press, 2000, 4th ed., 943 pages, ISBN 9780890420256

A comprehensive reference for psychiatric diagnostic criteria. Includes all existing psychiatric diseases defined by the American Psychiatric Association. Lacks discussion of etiologic bases and treatment, detracting from its utility as a clinical resource. Not a worthwhile purchase unless one is considering psychiatry as a career.

HANDBOOK/POCKETBOOK

Surgical Recall

$44.95

BLACKBOURNE

Lippincott Williams & Wilkins, 2008, 5th ed., 800 pages, Print ISBN 9780781770767, Audio ISBN 9780781766845

A practical and useful adjunct to a reference text, presented in a question-and-answer format typical of the *Recall* series. Excellent for wards pimping preparation and great to use in spare moments, especially before entering the OR. Covers a wide range of topics in the form of very high yield surgical pearls. Although its format makes for quick, easy reading, the text is insufficient for the shelf and board exams, as it covers topics superficially. Now also available in an audio version in downloadable MP3 files. Highly recommended for junior students seeking to survive the common pimp questions of a difficult rotation.

Current Essentials of Surgery

$34.95

DOHERTY

McGraw-Hill, 2005, 1st ed., 469 pages, ISBN 9780071423144

The counterpart to *Current Surgical Diagnosis & Treatment*, organized according to body part. Offers a quick review along with differentials, treatments, and pearls. Presented in a short, bulleted format. Not very comprehensive.

Mont Reid Surgical Handbook

$44.00

FISCHER

Elsevier, 2005, 5th ed., 848 pages, ISBN 9780323017046

A popular and great pocketbook designed for interns and junior surgical residents, but useful for motivated medical students as well. Decent for boards review, but best designed for rapid reading during the day with quick, easy-to-memorize facts for last-minute cramming. The outline format doesn't always provide adequate explanation of disease processes or operative procedures, and there is an insufficient number of tables and figures. The latest edition includes chapters on gynecologic acute abdomens, laparoscopic procedures, and transplant medicine.

Washington Manual of Surgery $49.95
KLINGENSMITH

Lippincott Williams & Wilkins, 2007, 5th ed., 736 pages,
ISBN 9780781774475

The counterpart to the *Washington Manual of Medical Therapeutics*, this text offers good coverage of basic general surgery as well as common problems in the surgical subspecialties. Practical chapters on day-to-day care of the surgical patient are also included. True to its title as a manual, the text may be more appropriate for residents and subinterns, as it offers little description of etiology, pathophysiology, and clinical features. The fifth edition includes updates on evidence-based guidelines and minimally invasive surgical techniques.

On Call Surgery $38.95
ADAMS

Elsevier, 2006, 3rd ed., 630 pages, ISBN 9781416024415

A compact guide with a format similar to that of *Surgery on Call*, addressing common problems surgeons confront while on call. Not comprehensive enough for wards preparation or study, but the pocketbook guides one's clinical thinking and approach toward emergent issues in a well-explained manner. Geared more toward residents on call than toward medical students.

Pocket Companion to Sabiston Textbook of Surgery $50.00
TOWNSEND

Elsevier, 2005, 17th ed., 1176 pages, ISBN 9780721604824

A condensed version of the parent book written in bulleted, outline format, allowing for easy access to information. Would benefit from more illustrations, but a better quick reference than Schwartz's *Companion Handbook*. Size is an issue, however, as the book is a tight fit for the coat pocket. Consider carrying in a backpack instead.

Current Clinical Strategies: Surgery $12.95
WILSON

Current Clinical Strategies, 2006, 6th ed., 112 pages,
ISBN 9781929622573

A compact, quick-reference pocketbook that addresses common surgical problems in outline format. Includes sample admission orders and operative notes. Also offers good, high-yield descriptions of etiology, pathophysiology, clinical features, diagnostic procedures, and treatment. Contains few tables and no pictures to illustrate anatomy or surgical techniques. A good overall value for its size and price.

Schwartz's Manual of Surgery
$54.95

BRUNICARDI

McGraw-Hill, 2006, 8th ed., 1008 pages, ISBN 9780071446884

A highly detailed handbook whose essay format lends itself more to in-depth review than to quick reference while on the wards. Includes discussions of basic anatomy and physiology. The new edition offers more comprehensive coverage of surgical techniques and includes more tables and illustrations than previous versions. A good supplement to the parent *Principles of Surgery* textbook. Too thick to fit in the coat pocket.

Surgery on Call
$39.95

LEFOR

McGraw-Hill, 2005, 4th ed., 492 pages, ISBN 9780071402545

A practical, quick-reference handbook of common problems encountered by the physician on call. Provides guidelines for initial evaluation, formulation of differentials, diagnostic workup, and management. Little discussion of pathophysiology is offered, and sections are divided according to patient complaint. More useful for working up "fresh" patients than for general review.

The Cleveland Clinic Guide to Surgical Patient Management
$45.00

PONSKY

Elsevier, 2002, 1st ed., 441 pages, ISBN 9780323017091

A comprehensive pocket guide that addresses common surgical problems with emphasis on surgical operations. Disease pathophysiology, typical presentations, clinical findings, and therapy are described in detail along with sample preoperative, postoperative, and discharge orders. The absence of illustrations makes it difficult to visualize anatomy and procedures. Geared more toward intern- and resident-level education.

Surgical Intern Pocket Survival Guide
$9.50

CHAMBERLAIN

International Medical Publishing, 1993, 1st ed., 74 pages, ISBN 9780963406354

A practical pocketbook detailing the basic logistics of day-to-day surgical life. Written for the intern, but can serve as a guide for subinterns as well. Outlines the approach toward the medical management of surgical patients, including sample orders and notes. Some parts may be too specific for beginning students, but most sections are useful. Some therapeutic measures are out of date. Sparse on topics other than common problems, but small, compact, and inexpensive.

A

Cope's Early Diagnosis of the Acute Abdomen

$34.50

SILEN

Oxford University Press, 2005, 21st ed., 298 pages,
ISBN 9780195175462

A classic, brief surgical textbook that every serious student of surgery should read. Offers an excellent exposition on differential diagnosis and physical examination, and helps students focus on the clinical skills they need to diagnose an acute abdomen using a readable, personable approach. A great text for knowledge and patient management, but not high yield for boards review.

A

First Aid for the Surgery Clerkship

$41.95

STEAD

McGraw-Hill, 2003, 1st ed., 529 pages, ISBN 9780071364225

A highly comprehensive overview of pertinent topics in surgery, written in outline format and intended for NBME shelf and USMLE Step 2 exam study. Covers essential high-yield information in a succinct, systematic manner. Includes well-organized tables as well as helpful figures. High-yield mnemonics and clinical scenarios are provided in the margins. Overall, an excellent review of the broad field of surgery. This publication is not affiliated with the authors of *First Aid for the Wards*.

A⁻

NMS Surgery Casebook

$39.95

JARRELL

Lippincott Williams & Wilkins, 2003, 1st ed., 420 pages,
ISBN 9780781732192

A great companion to any review book, with sections organized by organ system. Each section starts with case scenarios and is followed by a series of questions that prompt readers to think about the next step. Includes a detailed explanation for each case as well as figures and tables. Easy to read, and perfect for self-directed learning.

A⁻

Case Files Surgery
$29.95

TOY

McGraw-Hill, 2007, 2nd ed., 532 pages, ISBN 9780071463041

A compilation of more than 60 case series accompanied by extended discussions of each case, definitions of key terms, clinical pearls, a primer on how to approach problems, and a short section of USMLE-style questions. The format is similar to that of the *Underground Clinical Vignettes* series, but this book is much more comprehensive, placing greater emphasis on pathophysiology and management plans. Originally designed for USMLE Step 2 preparation, the book could also serve as a useful companion for the clerkship as well as a source of practice cases for the shelf exam. Does not include many figures or tables.

B⁺

NMS Surgery
$39.95

JARRELL

Lippincott Williams & Wilkins, 2007, 5th ed., 645 pages, ISBN 9780781759014

An overview of surgery presented in outline format that falls between a true reference and a handbook in its detail. Offers ample coverage of common diseases, but needs more illustrations and anatomy. Includes questions following each chapter as well as a comprehensive exam at the end. May be overly dense, but certainly provides a thorough review for shelf and USMLE Step 2 exam preparation. Not useful as a primary resource.

B⁺

In A Page Surgery
$32.95

KAHAN

Lippincott Williams & Wilkins, 2004, 1st ed., 288 pages, ISBN 9781405103657

A dry review of more than 150 diseases, organized by organ system. Each disease pathology is explained in one page, from etiology to prognosis with lists. Provides a big picture and high-yield information; best suited for quick review before seeing a patient or preparing for a pimp session. The book is thin but is not pocket-sized and also lacks figures and tables, so students will need to refer to other textbooks for more detailed information.

Underground Clinical Vignettes: Surgery

$22.95

KIM

Lippincott Williams & Wilkins, 2007, 4th ed., 167 pages,
ISBN 9780781768474

A well-organized review, with 76 cases following the typical clinical vignette format seen in this series. Includes a focused, high-yield discussion of pathogenesis, epidemiology, management, and complications. Black-and-white images are included where relevant. Insufficient for use in either clinical rotations or test preparation, but an easy-to-use supplement for either.

Introduction to Surgery

$45.95

LEVIEN

Elsevier, 1999, 3rd ed., 303 pages, ISBN 9780721676524

A clinically oriented, quick-review book written at a level appropriate for medical students. Each section begins with a clinical vignette followed by a well-written discussion of disease pathophysiology and management. Also offers helpful black-and-white illustrations of anatomy and surgical procedures. A good book to help guide the transition into clinical thinking, especially for students interested in surgery. Better for exam preparation than for rotation preparation.

General Surgery Review

$49.95

MAKARY

Ladner-Drysdale, 2008, 2nd ed., 582 pages, ISBN
9780976066224

A comprehensive review text with an easy-to-follow case-based format that makes use of more than 1000 clinical scenarios. Topics are nicely summarized without superfluous information, and exam pearls are interspersed throughout. Includes general as well as all major subspecialty reviews. Great for shelf as well as wards review. Available only online at www.shelfexam.com.

Blueprints in Surgery

$36.95

KARP

Lippincott Williams & Wilkins, 2006, 4th ed., 208 pages,
ISBN 9781405104999

A well-organized, short text review of general surgery with good, clear tables and diagrams. Easy to read, but with uneven coverage of high-yield topics. A brief question-and-answer section is included at the end of the text. Because it is geared toward study for the shelf and USMLE Step 2 exams, some of the information presented is oversimplified, especially with regard to surgical operations and procedures. Excellent for the basics, but students will need a more detailed reference for the rotation. Some students feel it is one of the weaker review books of the *Blueprints* series.

Colour Guide to Surgical Signs

$27.95

CAMPBELL

Elsevier, 1999, 2nd ed., 146 pages, ISBN 9780443061455

Concise text descriptions with associated radiographs and color photographs of manifestations of surgical disease. Good illustrations but not complete, limiting its usefulness on the wards.

Most Commons in Surgery

$29.95

GOLJAN

Elsevier, 2001, 1st ed., 658 pages, ISBN 9780721692913

A small reference book written in tabular format that describes the most common causes, manifestations, sites, signs or symptoms, complications, and management of all major surgical diseases. Also includes sections on subspecialties. The format is not particularly useful or well organized for study or review. Explanations to answers are minimal.

High-Yield Surgery

$26.95

NIRULA

Lippincott Williams & Wilkins, 2005, 2nd ed., 150 pages, ISBN 9780781776561

Part of a popular USMLE Step 1 prep series that offers a review book for each clerkship. Typical of its format, the book contains high-yield information in a clear and concise outline organized by organ system. However, this surgery book is probably too concise for shelf exam preparation. Best used for a quick preview reading before the rotation.

General Surgical Anatomy and Examination

$39.95

THOMPSON

Elsevier, 2002, 1st ed., 91 pages, ISBN 9780443063763

An illustrative text that integrates knowledge of normal anatomy with the physical examination of the surgical patient. Line drawings overlaid on color photographs highlight abnormal areas in a clear manner. Short, but generally accomplishes its goals. Not a long-term investment for the wards, but may be good for pre- or early-rotation preparation.

B+ | **Blueprints Clinical Cases in Surgery** | $29.95
LI

Lippincott Williams & Wilkins, 2007, 2nd ed., 304 pages,
ISBN 9781405104937

Organized by common presenting signs and symptoms, this book contains 60 symptom-based clinical cases accompanied by 200 USMLE-style questions. The format is similar to that of the *Case Files* series but places less emphasis on discussions and greater focus on questions.

B+ | **Blueprints Q&A Step 2 Surgery** | $19.95
NELSON

Lippincott Williams & Wilkins, 2005, 2nd ed., 184 pages,
ISBN 9781405103930

The new edition of this book contains more than 200 USMLE-style questions (increased from 100 from the previous edition) with explanations for both correct and incorrect answers, although the explanations are not as detailed and well referenced as those in the *PreTest* series. Originally designed for Step 2 preparation, but since the format of the shelf exam is similar, this would be a useful companion for clerkship preparation as well. The book is thin enough to carry in the pocket and could easily be read in a few days.

B | **Lange Q&A Surgery** | $39.95
CAYTEN

McGraw-Hill, 2007, 5th ed., 416 pages, ISBN 9780071475662

A question-and-answer book with more than 1000 questions organized under different topics. Provides detailed explanations of every answer. Includes a comprehensive practice exam with 100 questions at the end. Questions tend to focus on details. Best used as a supplement to the topic review books during the rotation.

B | **PreTest Surgery** | $26.95
KAO

McGraw-Hill, 2006, 11th ed., 384 pages, ISBN 9780071457705

A collection of 500 multiple-choice questions covering a wide range of topics in surgery. Includes clinical vignette–style questions and provides detailed paragraph-format explanations for each answer. Considered one of the weaker question books of the *PreTest* series.

REVIEW RESOURCES

SURGERY

Schwartz's Principles of Surgery

$160.00

SCHWARTZ

McGraw-Hill, 2005, 8th ed., 1950 pages, ISBN 9780071410908

A reference textbook for the serious surgery student, and probably the most widely used of the surgical textbooks. Well organized and comprehensive, with a good discussion of surgical disease processes and in-depth, complex explanations of the diagnosis and treatment of surgical problems. Expensive and requires considerable reading time, but a great investment for those considering a surgical career. A valuable reference for presentations and in-depth study. This edition has added a new focus on oncologic surgery and has strengthened the section on basic science.

Greenfield's Surgery: Scientific Principles and Practice

$199.00

MULHOLLAND

Lippincott Williams & Wilkins, 2005, 4th ed., 2100 pages, ISBN 9780781756266

Similar in style to the *Sabiston Textbook of Surgery*, this is another excellent reference with a heavy emphasis on integrating the principles of basic science with a discussion of surgical disease. Good photos and diagrams.

Sabiston Textbook of Surgery

$179.00

TOWNSEND

Elsevier, 2008, 18th ed., 2384 pages, ISBN 9781416036753

An excellent reference book and a good read for medical students entering a surgical career. Places greater emphasis on basic science than does *Principles of Surgery*, with a more extensive discussion of normal anatomy and physiology. Well organized with good coverage of surgical disease. Not quite as readable.

Current Surgical Therapy

$179.00

CAMERON

Elsevier, 2007, 9th ed., 1600 pages, ISBN 9781416034971

A highly detailed and technical surgical textbook designed for the practicing surgeon, with emphasis placed on evidence-based medicine. Highly comprehensive, with many high-yield images. Too much for even the dedicated surgical student, although those going into surgery may consider buying this later in their career.

REVIEW RESOURCES

SURGERY

B+

Current Surgical Diagnosis & Treatment

$64.95

DOHERTY

McGraw-Hill, 2005, 12th ed., 1468 pages, ISBN 9780071423151

A clinically practical, easy-to-read reference book that is geared toward residents but should also be useful for students considering surgery. Offers well-written explanations of the major diagnostic approaches toward and treatment options for surgical problems, but little information is given on operative procedures. This new edition has added more illustrations but is still heavy on text. Includes chapters on most surgical subspecialties.

B+

Essentials of General Surgery

$49.95

LAWRENCE

Lippincott Williams & Wilkins, 2005, 4th ed., 672 pages, ISBN 9780781750035

A basic introductory text to surgery that is written at the level of the junior medical student. Definitely an easy read, making it possible to cover the entire text within this busy rotation. Offers good pictorial and text reviews of pertinent anatomy and physiology, but lacks detail and depth in many areas. Weaker in its discussion of treatment and management, and does not cover subspecialties. Good questions and oral exam preparation are included at the end of each section. Appropriate as an introductory text for general surgery and for those who are not considering surgery as a career.

B+

Essentials of Surgical Specialties

$49.95

LAWRENCE

Lippincott Williams & Wilkins, 2006, 3rd ed., 544 pages, ISBN 9780781750042

A text presented in the same format as *Essentials of General Surgery*, except that this version discusses different surgical subspecialty topics. Refer to the review above for a more detailed evaluation.

APPENDIX

Abbreviations

Abbreviation	Meaning
A&O × 3	alert and oriented to person, place, and time
A&O × 4	alert and oriented to person, place, time, and situation
A&P	assessment and plan
A-a	alveolar-arterial (oxygen gradient)
AAA	abdominal aortic aneurysm
AAP	American Academy of Pediatrics
Ab	antibody
ABCs	airway, breathing, circulation
ABG	arterial blood gas
ABI	ankle-brachial index
ABPA	allergic bronchopulmonary aspergillosis
abx	antibiotics
ACA	anterior cerebral artery
ACC	American College of Cardiology
ACEI	angiotensin-converting enzyme inhibitor
ACG	American College of Gastroenterology
AChR	acetylcholine receptor
ACLS	advanced cardiac life support (protocol)
ACS	acute coronary syndrome, American Cancer Society
ACTH	adrenocorticotropic hormone
AD	Alzheimer's disease
ADA	American Diabetes Association
ADH	antidiuretic hormone
ADHD	attention-deficit hyperactivity disorder
AF	atrial fibrillation
AFI	amniotic fluid index
AFOSF	anterior fontanelle open, soft, and flat
AFP	α-fetoprotein
AG	anion gap
AH	auditory hallucinations
AHA	American Heart Association
AI	aortic insufficiency

Abbreviation	Meaning
AIDS	acquired immunodeficiency syndrome
AIN	acute interstitial nephritis
ALL	acute lymphocytic leukemia
ALS	amyotrophic lateral sclerosis
ALT	alanine transaminase
ANA	antinuclear antibody
ANCA	antineutrophil cytoplasmic antibody
AOM	acute otitis media
APD	afferent pupillary defect
aPTT	activated partial thromboplastin time
ARB	angiotensin receptor blocker
ARF	acute renal failure
AROM	artificial rupture of membranes
ARR	absolute risk reduction
AS	aortic stenosis
ASA	acetylsalicylic acid
5-ASA	5-aminosalicylic acid
ASCUS	atypical squamous cells of undetermined significance
ASD	atrial septal defect
ASO	antistreptolysin O
AST	aspartate transaminase
ATN	acute tubular necrosis
AV	arteriovenous, atrioventricular
AVM	arteriovenous malformation
AXR	abdominal x-ray
AZT	azidothymidine
BAD	bipolar affective disorder
BAL	2,3-dimercaptopropanol (dimercaprol)
BCG	bacille Calmette-Guérin
BID	twice a day
BMI	body mass index
BMP	basic metabolic panel
BNP	brain natriuretic peptide
BP	blood pressure
BPH	benign prostatic hypertrophy
bpm	beats per minute
BPP	biophysical profile
BPPV	benign paroxysmal positional vertigo

Abbreviation	Meaning	Abbreviation	Meaning
BR	bathroom	CTAB	clear to auscultation bilaterally
BRBPR	bright red blood per rectum	CV	cardiovascular
BS	bowel sounds	CVA	cerebrovascular accident,
BUN	blood urea nitrogen		costovertebral angle
BV	balloon valvuloplasty	CVS	chorionic villus sampling
BW	birth weight, body weight	c/w	consistent with
c̄	with	Cx	culture
CABG	coronary artery bypass grafting	CXR	chest x-ray
CAD	coronary artery disease	D&C	dilation and curettage
CaEDTA	calcium edetate	D4T	didehydrodeoxythymidine
CALLA	common ALL antigen	D5	5% dextrose
CAP	community-acquired pneumonia	D5W	dextrose in water
CBC	complete blood count	DBP	diastolic blood pressure
CBD	common bile duct	DC	direct current
CBT	cognitive-behavioral therapy	D/C	diarrhea/constipation, discontinuing
CC	chief complaint	d/c	discharge
C/C/E	clubbing/cyanosis/edema	DCIS	ductal carcinoma in situ
CCK	cholecystokinin	ddC	dideoxycytidine
CCP	cyclic citrullinated peptide	ddI	dideoxyinosine
CD	cluster of differentiation	DES	diethylstilbestrol
CDC	Centers for Disease Control and	DFA	direct fluorescent antibody
	Prevention	DHEAS	dehydroepiandrosterone sulfate
C/D/I	clean, dry, and intact	DIC	disseminated intravascular
CEA	carcinoembryonic antigen		coagulation
CF	cystic fibrosis	DKA	diabetic ketoacidosis
CFTR	cystic fibrosis transmembrane	DL_{CO}	diffusion capacity for carbon
	regulator		monoxide
CHD	congenital heart disease	DM	diabetes mellitus
CHF	congestive heart failure	DMARD	disease-modifying antirheumatic drug
CIN	cervical intraepithelial neoplasia	DNA	deoxyribonucleic acid
CJD	Creutzfeldt-Jakob disease	DNase	deoxyribonuclease
CK	creatine kinase	DNR	do not resuscitate
CKD	chronic kidney disease	d/o	disorder
CK-MB	creatine kinase, MB isoenzyme	DOA	day of admission
CLO	*Campylobacter*-like organism	DOE	dyspnea on exertion
CMP	complete metabolic panel	DRE	digital rectal exam
CMT	cervical motion tenderness	dsDNA	double-stranded DNA
CMV	cytomegalovirus	DSM	*Diagnostic and Statistical Manual*
CN	cranial nerve	DT	diphtheria and tetanus (vaccine)
CNS	central nervous system	DTaP	diphtheria, tetanus, acellular pertussis
c/o	complains of		(vaccine)
CO	carbon monoxide	DTs	delirium tremens
CO_2	carbon dioxide	DTRs	deep tendon reflexes
COMT	catechol-*O*-methyltransferase	DUB	dysfunctional uterine bleeding
COPD	chronic obstructive pulmonary	DVT	deep venous thrombosis
	disease	DWI	diffusion-weighted imaging
COX	cyclooxygenase	EBL	estimated blood loss
CPAP	continuous positive airway pressure	EBV	Epstein-Barr virus
CPP	cerebral perfusion pressure	ECG	electrocardiogram
CPR	cardiopulmonary resuscitation	ECT	electroconvulsive therapy
CrCl	creatinine clearance	ED	emergency department
CRP	C-reactive protein	EDC	estimated date of confinement
CSF	cerebrospinal fluid	EDD	estimated date of delivery
CT	computed tomography	EDTA	ethylenediamine tetraacetic acid

Abbreviation	Meaning
EEG	electroencephalogram
EF	ejection fraction
EFW	estimated fetal weight
EGD	esophagogastroduodenoscopy
ELISA	enzyme-linked immunosorbent assay
EM	emergency medicine
EMG	electromyogram
EOM	extraocular movement
EOMI	extraocular movements intact
EPS	extrapyramidal symptoms
ER	emergency room
ERCP	endoscopic retrograde cholangiopancreatography
ESR	erythrocyte sedimentation rate
EtOH	ethanol
Ext	extremities
FAST	focused abdominal sonography for trauma
F/C/S	fever/chills/sweating
Fe_{Na}	excreted fraction of filtered sodium
$FeSO_4$	ferrous sulfate
FEV_1	forced expiratory volume in 1 second
FFP	fresh frozen plasma
FH	family history
FHR	fetal heart rate
FHT	fetal heart tracing
FiO_2	fraction of inspired oxygen
FLAIR	fluid attenuation inversion recovery
FLM	fetal lung maturity
FM	fetal movement, fine motor
FNA	fine-needle aspiration
FSGS	focal segmental glomerulosclerosis
FSH	follicle-stimulating hormone
FT	fine touch
FTN	finger to nose
FTT	failure to thrive
FUO	fever of unknown origin
FVC	forced vital capacity
G6PD	glucose-6-phosphate dehydrogenase
GA	gestational age
GABA	gamma-aminobutyric acid
GAD	generalized anxiety disorder, glutamic acid decarboxylase
GAF	Global Assessment of Functioning
GB	gallbladder
GBM	glioblastoma multiforme
GBS	group B streptococcus, Guillain-Barré syndrome
GC	gonorrhea culture
GCS	Glasgow Coma Scale
GERD	gastroesophageal reflux disease
GETA	general endotracheal anesthesia
GFR	glomerular filtration rate
GGT	gamma-glutamyltransferase

Abbreviation	Meaning
GI	gastrointestinal
GM	gross motor
GN	glomerulonephritis
GNR	gram-negative rod
GnRH	gonadotropin-releasing hormone
GU	genitourinary
H&P	history and physical
HA	headache
HAART	highly active antiretroviral therapy
HACEK	*Haemophilus, Actinobacillus, Cardiobacterium, Eikenella, Kingella*
HAV	hepatitis A virus, hepatitis A vaccine
Hb	hemoglobin
HBsAg	hepatitis B surface antigen
HBV	hepatitis B virus, hepatitis B vaccine
HC	head circumference
HCC	hepatocellular carcinoma
hCG	human chorionic gonadotropin
Hct	hematocrit
HCV	hepatitis C virus
HD	hemodialysis, hospital day
HDL	high-density lipoprotein
HDV	hepatitis D virus
HEENT	head, eyes, ears, nose, and throat
HELLP	hemolysis, elevated liver (enzymes), low platelets
HEV	hepatitis E virus
HHNK	hyperosmolar hyperglycemic nonketotic coma
HHV	human herpesvirus
HI	homicidal ideation
Hib	*Haemophilus influenzae* type b (vaccine)
HIDA	hepato-iminodiacetic acid (scan)
HIV	human immunodeficiency virus
HLA	human leukocyte antigen
HNPCC	hereditary nonpolyposis colorectal cancer
h/o	history of
HOCM	hypertrophic obstructive cardiomyopathy
hpf	high-power field
HPI	history of present illness
HPO	hypertrophic pulmonary osteoarthropathy
HPV	human papillomavirus
HR	heart rate
HRT	hormone replacement therapy
HSM	hepatosplenomegaly
HSV	herpes simplex virus
5-HT	5-hydroxytryptamine (serotonin)
HTLV	human T-cell lymphotropic virus
HTN	hypertension

Abbreviation	Meaning
HTS	heel to shin
HUS	hemolytic-uremic syndrome
HVA	homovanillic acid
Hx	history
IBD	inflammatory bowel disease
IBS	irritable bowel syndrome
ICP	intracranial pressure
ICU	intensive care unit
ID	identification
IDDM	insulin-dependent diabetes mellitus
Ig	immunoglobulin
IIH	idiopathic intracranial hypertension
IM	intramuscular
INH	isoniazid
INR	International Normalized Ratio
I/O	intake/output
IOC	intraoperative cholangiogram
IPV	inactivated polio vaccine
ITP	idiopathic thrombocytopenic purpura
IUD	intrauterine device
IUGR	intrauterine growth retardation
IUP	intrauterine pregnancy
IUTD	immunizations up to date
IV	intravenous
IVC	inferior vena cava
IVDU	intravenous drug use
IVIG	intravenous immunoglobulin
JIA	juvenile idiopathic arthritis
JP	Jackson-Pratt (drain)
JVD	jugular venous distention
JVP	jugular venous pressure
KCl	potassium chloride
KOH	potassium hydroxide
KUB	kidney, ureter, bladder
KVO	keep vein open
L&D	labor and delivery
LAA	left atrial abnormality
LAD	lymphadenopathy
LBBB	left bundle branch block
LBO	large bowel obstruction
LCIS	lobular carcinoma in situ
LCPD	Legg-Calvé-Perthes disease
LDH	lactate dehydrogenase
LDL	low-density lipoprotein
LE	lower extremities
LEEP	loop electrosurgical excision procedure
LES	lower esophageal sphincter
LFT	liver function test
LGIB	lower gastrointestinal bleeding
LH	luteinizing hormone
LKM	liver-kidney microsome
LLE	left lower extremity
LLQ	left lower quadrant

Abbreviation	Meaning
LMN	lower motor neuron
LMP	last menstrual period
LMWH	low-molecular-weight heparin
LOC	loss of consciousness
LP	lumbar puncture
LR	lactated Ringer's solution
L/S	lecithin-to-sphingomyelin (ratio)
LUE	left upper extremity
LUQ	left upper quadrant
LV	left ventricle, left ventricular
LVEDP	left ventricular end-diastolic pressure
LVH	left ventricular hypertrophy
MAE	moves all extremities
MAO	monoamine oxidase
MAOI	monoamine oxidase inhibitor
MAP	mean arterial pressure
MAR	medication administration record
MCA	middle cerebral artery
MCTD	mixed connective tissue disorder
MCV	mean corpuscular volume
MCV4	meningococcal conjugate vaccine
MDD	major depressive disorder
MDE	major depressive episode
MDI	metered-dose inhaler
MELD	Model for End-Stage Liver Disease
$MgSO_4$	magnesium sulfate
MHA-TP	microhemagglutination assay— *Treponema pallidum*
MI	myocardial infarction
MIBI	methoxyisobutyl isonitrile (stress test)
MLF	medial longitudinal fasciculus
MMM	mucous membranes moist
MMR	measle, mumps, rubella (vaccine)
MMSE	mini-mental status exam
6-MP	6-mercaptopurine
MPO	myeloperoxidase
MPSV4	meningococcal polysaccharide vaccine
MPTP	1-methyl-4-phenyl-tetrahydropyridine
MR	mitral regurgitation
MRA	magnetic resonance angiography
MRCP	magnetic resonance cholangiopancreatography
M/R/G	murmurs/rubs/gallops
MRI	magnetic resonance imaging
MRSA	methicillin-resistant *Staphylococcus aureus*
MS	mental status, mitral stenosis, multiple sclerosis, musculoskeletal
MS-1, 2, etc.	medical student (and year)
MS-AFP	maternal serum α-fetoprotein
MSE	mental status examination
MuSK	muscle-specific kinase
MVI	multivitamin infusion

Abbreviation	Meaning
MVP	mitral valve prolapse
NABS	normoactive bowel sounds
NAD	no acute distress
NAG	non–anion gap
NBME	National Board of Medical Examiners
NBNB	nonbilious, nonbloody
NC	nasal cannula
NC/AT	normocephalic/atraumatic
ND	nondistended
NDDG	National Diabetes Data Group
NG	nasogastric
NICU	neonatal intensive care unit
NIDDM	non-insulin-dependent diabetes mellitus
NIH	National Institutes of Health
NKDA	no known drug allergies
nl	normal
NMDA	N-methyl-D-aspartate
NNT	number needed to treat
NOS	not otherwise specified
NPO	nil per os (nothing by mouth)
NR	normal range
NS	normal saline
NSAID	nonsteroidal anti-inflammatory drug
NSCLC	non–small cell lung carcinoma
NST	nonstress test
NSTEMI	non-ST-elevation myocardial infarction
NSVD	normal spontaneous vaginal delivery
NT	nontender
N/V	nausea/vomiting
NVE	native valve endocarditis
NYHA	New York Heart Association
O&P	ova and parasites
OB/GYN	obstetrics and gynecology
OCD	obsessive-compulsive disorder
OCP	oral contraceptive pill
OOB	out of bed
O/P	oropharynx
OR	operating room
o/w	otherwise
P	pulse
PA	posteroanterior
$PaCO_2$	partial pressure of carbon dioxide in arterial blood
PaO_2	partial pressure of oxygen in arterial blood
PAO_2	alveolar oxygen pressure
PCA	patient-controlled analgesia, posterior cerebral artery
PCO_2	partial pressure of carbon dioxide

Abbreviation	Meaning
PCOS	polycystic ovarian syndrome
PCP	phencyclidine ("angel dust"), *Pneumocystis carinii* (now *jiroveci*) pneumonia
PCV	pneumococcal conjugate vaccine
PD	peritoneal dialysis
PDA	patent ductus arteriosus, personal digital assistant
PDD	pervasive developmental disorder
PDS	polydioxanone (sutures)
PE	physical examination, pulmonary embolism
PEF	peak expiratory flow
PERRL	pupils equal, round, and reactive to light
PET	positron emission tomography
PFT	pulmonary function test
PG	plasma glucose, prostaglandin
PGY	postgraduate year
PID	pelvic inflammatory disease
PIV	parainfluenza virus
PMH	past medical history
PMI	point of maximal impulse
PML	progressive multifocal leukoencephalopathy
PMN	polymorphonuclear (leukocytes)
PNL	prenatal labs
PNV	prenatal vitamins
PO	per os (by mouth)
PO_2	partial pressure of oxygen
PO_4	phosphate
POD	postoperative day
PORT	Patient Outcomes Research Team (score)
PP	pin prick
ppd	pack per day
PPD	postpartum day, purified protein derivative (of tuberculin)
PPI	proton pump inhibitor
PPROM	premature preterm rupture of membranes
PPV	pneumococcal polysaccharide vaccine
PR	per rectum
PRN	pro re nata (as needed)
PSH	past surgical history
PT	prothrombin time
PTA	prior to admission
PTCA	percutaneous transluminal coronary angioplasty
PTHrP	PTH-related peptide
PTSD	post-traumatic stress disorder
PTT	partial thromboplastin time
PUD	peptic ulcer disease

Abbreviation	Meaning
PVE	prosthetic valve endocarditis
QAM	every morning
QD	every day
QHS	every night
QID	four times a day
RA	rheumatoid arthritis, room air
RAA	right atrial abnormality
RAM	rapid alternating movements
RAS	renal artery stenosis
RBBB	right bundle branch block
RBC	red blood cell
RCT	randomized controlled trial
RDS	respiratory distress syndrome
RF	radio frequency, rheumatoid factor
RLE	right lower extremity
RLQ	right lower quadrant
RNA	ribonucleic acid
r/o	rule out
ROM	range of motion, rupture of membranes
ROS	review of systems
RPR	rapid plasma reagin (test)
RR	red reflex, respiratory rate
RRR	regular rate and rhythm, relative risk reduction
RRT	renal replacement therapy
RSV	respiratory syncytial virus
RT	recreational therapist
RTA	renal tubular acidosis
RUA	routine urinalysis
RUE	right upper extremity
RUQ	right upper quadrant
RV	residual volume
RVH	right ventricular hypertrophy
SA	sinoatrial
SAAG	serum-ascites albumin gradient
SAB	spontaneous abortion
SAD	schizoaffective disorder
SAH	subarachnoid hemorrhage
SaO_2	arterial oxygen saturation
Sat	oxygen saturation
SBO	small bowel obstruction
SBP	systolic blood pressure
SCD	sequential compression device
SCFE	slipped capital femoral epiphysis
SCLC	small cell lung carcinoma
SCM	sternocleidomastoid
SEM	systolic ejection murmur
SES	socioeconomic status
SGOT	serum glutamic oxaloacetic transaminase
SH	social history
SI	suicidal ideation
SIADH	syndrome of inappropriate secretion of ADH

Abbreviation	Meaning
SIDS	sudden infant death syndrome
SIRS	systemic inflammatory response syndrome
SLE	systemic lupus erythematosus
SOAP	subjective (data), objective (data), assessment, and plan
SOB	shortness of breath
s/p	status post (postoperative)
SPEP	serum protein electrophoresis
SQ	subcutaneous
SSE	sterile speculum exam
SSI	sliding-scale insulin
SSRI	selective serotonin reuptake inhibitor
STD	sexually transmitted disease
SVC	superior vena cava
SVE	sterile vaginal exam
SVR	systemic vascular resistance
SVT	supraventricular tachycardia
T	temperature
TAB	therapeutic abortion
TAH-BSO	total abdominal hysterectomy/ bilateral salpingo-oophorectomy
TB	tuberculosis
TBSA	total body surface area
TBW	total body water
3TC	dideoxythiacytidine
Tc	technetium
T_c	current temperature
TCA	tricyclic antidepressant
TED	thromboembolic deterrent (stockings)
T/E/D	tobacco/EtOH (alcohol)/drugs
TEE	transesophageal echocardiography
TFT	thyroid function test
TG	triglyceride
TH	tactile hallucinations
TIA	transient ischemic attack
TIBC	total iron-binding capacity
TID	three times a day
TIPS	transjugular intrahepatic portosystemic shunt
TLC	total lung capacity
TM	tympanic membrane
T_m	maximum temperature
TMP-SMX	trimethoprim-sulfamethoxazole
TN	trigeminal neuralgia
TNF	tumor necrosis factor
TNM	tumor, node, metastasis (staging)
TOA	tubo-ovarian abscess
TOC	test of cure
ToRCHeS	toxoplasmosis, rubella, cytomegalovirus, herpes simplex, syphilis

Abbreviation	Meaning
tPA	tissue plasminogen activator
TPAL	term, preterm, abortion, living
TPN	total parenteral nutrition
TSH	thyroid-stimulating hormone
TTE	transthoracic echocardiography
TTP	thrombotic thrombocytopenic purpura
TUR	transurethrally resected
UA	urinalysis
UC	uterine contraction
UE	upper extremities
UGIB	upper gastrointestinal bleeding
UMN	upper motor neuron
UO	urine output
UPEP	urine protein electrophoresis
URI	upper respiratory infection
USMLE	United States Medical Licensing Examination
USOH	usual state of health
USPTF	United States Preventive Services Task Force
UTI	urinary tract infection

Abbreviation	Meaning
VA	Department of Veterans Affairs
VB	vaginal bleeding
VC	vital capacity
VCUG	voiding cystourethrogram
VDRL	Venereal Disease Research Laboratory (test)
VF	ventricular fibrillation
VH	visual hallucinations
VIP	vasoactive intestinal peptide
VMA	vanillylmandelic acid
VOR	vestibulo-ocular reflex
V/Q	ventilation-perfusion (ratio)
VS	vital signs
VSD	ventricular septal defect
VT	ventricular tachycardia
VZIG	varicella-zoster immune globulin
VZV	varicella-zoster virus
WBC	white blood cell, white blood cell count
WD/WN	well developed and well nourished
WHO	World Health Organization
W/R/R	wheezes/rhonchi/rales

INDEX

Depakote (valproate), 351
Depersonalization, 353
Derealization, 353
Dermatomyositis, 124
Diabetes mellitus (DM), 151–155
  diagnostic criteria for, 152
    type 1, 152–154
    type 2, 152–154
Diabetic ketoacidosis (DKA), 151
Diabetic nephropathy, 135, 154
Diabetic retinopathy, 220
Diagnostic and Statistical Manual of Mental Disorders, 4th edition (DSM-IV), 337
  classification, 337
Dialysis, indications for, 132
Diaper rash, 290–291
Diarrhea, 143–144
  acute, 144
  chronic, 144, 156
  malabsorptive, 143
  osmotic, 143, 144
  secretory, 143
Diastolic dysfunction, 108
  treatment of, 111
Diffusion-weighted imaging (DWI), 182
Diplopia, horizontal, 202
Disseminated intravascular coagulation (DIC), 124
Diverticular disease, 405
Diverticulitis, 399
  diverticulosis vs., 406
  right-sided, 139
Diverticulosis, 402
  vs. diverticulitis, 406
Dix-Hallpike maneuver, 198
Down syndrome (trisomy 21), 294
Droperidol, 356
Drug fever, 155
Dysequilibrium, 196–199
  central vs. peripheral, 197
  etiologies of peripheral and central, 198
  neurologic causes, 197
    benign paroxysmal positional vertigo (BPPV), 197
    Ménière's disease, 197
  non-neurologic causes, 196
Dysthymic disorder, 348–349

E

Echolalia, 353
Eclampsia, 239
  management of, 240

Ectopic pregnancy, 139
  ruptured, 399
Edwards' syndrome (trisomy 18), 294
Ehlers-Danlos syndrome, 119
Eikenella, 114
Electrocardiogram (ECG), reading, 37–38
  interpretation, 38–39
Electrocardioversion, 106–107
Electroconvulsive therapy (ECT), 348
Electrolytes, 50
  requirements, 43
Emergencies, patient, 48–50
  cardiopulmonary arrest, 48–50
Emphysema, 121
Endocarditis, infective. *See* Infective endocarditis
Endocrinology, 151–155
  diabetes mellitus (DM), 151–155
Endometrial cancer, 269
Endometriosis, 254–255
Enterobacter, 130, 160, 310, 415
Enterococcus, 114
Enterococcus faecalis, 160
Enterovirus, 307
Enzyme-linked immunosorbent assay (ELISA), 156, 158
Ependymoma, 204
Epididymitis, 139
Epiglottitis, characteristics of, 325
Epiphyseal fractures, 320
  Salter-Harris classification of, 320
Erythema infectiosum (fifth disease), 292
Escherichia coli, 130, 160, 265, 303, 310, 415
  O157:H7, 144
Esophageal varices, 402
Esophagitis, 399, 400
  candidal, 156
  herpes simplex virus (HSV), 156
Essential tremor, 205
  vs. Parkinson's disease, 206
Ewing's sarcoma, 319

F

Factitious disorder (Munchausen syndrome), 380
Factitious fever, 155
Febrile seizures, 316–317
  simple vs. complex, 316

Ferning test, 247
Fetal heart rate (FHR) monitoring, 249–251
  patterns, 250
  tracings, 250
Fever management, 301–302
  febrile child 3–36 months old without a source, 302
  febrile infant < 28 days old, 301–302
  febrile infant 28–90 days old without a source, 302
Fifth disease (erythema infectiosum), 292
First-trimester bleeding, 240
Fitz-Hugh–Curtis syndrome, 266, 267, 398
Flight of ideas, 353
Fluid attenuation inversion recovery (FLAIR) imaging, 182
Fluid compartments, 40
Fluids and electrolytes, 38, 40–45
  fluid compartments, 40
  intravenous (IV) fluids, 40–41
  therapy, 41–45
    deficit therapy, 44–45
    fluid resuscitation, 41–42
    maintenance fluids, 42–43
    replace ongoing losses, 44
  total body water, 40
Fluids, components of common, 41
Fluphenazine (Prolixin), 356
Focal segmental glomerulosclerosis (FSGS), 135
Fractures, pediatric, 320
  epiphyseal, 320
    Salter-Harris classification of, 320
  greenstick, 320
  torus, 320
Fragile X syndrome, 375

G

Gallavardin phenomenon, 118
Gallstone ileus, 403, 404
Gallstones, 413
Gardnerella, 262
Gastritis, 139, 144–145, 399
  acute "stress," 144
  chronic "nonerosive," 144
    decision diagram for diagnosis of causes of, 145
Gastroenteritis, 139, 399

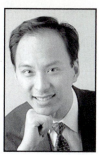

Tao Le, MD, MHS

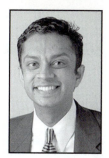

Vikas Bhushan, MD

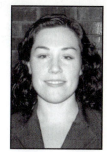

Julia Skapik, MD, MPH

Tao Le, MD, MHS

Tao has been a well-recognized figure in medical education for the past 15 years. As senior editor, he has led the expansion of *First Aid* into a global educational series. In addition, he is the founder of the *USMLERx* online test bank series as well as a cofounder of the *Underground Clinical Vignettes* series. As a medical student, he was editor-in-chief of the University of California, San Francisco *Synapse*, a university newspaper with a weekly circulation of 9000. Tao earned his medical degree from the University of California, San Francisco in 1996 and completed his residency training in internal medicine at Yale University and allergy and immunology fellowship training at Johns Hopkins University. At Yale, he was a regular guest lecturer on the USMLE review courses and an adviser to the Yale University School of Medicine curriculum committee. Tao subsequently went on to cofound Medsn and served as its chief medical officer. He is currently pursuing research in asthma education at the University of Louisville.

Vikas Bhushan, MD

Vikas is an author, editor, entrepreneur, and roaming teleradiologist who divides his days between Los Angeles, Maui, and balmy remote locales with abundant bandwidth. In 1992 he conceived and authored the original *First Aid for the USMLE Step 1*, and in 1998 he originated and coauthored the *Underground Clinical Vignettes* series. His entrepreneurial adventures include a successful software company; a medical publishing enterprise (S2S); an e-learning company (Medsn); and, most recently, an ER teleradiology venture (24/7 Radiology). His eclectic interests include medical informatics, independent film, humanism, Urdu poetry, world music, South Asian diasporic culture, and avoiding a day job. He has also coproduced a music documentary on qawwali; coproduced and edited *Shabash 2.0: The Hip Guide to All Things South Asian in North America*; and is now completing a CD/book project on Sufi poetry translated into four languages. Vikas completed a bachelor's degree in biochemistry from the University of California, Berkeley; an MD with thesis from the University of California, San Francisco; and a radiology residency from the University of California, Los Angeles.

Julia Skapik, MD, MPH

Julia is a resident in internal medicine at the University of Pittsburgh Medical Center. She holds an MPH from the Johns Hopkins Bloomberg School of Public Health and an MD from the Johns Hopkins School of Medicine. Originally from Licking County, Ohio, she attended New College of Florida, graduating with dual BAs in biology and psychology in 2001. Subsequently, she spent a year at the FDA in Bethesda performing viral and vaccine neurovirulence research. Since then, she has worked on many research projects, primarily examining medical errors. She is also the author of the chapter "Psychotic Disorders, Severe Mental Illness, and HIV Infection" in the *Comprehensive Textbook of AIDS Psychiatry* and has authored several other articles in the areas of mental health and health quality. She was also an editor of the sixth edition of *First Aid for USMLE Step 2 CK*.

ABOUT THE AUTHORS

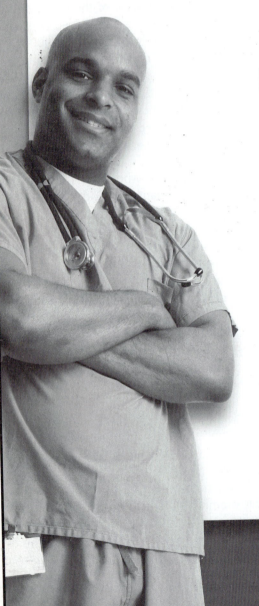